A Guide to Oncology Symptom Management

Edited by

Carlton G. Brown, PhD, RN, AOCN®

Oncology Nursing Society
Pittsburgh, Pennsylvania

ONS Publishing Division
Publisher: Leonard Mafrica, MBA, CAE
Director, Commercial Publishing: Barbara Sigler, RN, MNEd
Managing Editor: Lisa M. George, BA
Technical Content Editor: Angela D. Klimaszewski, RN, MSN
Staff Editor: Amy Nicoletti, BA
Copy Editor: Laura Pinchot, BA
Graphic Designer: Dany Sjoen

A Guide to Oncology Symptom Management

First printing, September 2009
Second printing, October 2010
Third printing, June 2011

Library of Congress Control Number: 2009935534

ISBN: 978-1-890504-89-2

Publisher's Note

This book is published by the Oncology Nursing Society (ONS). ONS neither represents nor guarantees that the practices described herein will, if followed, ensure safe and effective patient care. The recommendations contained in this book reflect ONS's judgment regarding the state of general knowledge and practice in the field as of the date of publication. The recommendations may not be appropriate for use in all circumstances. Those who use this book should make their own determinations regarding specific safe and appropriate patient-care practices, taking into account the personnel, equipment, and practices available at the hospital or other facility at which they are located. The editor and publisher cannot be held responsible for any liability incurred as a consequence from the use or application of any of the contents of this book. Figures and tables are used as examples only. They are not meant to be all-inclusive, nor do they represent endorsement of any particular institution by ONS. Mention of specific products and opinions related to those products do not indicate or imply endorsement by ONS. Web sites mentioned are provided for information only; the hosts are responsible for their own content and availability. Unless otherwise indicated, dollar amounts reflect U.S. dollars.

ONS publications are originally published in English. Publishers wishing to translate ONS publications must contact the ONS Publishing Division about licensing arrangements. ONS publications cannot be translated without obtaining written permission from ONS. (Individual tables and figures that are reprinted or adapted require additional permission from the original source.) Because translations from English may not always be accurate or precise, ONS disclaims any responsibility for inaccuracies in words or meaning that may occur as a result of the translation. Readers relying on precise information should check the original English version.

Printed in the United States of America

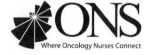

Oncology Nursing Society
Integrity • Innovation • Stewardship • Advocacy • Excellence • Inclusiveness

This textbook is dedicated to the patients and families with cancer who taught us all inexplicable lessons about the cancer journey and to the oncology nurses who have provided care for those patients.

Personally, I dedicate this textbook to the memory of my mother, Maria Bakker Brown, and to my nephew Aidan Brown, who has given me a renewed sense of hope for the future.

Contributors

Editor

Carlton G. Brown, PhD, RN, AOCN®
Assistant Professor
University of Delaware, School of Nursing
Newark, Delaware
Chapter 12. Electrolyte Imbalances, Tumor Lysis Syndrome, and Syndrome of Inappropriate Antidiuretic Hormone; Chapter 16. Oral Mucositis

Authors

Ann M. Berger, PhD, RN, AOCN®, FAAN
Dorothy Hodges Olson Endowed Chair in Nursing
Professor and Advanced Practice Nurse, Oncology
University of Nebraska Medical Center, College of Nursing
Omaha, Nebraska
Chapter 23. Sleep-Wake Disturbances

Barbara A. Biedrzycki, MSN, CRNP, AOCNP®
Clinical Research Associate
Sidney Kimmel Comprehensive Cancer Center at Johns Hopkins
Baltimore, Maryland
Chapter 20. Peripheral Neuropathy

JoAnn Coleman, RN, MS, AOCN®, ACNP
Coordinator
Pancreas Multidisciplinary Cancer Clinic
Sidney Kimmel Comprehensive Cancer Center at Johns Hopkins
Baltimore, Maryland
Chapter 10. Diarrhea

Megan Dunne, RN, MA, ANP-BC, AOCN®
Nurse Practitioner for Clinical Trials
Memorial Sloan-Kettering Cancer Center
New York, New York
Chapter 22. Skin and Nail Alterations

Beth Eaby, MSN, CRNP, OCN®
Nurse Practitioner
Hospital of the University of Pennsylvania, Abramson Cancer Center
Philadelphia, Pennsylvania
Chapter 6. Chemotherapy-Induced Nausea and Vomiting

Christine Engstrom, PhD, CRNP, AOCN®
Oncology Clinical Nurse Advisor
Veterans Affairs Central Office
Office of Nursing Services
Washington, District of Columbia
Chapter 14. Hot Flashes

Jeanne Erickson, PhD, RN, AOCN®
Assistant Professor of Nursing
University of Virginia School of Nursing
Charlottesville, Virginia
Chapter 23. Sleep-Wake Disturbances

Sylvia C. Fairclough, RN, BSN, OCN®
Washington, District of Columbia
Chapter 12. Electrolyte Imbalances, Tumor Lysis Syndrome, and Syndrome of Inappropriate Antidiuretic Hormone

Cathy Fortenbaugh, RN, MSN, AOCN®
Oncology Clinical Nurse Specialist
Capital Health System
Trenton, New Jersey
Chapter 8. Constipation

Clara Granda-Cameron, RN, BSN, MSN, CRNP, AOCN®, ANCC
Coordinator, Pain and Supportive Care Program
Joan Karnell Cancer Center at Pennsylvania Hospital
Philadelphia, Pennsylvania
Chapter 5. Cancer Cachexia

Margaret M. Joyce, PhD(c), RN, AOCN®
Advanced Practice Nurse
Cancer Institute of New Jersey
New Brunswick, New Jersey
Chapter 11. Dyspnea

Cheryl Lacasse, RN, MS, OCN®
Clinical Professor
College of Nursing
University of Arizona
Tucson, Arizona
Chapter 1. Symptoms in Older Adults

Frances Lee-Lin, RN, PhD, OCN®, CNS
Assistant Professor
Oregon Health & Science University School of
   Nursing
Portland, Oregon
Chapter 2. Alopecia

Mary Pat Lynch, CRNP, MSN, AOCN®
Cancer Center Administrator
Joan Karnell Cancer Center at Pennsylvania Hospital
Philadelphia, Pennsylvania
Chapter 5. Cancer Cachexia

Debra D. Mark, RN, PhD
Assistant Professor
Director, Office of Research and Extramural
   Programming
University of Hawaii School of Nursing and Dental
   Hygiene
Honolulu, Hawaii
Chapter 21. Altered Sexuality Patterns

Joyce A. Marrs, MS, FNP-BC, AOCNP®
Nurse Practitioner
Dayton Physicians, Hematology & Oncology
Dayton, Ohio
Chapter 15. Lymphedema

Christine Miaskowski, RN, PhD, FAAN
Professor and Associate Dean
University of California
San Francisco, California
Chapter 19. Cancer Pain

Sheryl Miller, RN, MSN, MBA, OCN®
Field Manager
Innovex
Lancaster, Ohio
Chapter 3. Anemia

Sandra A. Mitchell, PhD, CRNP, AOCN®
Nurse Scientist
Clinical Center, National Institutes of Health
Bethesda, Maryland
Chapter 13. Cancer-Related Fatigue

Tamsin J. Mulrooney, ARNP, PhD, OCN®, CBCN
Oncology Clinical Coordinator
Genentech BioOncology
South San Francisco, California
Chapter 7. Cognitive Impairment

Lillian Nail, PhD, RN, FAAN
Rawlinson Professor and Senior Scientist
Oregon Health & Science University School of
   Nursing
Portland, Oregon
Chapter 2. Alopecia

Patricia W. Nishimoto, RN, DNS, FAAN
Adult Oncology Clinical Nurse Specialist
Tripler Army Medical Center
Honolulu, Hawaii
Chapter 21. Altered Sexuality Patterns

Colleen O'Leary, RN, MSN, AOCNS®
Oncology Clinical Nurse Specialist
Good Samaritan Hospital
Downer's Grove, Illinois
Chapter 17. Neutropenia and Infection

Kathy Sharp, MSN, FNP-BC, AOCNP®
Oncology Nurse Practitioner
Blue Ridge Medical Specialists, P.C.
Bristol, Tennessee
Chapter 9. Depression

Lisa Kennedy Sheldon, PhD, APRN, AOCNP®
Oncology Nurse Practitioner
St. Joseph Hospital
Nashua, New Hampshire
Assistant Professor
University of Massachusetts–Boston
Boston, Massachusetts
Chapter 4. Anxiety and People With Cancer

Carrie Tompkins Stricker, PhD, CRNP, AOCN®
Director of Nursing
Division of Hematology/Oncology
Clinical Assistant Professor of Nursing
University of Pennsylvania
Philadelphia, Pennsylvania
*Chapter 6. Chemotherapy-Induced Nausea and
    Vomiting; Chapter 18. Osteoporosis and Bone
    Health*

Susan Tinley, PhD, RN
Associate Professor
Creighton University, School of Nursing
Omaha, Nebraska
Chapter 24. Spiritual Care From the Oncology Nurse

Disclosure

Editors and authors of books and guidelines provided by the Oncology Nursing Society are expected to disclose to the participants any significant financial interest or other relationships with the manufacturer(s) of any commercial products.

A vested interest may be considered to exist if a contributor is affiliated with or has a financial interest in commercial organizations that may have a direct or indirect interest in the subject matter. A "financial interest" may include, but is not limited to, being a shareholder in the organization; being an employee of the commercial organization; serving on an organization's speakers bureau; or receiving research from the organization. An "affiliation" may be holding a position on an advisory board or some other role of benefit to the commercial organization. Vested interest statements appear in the front matter for each publication.

Contributors are expected to disclose any unlabeled or investigational use of products discussed in their content. This information is acknowledged solely for the information of the readers.

The contributors provided the following disclosure and vested interest information:
Megan Dunne, RN, MA, ANP-BC, AOCN®, Institute for Medical Education and Research, faculty
Beth Eaby, MSN, CRNP, OCN®, Merck and Co., speakers bureau, advisory board
Joyce A. Marrs, MS, FNP-BC, AOCNP®, Genentech, Inc., Pfizer Inc., speakers bureaus
Christine Miaskowski, RN, PhD, FAAN, Endo Pharmaceuticals, PriCara, Purdue Pharma L.P., Wyeth Pharmaceuticals, consultant
Carrie Tompkins Stricker, PhD, CRNP, AOCN®, Merck and Co., Roche Pharmaceuticals, speakers bureaus

Contents

Foreword

Oncology nurses around the world care for people who experience multiple and varied symptoms and conditions that are cancer-related, treatment-related, or related to non-cancer issues. These nurses require information that is based on highest-level evidence and focused on responses to these symptoms. They will benefit from the thorough coverage of symptoms and conditions in *A Guide to Oncology Symptom Management*. From the book's first chapter with its evaluation of the unique experiences of older adults with cancer through the final chapter that covers spiritual needs of patients with cancer, this book offers an excellent overview of common symptoms and problems that affect individuals with cancer.

Major symptoms and conditions are addressed thoroughly. Each chapter offers incidence and prevalence information along with an explanation of pathophysiology related to the topic. This background information informs the reader about elements of the unique case study that begins and ends each chapter. Appropriate evidence-based assessment and treatment strategies—both medical and nursing—are discussed from a nursing perspective. All chapters focus on human responses to the symptom or condition. For each topic, clinical practice recommendations and major patient teaching points stemming from the evidence are included. Outcomes to be expected from optimal management are delineated clearly.

This book evolved naturally from the Oncology Nursing Society's (ONS's) forward-thinking initiatives related to evidence-based practice. From the Fatigue Initiative Through Research and Education (FIRE®) and the subsequent Priority Symptom Management (PRISM) project (Ropka & Spencer-Cisek, 2001), ONS spearheaded development of the online Evidence-Based Practice Resource Area in 2002 (http://onsopcontent.ons.org/toolkits/evidence). In 2003, a Steering Council Project Team developed a definition of oncology nursing-sensitive patient outcomes based on a review of models and literature and proposed definitions and an organizing framework. Following this, researchers developed evidence-based summaries of select patient outcomes (e.g., lymphedema, nausea and vomiting, pain) that were used in published studies. These are found in the Outcomes Resource Area of the ONS Web site (www.ons.org/outcomes/measures/summaries.shtml). A natural spin-off, the Putting Evidence Into Practice (PEP) project aims to improve oncology nursing-sensitive patient outcomes through resources that provide evidence-based interventions. Between 2006 and 2008, groups of clinicians and researchers developed literature syntheses that led to 16 PEP resources. Each resource provides evidence-based interventions for patient care and teaching that are color-coded based on strength of evidence (Doorenbos et al., 2008). Literature syntheses and a toolkit developed for use by ONS chapters are available on the ONS Web site. A compilation of updated PEP resources (Eaton & Tipton, 2009) contains assessment and measurement tools as well as ideas for patient care and organizational use, along with case studies to illustrate application of the tools. Each sponsored effort has involved delineation of the current state of the knowledge on particular oncology-related topics and subsequently has supported education programs for oncology nurses and the public.

A Guide to Oncology Symptom Management contains useful and evidence-based nursing information focused on important oncology-specific symptoms and conditions. Nurses will recognize signs and symptoms experienced by real patients and can be confident that the assessment and treatment strategies recommended are based on best evidence and are feasible in real-world settings. They will discover that each chapter considers psychological, physiologic, sociologic, and spiritual needs of patients experiencing symptoms and that implementation of recommended management will assist in enhancing their patients' quality of life. This book is an important acknowledgment of the important part that nurses play in helping people with cancer to manage the often devastating symptoms and problems related to their disease. It is an important and timely contribution to the oncology nursing literature.

Dana N. Rutledge, RN, PhD
Professor, Department of Nursing, California State University, Fullerton
Nursing Research Facilitator, St. Joseph Hospital
Orange, California

References

Doorenbos, A.Z., Berger, A.M., Brohard-Holbert, C., Eaton, L., Kozachik, S., LoBiondo-Wood, G., et al. (2008). Oncology Nursing Society Putting Evidence Into Practice Resources: Where are we now and what is next? *Clinical Journal of Oncology Nursing, 12*(6), 965–970.

Eaton, L.H., & Tipton, J.M. (Eds.). (2009). *Putting evidence into practice: Improving oncology patient outcomes.* Pittsburgh, PA: Oncology Nursing Society.

Ropka, M.E., & Spencer-Cisek, P. (2001). PRISM: Priority Symptom Management Project phase I: Assessment. *Oncology Nursing Forum, 28*(10), 1585–1594.

Acknowledgments

A textbook of this size and stature doesn't come together without lots of persistent assistance and encouragement. I'd like to thank the authors of the chapters herein, who provided their special nursing expertise to these pages through their focus on the symptoms that affect patients with cancer. I'd like to thank Barbara Sigler from ONS Publishing for her vision of this textbook and for her encouragement across every step of the process. To the ONS Publishing Team—Judy Holmes, Lisa George, and especially Amy Nicoletti—for their ongoing dedication to the success of this publication. Finally, I'd like to thank Sylvia Fairclough and Deborah Mayer, two incredibly gifted oncology nurses, for their subtle nudges and ongoing words of support.

CHAPTER 1

Symptoms in Older Adults

Cheryl Lacasse, MS, RN, OCN®

Case Study

M.F. is a 73-year-old man with recurrent colorectal cancer with metastases to the small bowel, liver, lungs, and thoracic spine area and is admitted for pneumonia in the right lower and mid lobe with pleural effusion. His medical history includes osteoarthritis diagnosed 12 years ago, cardiovascular disease (hypertension and congestive heart failure after a myocardial infarction two years ago), type 2 diabetes diagnosed seven years ago, and postoperative deep vein thrombosis after colectomy surgery. Past cancer history includes prostate cancer diagnosed three years ago, treated with radical retroperitoneal prostatectomy with lymph node dissection and follow-up radiation therapy, and colon cancer diagnosed four months ago treated with a total colectomy. He is currently receiving oxaliplatin and 5-fluorouracil, but his treatment has been complicated by bone marrow suppression and altered nutrition. Current medications include ceftriaxone IV, gentamicin IV, prednisone for five days, digoxin, furosemide, potassium chloride, lisinopril, atenolol, Humalog® (Eli Lilly and Co.) insulin subcutaneous injection on sliding scale, citalopram, vitamin K, and a multivitamin. Medications prescribed as needed include acetaminophen, hydrocodone and acetaminophen, albuterol nebulizers, and ibuprofen. A comprehensive symptom assessment reveals achy pain in the thoracic and lumbar spine area rated as 7 on a 0–10 pain scale, occasional sharp pain in his right knee, headache, nausea, dyspnea on exertion, sharp pain with inspiration, fatigue rated as 6 on a 0–10 scale, insomnia, petechiae on abdomen and lower extremities, anorexia with a 30-pound weight loss since diagnosis of colon cancer, and sadness because of the diagnosis, disease progression, and loss of previous good health and active lifestyle. M.F. has been married for 47 years, and his wife is his primary caregiver and has several comorbidities herself.

Overview

In 2006, adults age 65 and older accounted for just more than 12% of the total U.S. population (Federal Interagency Forum on Aging-Related Statistics, 2008). It is projected that by 2030, 20% of the U.S. population will be age 65 years and older as the baby boomer generation ages (Federal Interagency Forum on Aging-Related Statistics). In addition, the group of older adults age 85 years and older is projected to grow rapidly after 2030 as the baby boomers enter the oldest-old population group (Federal Interagency Forum on Aging-Related Statistics). Older adults are one of the most vulnerable and rapidly growing populations with cancer. More than three-quarters of all cancers are diagnosed in individuals age 55 years and older. Cancer and heart disease are the leading causes of death in adults age 65 and older (Jemal et al., 2009). Men age 70 years and older have a one-in-three probability of developing cancer, with the most common cancers being prostate, lung and bronchus, colon and rectum, and urinary bladder (Jemal et al.). Women age 70 years and older have a one-in-four chance of developing cancer, with the most common cancers being breast, lung and bronchus, colon and rectum, and uterine (Jemal et al.). Many issues are unique to the aging population and may have an overall effect on symptom management in this population. These include the changes of normal aging, common health issues in the aging population such as chronic illnesses, frailty, polypharmacy, and complex symptom relationships, which include groups of symptoms attributed to aging and chronic illness.

Overview of Normal Aging

Most individuals who are age 65 and older experience normal physiologic changes, which may have an effect on the manifestation of cancer-related symptoms and their treatment. Table 1-1 includes normal physiologic changes of aging and considerations for symptom assessment and management in older adults. Aging skin has thinner layers because of the loss of cutaneous and subcutaneous tissue, fewer blood vessels and nerves, and less elasticity. Bone loss is a common occurrence in aging individuals and may occur as a result of altered calcium metabolism. In addition, loss of soft tissue function, including muscle atrophy and slowing of the nervous system, may affect overall physical functioning and independence. Sensory loss and altered cognitive functioning may have an impact on overall functioning and successful pharmacologic and nonpharmacologic symptom management modalities.

TABLE 1-1	Physiologic Changes of Aging and Their Relationship to Symptom Management
Physiologic Change	**Potential Impact on Symptom Management**
Skin	
Decreased cutaneous layers and thinned subcutaneous tissue	Can increase risk for effects of anorexia and cachexia
Decreased blood vessels	May alter absorption of transdermal medications; may decrease ability to use IV route for symptom management
Decreased nerves	May alter pain sensation
Decreased elasticity	Increases risk for skin tears
Bones	
Altered calcium metabolism leading to bone loss	Increases risk for bone instability with metastatic bone disease
Tooth loss	Increases risk for malnutrition during therapy and subsequent nutrition-related symptoms such as anemia, mucous membrane and skin breakdown, and electrolyte disturbances
Soft Tissue	
Muscle atrophy	Decreases strength and endurance, which may increase fatigue
Nervous system slowing	Decreases fine motor control, which may have an impact on implementing symptom management strategies
Increased body fat	May have an impact on drug metabolism

(Continued on next page)

TABLE 1-1	Physiologic Changes of Aging and Their Relationship to Symptom Management *(Continued)*
Physiologic Change	**Potential Impact on Symptom Management**

Sensory Loss	
Hearing	May have an impact on communication of patient education information for symptom management
Vision	May have an impact on communication of patient education information for symptom management
Smell	May have an impact on successful treatment of anorexia or cachexia
Hematology and Immunology	
Decreased bone marrow reserve	May have delayed response to infection and anemia
Anemia related to decreased intrinsic factor production and decreased iron metabolism	May contribute to cancer-related fatigue
Increased clotting caused by increased platelet adhesion	May contribute to perfusion issues and lead to vague, non-cancer-related symptoms
Circulation	
Enlargement of heart Slowing of electrical activity Changes in collagen in arteries, causing stiffness and thickening	Caution should be used with symptom management drugs that may affect cardiac function, such as medications used for treating neuropathic pain.
Pulmonary	
Decreased oxygen and carbon dioxide exchange because of decreased elasticity of lung tissue and alveoli enlargement	Caution should be used with medications that have a direct effect on pulmonary functioning, such as benzodiazepines or opioids.
Decreased cough reflex and ciliary function	May increase risk of decreased airway clearance
Gastrointestinal	
Decline in small intestinal absorption of vitamins D and B$_{12}$ and folic acid	Increases risk for developing anemia and bone loss
Thinning of intestinal lining, decreased mucus production, and weaker intestinal muscles	Increases risk for constipation
Diminished liver function because of circulatory and metabolic changes	May have an impact on drug metabolism by slowing drug metabolism and leading to increased drug toxicity
Urinary	
Decreased renal perfusion beginning at age 40	Increases risk for developing drug toxicity, especially with nonsteroidal anti-inflammatory drugs and diuretics
Decreased number of nephrons and glomeruli with decreased glomerular filtration rate	May increase risk for dehydration or fluid overload
Decreased adaptability of kidneys to handle stress	Altered potassium regulation
Decreased bladder capacity and tone; decreased tone of pelvic floor	May lead to urinary incontinence
Enlargement of prostate	Eventually leads to lower urinary tract symptoms
Cognitive	
Decrease in short-term memory	May decrease ability to remember details of symptom onset, duration, and treatment

Note. Based on information from Aldwin & Gilmer, 2004; Tabloski, 2006.

An altered hematopoietic system in the older adult may lead to a delayed response of bone marrow to therapy-induced bone marrow suppression and may increase the risk of infection and anemia (Tabloski, 2006). In addition, the older adult may have an altered production and metabolism of intrinsic factor and iron. Alterations in the cardiopulmonary systems may increase the adverse effects of symptom management medications. Alterations in the gastrointestinal system may affect multiple systems, such as vitamins D and B_{12} and folic acid absorption; bowel elimination; and hepatic metabolism of pharmacologic agents (Tabloski). Changes in urinary elimination may have a major impact on drug metabolism via the kidneys, hydration status, and urinary continence. Cognitive changes usually are subtle and affect short-term memory acuity.

Common Health Issues in the Aging Population

Chronic Illnesses and Conditions

Most individuals older than 65 years of age have at least one chronic illness, and many of them have two or more (Yancik, 1997). The average number of comorbidities stratified by age in the older adult oncology population range from two to three comorbidities for 55–64-year-olds to three to four comorbidities for those age 75 and older (Yancik). The most prevalent chronic conditions reported by the Federal Interagency Forum on Aging-Related Statistics (2008) are hypertension, arthritis, heart disease, cancer, diabetes, and chronic respiratory illnesses. The same agency lists the following chronic diseases as the leading causes of death in people 65 years or older: heart disease, cancer, cerebrovascular disease, chronic lower respiratory diseases, influenza and pneumonia, diabetes, and Alzheimer disease. In addition, individuals age 65 years and older have hearing trouble (41.5%), trouble with vision (approximately 17%), and issues with dentition, with about 26% having no natural teeth (Federal Interagency Forum on Aging-Related Statistics). Comorbidities and their symptoms add to the complexity of cancer-related symptom identification and treatment. For example, an older adult with significant cardiac disease and lung cancer may have overlapping symptoms of chest pain, shortness of breath, fatigue, and cough, which may require simultaneous oncology and cardiopulmonary-related treatments.

In addition, the "normal" symptom experience may be correlated with aging or chronic illness but not cancer or its treatment. The traditional retirement age has been suggested to be a developmental marker for changes in symptom perception from abnormal to a normal expectation that comes with age (Williamson & Schulz, 1995). Altered symptom perception may affect "normal signals" to seek treatment if symptoms are perceived to be part of the aging process or attributable to comorbidities. For example, an older adult experiencing chronic fatigue may attribute it to old age or heart disease when in fact it is a serious symptom of chronic leukemia or multiple myeloma. Several studies that have assessed symptoms by self-report have suggested that older adults experience less symptom severity and symptom distress than younger populations (Degner & Sloan, 1995; McMillan, 1989; Williamson & Schulz). When assessing symptoms of older adults by self-report, healthcare providers should consider that symptoms are either experienced less overall, are "normalized" within the context of a person's chronic illness experience, or do not have a profound impact on overall functioning. Further research is needed to determine if older adults perceive symptoms the same way as younger populations.

Polypharmacy

The use of multiple medications to treat health-related conditions generally is considered polypharmacy; however, multiple definitions are used in the literature (Fulton & Allen, 2005). Williams (2002) reported that an estimated 61% of individuals age 65 years and older take at least one medication. In addition, Williams reported that most of these older individuals take an average of three to five prescription medications per day, not including over-the-counter and herbal medications. Many factors contribute to the cause of polypharmacy, including (a) multiple chronic conditions, (b) age-related physiologic changes, (c) lack of knowledge about the use of multiple medications, (d) increased use of complementary therapies, (e) self-medication with over-the-counter medications, and (f) use of multiple healthcare providers (Fulton & Allen). The issue of polypharmacy has major implications for the use of pharmacologic methods of symptom management in older adults.

Adverse drug reactions are a concern with older adults with multiple chronic conditions and symptoms who are taking multiple medications. For example, an 82-year-old with metastatic breast cancer, hypertension, congestive heart failure, and gastroesophageal reflux disease may be on multiple medications to manage her chronic conditions and their symptoms, such as multiple antihypertensives, a proton pump inhibitor, a diuretic, and oral chemotherapy. Pain management that includes a nonsteroidal anti-inflammatory drug may be contraindicated because of the risk for increased gastrointestinal irritation, increased risk of renal toxicity, and altered therapeutic effect of antihypertensives. Generally, the potential for an individual to have adverse drug reactions increases with the number of medications taken. Gurwitz et al. (2003) suggested that the rate of adverse drug reaction is 50% when an individual is on five drugs together, and 100% when an individual is taking eight or more medications together. Overall negative outcomes of polypharmacy may include drug-drug interactions that either enhance a drug's potency or diminish its therapeutic effect, thus leading to further symptoms. Multiple drugs may cause a cumulative toxic effect on the chemoreceptor trigger zone, leading to nausea, vomiting, and altered nutritional intake. Adverse effects of multiple drugs also can lead to an increase in delirium and falls in older adults (Gurwitz et al.).

Frailty

In addition to normal changes that occur in aging, older adults with cancer and multiple medical illnesses may experience loss of organ function, decrease in physical function reserve, and overall health decline. The term *frail elders* has been applied to older populations who have decreased physical, cognitive, and social functioning leading to overall disability. Frailty has been defined as a multidimensional phenomenon that includes a decline in daily physical functioning, imbalanced nutrition, cognitive decline, and sensory impairment (Strawbridge, Shema, Balfour, Higby, & Kaplan, 1998). The concept of frailty may be defined as a clinical syndrome that includes the following characteristics: decreased physiologic and psychological homeostasis, chronic malnutrition (unintentional weight loss of 10 pounds or more in the past year, self-report of exhaustion, weakness), and sarcopenia (leading to slow walking speed and minimal physical activity) (Fried et al., 2001). A comprehensive geriatric assessment (CGA) can screen for frailty in the older adult oncology population and may yield valuable information for healthcare providers to use when making treatment-related decisions (Ferrucci et al., 2003). Symptom assessment and management in the frail elder population is very challenging and requires careful consideration of appropriate pharmacologic and nonpharmacologic symptom management approaches and their overall impact on functioning and quality of life.

Cancer-Related Symptom Issues

Assessment

Because most cancers occur in the older adult population, symptom assessment needs to include a broad approach, as members of this population are likely to have complex medical histories that include multiple chronic illnesses with concurrent symptoms and their treatments. The presence of oncology-related symptoms should be explored in context with the patient's medical and surgical histories and current medical and surgical treatments. Maas, Janssen-Heijnen, Olde Rikkert, and Machteld Wymenga (2007) suggested that a multidisciplinary CGA is instrumental in collecting valuable data for determining specific clinical interventions and their practical outcome end points. Typically, a CGA includes a medical history, physical and cognitive functional assessment (focused on activities of daily living, instrumental activities of daily living, and sensory function), psychological and social functioning, socioeconomic environment, nutrition, and polypharmacy (Effingham, Meyer, & Balducci, 2003; Ferrucci et al., 2003; Maas et al.). In addition, the CGA screens older adults for the presence of geriatric syndromes, including pressure sores, history of falls, incontinence, delirium, depression, dementia, and functional decline (Maas et al.; Tabloski, 2006). Commonly used CGA screening tools are listed in Table 1-2 and can be found online at the Hartford Institute for Geriatric Nursing ConsultGeriRN.org Web site (www.consultgerirn.org/resources), which provides evidence-based online resources for nurses to enhance the clinical care of the older adult population with a variety of complex needs.

TABLE 1-2	Commonly Used Assessment Tools in a Comprehensive Geriatric Assessment
Focus of Assessment	**Assessment Tools**
Physical	Katz Index of Independence in Activities of Daily Living*
Comorbidity	Number of comorbid conditions
Cognitive	The Mini-Cog Confusion Assessment Method*
Psychological	Geriatric Depression Scale*
Nutrition	Mini Nutritional Assessment*
Polypharmacy	Chart review and medication count
Independent living skills	Lawton Instrumental Activities of Daily Living (IADL) Scale*
Falls	Hendrich II Fall Risk Model*
Skin breakdown	Braden Scale*
Incontinence	Urinary Incontinence Assessment*
Elder abuse	Elder Mistreatment Assessment*
Caregiver burden	Caregiver Strain Index*

* These tools are available with a brief description on the *Try This: Best Practices in Nursing Care to Older Adults* Web site (http://www.consultgerirn.org/resources, accessed June 1, 2008) from the Hartford Institute for Geriatric Nursing, New York University, College of Nursing.

Note. Based on information from Effingham et al., 2003.

Heidrich, Egan, Hengudomsub, and Randolph (2006) studied symptoms, beliefs about symptoms, and quality of life in older breast cancer survivors and found that many participants attributed their symptoms to aging and chronic health problems. Symptoms attributed to chronic illness or cancers were related to increased pain, depression, impaired role function, and poor mental health. Individuals who did not know the cause of their symptoms had poorer social functioning, poorer mental health (depression and anxiety), and increased fatigue. This study suggests that broad symptom assessment and CGA may be important for planning comprehensive symptom management.

Symptom Perception

Symptoms in older adults may be complex in origin, and symptom perception of chronic illness, presenting symptoms of cancer, symptoms of disease exacerbation, and symptoms caused by treatment of disease may be blurred. Table 1-3 lists presenting symptoms of the most common cancers in older adults (prostate, breast, lung and bronchus, and colorectal cancers) and common chronic conditions in older adults, which have overlapping symptoms. The symptoms of prostate cancer are very similar to the presenting symptoms of benign prostatic hypertrophy, which is an expected condition of aging males. In the absence of mam-

TABLE 1-3	Comparison of Presenting Symptoms of Common Cancers and Chronic Conditions Diagnosed at Age 60 or Older
Diagnosis/Chronic Condition	**Common Presenting Symptoms**
Breast cancer	Abnormal mammography, painless lump (American Cancer Society [ACS], 2009)
Prostate cancer	Early disease: No symptoms Advanced disease: Weak or interrupted urinary flow, difficulty starting or stopping urinary stream, nocturnal urinary frequency, blood in urine, pain or burning with urination (ACS, 2009) Metastatic disease: Continual pain in lower back, pelvis, and upper thighs
Benign prostatic hypertrophy	Increasing intensity of lower urinary tract symptoms (nocturia, daytime urinary frequency, urgency, urinary hesitancy, weak urinary stream) (Gray, 2005)
Cancers of the lung and bronchus	Persistent cough, blood-streaked sputum, chest pain, voice change, recurrent pulmonary infections (ACS, 2009)
Chronic lung disease	Productive cough, decreased exercise tolerance, wheezing, shortness of breath, prolonged expiration, dyspnea on exertion or at rest (Cronin & Miracle, 2005)
Chronic cardiac disease	Chest pain, palpitations, dyspnea, orthopnea, cough, wheezing, cyanosis, hemoptysis, tachypnea, fatigue, muscle weakness, syncope, weight gain, dependent edema, anxiety, confusion, insomnia, decreased exercise tolerance (Tazbir & Keresztes, 2005)
Cancers of the colon and rectum	Early stage: Minimal symptoms Metastatic disease: Continual pain in lower back, pelvis, and upper thighs
Diverticulitis	Steady left lower quadrant or mid-abdominal pain, altered bowel habits (diarrhea, constipation, or both), increased flatus, anorexia, low-grade fever, trace blood or mucus in stool (Rogers, 2005)

mography, the presenting symptoms of breast cancer may be mistaken as normal changes of aging breast tissue. Symptoms of lung and bronchus cancer are somewhat similar to symptoms of chronic lung diseases. Colorectal cancer symptoms may mimic symptoms of a wide variety of gastrointestinal diseases. Clinicians must consider the symptoms of chronic illnesses, primary cancer, and treatments when performing a comprehensive symptom assessment on older adults. Oncology nurses have a distinct opportunity to detect potential cancers or cancer-related complications in older adults because their symptoms may be intertwined with chronic illness symptoms and perceived symptoms of normal aging.

Symptoms and Their Relationships

The symptom of pain is well studied in the older adult population. The multiple dimensions of the pain experience of older adults with cancer include the physiologic, psychological, spiritual, affective, and contextual dimensions and require careful assessment. The physiologic sensation of pain in older adults is very complex and may be affected by symptoms of multiple chronic illnesses and their treatments and specific values and beliefs about the origin of the pain, its meaning, and past pain experiences (Ray, 2002). The affective dimension of pain integrates sympathetic sensation, cognitive appraisal (what type of threat is the pain), and the perceived meaning of pain. The contextual meaning of pain includes sociocultural values and beliefs and perceptions of disease (both cancer and other chronic illnesses). A recent interdisciplinary review of pain assessment in older adults reported a comprehensive consensus statement including recommendations for physical evaluation, use of self-report, assessment of older adults with dementia, functional status evaluation, emotional functioning evaluation, and medication history (Hadjistavropoulos et al., 2007). This group represented the disciplines of medicine, nursing, pharmacy, psychology, occupational therapy, physiotherapy, neurology, and gerontology. The group provided a critical review of the most common assessment tools in pain management of older adults and suggested that the client's ability to report pain is an important factor in selecting a pain assessment method and tool (Hadjistavropoulos et al.). Over the past decade, scientific knowledge has begun to expand the understanding of differences in pain perception between younger and older individuals. Some evidence has suggested that pain perception may steadily increase until the seventh decade and then begins to decline, possibly because of altered neurologic functioning in peripheral and central pathways caused by aging (Gibson & Helme, 2001). Oncology nurses need to carefully assess the current pain of older adults within the context of physiologic age and condition and general pain experience.

Pain also has been studied in relationship to other cancer-related symptoms, such as fatigue and depression. Chang, Hwang, Feuerman, and Kasimis (2000) studied symptom prevalence, distress, and intensity in older adults with cancer and found that patients with moderate or severe pain and fatigue had an increased number of reported symptoms and a high level of symptom distress. Given, Given, Azzouz, and Stommel (2001) found that patients who were most likely to report pain and fatigue were those with three or more chronic illnesses, lung cancer, and late-stage cancer.

Other studies also have suggested a strong relationship between the symptoms of pain and fatigue, along with their contribution to decline in physical functioning (Bennett, Stewart, Kayser-Jones, & Glaser, 2002; Dodd, Miaskowski, & Paul, 2001; Given, Given, Azzouz, Kozachik, & Stommel, 2001; Hodgson & Given, 2004). Additionally, researchers have explored the relationship among symptoms (including pain and fatigue), physical functioning, and depression in older adults. Generally, research has supported that increased symptom severity and decreased physical functioning may lead to depressive symptoms in older adults (Geerlings, Twisk, Beekman, Deeg, & van Tilburg, 2002; Kurtz, Kurtz, Stommel, Given, & Given, 2001; Williamson & Schulz, 1995). This evidence suggested that the decline in physical functioning caused by symptoms may have a profound effect on the psychological and social well-being of older adults. The implications for nursing symptom management include focusing on symptoms that have a negative impact on physical functioning, such as pain or fatigue, using client-centered goal setting to plan care, and critically evaluating the impact of symptom management strategies on patients' quality of life.

In addition, the exploration of symptom clusters in individuals with chronic diseases and cancer may further illuminate the complexity of symptoms in older adults with multiple chronic illnesses.

> A symptom cluster consists of 2 or more symptoms that are related to each other and that occur together. Symptom clusters are composed of stable groups of symptoms, are relatively independent of other clusters, and may reveal specific underlying dimensions of symptoms. Relationships among symptoms within a cluster should be stronger than relationships among symptoms across different clusters. Symptoms in a cluster may or may not share the same etiology. (Kim, McGuire, Tulman, & Barsevick, 2005, p. 278)

In an overview of symptom clusters related to specific cancers, Gift (2007) concluded that a cluster of symptoms commonly is found in many different types of cancers and includes (but is not limited to) pain, fatigue, sleep disruptions, depression, and weakness. Gift also suggested that symptoms be viewed in the context of the type of cancer and its treatment, comorbidities, duration and interpretation of symptoms, and changes over time. Bender et al. (2008) suggested that symptom clusters in older adults may be unique to chronic health problems and comorbidities within the context of the cancer experience.

Pharmacologic Management

Pharmacologic intervention for oncology symptom management of older adults requires the consideration of current health status, the medical treatment regimen, and physical and mental functioning. For example, a 78-year-old with metastatic colon cancer to the liver and a history of stroke and multi-infarct dementia may be challenging to assess for symptom presence and distress, treat with appropriate medications for symptom control, and evaluate the outcome of symptom management. Care should be taken to avoid the use of medications that may cause severe toxicities in the older adult. Fick et al. (2003) used a panel of nationally recognized experts in geriatric care, clinical pharmacology, and psychopharmacology to reach a consensus about potentially inappropriate medications for older adults. The results of this study were used to revise the original criteria that had guided physicians for more than 10 years when they were prescribing and working with adults age 65 and older.

Laroche, Charmes, and Merle (2007) completed a study in France using an expert panel consensus format, which yielded similar results. Both sets of researchers cautioned clinicians to use their list of criteria as a general guide for determining the appropriateness of pharmacologic treatments in the older adult population. Table 1-4 has a comprehensive list of medications and their potential toxicities related to oncology symptom management in the older adult population. When determining the appropriate pharmacologic management for cancer-related symptoms in older adults, clinicians should consider the individual's clinical condition, functional status (both physical and cognitive), current comprehensive drug list (both oncology-related and general), and overall prognosis.

TABLE 1-4	Potentially Inappropriate Symptom Management Medications for Older Adults
Drug	**Description of Potential Toxicities**
Nonsteroidal Anti-Inflammatory Drugs (NSAIDs)	May cause or exacerbate gastric or duodenal ulcers* Prolonged clotting time and international normalized ratio* Decreased platelet function*
Indomethacin	Central nervous system (CNS) effects (highest of all NSAIDs)*
Ketorolac	Asymptomatic gastrointestinal conditions, such as ulcers*
Aspirin (> 325 mg)	Asymptomatic gastrointestinal conditions, such as ulcers*
Naproxen	Gastrointestinal bleeding* Renal failure* High blood pressure* Heart failure*
Opioids	
Meperidine	Has an intense side effect profile for adverse effects, especially CNS effects such as seizures; most critical in individuals with renal compromise*
Morphine, hydromorphone, fentanyl	Has an intense side effect profile at higher doses, especially CNS effects (such as somnolence, respiratory depression, and delirium)*
Adjuvant Drugs	
Muscle relaxants (methocarbamol, carisoprodol, chlorzoxazone, metaxalone, cyclobenzaprine, baclofen)	Anticholinergic effects*† Sedation* Weakness* Cognitive impairment*
Tricyclic antidepressants (amitriptyline and amitriptyline compounds)	Strong anticholinergic effects*† May lead to ataxia, impaired psychomotor function, syncope, and falls Cardiac arrhythmias (QT interval changes)* May produce polyuria or lead to urinary incontinence* May exacerbate chronic constipation
Doxepin	Cardiac arrhythmias* May produce polyuria or lead to urinary incontinence* May exacerbate chronic constipation
Antihistamines (diphenhydramine, hydroxyzine, promethazine)	Potent anticholinergic properties*† May lead to confusion and sedation
Benzodiazepines	Increased sensitivity at higher doses with prolonged sedation and increased risk for falls
• Short acting (lorazepam ≥ 3 mg, oxazepam ≥ 60 mg, alprazolam ≥ 2 mg)	May produce or exacerbate depression Smaller doses may be both effective and safer.
• Long acting (diazepam)	CNS effects* May cause or exacerbate respiratory depression in chronic obstructive pulmonary disease* May produce polyuria or lead to urinary incontinence*

(Continued on next page)

TABLE 1-4	Potentially Inappropriate Symptom Management Medications for Older Adults *(Continued)*
Drug	**Description of Potential Toxicities**
Selective serotonin reuptake inhibitor antidepressants (fluoxetine, citalopram, paroxetine, sertraline)	May produce CNS stimulation, sleep disturbances, and increasing agitation* May exacerbate or cause syndrome of inappropriate secretion of antidiuretic hormone or hyponatremia
Decongestants	High level of CNS stimulation, which may lead to insomnia*
CNS stimulants (methylphenidate)	Altered CNS function, leading to cognitive impairment* Appetite-suppressing effect*

*High severity rating
†Anticholinergic effects include some of the following symptoms: blurred vision, constipation, drowsiness, sedation, dry mouth, tachycardia, urinary retention, confusion, disorientation, memory impairment, dizziness, nausea, nervousness, agitation, anxiety, facial flushing, weakness, and delirium.

Note. Based on information from Fick et al., 2003; Laroche et al., 2007.

In general, symptoms in older adults can be managed effectively with conservative pharmacologic therapies. Adult dosing of medications generally is safe for older adults, but clinicians must seriously consider the patient's size, nutritional status (i.e., serum albumen level, as some drugs are protein bound), renal and hepatic function, lifestyle and life responsibilities, and economic issues. The general rule of "start low and go slow" with regard to dosing symptom management medications is especially important in the older adult population. Comprehensive evidence-based clinical guidelines for treating older adults with cancer and complex symptoms such as pain are available to clinicians and can assist in critical clinical decision making about the application of symptom management strategies (American Geriatrics Society [AGS] Panel on Persistent Pain in Older Persons, 2002; National Comprehensive Cancer Network, 2009).

Nonpharmacologic Management

Many of the nonpharmacologic techniques generally used for cancer symptom management can be used with the older adult population. Care must be taken to adapt these interventions to the limitations of the patients and their individualized responses. Physical activity (exercise and strength training) is one evidence-based intervention that is effective in many chronic illness populations and older adults with cancer. A recent review of the use of physical activity in older people with cancer suggested that this intervention decreases fatigue, elevates mood, improves physical functioning, decreases role limitations, decreases falls, and modifies cardiovascular risk factors (Penedo, Schneiderman, Dahn, & Gonzalez, 2004). Benefits to using physical activity as an intervention for cancer-related symptoms in older adults with cancer may include decreased pain, fall risk, depression, and fatigue and increased appetite and sense of well-being (AGS Panel on Persistent Pain in Older Persons, 2002). However, this intervention needs to be tailored to the individual's physical and cognitive limitations.

Considering the symptom of pain, older adults are reported to use multiple nonpharmacologic methods, and many perceive these therapies to be effective in managing their pain (Barry, Gill, Kerns, & Reid, 2005; Jakobsson, Hallberg, & Westergren, 2004). Several nonpharmacologic techniques frequently used by older adults to treat their pain include physical therapies (heat, massage, stretching, and muscle release), cognitive-behavioral therapies (distraction, imagery, relaxation exercises), assistive devices (canes, walkers, raised toilet seats and chairs, large-grip utensils), and complementary therapies (therapeutic touch, music therapy, exercise, reminiscence therapy) (AGS Panel on Persistent Pain in Older Persons, 2002; Barry et al.; Coyle & Derby, 2006; Jakobsson et al.; Weiner & Hanlon, 2001). Many of these techniques may be used for management of other cancer-related symptoms, such as fatigue, depression, anxiety, and functional decline. However, the current evidence for use of these interventions in the older adult cancer population is minimal.

Symptom Management Outcomes

Quality symptom management is a key to enhancing the overall quality of life and optimal functioning of older adults with cancer-related symptoms. General cancer symptom management principles may be safely applied to the gero-oncology population with careful consideration of the physiologic changes of aging. Clinical research in symptom management interventions for older adults with cancer is very sparse and needs to be the focus of interdisciplinary research teams. The incorporation of an abbreviated CGA for each individual with cancer who is age 65 and older may provide valuable insights into the most appropriate holistic symptom management to implement. General knowledge of the normal changes that occur with aging also may assist members of the healthcare team to be more vigilant in assessing for positive and negative patient responses to therapy. In addition, this knowledge will aid in the planning and implementation of age-specific education about symptom management therapies. Maintaining a caring partnership with older adults with cancer and their families will provide the best possible symptom management outcomes and will lead to higher levels of functioning and better overall quality of life.

Need for Future Research

Further studies need to be done to explicate the symptoms of older cancer survivors with multiple chronic illnesses. Generally, symptoms that are common in the oncology population are also common in the older adult population, but more research is needed regarding the appropriate assessment of symptoms, prevalence of these symptoms, distress and intensity of symptoms, their overlap with common symptoms in chronic illness, and symptom management within the older population.

Conclusion of Case Study

Factors to Consider for This Patient

Assessment

A screening of the functional status of this older adult indicates that he is at risk for functional decline because of symptoms related to cancer and other comorbidities, nutritional deficits, chemotherapy-related bone marrow depression, and reactive depression. The patient also is currently at risk for falls because of spine pain and its effect on safe movement, and for skin breakdown because of nutritional deficits, diabetes, and prednisone therapy. An assessment of laboratory values reveals decreased renal and hepatic function beyond the expected decline with aging and chemotherapy-induced pancytopenia. Functional decline may be the most important factor to address in achieving optimal symptom control. The patient clearly verbalizes that quality of life is more important than quantity of life. The patient defines quality of life as having enough symptom control to have clear thinking and spend time with his close friends and family.

Goal of Care

Collaborative goal setting is a key component in achieving optimal symptom management outcomes, which is defined by M.F. as quality of life.

Planning Comprehensive Symptom Management

Pharmacologic management requires careful consideration of comorbidities and drug-drug interactions with cardiac, pulmonary, arthritis, diabetes, and pneumonia-related medications. The symptom of pain may be the most challenging to treat because multiple sources of pain exist related to the cancer and acute and chronic illnesses. Although acetaminophen is the drug of choice for pain management in older adults, this patient reports significant pain, which may not be responsive to acetaminophen, and also has decreased hepatic function. Ibuprofen may be the drug of choice for bone pain, but this medication may cause further renal impairment, exacerbate nausea, increase the risk of bleeding (especially gastrointestinal bleeding), and decrease the therapeutic effect of the patient's antihypertensives. Opioids such as morphine may be an alternative to treat this patient's pain and dyspnea; however, low doses should be used, and the patient should be monitored carefully for adverse effects such as delirium. A medication with a low adverse effect profile, such as low doses of a selective 5-HT_3 receptor blocker (i.e., ondansetron), should be used to treat nausea. Treatment of fatigue should consist of nutritional support and hematopoietic growth factors.

The most appropriate nonpharmacologic therapy for this patient should include patient and family education, relaxation exercises such as music therapy, and gentle physical activity when the patient has recuperated from the pneumonia. Progressive physical activity is important in assisting this patient to treat his fatigue and attain his maximum level of functioning and may have a profound effect on his ability to cope with the disease process.

Evaluation of Symptom Management

Evaluation of the symptom management plan and implementation should be done with respect to the effect of treatment on the symptoms themselves, the stability of the patient's chronic illnesses, the caregiver's perspective, and the patient's overall quality of life as he defines it.

Conclusion

Approximately 20% of the U.S. population will be age 65 and older by 2030, and nurses will be challenged to care for a population with multiple complex healthcare needs, including those with cancer. The intertwined nature of symptoms related to cancer and its treatment, chronic illnesses, and an individual's perception of normal aging presents a challenge for optimal symptom management in the gero-oncology population. Nurses must utilize evidence-based practices in oncology and geriatric care to ensure quality care for older adults with cancer. These practices include comprehensive assessment of health issues that are common to older patients with cancer, such as frailty, polypharmacy, and physical, cognitive, and social functioning, along with comprehensive management of each. Nurses are essential members of the interdisciplinary cancer care team and are responsible for ensuring the best possible symptom management outcomes without compromising the quality of life of the gero-oncology population.

References

Aldwin, C.M., & Gilmer, D.F. (2004). *Health, illness, and optimal aging.* Thousand Oaks, CA: Sage.

American Cancer Society. (2009). *Cancer facts and figures 2009.* Atlanta, GA: American Cancer Society.

American Geriatrics Society (AGS) Panel on Persistent Pain in Older Persons. (2002). The management of persistent pain in older persons. *Journal of the American Geriatrics Society, 50*(Suppl. 6), S205–S224.

Barry, L., Gill, T., Kerns, R., & Reid, C. (2005). Identification of pain-reduction strategies used by community-dwelling older persons. *Journal of Gerontology: Medical Sciences, 60A*(12), 1569–1575.

Bender, C.M., Engberg, S.J., Donovan, H.S., Cohen, S.M., Houze, M.P., Rosenzweig, M.Q., et al. (2008). Symptom clusters in adults with chronic health problems and cancer as a comorbidity [Online exclusive]. *Oncology Nursing Forum, 35*(1), E1–E11. Retrieved March 20, 2008, from http://ons.metapress.com/content/t72708g317225271/fulltext.pdf

Bennett, J.A., Stewart, A.L., Kayser-Jones, J., & Glaser, D. (2002). The mediating effect of pain and fatigue on level of functioning in older adult. *Nursing Research, 51*(4), 254–265.

Chang, V.T., Hwang, S.S., Feuerman, M., & Kasimis, B.S. (2000). Symptom and quality of life survey of medical oncology patients at a Veterans Affairs medical center: A role for symptom assessment. *Cancer, 88*(5), 1175–1183.

Coyle, N., & Derby, S. (2006). Symptom management of pain. In D. Cope & A. Reb (Eds.), *An evidence-based approach to the treatment and care of the older adult with cancer* (pp. 397–438). Pittsburgh, PA: Oncology Nursing Society.

Cronin, S.N., & Miracle, K. (2005). Management of clients with lower airway and pulmonary vessel disorders. In J.M. Black & J.H. Hawks (Eds.), *Medical-surgical nursing: Clinical management for positive outcomes* (pp. 1807–1836). St. Louis, MO: Elsevier Saunders.

Degner, L.F., & Sloan, J.A. (1995). Symptom distress in newly diagnosed ambulatory cancer patients and as a predictor of survival in lung cancer. *Journal of Pain and Symptom Management, 10*(6), 423–431.

Dodd, M.L., Miaskowski, C., & Paul, S. (2001). Symptom clusters and their effect on the functional status of patients with cancer. *Oncology Nursing Forum, 28*(3), 465–470.

Effingham, K., Meyer, J., & Balducci, L. (2003). Obtaining a comprehensive geriatric assessment. In J. Overcash & L. Balducci (Eds.), *The older cancer patient: A guide for nurses and related professionals* (pp. 86–106). New York: Springer.

Federal Interagency Forum on Aging-Related Statistics. (2008). *Older Americans 2008: Key indicators of well-being.* Washington, DC: U.S. Government Printing Office.

Ferrucci, L., Guralnik, J.M., Cavazzini, C., Bandinelli, S., Lauretani, F., Bartali, B., et al. (2003). The frailty syndrome: A critical issue in geriatric oncology. *Critical Reviews in Oncology/Hematology, 46*(2), 127–137.

Fick, D.M., Cooper, J.W., Wade, W.E., Waller, J.L., Maclean, J.R., & Beers, M.H. (2003). Updating the Beers criteria for potentially inappropriate medication use in older adults: Results of a US consensus panel of experts. *Archives of Internal Medicine, 163*(22), 2716–2724.

Fried, L.P., Tangen, C.M., Walston, J., Newman, A.B., Hirsch, C., Gottdiener, J., et al. (2001). Frailty in older adults: Evidence for a phenotype. *Journal of Gerontology: Medical Sciences, 56A*(3), M146–M156.

Fulton, M.M., & Allen, E.R. (2005). Polypharmacy in the elderly: A literature review. *Journal of the American Academy of Nurse Practitioners, 17*(4), 123–132.

Geerlings, S.W., Twisk, J.W., Beekman, A.T., Deeg, D.J., & van Tilburg, W. (2002). Longitudinal relationship between pain and depression in older adults: Sex, age and physical disability. *Social Psychiatry and Psychiatric Epidemiology, 37*(1), 23–30.

Gibson, S.J., & Helme, R. (2001). Age-related differences in pain perception and report. *Clinics in Geriatric Medicine, 17*(3), 433–456.

Gift, A.G. (2007). Symptom clusters related to specific cancers. *Seminars in Oncology Nursing, 23*(2), 136–141.

Given, B., Given, C.W., Azzouz, F., & Stommel, M. (2001). Physical functioning of elderly cancer patients prior to diagnosis and following initial treatment. *Nursing Research, 50*(4), 222–232.

Given, C.W., Given, B., Azzouz, F., Kozachik, S., & Stommel, M. (2001). Predictors of pain and fatigue in the year following diagnosis among elderly cancer patients. *Journal of Pain and Symptom Management, 21*(6), 456–466.

Gray, M. (2005). Management of men with reproductive disorders. In J.M. Black & J.H. Hawks (Eds.), *Medical-surgical nursing: Clinical management for positive outcomes* (pp. 1013–1052). St. Louis, MO: Elsevier Saunders.

Gurwitz, J.H., Field, T.S., Harrold, L.R., Rothschild, J., Debellis, K., Seger, A.C., et al. (2003). Incidence and preventability of adverse drug events among older persons in the ambulatory setting. *JAMA, 289*(9), 1107–1116.

Hadjistavropoulos, T., Herr, K., Turk, D.C., Fine, P.G., Dworkin, R.H., Helme, R., et al. (2007). An interdisciplinary expert consensus statement on assessment of pain in older persons. *Clinical Journal of Pain, 23*(1), S1–S43.

Heidrich, S.M., Egan, J.J., Hengudomsub, P., & Randolph, S.M. (2006). Symptoms, symptom beliefs, and quality of life of older breast cancer survivors: A comparative study. *Oncology Nursing Forum, 33*(2), 315–322.

Hodgson, N.A., & Given, C.W. (2004). Determinants of functional recovery in older adults surgically treated for cancer. *Cancer Nursing, 27*(1), 10–16.

Jakobsson, U., Hallberg, I.R., & Westergren, A. (2004). Pain management in elderly persons who require assistance with activities of daily living: A comparison of those living at home with those in special accommodations. *European Journal of Pain, 8*(4), 335–344.

Jemal, A., Siegel, R., Ward, E., Hao, Y., Xu, J., & Thun, M.J. (2009). Cancer statistics, 2009. *CA: A Cancer Journal for Clinicians, 59*(4), 225–249.

Kim, H.J., McGuire, D.B., Tulman, L., & Barsevick, A.M. (2005). Symptom clusters: Concept analysis and clinical implications for cancer nursing. *Cancer Nursing, 28*(4), 270–282.

Kurtz, M.E., Kurtz, J.C., Stommel, M., Given, C.W., & Given, B. (2001). Physical functioning and depression among older persons with cancer. *Cancer Practice, 9*(1), 11–18.

Laroche, M.L., Charmes, J.P., & Merle, L. (2007). Potentially inappropriate medications in the elderly: A French consensus panel. *European Journal of Clinical Pharmacology, 63*(8), 725–731.

Maas, H.A., Janssen-Heijnen, M.L., Olde Rikkert, M.G., & Machteld Wymenga, A.N. (2007). Comprehensive geriatric assessment and its clinical impact in oncology. *European Journal of Cancer, 43*(15), 2161–2169.

McMillan, S. (1989). The relationship between age and intensity of cancer-related symptoms. *Oncology Nursing Forum, 16*(2), 237–241.

National Comprehensive Cancer Network. (2009). *NCCN Clinical Practice Guidelines in Oncology™: Senior adult oncology* [v.1.2009]. Retrieved April 2, 2009, from http://www.nccn.org/professional/physician_gls/PDF/senior.pdf

Penedo, F.J., Schneiderman, N., Dahn, J.R., & Gonzalez, J.S. (2004). Physical activity interventions in the elderly: Cancer and comorbidity. *Cancer Investigation, 22*(1), 51–67.

Ray, A. (2002). Pain perception. *Clinical Geriatrics, 10*(3), 38–43.

Rogers, H.M. (2005). Management of clients with intestinal disorders. In J.M. Black & J.H. Hawks (Eds.), *Medical-surgical nursing: Clinical management for positive outcomes* (pp. 807–856). St. Louis, MO: Elsevier Saunders.

Strawbridge, W.J., Shema, S.J., Balfour, J.L., Higby, H.R., & Kaplan, G.A. (1998). Antecedents of frailty over three decades in an older cohort. *Journal of Gerontology: Social Sciences, 53B*(1), S9–S16.

Tabloski, P.A. (2006). *Gerontological nursing.* Upper Saddle River, NJ: Pearson Prentice Hall.

Tazbir, J., & Keresztes, P.A. (2005). Management of clients with functional cardiac disorders. In J.M. Black & J.H. Hawks (Eds.), *Medical-surgical nursing: Clinical management for positive outcomes* (pp. 1627–1670). St. Louis, MO: Elsevier Saunders.

Weiner, D., & Hanlon, J. (2001). Pain in nursing home residents: Management strategies. *Drugs and Aging, 18*(1), 13–29.

Williams, C. (2002). Using medications appropriately in older adults. *American Family Physician, 66*(10), 1917–1924.

Williamson, G.M., & Schulz, R. (1995). Activity restriction mediates the association between pain and depressed affect: A study of younger and older adult cancer patients. *Psychology and Aging, 10*(3), 369–378.

Yancik, R. (1997). Cancer burden in the aged: An epidemiologic and demographic overview. *Cancer, 80*(7), 1273–1283.

CHAPTER 2

Alopecia

Lillian M. Nail, PhD, RN, CNS, FAAN,
and Frances Lee-Lin, PhD, RN, OCN®, CNS

Case Study

P.W. is a 47-year-old woman diagnosed with node-positive breast cancer. She underwent a left mastectomy with immediate reconstruction and is scheduled to begin chemotherapy. The regimen begins with doxorubicin 60 mg/m² IV plus cyclophosphamide 600 mg/m² IV every 21 days for four cycles. While she was waiting for her postoperative healing to reach the level where she could begin chemotherapy, P.W. attended a chemotherapy orientation class. The progress note in her chart from the nurse who led the class indicates that the patient was very concerned about hair loss and had difficulty focusing on any of the other topics discussed during the class. When the nurse goes into the waiting room to introduce herself to the patient, she notices that the patient is a well-dressed woman in a business suit, sitting by herself at the far end of the room and staring at the other people in the room. The nurse introduces herself to the patient and escorts her to a private room in the treatment area. As part of the pretreatment assessment, the nurse asks the patient if she has any questions about her chemotherapy and also offers to review the relevant components of the orientation class. P.W. replies that she thinks the chemotherapy regimen that has been prescribed is the wrong one for her. She tells the nurse that she knows that some people with cancer do not lose their hair, and she wants the treatment they are getting rather than any of the choices that were presented to her.

Overview

Hair loss is a common side effect of many chemotherapy drugs used in cancer treatment. It also occurs in areas of the body treated with radiation and can be a result of treatments that alter the body's hormone environment. Despite the high rate of alopecia with commonly used chemotherapy drugs and radiation, research is limited regarding mechanisms of hair loss, human responses to potential or actual hair loss, strategies for preventing hair loss, and approaches to promoting hair regrowth in people with cancer. This chapter reviews each of these topics and summarizes current clinical practice recommendations for the care of people who are at risk for or are experiencing alopecia.

The characteristics, functions, and patterns of distribution of mammalian hair vary by species. Compared to the hair of most mammals, human hair provides little protection from the cold and is dense on only a few locations of the body. In humans, the primary use of hair is to communicate social and sexual identity. In other mammals, hair has additional functions relevant to survival, such as hiding the animal from predators, serving as a sensory organ used in communication or locating predators and prey, and deterring predators (e.g., quills) (Messenger, 2003). Although humans do not depend on hair for personal protection, hair is an important element of appearance and identity. Over the course of human history, complete loss of scalp hair has been associated with disease, louse infestation, submission, incarceration, and loss of self in images of war, plague, crime, and poverty. In contrast, contemporary images of completely shaved heads in Western society are associated with specific political views, rebellion against authority, physical strength, and toughness.

Pathophysiology

Hair Growth Phases

Each hair develops within a hair follicle that provides the environment for the initiation, maturation, shedding, and eventual replacement of the hair. The life of an individual hair has three phases: anagen, catagen, and telogen. The length of the active growth phase, the anagen phase, determines the maximum length of the hair. During the catagen phase, the hair is no longer growing, the base of the hair shaft becomes firm, and the bottom of the hair follicle moves closer to the surface of the skin. At this point, the base of the shaft is basically free of the follicle. In the telogen, or resting, phase, the hair shaft can be shed, but it may not fall out until the anagen phase is reestablished and the new hair pushes the firm base of the original hair to the skin surface. Both the anagen and telogen phases overlap the catagen phase, so the catagen phase usually is not addressed separately from the anagen and telogen phases of hair growth (Messenger, 2003; Tomlinson & McIntosh, 2005; Wang, Lu, & Au, 2006).

In humans, both the duration of the anagen phase and the proportion of hairs in the anagen phase at any given time vary by anatomic location. Scalp hair is in the anagen phase for two to six years, and 85%–90% of scalp hairs are in the anagen phase at any one time. In contrast, eyebrow hairs have a much shorter anagen phase of one to two months, with 6%–15% of hairs estimated to be in the anagen phase at any one time. Because the scalp has the highest percentage of hairs in the anagen phase at any single point in time, the effects of systemic cancer treatments that interfere with hair growth will appear in scalp hair before they are seen in other types of human hair (Messenger, 2003).

Control of Hair Growth

Researchers have explored the control of hair growth in animal and human studies, but the precise mechanism responsible for switching hair growth on and off has not been identified. Much research has been done on the role of androgen in stimulating both hair growth and hair loss. Many molecular mediators of the hair growth cycle have been identified, including estrogen receptors, vascular endothelial growth factor, epidermal growth factor, tumor necrosis factor alpha, mast cells, and interleukin-1. Specific cells, such as the cells of the dermal papilla at the base of the hair follicle and hair follicle stem cells alone or in interaction with other cells, also may contribute to the control of hair growth (Botchkarev, 2003; Botchkarev et al., 2000; Messenger, 2003; Sharov et al., 2003; Tomlinson & McIntosh, 2005; Wyatt, Leonard, & Sachs, 2006).

Hair Loss During Cancer Treatment

Types of Hair Loss

Anagen Hair Loss

Anagen hair loss is caused by disruption in hair growth and is the type of hair loss induced by cancer chemotherapy and radiation because both treatment modalities target rapidly dividing cells. Exposure to the drug or to radiation interferes with hair growth, producing a weak or narrowed area in the hair shaft where the hair breaks off or causes cells surrounding the hair root to die so the hair is able to fall out. Cyclic chemotherapy causes successive areas of narrowing on hair that does not break at the first exposure to the treatment. These hairs exhibit a second area of narrowing following the second treatment (Sinclair, Grossman, & Kvedar, 2003).

With repeated doses of radiation delivered five days per week, hair in the irradiated area becomes progressively narrower and eventually breaks (Sinclair et al., 2003). High radiation doses delivered over short periods of time can permanently destroy hair follicles (Kondziolka, Niranjan, Flickinger, & Lunsford, 2005).

Telogen Hair Loss

Several acute, long-lasting, and late effects of cancer treatment, as well as complications of cancer, can cause hair loss during the telogen phase. Hypothyroidism, cessation or initiation of hormonal contraceptives in women, some hormone replacement therapy in women, decreased caloric intake, protein-calorie deficiency, iron deficiency (e.g., dietary, blood loss), deficiencies in essential fatty acids, zinc deficiency, biotin deficiency, liver disease, fever, and injuries or medical procedures that lead to pressure-induced ischemia are all believed to cause hair loss during the telogen phase (Fiedler & Gray, 2003).

Some drugs used in cancer treatment, cancer supportive care, or the management of comorbid conditions also are associated with telogen hair loss. Methotrexate, interferon alfa, and interferon gamma are examples of cancer treatments that cause telogen hair loss. Supportive care drugs that produce telogen hair loss include high doses of some antifungals, octreotide, amphetamines, and androgens. Anticoagulants, propranolol, allopurinol, and cimetidine are examples of drugs that may be used in the management of comorbid illnesses in adults with cancer and cause telogen hair loss (Fiedler & Gray, 2003). When the drug causing hair loss is discontinued or the underlying deficiency state is corrected, telogen hair loss resolves.

Pattern of Hair Loss and Regrowth

The severity and incidence of hair loss associated with specific cancer treatment regimens are established during treatment trials through the documentation of side effects using toxicity rating instruments such as the National Cancer Institute's (NCI's) adverse event scoring system. Unlike other side effects, which are scored on a five-point (1–5) scale with the highest score indicating a life-threatening event, hair loss is scored using a more restricted range: hair loss of up to 50% that is not obvious from a distance (grade 1) to loss of more than 50% that is readily apparent to others (grade 2) (NCI Cancer Therapy Evaluation Program, 2009). The incidence rate and severity of drug-induced hair loss are reported in the studies used to support U.S. Food and Drug Administration (FDA) approval of new cancer treatment drugs and new indications for existing drugs. When new drugs are tested in combination with established chemotherapy drugs rather than as single agents, the new drug's contribution to hair loss is seen in the difference between the rate and severity with the established regimen compared to the rate and severity of hair loss reported for the new combination regimen. When the established regimen includes chemotherapy drugs that cause high rates of hair loss, the new drug's potential to cause hair loss if used alone or in a different drug combination may be obscured by the effects of other drugs in the treatment regimen.

The variation in the proportion of individual hairs in the anagen phase in different types of body hair explains the pattern of progression of hair loss during cancer chemotherapy. Generally, scalp hair disappears first, body hair follows, and eyebrow hairs are lost last. Scalp hair may begin to grow between treatments depending upon the drug, dose, frequency of treatment, and characteristics of the individual's hair. Some people experience patchy hair loss initially, others may retain isolated hairs on the scalp and never lose all of their body hair, and some may lose all of the hair on their body. Chemotherapy-induced hair loss with standard-dose therapies is temporary, and extensive regrowth is apparent within the first months after completion of treatment. Patchy hair regrowth and permanent alopecia have been reported following bone marrow or stem cell transplantation and may be seen with some hormonal therapies that begin or continue following the completion of chemotherapy.

Except for whole body irradiation, hair loss during external radiation treatment is limited to the treatment field. The area of hair loss follows the shape of the treatment field. Regrowth depends upon the dose such that higher doses increase the likelihood of permanent hair loss (Kondziolka et al., 2005). People who had mantle field irradiation for Hodgkin disease often have a higher than normal, perfectly straight hairline at the base of their skull. This unusual hairline corresponds with the upper border of the treatment field. When hair regrows in a treated area, regrowth may be concentrated along the outer edge of a treatment field and may be gradual so that the definition of the edge of the field softens over the years and less regrowth occurs in the central part of the field. Whether this is a result of dose variation at the edge of the treatment field or is caused by some sort of biologic process linked to nearby unaffected hair follicles is unclear.

Preventing Hair Loss

Decreasing Blood Flow to the Scalp

A variety of strategies for preventing or delaying hair loss have been proposed, and a few have been studied. In the 1980s, interest emerged in restricting blood flow to the scalp by using scalp cooling (hypothermia) or scalp tourniquets alone or in combination. The rationales for this practice were that decreasing blood flow would decrease the amount of cytotoxic drug exposure at the level of the hair follicle and, in the case of scalp cooling, that cooling also would decrease biochemical activity in the scalp and consequently decrease susceptibility to damage from cancer chemotherapy (Christodoulou, Tsakalos, Galani, & Skarlos, 2006; Grevelman & Breed, 2005). Because of the concern about the possibility of increasing the risk of scalp metastases or recurrence if cancer cells were among the cells protected and the lack of support for efficacy, no devices have received FDA approval for scalp cooling for prevention of chemotherapy-induced alopecia (FDA Center for Devices and Radiological Health, n.d.). Scalp cooling continues to be studied and used outside the United States.

A recent review of research on scalp cooling (Grevelman & Breed, 2005) analyzed 53 published reports and three personal communications. The reviewers concluded that scalp cooling is helpful in preventing hair loss but that the quality of the studies was low and that safety issues exist in patients receiving treatment for hematologic malignancies. They identified several important issues requiring further research in multicenter studies, including safety, efficacy, the optimum approach to scalp cooling, the duration of cooling following the completion of the chemotherapy infusion, patient tolerance of the procedure, and the extent to which the categorization of results as "good" reflected the patient's report of acceptability of hair preservation (Grevelman & Breed).

Pharmacologic Therapies

A wide range of pharmacologic approaches to chemotherapy-induced hair loss have been tried, but few have progressed to human trials. Topical minoxidil, which is indicated for treating androgenic hair loss and alopecia areata, has decreased the duration of hair loss in women receiving adjuvant chemotherapy for breast cancer and gynecologic cancer (Wang et al., 2006). Because some of the chemotherapy regimens used during these studies have been replaced, the results may not apply to current adjuvant therapy for these cancers.

Topical antibodies to specific chemotherapy drugs, such as doxorubicin, have shown promise in animals for single-agent chemotherapy but are not expected to be useful in combination chemotherapy because each antibody only targets one drug. Initial animal studies using several different cytokines or growth factors to prevent hair loss from cytarabine and cyclophosphamide showed an effect for cytarabine only, again raising concern about its usefulness in multidrug regimens. Cyclosporine A, an immunosuppressant that also stimulates hair growth, has shown positive results when used topically or systemically in rodent tests of several different cancer chemotherapy drugs, but increasing immunosuppression poses safety issues that argue against pursuing this approach in humans (Wang et al., 2006).

Topical calcitriol (vitamin D_3) showed positive effects with a variety of commonly used chemotherapy agents. Enthusiasm for using topical calcitriol, however, decreased when it was ineffective in preventing hair loss caused by 5-fluorouracil, doxorubicin, and cyclophosphamide in women with breast cancer, along with causing contact dermatitis (Bleiker, Nicolaou, Traulsen, & Hutchinson, 2005). Additional approaches being tested for preventing hair loss in cancer chemotherapy include the use of parathyroid hormone and parathyroid hormone–related peptide agonists and antagonists, *p53* inhibitors, selenium, and a mushroom extract (*Agaricus blazei* Murill Kyowa) (Ahn et al., 2004; Sieja & Talerczyk, 2004; Wang et al., 2006).

Radioprotectors (drugs that protect normal cells from radiation damage) are expected to protect against hair loss in patients receiving radiation to the scalp, but few studies have been done of alopecia prevention strategies in whole brain irradiation or other forms of external radiation treatments that include scalp hair in the treatment field. A pilot study of topical tempol in patients receiving whole brain radiation therapy for brain metastases showed that the drug prevented hair loss and was associated with rapid hair regrowth when drug-treated patients were compared to controls (Metz et al., 2004). In addition, amifostine may be useful in preserving scalp hair, but limited published data exist on its effects (Kouloulias et al., 2004).

Hair Care Techniques

A variety of self-care strategies focused on preventing or delaying scalp hair loss caused by cancer chemotherapy appear in the patient education and professional literature. These include cutting hair short prior to beginning treatment, using a satin pillowcase on the bed pillow, brushing hair gently, not using high heat on hair dryers, avoiding curling irons and curlers, avoiding hair dyes and permanent waves, not braiding the hair, and using a neutral pH shampoo (NCI, 2007). Many of these suggestions, such as brushing hair gently, cutting hair short, avoiding braiding, and using a satin pillowcase, appear to decrease traction on hair to preserve damaged hairs that could be susceptible to breaking with higher traction. Others, such as the avoidance of high temperatures and chemicals, suggest that the recommendation is based on concern about skin irritation around the hair shaft. None of the suggested self-care strategies have a research base.

Human Responses to Hair Loss

Many studies have documented the distress associated with both the anticipation of scalp hair loss and the experience of living with scalp hair loss as a side effect of cancer chemotherapy (Boehmke & Dickerson, 2005; Browall, Gaston-Johansson, & Danielson, 2006; Carpenter & Brockopp, 1994; Fallowfield, McGurk, & Dixon, 2004; Forrest, Plumb, Ziebland, & Stein, 2006; Freedman, 1994; Frith, Harcourt, & Fussell, 2007; Hofman et al., 2004; Lloyd, Nafees, Narewska, Dewilde, & Watkins, 2006; McGarvey, Baum, Pinkerston, & Rogers, 2001; Munstedt, Manthey, Sachsse, & Vahrson, 1997; Rosman, 2004; Williams, Wood, & Cunningham-Warburton, 1999). Most of these studies explored the experience of cancer treatment in general. Although responses to hair loss are not a specific focus of most work, results of the studies of the cancer treatment experience are consistent. The loss of scalp hair is feared; the likelihood of scalp hair loss is considered during treatment decision making; a variety of concrete strategies are used to deal with hair loss (going bald, using a wig, using other head coverings); and scalp hair loss may be viewed as a stigma (Boehmke & Dickerson; Carpenter & Brockopp; Cash, 2001; Fallowfield et al.; Freedman; Frith et al.; McGarvey et al.; Munstedt et al.; Rosman). In general, men report less distress from hair loss than women and are less likely than women to use a wig or head covering (Rosman).

Little data exist on the responses of others to an individual's hair loss. Reports of qualitative studies imply that the decision by women to display a bald head is one that they consider carefully and that family members, including children, become accustomed to the change in the woman's appearance over time (Williams, Piamjariyakul, et al., 2006). However, the responses of others to unexpected baldness is often one of shock. Women have reported feeling as though people view them differently because of their hair loss and have expressed concern about the impact of hair loss on the way people think about and act toward them (Rosman, 2004).

The research focusing on hair loss reveals a wide range of responses to both the prospect of and the reality of hair loss. For some, hair loss is the concrete evidence of cancer. Others view it as a sign that they are moving forward by being treated. Cultural differences in the meaning of hair and hair loss are critical to the meaning that people ascribe to the experience. For example, some Native Americans view long hair as a sign of respect for motherhood. Some collect shed hairs in a pillow for their entire lifetime as part of a practice of keeping one's body intact. Others view loss of hair as shameful (Native American Cancer Research, 2008). Whether one's interpretation of the hair loss drives decisions about what action to take in managing it is unknown, and the range of behaviors used to camouflage hair loss is broad (Forrest et al., 2006; Freedman, 1994; Frith et al., 2007; McGarvey et al., 2001; Munstedt et al., 1997; Rosman, 2004; Ucok, 2007). Some people experiencing scalp hair loss with cancer treatment choose to make a statement of identity by going bald. Others have created one or more "new" identities based on wigs, scarves, hats, and going bald. Some have had their scalps adorned with tattoos (permanent or temporary). Those who want to look about the same as they always have seek out wigs that match their own hair color and style, whereas others seek out new colors and styles. Some people who acquire wigs find that wearing the wig is not tolerable because it is too hot, is too itchy (even with a wig cap placed on the scalp before the wig is put on), does not fit well, or is burdensome to care for. Others wear a wig at all times, even while asleep. Children with cancer treatment–related alopecia often wear baseball caps or go bald, whereas female adolescents seem to use the same range of behaviors as adult women (Williams, Schmideskamp, Ridder, & Williams, 2006).

Some people clip or shave off their scalp hair when it becomes apparent to others that they are losing their hair or before they begin to lose hair to avoid having to deal with shedding and thinning. A family member, friend, or group of supporters may be recruited to participate in the clipping, with some approaching this event as a formal rite of passage with a celebratory component. The process of dealing with scalp hair regrowth is less apparent in the research, clinical literature, and reports of personal experiences with cancer treatment. Some people have difficulty acknowledging their new hair and show the same reluctance to expose the new hair as they had in showing their bald head (Rosman, 2004).

Almost no research has been done on the impact of hair loss in anatomic locations other than the scalp in people undergoing cancer treatment. Pubic hair is part of adult identity and sexual identity, and the loss of pubic hair can produce feelings of regression to a child-like state. The loss of visible body hair may be viewed as a positive or negative aspect of the cancer treatment experience depending upon individual body image beliefs, gender, and cultural norms. Responses to loss of hair other than scalp hair have not been studied and rarely are addressed in educational materials for cancer care providers or people with cancer. Although some patient education materials suggest that regrown scalp hair will differ from the original scalp hair in color and texture, this idea has limited research support. Whether the characteristics of regrown hair vary according to the type of cancer treatment or other variables, such as shifts in the hormone environment or damage to hair follicles, is unclear.

Clinical Practice Recommendations

When interactions with healthcare providers are part of the research, the typical finding is that providers do not appreciate the psychosocial impact of hair loss. Clinicians need to be aware of the variation in responses to hair loss along with the need for adequate preparation. They also must correct misconceptions and avoid minimizing the concerns expressed by people facing or experiencing hair loss.

Preparing People for Hair Loss

Accurate information about the likelihood and nature of hair loss is a key element of preparing people for cancer treatment. Public awareness of hair loss as a side effect of treatment is widespread and has produced some misconceptions about who is likely to experience hair loss. People beginning radiation treatment to an anatomic site other than the head commonly think that they will lose their scalp hair. Similarly, the variation in rates of hair loss associated with different types of chemotherapy or biologic therapies may not be understood. Clinicians must clarify what is expected for specific treatments while acknowledging that a range of individual variation exists.

When the treatment being used is one that is likely to cause hair loss, being clear that all hair, not just scalp hair, may be lost and that these losses may not occur at the same time will help patients to plan for and interpret their experience. Providing information about the variety of hair loss management options available, including the information that a bald head can get cold (wear a fleece cap) and that a runny nose may drip more suddenly than usual (carry tissues), helps people to prepare responses for these new experiences. Acknowledging that hair loss can be distressing, that it may have special meaning to an individual that others do not appreciate, and that it will have an impact on family members and friends, as well as providing information about resources for dealing with these concerns, are important parts of preparing people for the experience of hair loss.

Preventing Scalp Problems

Specific instructions for preventing scalp problems vary according to the type of treatment and should be provided to all patients. Scalp care during whole brain irradiation often includes restrictions on and suggestions for the use of lotions, creams, and ointments, which are specific to each radiation treatment department. Scalp care during cancer chemotherapy is less complicated and addresses a few general principles, including protecting skin from the sun and preventing injury to the scalp because of the loss of local protection from scalp hair. Instructions to inspect the scalp, including the back of the head, for rashes, sunburn, and scratches or blisters from wigs, hats, or decorations on scarves are important as part of the general recommendations for preventing and recognizing infection and maintaining skin integrity.

Head Coverings

People who want a wig that matches their own hair color and style should select the wig while they still have their hair to achieve the best possible match. Some may choose to use a scarf or hat in combination with hairpieces designed as bangs, ponytails, sideburns, or a fall of long hair under the sides and back of a hat or scarf, whereas others may use scarves or hats without any hairpiece. Cancer care providers need to recognize that most head covering strategies result in some out-of-pocket expense and maintenance challenges. Health insurance may cover at least part of the expense of a wig if the patient has a prescription for a hair prosthesis. High-quality synthetic hair wigs, which are easier to care for than a human hair wig, cost approximately $200, and high-quality human hair wigs generally are more expensive. A simple cotton or silk head scarf or head covering often costs $35–$50, and hats can range in cost from a few dollars for a simple baseball cap to more than $500 for women's fashion hats. Those who want variety in color or style of scarves and hats can easily spend more than the cost of a high-quality wig.

Appearance programs for people with cancer include the "Look Good . . . Feel Better" program as well as local programs developed by individual healthcare systems as part of their cancer program or by retailers who stock products used by people with cancer. *Look Good . . . Feel Better* is a brand-neutral program that addresses a combination of skin care, makeup, and head covering strategies and targets women as the primary audience (American Cancer Society, 2007). A companion self-help brochure and Web site (www.lookgoodfeelbetterformen .org) also are available for men.

Conclusion of Case Study

P.W. agrees to receive the planned chemotherapy following a careful, individualized explanation of the reason why different types of chemotherapy or other treatment modalities are recommended for different types of cancer. Because her attention during the chemotherapy orientation class had been focused on her concerns about hair loss, the nurse reviews key material from the class with her individually before administering the first cycle of chemotherapy. The nurse makes several follow-up telephone calls over the next three weeks. During that time period, the nurse arranges for P.W. to meet some women who worked during their treatment to talk about their experience with hair loss in the workplace, as that was one of the patient's primary concerns. P.W. also asks about strategies for preventing hair loss. The nurse reviews the materials P.W. had found that promoted hair care products and nutritional supplements as helpful in preventing hair loss and discusses these with her in relation to the research on hair loss and recommendations for the use of vitamins and supplements during cancer treatment.

During a recent telephone conversation, P.W. tells the nurse that it was helpful to meet others who had gone through the same thing but that she was not going to use scarves or hats or go bald and that she would be working on maintaining her "normal" appearance. By the time of her second treatment, she had purchased two identical wigs and had each styled to match her own hairstyle. She explains that she needs two so that she always has a wig to wear, even while one was at the salon being shampooed and styled. She also tells the nurse that she began wearing a wig all the time while she still had her own hair so that none of her coworkers would see her hair falling out or notice any thinning.

The nurse's plan of care for P.W. includes consistently complimenting her on her appearance, avoiding suggesting that her coworkers might be a source of support or aid for her during treatment, as she has not shared her diagnosis with anyone at work, and always structuring her visits that include physical examinations so that she has sufficient private time to adjust or replace her wig in case it is dislodged in the process of changing into or out of an examination gown. During the months following the completion of her chemotherapy, the nurse provides support to her in her decision to continue wearing a wig until she is confident that her own hair can be styled to closely resemble the wig.

Conclusion

Hair loss continues to be part of the cancer treatment experience for many people with cancer. What impact new cancer treatment approaches, such as targeted therapies, will have on this side effect is unclear. Recent interest in understanding the basic biology of hair loss as a side effect of cancer treatment may lead to translational studies of novel prevention strategies. Current clinical practice recommendations focus on recognizing the importance of the problem to people with cancer, respecting the concerns and responses of individuals who are anticipating or experiencing hair loss, delivering appropriate preparation for the experience of hair loss, and providing support to people dealing with changes in self-image and identity as a result of hair loss.

References

Ahn, W.S., Kim, D.J., Chae, G.T., Lee, J.M., Bae, S.M., Sin, J.I., et al. (2004). Natural killer cell activity and quality of life were improved by consumption of a mushroom extract, *Agaricus blazei Murill* Kyowa, in gynecological cancer patients undergoing chemotherapy. *International Journal of Gynecological Cancer, 14*(4), 589–594.

American Cancer Society. (2007, December 11). *Look good . . . feel better.* Retrieved April 20, 2008, from http://www.cancer.org/docroot/ESN/content/ESN_3_1X_Look_Good_Feel_Better.asp

Bleiker, T.O., Nicolaou, N., Traulsen, J., & Hutchinson, P.E. (2005). Atrophic telogen effluvium from cytotoxic drugs and a randomized controlled trial to investigate the possible protective effect of pretreatment with a topical vitamin D analogue in humans. *British Journal of Dermatology, 153*(1), 103–112.

Boehmke, M.M., & Dickerson, S.S. (2005). Symptom, symptom experiences, and symptom distress encountered by women with breast cancer undergoing current treatment modalities. *Cancer Nursing, 28*(5), 382–389.

Botchkarev, V.A. (2003). Molecular mechanisms of chemotherapy-induced hair loss. *Journal of Investigative Dermatology: Symposium Proceedings, 8*(1), 72–75.

Botchkarev, V.A., Komarova, E.A., Siebenhaar, F., Botchkareva, N.V., Komarov, P.G., Maurer, M., et al. (2000). p53 is essential for chemotherapy-induced hair loss. *Cancer Research, 60*(18), 5002–5006.

Browall, M., Gaston-Johansson, F., & Danielson, E. (2006). Postmenopausal women with breast cancer: Their experiences of the chemotherapy treatment period. *Cancer Nursing, 29*(1), 34–42.

Carpenter, J.S., & Brockopp, D.Y. (1994). Evaluation of self-esteem of women with cancer receiving chemotherapy. *Oncology Nursing Forum, 21*(4), 751–757.

Cash, T.F. (2001). The psychology of hair loss. *Clinics in Dermatology, 19*(2), 161–166.

Christodoulou, C., Tsakalos, G., Galani, E., & Skarlos, D.V. (2006). Scalp metastases and scalp cooling for chemotherapy-induced alopecia prevention. *Annals of Oncology, 17*(2), 350.

Fallowfield, L., McGurk, R., & Dixon, M. (2004). Same gain, less pain: Potential patient preferences for adjuvant treatment in premenopausal women with early breast cancer. *European Journal of Cancer, 40*(16), 2403–2410.

Fiedler, V.C., & Gray, A.C. (2003). Diffuse alopecia: Telogen hair loss. In E.A. Olsen (Ed.), *Disorders of hair growth: Diagnosis and treatment* (2nd ed., pp. 303–320). New York: McGraw-Hill.

Forrest, G., Plumb, C., Ziebland, S., & Stein, A. (2006). Breast cancer in the family—children's perceptions of their mother's cancer and its initial treatment: Qualitative study. *BMJ, 332*(7548), 998–1003.

Freedman, T. (1994). Social and cultural dimensions of hair loss in women treated for breast cancer. *Cancer Nursing, 17*(4), 334–341.

Frith, H., Harcourt, D., & Fussell, A. (2007). Anticipating an altered appearance: Women undergoing chemotherapy treatment for breast cancer. *European Journal of Oncology Nursing, 11*(5), 385–391.

Grevelman, E.G., & Breed, W.P. (2005). Prevention of chemotherapy-induced hair loss by scalp cooling. *Annals of Oncology, 16*(3), 352–358.

Hofman, M., Morrow, G.R., Roscoe, J.A., Hickok, J.T., Mustian, K.M., Moore, D.F., et al. (2004). Cancer patients' expectations of experiencing treatment-related side effects: A University of Rochester Cancer Center—Community Clinical Oncology Program study of 938 patients from community practices. *Cancer, 101*(4), 851–857.

Kondziolka, D., Niranjan, A., Flickinger, J.C., & Lunsford, L.D. (2005). Radiosurgery with or without whole-brain radiotherapy for brain metastases: The patients' perspective regarding complications. *American Journal of Clinical Oncology, 28*(2), 173–179.

Kouloulias, V.E., Kouvaris, J.R., Kokakis, J.D., Kostakopoulos, A., Mallas, E., Metafa, A., et al. (2004). Impact on cytoprotective efficacy of intermediate interval between amifostine and radiotherapy: A retrospective analysis. *International Journal of Radiation Oncology, Biology, Physics, 59*(4), 1148–1156.

Lloyd, A., Nafees, B., Narewska, J., Dewilde, S., & Watkins, J. (2006). Health state utilities for metastatic breast cancer. *British Journal of Cancer, 95*(6), 683–690.

McGarvey, E.L., Baum, L.D., Pinkerston, R.C., & Rogers, L.M. (2001). Psychological sequelae and alopecia among women with cancer. *Cancer Practice, 9*(6), 283–289.

Messenger, A. (2003). The control of hair growth and pigmentation. In E.A. Olsen (Ed.), *Disorders of hair growth: Diagnosis and treatment* (2nd ed., pp. 49–74). New York: McGraw-Hill.

Metz, J.M., Smith, D., Mick, R., Lustig, R., Mitchell, J., Cherakuri, M., et al. (2004). A phase I study of topical tempol for the prevention of alopecia induced by whole brain radiotherapy. *Clinical Cancer Research, 10*(19), 6411–6417.

Munstedt, K., Manthey, N., Sachsse, S., & Vahrson, H. (1997). Changes in self-concept and body image during alopecia induced cancer chemotherapy. *Supportive Care in Cancer, 5*(2), 139–143.

National Cancer Institute. (2007, June 29). *Chemotherapy and you: Support for people with cancer.* Retrieved September 15, 2007, from http://www.cancer.gov/cancertopics/chemotherapy-and-you

National Cancer Institute Cancer Therapy Evaluation Program. (2009). *Common terminology criteria for adverse events* (version 4.0). Retrieved July 24, 2009, from http://ctep.cancer.gov/protocolDevelopment/electronic_applications/docs/ctcaev4.pdf

Native American Cancer Research. (2008). *Native American cancer research: Survivors: Side effects: Hair loss.* Retrieved November 24, 2008, from http://natamcancer.org/hairloss.html

Rosman, S. (2004). Cancer and stigma: Experience of patients with chemotherapy-induced alopecia. *Patient Education and Counseling, 52*(3), 333–339.

Sharov, A.A., Li, G.Z., Palkina, T.N., Sharova, T.Y., Gilchrest, B.A., & Botchkarev, V.A. (2003). Fas and c-kit are involved in the control of hair follicle melanocyte apoptosis and migration in chemotherapy-induced hair loss. *Journal of Investigative Dermatology, 120*(1), 27–35.

Sieja, K., & Talerczyk, M. (2004). Selenium as an element in the treatment of ovarian cancer in women receiving chemotherapy. *Gynecologic Oncology, 93*(2), 320–327.

Sinclair, R., Grossman, K.L., & Kvedar, J.C. (2003). Anagen hair loss. In E.A. Olsen (Ed.), *Disorders of hair growth: Diagnosis and treatment* (2nd ed., pp. 275–302). New York: McGraw-Hill.

Tomlinson, D., & McIntosh, N. (2005). Skin: Cutaneous toxicities. In D. Tomlinson & N.E. Kline (Eds.), *Pediatric oncology nursing: Advanced clinical handbook* (pp. 355–364). New York: Springer.

Ucok, O. (2007). The fashioned survivor: Institutionalized representations of women with breast cancer. *Communication and Medicine, 4*(1), 67–78.

U.S. Food and Drug Administration Center for Devices and Radiological Health. (n.d.). *Products classification database.* Retrieved November 24, 2008, from http://www.accessdata.fda.gov/scripts/cdrh/cfdocs/cfPCD/PCDSimpleSearch.cfm

Wang, J., Lu, Z., & Au, J. (2006). Protection against chemotherapy-induced alopecia. *Pharmaceutical Research, 23*(11), 2505–2514.

Williams, J., Wood, C., & Cunningham-Warburton, P. (1999). A narrative study of chemotherapy-induced alopecia. *Oncology Nursing Forum, 26*(9), 1463–1468.

Williams, P.D., Piamjariyakul, U., Ducey, K., Badura, J., Boltz, K.D., Olberding, K., et al. (2006). Cancer treatment, symptom monitoring, and self-care in adults: Pilot study. *Cancer Nursing, 29*(5), 347–355.

Williams, P.D., Schmideskamp, J., Ridder, E.L., & Williams, A.R. (2006). Symptom monitoring and dependent care during cancer treatment in children: Pilot study. *Cancer Nursing, 29*(3), 188–197.

Wyatt, A.J., Leonard, G.D., & Sachs, D.L. (2006). Cutaneous reactions to chemotherapy and their management. *American Journal of Clinical Dermatology, 7*(1), 45–63.

CHAPTER 3

Anemia

Sheryl Miller, RN, MSN, MBA, OCN®

Case Study

T.C. is a 62-year-old female with a two-month history of dry cough, mild dyspnea with exertion, and complaint of fatigue rated as 6 on a scale of 0–10. T.C. states that she believes she has lost weight in the past few months. She is a nonsmoker but reports that her spouse smokes one pack per day. T.C. is retired and cares for her two young grandchildren two days a week.

T.C.'s medical history includes coronary artery disease and controlled hypertension. Baseline laboratory values reveal the following: white blood cell count is 4,000/mm^3, absolute neutrophil count is 2,400/mm^3, red blood cell (RBC) count is 5.1×10^6/mm^3, hemoglobin (Hgb) is 10.5 g/dl, hematocrit is 34%, ferritin is 120 ng/ml, and serum iron, vitamin B$_{12}$, folate, and chemistry are within normal limits. Computed tomography scan reveals a 4 cm mass in the right upper lung. Needle biopsy confirms an adenocarcinoma, non-small cell lung cancer. Mediastinoscopy reveals N2 disease (single-level ipsilateral mediastinal node involvement). T.C. is scheduled for neoadjuvant chemoradiation, followed by surgical resection. Is T.C. at risk for anemia?

Overview

Anemia is a problem common to patients with cancer and is a symptom that oncology nurses address almost daily in practice. The incidence of anemia varies widely with the type of malignancy and extent of disease. Recent research reveals a high prevalence of anemia (30%–90%) in patients with cancer who are not receiving treatment and an even higher rate of anemia in patients who are undergoing chemotherapy or radiation therapy (Knight, Wade, & Balducci, 2004). As cancer progresses, the prevalence of anemia increases, creating a challenge for the healthcare team in distinguishing the effects of disease from the symptoms of anemia (Knight et al.; Schwartz, 2007).

A review of published chemotherapy trials, including those done on single agents and combination therapies, validated a significant incidence of chemotherapy-induced anemia across many tumor types. Patients with lung, gynecologic, and genitourinary tumors and lymphoma were found to have the greatest incidence of anemia that necessitated transfusion (Groopman & Itri, 1999). Among the tumor types studied, a high incidence of mild-to-moderate anemia also was identified (Groopman & Itri). A more recent study (Knight et al., 2004) found a high incidence of anemia across numerous tumor types, including lung (8%–84%), colon

(30%–67%), breast (41%–82%), head and neck (16%–65%), gynecologic (26%–85%), bone (78%), brain (59%), pancreatic (93%), and hematologic malignancies (32%–100%). Furthermore, the authors identified 18 studies reporting a relationship between anemia and diminished survival or increased mortality (Knight et al.).

The European Cancer Anaemia Survey studied the prevalence and incidence of anemia in more than 15,000 patients with cancer. The researchers found a 39.3% prevalence of anemia at enrollment in the survey, a 53% incidence of anemia, and a statistically significant correlation between decreased Hgb levels and poor performance scores (Birgegard, Gascon, & Ludwig, 2006). Therefore, as the patient's Hgb decreased, the patient's performance status worsened.

Caro, Salas, Ward, and Goss (2001) completed a review of the literature and found a 20%–43% reduction in median survival in patients with cancer who were diagnosed with anemia. All of the 60 studies in the review reported a longer median survival in patients who were not anemic. For example, the relative risk of death in patients with lung cancer who were anemic increased by 19% compared to those without anemia. For anemic patients with head and neck cancer, the risk of death increased by 75%, and for those with lymphoma, by 67% (Caro et al.).

Although the significant incidence of anemia in patients with cancer has driven progress in toxicity management, anemia nonetheless often is underdiagnosed and undertreated (Hurter & Bush, 2007; Loney & Chernecky, 2000). One reason for this problem is the lack of a standard, universal definition of anemia (Hurter & Bush; Knight et al., 2004). Another issue is the importance that healthcare professionals place on quantitative measures when assessing for anemia, while patient symptoms and quality-of-life (QOL) concerns often go unnoticed. The impact of anemia is profound and negatively affects patients' QOL, functional status, and survival (Mock & Olsen, 2003). Oncology nurses are ideally situated to identify patient symptoms and functional status changes early in the patient's care and serve as a patient advocate consistently over the course of treatment and beyond (Foubert, 2006).

Pathophysiology

Anemia is defined as a reduction in the number of circulating RBCs, the amount of Hgb, or volume of hematocrit, causing a reduction in the oxygen-carrying capacity of the body (Pagana & Pagana, 2002; Porth, 1994). In patients with malignancies, anemia may result from a number of causes, including blood loss, increased RBC destruction, or decreased RBC production (Loney & Chernecky, 2000; Porth). To fully appreciate the symptom of anemia, an understanding of the normal process of erythropoiesis is needed.

RBCs are produced in almost all bones until age 20, after which they originate primarily in the vertebrae, sternum, ribs, and pelvis (Porth, 1994). Erythroblasts develop into RBCs after a series of divisions, but it is during the erythroblast phase that Hgb synthesis begins. The mature RBC, or erythrocyte, serves mainly as a vehicle for Hgb transport, carrying oxygen to the tissues and binding carbon dioxide for transport from the tissues to the lungs (Loney & Chernecky, 2000; Porth). RBCs have a biconcave disk shape to allow greater surface area for the Hgb and oxygen to combine, and they can change shape as needed in order to pass through small capillaries (Pagana & Pagana, 2002).

The production of RBCs is regulated by tissue oxygen needs. The kidneys release erythropoietin in response to hypoxia, sending a signal to the progenitor cells in the bone marrow to produce more RBCs. The RBCs develop and mature in approximately five to seven days and then are released into the bloodstream, where they typically survive for 120 days. Once oxygen levels recover, erythropoietin production is downregulated (Schwartz, 2007). To replace the old RBCs destroyed by phagocytic cells in the spleen, the body must produce 20 ml of RBCs every two days (Loney & Chernecky, 2000).

As mentioned, hypoxia triggers the body processes that lead to the production of new RBCs. Hypoxia has been found to stimulate angiogenesis, increase resistance of cells to apoptosis, and increase gene mutation. Furthermore, anemia in patients with cancer is thought to result in tumor hypoxia, angiogenesis, and resistance to therapy (Varlotto & Stevenson, 2005).

In patients with malignancies, multiple factors can cause anemia. Anemia caused by relative loss of RBCs and circulating volume can result from surgical blood loss, acute or chronic gastrointestinal hemorrhage, excessive diagnostic phlebotomy, or disseminated intravascular coagulation. Increased RBC destruction can cause various types of hemolytic anemia and cold agglutinin disease (a syndrome in which antibodies adhere to RBCs at low temperatures, causing hemolysis). Anemia resulting from decreased RBC production can be caused by treatment-induced myelosuppression, renal impairment, nutritional deficiencies, anemia of chronic disease, or tumor infiltration of the bone marrow (Hurter & Bush, 2007; Langer, Choy, Glaspy, & Colowick, 2002; Loney & Chernecky, 2000). Therefore, the patient with cancer who is receiving platinum-based chemotherapy, which is associated with significant renal toxicity, has twice the risk of anemia.

The best way to determine the cause of anemia is to evaluate the RBC size. The RBC indices reveal the size of the RBC and its Hgb content and comprise the mean corpuscular volume (MCV), mean corpuscular hemoglobin concentration (MCHC), and the red cell size distribution width (RDW). The MCV identifies the average size of the RBC and assists in the classification of anemia as microcytic (low MCV), normocytic (normal MCV), or macrocytic (high MCV). The mean corpuscular hemoglobin (MCH) measures the average Hgb weight in each RBC. The level is increased in macrocytic anemia and decreased in microcytic anemia. The MCHC measures the amount of Hgb in each RBC and leads to further classification of anemia as hypochromic, normochromic, or hyperchromic. It is useful for monitoring response to anemia treatment. The RDW looks at the degree of variation in RBC size and may help to differentiate anemia of chronic disease from iron-deficiency anemia (Hurter & Bush, 2007; Pagana & Pagana, 2002).

In addition to the RBC indices, standard tests in the laboratory workup for anemia include Hgb and hematocrit, reticulocyte count, and iron studies. A reticulocyte is an immature RBC. The reticulocyte count measures the effectiveness of the bone marrow in producing RBCs. A low reticulocyte count denotes decreased production of RBCs in the bone marrow in spite of the patient's anemic condition. In contrast, a high reticulocyte count indicates an increased production of RBCs in the bone marrow in response to the loss or destruction of RBCs (Hurter & Bush, 2007; Pagana & Pagana, 2002). Table 3-1 lists the classifications of common cancer-related anemias.

Iron studies are important in the differential diagnosis of anemia, as iron is essential for Hgb production. Iron deficiency can promote anemia or be its primary cause, and it can reduce the effectiveness of anemia treatment. Serum ferritin, transferrin saturation, and total iron-binding capacity (TIBC) are included in iron studies. Together, they measure the body's ability to store and transport iron. Serum ferritin alone is an insufficient measure, as certain malignancies (e.g., hematologic, breast) cause increased ferritin values (Henry, Dahl, Auerbach, Tchekmedyian, & Laufman, 2007; Pagana & Pagana, 2002; Schwartz, 2007).

Vitamin B_{12} and folate are necessary for the production of RBCs, and folate is essential for normal blood cell function. They often are tested in conjunction to help to determine the cause if a macrocytic anemia is present. Elevated vitamin B_{12} can be caused by certain

TABLE 3-1	Classifications of Common Cancer-Related Anemias	
Anemia Type	**Description**	**Differential Diagnosis**
Microcytic	Decreased mean corpuscular volume (MCV) (< 80 fl) Red blood cells (RBCs) small in size	Iron deficiency Anemia of chronic disease Thalassemia minor Sideroblastic anemia
Normocytic	Normal MCV (80–100 fl) RBCs normal in size	Anemia of chronic disease Hemolytic anemia Aplastic anemia Renal failure
Macrocytic	Increased MCV (> 100 fl) RBCs large in size	B_{12} deficiency Folate deficiency Myelodysplastic syndromes
Low reticulocyte count	Decreased RBC production < 0.5%–1.5% of erythrocytes	Anemia of chronic disease Aplastic anemia Iron deficiency Vitamin B_{12} deficiency Folate deficiency Bone marrow suppression or infiltration
High reticulocyte count	Increased RBC destruction > 0.5%–1.5% of erythrocytes	Hemolysis Chemotherapy-induced Autoimmune

Note. Based on information from Loney & Chernecky, 2000; Lynch, 2006.
From "Cancer-Related Anemia: Clinical Review and Management Update," by B. Hurter and N.J. Bush, 2007, *Clinical Journal of Oncology Nursing, 11*(3), p. 350. Copyright 2007 by Oncology Nursing Society. Reprinted with permission.

leukemias, such as chronic granulocytic leukemia and myelomonocytic leukemia, as well as cancers with liver metastasis. Decreased vitamin B_{12} levels occur in macrocytic anemia and iron and folic acid deficiencies. Decreased folate levels are associated with macrocytic anemia, folic acid deficiency, hemolytic anemia, acute leukemia, and metastatic carcinomas (Pagana & Pagana, 2002). See Figure 3-1 for a decision-making guide for identifying sources of anemia.

Anemia of chronic disease (ACD) is thought to be the primary reason for the underlying cause of cancer-related anemia (Langer et al., 2002). It is a state of impaired iron utilization in which Hgb is decreased but ferritin is normal or high. ACD is a condition of insufficient erythropoietin production and weakened bone marrow response to erythropoietin (Langer et al.). In ACD, the reticulocyte count is low, signaling a decreased production of RBCs. Reduced levels of iron and transferrin saturation occur in this normocytic, normochromic anemia (Weiss & Goodnough, 2005).

The prevalence of ACD in patients with cancer ranges from 30%–77% (Weiss & Goodnough, 2005). Results from animal studies suggest that inflammation plays a role in ACD and that hepcidin, a protein regulated by iron, also is an essential factor in its development (Weiss & Goodnough). Figure 3-2 depicts the pathophysiologic mechanisms underlying ACD. The development of malignant cells leads to activation of T cells and monocytes, which drive immune effector functions. This results in the production of cytokines (i.e., interferon, tumor necrosis factor [TNF], interleukin [IL]-1, IL-6, and IL-10), which stim-

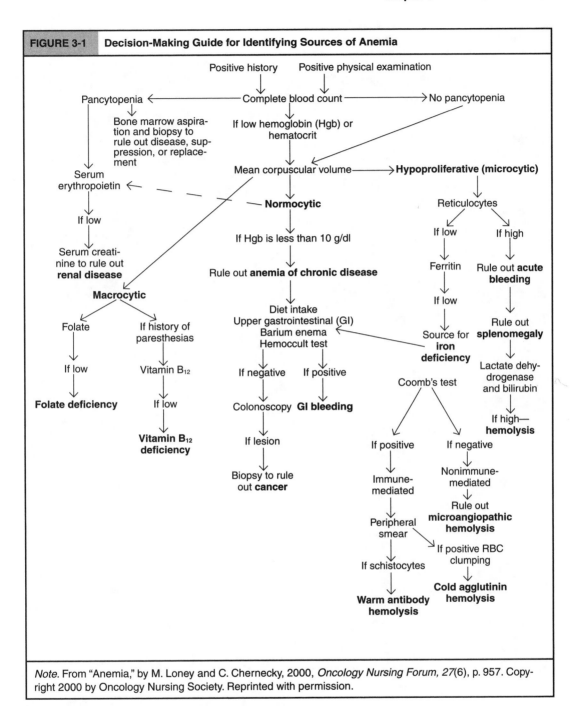

FIGURE 3-1   Decision-Making Guide for Identifying Sources of Anemia

Note. From "Anemia," by M. Loney and C. Chernecky, 2000, *Oncology Nursing Forum, 27*(6), p. 957. Copyright 2000 by Oncology Nursing Society. Reprinted with permission.

ulate the liver to produce hepcidin. Iron absorption in the duodenum is decreased, leading to an uptake of ferrous iron. Interferon prevents the release of iron from macrophages, whereas TNF, IL-1, IL-6, and IL-10 stimulate iron storage and retention within macrophages. Serum iron concentration is decreased, as is the kidneys' production of erythropoietin (Weiss & Goodnough).

FIGURE 3-2 | **Pathophysiologic Mechanisms Underlying Anemia of Chronic Disease**

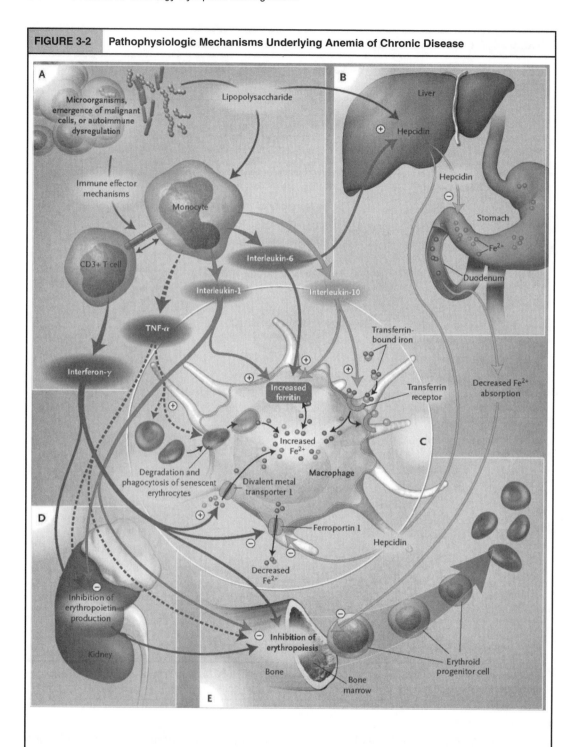

Note. From "Medical Progress: Anemia of Chronic Disease," by G. Weiss and L.T. Goodnough, 2005, *New England Journal of Medicine, 352*(10), p. 1013. Copyright 2005 by Massachusetts Medical Society. All rights reserved. Reprinted with permission.

Assessment

Although objective findings are essential to the differential diagnosis of anemia, subjective information is beneficial in planning interventions to enhance patient QOL. Anemia can cause a wide range of symptoms that can affect the function of almost every organ and tissue in the body. Severity of symptoms depends on the degree of anemia, rapidity of onset, the body's ability to compensate, comorbidities, and physiologic status of the patient (Hurter & Bush, 2007; National Comprehensive Cancer Network [NCCN], 2008).

A comprehensive assessment of anemia includes a detailed history and physical examination. The history begins with a risk assessment. NCCN (2008) guidelines list the risk factors for anemia as blood transfusion in the past six months, history of prior myelosuppressive therapy or radiotherapy to greater than 20% of the skeleton, current therapy with known myelosuppression potential, comorbidities, and low Hgb level at baseline. When taking a patient's history, the medical, surgical, and oncologic history must be included. Cancer diagnosis, stage, treatment, response, and treatment-related side effects are important components. The patient's current health status, including diseases, recurrent illnesses or infections, medications, symptoms, diet, and functional changes (i.e., ability to complete activities of daily living) are vital to a differential diagnosis of anemia (Loney & Chernecky, 2000).

The physical examination should be exhaustive, as cancer-related anemia can affect almost every body system (Hurter & Bush, 2007). Many of the symptoms of anemia arise from the body's inability to compensate adequately for chronic oxygen deficiency. In the majority of patients, anemia develops gradually, and the body may compensate so well that symptoms are not observable. However, patients may be aware of subtle changes in their ability to tolerate activity and may notice mild shortness of breath following activity or increased fatigue. The nurse's detailed history and physical examination may reveal these subtle changes (Mock & Olsen, 2003; Worrall, Tompkins, & Rust, 1999).

Physical examination in a patient with mild to moderate anemia may reveal pallor, shortness of breath on exertion, and manifestations of fatigue. In patients with severe anemia, dyspnea may occur at rest, cardiovascular symptoms may manifest, and debilitating fatigue often is present. These symptoms are a result of the decreased oxygenation of Hgb, which leads to hypoxia and increased cardiac output. The reduction in the number of RBCs also affects the blood's consistency and volume, thus causing the blood to flow faster and more fiercely. Signs of this low blood viscosity include systolic murmurs and bruits (Mock & Olsen, 2003; Worrall et al., 1999). Figure 3-3 illustrates the signs and symptoms of anemia.

A number of standard toxicity criteria for anemia exist, the most common of which are the World Health Organization and the National Cancer Institute grading systems (see Table 3-2). Research studies often highlight severe toxicities (grades 3 and 4) while failing to recognize those that are mild to moderate (grades 1 and 2). Yet, mild to moderate anemia may significantly reduce the QOL and functional status of patients and can be correlated with decreased survival (Mock & Olsen, 2003). Grading systems rely solely on the objective measure of anemia (Hgb level) and fail to associate patient symptoms and QOL with anemia (Groopman & Itri, 1999).

The NCCN (2008) guidelines offer evidence-based strategies for screening, assessing, and managing patients with cancer-related anemia. NCCN updates the guidelines frequently, and they can be accessed online and downloaded free of charge. Although the NCCN guidelines serve as an excellent resource, they are general and must be customized to meet the needs of the patient population and the oncology institution or practice (Schwartz, 2007). The American Society of Clinical Oncology (www.asco.org) and the American Society of Hema-

---

FIGURE 3-3 | **Signs and Symptoms of Anemia**

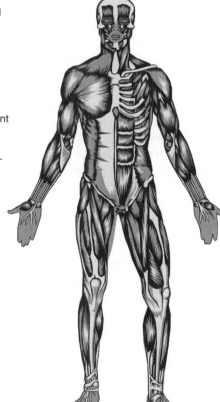

General
Fatigue, lethargy, apathy, fever

Immune System
Weakened macrophage and
   T-cell function

Central Nervous System
Headaches
Vertigo, dizziness
Irritability
Confusion, impaired judgment
Ataxia, weakness
Retinal hemorrhage
Loss of sensation or proprio-
   ception
Spasticity

Respiratory System
Tachypnea
Dyspnea
Pulmonary edema

Genitourinary System
Proteinuria
Water retention
Menorrhagia
Amenorrhea
Reduced libido
Impotence

Hematologic System
Generalized lymphadenopathy

Cardiovascular System
Tachycardia
Angina, palpitations
Dysrhythmias
Systolic murmur
Bruit
Postural hypotension

Gastrointestinal System
Indigestion
Irregular bowel movements
Stomatitis
Occult blood loss
Ascites
Hepatosplenomegaly
Abdominal distention

Peripheral Vascular System
Cold skin
Swelling in calves, legs, feet

Musculoskeletal System
Decreased muscular resis-
   tance
Bone pain

Integumentary System
Pallor
Blue, pale, or white sclera
Brittle, broken nails
Poor skin turgor
Dry, brittle, and thinning hair
Ecchymosis, petechiae, nasal/gingival bleeding
Poor wound healing, skin ulcerations

Note. Based on information from Ludwig & Strasser, 2001; Mock & Olsen, 2003; Worrall et al., 1999.

---

tology (www.hematology.org) adopted joint guidelines for anemia in 2002, but they are not updated as frequently as the NCCN guidelines (see Rizzo et al., 2002, for a detailed discussion of these guidelines).

Recommended assessment tools for anemia include the Functional Assessment of Cancer Therapy–Anemia subscale (FACT-An), the Brief Fatigue Inventory (BFI), the Linear Analog

TABLE 3-2	Grading Systems for Anemia					
Severity	**WHO**	**NCI**	**ECOG**	**SWOG**	**CALGB**	**GOG**
Grade 0 (WNL)*	≥ 11.0 g/dl	WNL	WNL	WNL	WNL	WNL
Grade 1 (mild)	9.5–10.9 g/dl	10.0 g/dl to WNL	10.0 g/dl to WNL	10.0 g/dl to WNL	10.0 g/dl to WNL	10.0 g/dl to WNL
Grade 2 (moderate)	8.0–9.4 g/dl	8.0–10.0 g/dl	8.0–10.0 g/dl	8.0–9.9 g/dl	8.0–10.0 g/dl	8.0–10.0 g/dl
Grade 3 (serious/severe)	6.5–7.9 g/dl	6.5–7.9 g/dl	6.5–7.9 g/dl	6.5–7.9 g/dl	6.5–7.9 g/dl	6.5–7.9 g/dl
Grade 4 (life threatening)	< 6.5 g/dl	< 6.5 g/dl	< 6.5 g/dl	< 6.5 g/dl	< 6.5 g/dl	< 6.5 g/dl

* WNL hemoglobin values are 12.0–16.0 g/dl for women and 14.0–18.0 g/dl for men.

CALGB—Cancer and Leukemia Group B; ECOG—Eastern Cooperative Oncology Group; GOG—Gynecologic Oncology Group; NCI—National Cancer Institute; SWOG—Southwest Oncology Group; WHO—World Health Organization; WNL—within normal limits

Note. From "Chemotherapy-Induced Anemia in Adults: Incidence and Treatment," by J.E. Groopman and L.M. Itri, 1999, *Journal of the National Cancer Institute, 91*(19), p. 1617. Copyright 1999 by Oxford University Press. Reprinted with permission.

Scale Assessment (LASA), and the SF-36®. The FACT-An is a scale with 55 questions specific to cancer, including 13 questions regarding fatigue and 7 related to anemia. The BFI includes four questions and asks patients to rate the impact of fatigue on their daily functioning in the past 24 hours. Patients can use the LASA scale to self-measure energy level, ability to complete activities of daily living, and QOL using a range of 0–100. The SF-36 is a non–cancer-specific 11-question scale focused on the mental and physical aspects of QOL (NCCN, 2007; Schwartz, 2007).

Assessment of fatigue is essential when completing a comprehensive assessment of anemia. Fatigue continues to be the most common symptom of cancer and cancer treatment and is the most frequently reported symptom of cancer-related anemia. Fatigue is multidimensional, and treatment is determined by identifying and managing the underlying cause (Foubert, 2006; Mock & Olsen, 2003). See Chapter 13 for a more detailed discussion of fatigue.

Evidence-Based Interventions

The primary treatments for cancer-related anemia include blood transfusions and erythropoietic therapy. In addition, iron supplementation may be a necessary adjunct to treatment with an erythropoietin-stimulating therapy. The expected outcomes of treatment are an increase in Hgb to the patient's normal level, the resolution of symptoms, an increase in the patient's QOL, and the ability to complete the treatment course without interruption.

Blood Transfusions

Transfusions of packed RBCs typically are administered when immediate and rapid correction of the anemia is needed because of a low Hgb level or the presence of severe symptoms (NCCN, 2008; Varlotto & Stevenson, 2005). However, transfusions provide temporary results and may be harmful to patients with cancer. Transfusions have been associated with an increase in cancer recurrence, decrease in overall survival, and a poorer cancer prognosis (Varlotto & Stevenson; Ward & Levy, 2004). The immunosuppressive effects of blood transfusions are still under investigation, but studies have found increased IL-10 levels and decreased natural killer cells and T cells following transfusion (Varlotto & Stevenson).

In considering transfusions, understanding the process of RBC storage and how this may translate to a transfusion providing minimal benefit to the patient is important. When blood is donated for clinical use, it typically is stored for 35–42 days (Hovav, Yedgar, Manny, & Barshtein, 1999). The shelf-life of a unit of packed RBCs is 42 days (six weeks), and most blood is given between days 21 and 42. Research by Hovav et al. has revealed that during storage, RBCs change from their normal shape to a dented or shriveled structure. The shape of the RBC is important to its ability to carry out normal functions, especially oxygen transport.

In addition, RBCs contain the metabolite 2,3-diphosphoglycerate (DPG). The oxygen-releasing function of RBCs is impaired when 2,3-DPG levels are low. Within two weeks of storage, RBCs completely lose 2,3-DPG. Therefore, not surprisingly, transfusions have not been found to increase oxygen consumption in critically ill patients with sepsis. Researchers currently are trying to develop storage solutions that will maintain the functional properties of RBCs (Elfath, 2006; Madjdpour & Spahn, 2005).

Prior to the 1980s, blood transfusions often were given to patients when the Hgb dropped below 10 g/dl (NCCN, 2007). After the development of erythropoietic therapies, and because of the identification of HIV transmission via transfusions, the threshold was lowered to 8 g/dl. Over the past decade, the growing shortage of blood worldwide and the awareness of new risks associated with transfusion have led many institutions to lower their threshold for transfusion to 7 g/dl (NCCN, 2007; Schwartz, 2007). The *Circular of Information for the Use of Human Blood and Blood Components* (American Association of Blood Banks, 2002) recommends the use of alternatives to blood transfusions whenever possible. Alternatives include iron, vitamin B_{12}, folic acid, and erythropoietin.

The most serious risks of blood transfusions include mistransfusion and transfusion-related acute lung injury (TRALI). Although the public is now aware of the dangers of transmitting infection through blood transfusions, a general lack of awareness exists regarding the risk of mistransfusion (Brooks, 2005). Approximately 1 in 14,000 units of blood in the United States is transfused to someone other than the intended recipient. For example, Patient A and Patient B have the same last name but different blood types, and both are receiving two units of packed RBCs on the oncology unit on the same day. Patient A receives the unit of blood intended for Patient B. Sixty-six percent of errors occur from improper identification of patients or mislabeling of samples during phlebotomy, and an estimated 30% of errors occur in the laboratory (Goodnough, 2005).

TRALI is another serious risk of blood transfusions and occurs in approximately 1 in 5,000 transfusions in the United States. It is an acute respiratory distress syndrome that can occur from an antibody-mediated reaction or the accumulation of lipid products from donor blood cell membranes during blood storage (Gajic & Moore, 2005; Goodnough, 2005; Madjdpour & Spahn, 2005). Symptoms usually appear within six hours of the start of the transfusion and include dyspnea, tachypnea, hypotension, fever, and frothy sputum. TRALI is difficult to diagnose because no single test exists for it and the symptoms are similar to other conditions, such as adult respiratory distress syndrome. Treatment consists of supportive care, and although most patients recover within one to two days, some require mechanical ventilation, and all receive intensive care treatment (Gajic & Moore).

Implications for nurses with regard to the administration of blood include the recognition that transfusions provide a temporary benefit and may be detrimental for patients with cancer. Nurses should be aware that the most serious risk associated with blood transfusion is mistransfusion, of which the most common issue is proper patient identification. Transfusions are beneficial for patients who are in need of rapid correction of Hgb, but in light of the risks, alternatives to transfusion should be chosen whenever feasible.

Erythropoietic Therapy

As an alternative to blood transfusion, two products are available in the United States: epoetin alfa (Procrit®, Ortho Biotech Products, L.P.; Epogen®, Amgen Inc.) and darbepoetin alfa (Aranesp®, Amgen Inc.). The U.S. indications for epoetin alfa include the treatment of anemia in patients with nonmyeloid malignancies who are receiving concomitant chemotherapy, anemic patients with chronic renal disease, zidovudine-treated patients with HIV and anemia, and anemic patients undergoing elective, noncardiac, nonvascular surgery (Ortho Biotech Products, L.P., 2007). Darbepoetin alfa is indicated in the United States for the treatment of anemia associated with chronic renal failure and in patients with nonmyeloid malignancies receiving concomitant chemotherapy (Amgen Inc., 2007).

The NCCN (2008) guidelines recommend considering erythropoietic therapy when the patient has an Hgb level of less than 11 g/dl and is symptomatic or when the patient is asymptomatic but has risk factors present. If the patient does not experience a 1 g/dl rise in Hgb by four weeks of therapy with epoetin alfa or six weeks of therapy with darbepoetin alfa, a dose increase is indicated. If no Hgb response occurs by 8–12 weeks, erythropoietic therapy should be discontinued and transfusion should be considered if needed. If dose titration produces a response, erythropoietic therapy should be continued to maintain an optimal Hgb level of 11–12 g/dl until six weeks after the completion of chemotherapy, at which time it should be discontinued. **For an Hgb rise of more than 1 g/dl in a two-week period, the erythropoietin dose should be reduced by 25%–50%, and if the Hgb rises above 12 g/dl, therapy should be withheld until the Hgb drops below 12 g/dl and restarted at a 25% dose reduction** (Amgen Inc., 2007; NCCN, 2008; Ortho Biotech Products, L.P., 2007).

NCCN guidelines provide dosing recommendations for both epoetin alfa and darbepoetin alfa. Initial dosing, following the package insert dosing schedule, is a choice of epoetin alfa 150 units/kg administered subcutaneously three times weekly or epoetin alfa 40,000 units administered subcutaneously every week. Doses are titrated to 300 units/kg or 60,000 units, respectively, for no response. Darbepoetin initial dosing is 2.25 mcg/kg administered subcutaneously weekly, titrated to 4.5 mcg/kg for no response, or darbepoetin 500 mcg given subcutaneously every three weeks (NCCN, 2008). The most common dosing schedule of epoetin alfa for patients with cancer who are receiving chemotherapy is 40,000 units given subcutaneously once weekly. The dose of darbepoetin alfa commonly used in the oncology setting is 500 mcg given subcutaneously every three weeks.

Alternative regimens were added to the NCCN guidelines in 2007, including darbepoetin 100 mcg fixed dose subcutaneously every week, titrated to 150–200 mcg for no response; darbepoetin 200 mcg fixed dose subcutaneously every two weeks, titrated to 300 mcg for no response; and darbepoetin 300 mcg fixed dose subcutaneously every three weeks, titrated to 500 mcg for no response. In addition, epoetin alfa 80,000 units every two weeks subcutaneously and epoetin alfa 120,000 units subcutaneously every three weeks were included as alternative regimens (NCCN, 2007).

Many studies have reported that treatment with erythropoietic therapy increases Hgb levels, decreases the need for transfusions, and improves QOL and functional status in patients with cancer who have chemotherapy-induced anemia (Demetri, Kris, Wade, Degos, & Cella, 1998; Glaspy, 1997; Glaspy et al., 2003; Shasha, George, & Harrison, 2003; Witzig et al., 2005). Bohlius et al. (2006) completed a systematic literature review of 57 randomized controlled trials of 9,353 patients to determine the effects of erythropoietic therapy for the prevention or treatment of cancer-related anemia. The researchers found that erythropoietic therapy reduced the risk for blood transfusions by 36% (95% confidence interval [CI]) and improved hematologic response. However, erythropoietic therapy increased the risk of thrombotic and vascular events by 67% (95% CI), and its effects on overall survival were inconclusive (Bohlius et al.).

In comparing the two therapies, a systematic literature review of 40 studies including 21,378 patients was conducted to assess the clinical benefits and risks associated with epoetin and darbepoetin alfa and found no clinically relevant differences between the two drugs (Ross et al., 2006). Two additional studies compared darbepoetin alfa 200 mcg every two weeks with epoetin alfa 40,000 units weekly to assess the efficacy and safety of both agents. The researchers found similar clinical effectiveness between the two therapies (Glaspy et al., 2006; Herrington et al., 2005).

The U.S. Food and Drug Administration (FDA) revised the labeling of erythropoietic therapies in March 2007 after studies revealed a greater possibility of serious to life-threatening side effects (e.g., serious cardiovascular and thromboembolic events, tumor progression) or death when using epoetin alfa and darbepoetin alfa. An important note is that patients participating in these studies were not receiving chemotherapy. **Concerns included an increased risk of serious cardiovascular events in patients with chronic renal failure receiving erythropoietic therapies dosed to target an Hgb level of greater than 12 g/dl, risk of thrombosis in patients treated with erythropoietic therapies before surgery, and possible enhancement of tumor growth rate in patients with breast, non-small cell lung, head and neck, lymphoid, and cervical cancers with the use of erythropoietic therapies dosed to achieve an Hgb level greater than 12 g/dl** (Lappin, Maxwell, & Johnston, 2007; Ortho Biotech Products, L.P., 2007). The FDA recommends using the lowest possible dose of erythropoietic agents to raise the Hgb level and avoid transfusion (FDA, 2007; NCCN, 2008).

Nursing implications for the administration of erythropoietic agents includes the need for nurses to keep abreast of current studies assessing the efficacy of these treatments now that studies have shown erythropoietic therapy to be potentially beneficial and harmful for patients. Nurses must advocate for patients to receive the lowest dose possible that is able to increase the Hgb level and avoid transfusion, remain aggressive in monitoring Hgb two times weekly for two to six weeks following dose adjustments to ensure stabilization of Hgb, and diligently withhold erythropoietic therapy if the Hgb level is greater than 12 g/dl (NCCN, 2008).

Some patients report discomfort from the subcutaneous injection of epoetin alfa, which results from the citrate buffer in single-dose vials of the drug. Epoetin alfa should be warmed to room temperature before administration to decrease the likelihood of stinging with injection. Topical anesthetics or ice applied to the site can reduce discomfort, and the drug should be given slowly. Other strategies include using a smaller-gauge needle to administer epoetin alfa and rotating injection sites to alleviate discomfort (Buchsel, Murphy, & Newton, 2002).

Iron Supplementation

Iron supplementation is necessary in the majority of patients receiving erythropoietic therapy because of the eventual development of functional iron deficiency, defined as a serum ferritin concentration of less than 300 ng/ml or transferrin saturation of less than 20% (NCCN, 2008). In functional iron deficiency, storage iron cannot be activated, whereas in absolute iron deficiency, patients have deficient iron stores (Henry et al., 2007). Reduction in iron stores may result from ACD, nutritional deficiencies, or chronic blood loss (Schwartz, 2007). Supplementation with usable iron is required in patients with functional iron deficiency to enhance the patient's response to erythropoietin therapy (Henry et al.).

Once erythropoietic therapy is warranted, iron studies should be completed before initiating therapy. If the patient has absolute iron deficiency, defined as serum ferritin less than 30 ng/ml or transferrin saturation less than 15%, iron supplementation is indicated. If the Hgb does not increase, the patient should be evaluated for functional iron deficiency. Although the primary route of iron supplementation has been oral therapy, recent data indicate that IV iron may have a greater efficacy (NCCN, 2008).

The objective of oral iron supplementation is to administer 200 mg daily. Multiple preparations of oral iron are available with varying amounts of elemental iron in each tablet. Gastrointestinal side effects, such as abdominal pain, nausea, vomiting, and constipation, are common with oral iron treatment and can result in patient noncompliance. Taking the supplement with food reduces the severity of side effects, but it also can reduce iron absorption (NCCN, 2007). As mentioned earlier, ACD, which is prevalent in patients with cancer, causes decreased oral iron absorption.

Available parenteral iron preparations include iron dextran, ferric gluconate, and iron sucrose. Iron dextran is not as safe as the other parenteral iron options, and test doses are required. Hypersensitivity to iron dextran usually occurs in the first few minutes after administering treatment and may include symptoms of urticaria, skin rash, allergic purpura, pruritus, fever, chills, dyspnea, arthralgia, myalgia, and anaphylaxis (Wilson, Shannon, & Stang, 2006). The NCCN (2008) guidelines strongly recommend test doses when administering ferric gluconate or iron sucrose to patients who are sensitive to iron dextran and those who have allergies to other medications. In addition, patients should be premedicated with diphenhydramine and acetaminophen prior to IV iron administration.

The NCCN (2008) recommendations for parenteral iron administration include
- Iron dextran: A test dose of 25 mg slow IV push is required; treatment is 100 mg IV over five minutes, but higher doses can be given over a few hours.
- Ferric gluconate: A test dose of 25 mg slow IV push or infusion is recommended; treatment is 125 mg IV injection or infusion over 60 minutes.
- Iron sucrose: A test dose of 25 mg slow IV push is recommended; treatment is 200 mg IV injection or infusion over 60 minutes.

Henry et al. (2007) conducted a study of 187 patients with chemotherapy-induced anemia to determine the safety and efficacy of IV ferric gluconate, oral ferrous sulfate, or no iron to improve the Hgb level in anemic patients receiving chemotherapy and epoetin alfa. Patients were randomized to eight weeks of therapy with either 125 mg of IV ferric gluconate weekly, 325 mg of oral ferrous sulfate three times daily, or no iron treatment. Epoetin alfa was administered for 12 weeks beginning at the first clinic visit. The researchers found that IV ferric gluconate significantly improved the response to epoetin alfa (p = 0.0092). The Hgb response rate for patients receiving IV ferric gluconate was 73%, compared to 45% and 41% for patients receiving oral iron and no iron, respectively. Of the 50 patients in this study with a baseline transferrin saturation of less than 20%, the Hgb response rate for patients receiving IV ferric gluconate was 81%, compared to 37% and 27% in those receiving oral iron or no iron, respectively. The response rates for the oral iron and no iron groups were so similar that it raises the question of whether oral iron should even be an option for patients with cancer who are receiving erythropoietic therapy (Henry et al.).

Nursing implications for the administration of iron supplementation includes continuous monitoring of iron status and appropriate patient teaching based on the route of administration. Patients should be taught to take oral iron supplements on an empty stomach, as it increases absorption, and to report gastrointestinal symptoms promptly so that interventions can be implemented. In administering IV iron, nurses should be cognizant of the importance of test doses and premedication with diphenhydramine and acetaminophen (NCCN, 2008).

Standing Orders

Currently, the Oncology Nursing Society does not have a Putting Evidence Into Practice resource related to anemia. However, one strategy that nurses can promote within their practice settings to encourage consistent evidence-based practice is the development and implementation of standing orders. Although they are not currently a standard practice in all oncology settings, standing orders are becoming more common, especially in academic cancer centers and large oncology practices. As explained by Mickle and Reinke (2007), "standing orders, when written by a multidisciplinary team that includes physicians, nurses, and pharmacists, allow nurses to initiate and discontinue drugs more autonomously within the scope of their expertise and knowledge" (p. 534). One of the greatest benefits of standing orders is that they reduce delays in patient interventions. In addition, they verify that practice standards are being used and establish consistency in patient care (Mickle & Reinke). Figure 3-4 is an example of a standing order algorithm for anemia.

Expected Outcomes

In review, the goals of anemia management are to increase the Hgb level to the patient's normal level, resolve symptoms, improve the patient's QOL, and allow the patient to complete the treatment course uninterrupted. A key study that researched the Hgb level at which the greatest effect on QOL is realized was an incremental analysis conducted by Cleeland et al. (1999). The researchers found that the largest improvement in QOL occurred when the patient's Hgb level increased from 11 g/dl to 12 g/dl and that QOL benefits were more significant in patients with mild anemia than in those with moderate to severe anemia (Cleeland et al.). Crawford et al. (2002) confirmed these results, finding the greatest gain in QOL to occur at an Hgb level of 11–13 g/dl upon analyzing the same community-based studies as Cleeland et al. Lyman and Glaspy (2006) conducted a systematic literature review to detect whether benefits exist for early intervention with erythropoietic therapy to treat chemotherapy-induced anemia. The researchers concluded that patients receive the greatest clinical benefit from erythropoietic therapy when treatment is begun early, defined as an Hgb level greater than 10 g/dl.

These studies were important in that they identified strategies to enhance patients' QOL, including initiating treatment early and maintaining the patient's Hgb level between 11 g/dl and 12 g/dl. Nurses should strive to identify anemia early and begin treatment promptly to prevent the development of moderate to severe anemia. Nurses must recognize that even moderate anemia has been associated with decreased survival in patients with cancer. Anticipating anemia, comprehensively assessing the problem, and ad-

FIGURE 3-4	Sample Standing Order Algorithm

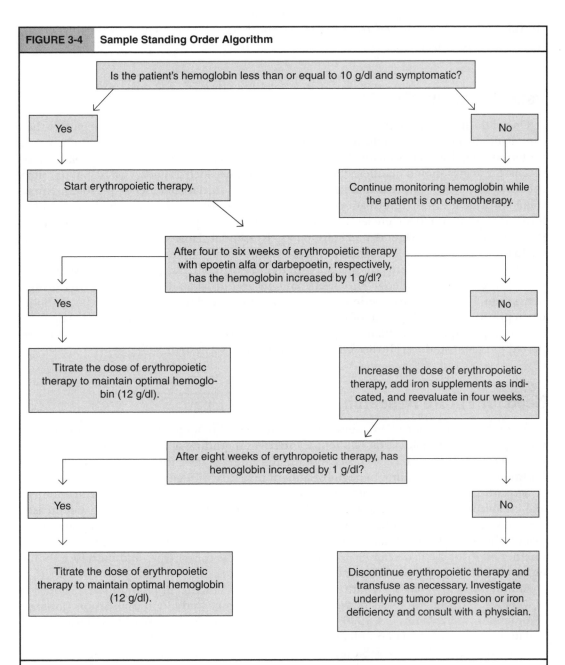

Note. Documentation required by Medicare: serum iron ÷ total iron-binding capacity = transferrin saturation; transferrin saturation (must be 20% or higher); serum ferritin (must be 100 ng/ml or higher); hemoglobin (< 12 g/dl); hematocrit (lower than 36%–40%); serum creatinine

Note. In patients with hemoglobin concentration < 12 g/dl that has never fallen below 10 g/dl, clinical circumstance should dictate whether to implement erythropoietic treatment immediately or to continue observation.

Note. Based on information from National Comprehensive Cancer Network, 2007; Rizzo et al., 2002. From "A Review of Anemia Management in the Oncology Setting: A Focus on Implementing Standing Orders," by J. Mickle and D. Reinke, 2007, *Clinical Journal of Oncology Nursing, 11*(4), p. 538. Copyright 2007 by Oncology Nursing Society. Reprinted with permission.

vocating for evidence-based treatments are the keys for oncology nurses in providing high-quality patient care.

Patient Teaching Points

One of the most crucial roles of the oncology nurse is to instruct patients with regard to their care. Patients must be fully educated about anemia. At diagnosis, nurses can define anemia for the patient, discuss risk factors for and causes of anemia, list symptoms, and explain blood counts. Strategies should be offered for managing fatigue, such as energy conservation, sleep routines, distraction, exercise, and keeping a symptom journal (Buchsel et al., 2002). Nurses should provide nutrition information, including suggestions for energy-boosting foods and information on vitamin deficiencies. For patients taking iron supplements, education regarding the prevention and management of constipation is essential (Hurter & Bush, 2007). See Chapter 13 for a more detailed discussion of fatigue management strategies.

Education fosters patient compliance with treatment and allows patients to actively participate in their care. Knowledge empowers patients and provides a sense of control during a time in which they may be experiencing significant losses and fears. Education ideally should begin prior to the development of symptoms. Nurses should encourage patients to report all symptoms promptly and explain the potential benefits of early intervention for anemia as reported in recent studies (Hurter & Bush, 2007; Lyman & Glaspy, 2006).

Need for Future Research

A number of questions and issues remain with regard to anemia and its treatment. First, with regard to the classification of anemia, the current grading systems do not consider gender differences (Schwartz, 2007). Because the normal Hgb level for men is higher than that for women, the optimal time to begin treatment may vary with gender.

Second, erythropoietin receptors have been found on tumor cells, such as head and neck and breast tumor cells (De Los Santos & Thomas, 2007). Studies have reported a decreased survival in patients treated with erythropoietic agents while receiving chemotherapy or radiation therapy (Henke et al., 2003; Leyland-Jones et al., 2005). This raises the question of whether erythropoietic therapy is detrimental for specific tumor types and therefore should be avoided (De Los Santos & Thomas).

Another issue that has been addressed in older studies but needs revisiting is the question of whether a correlation exists between cancer recurrence and blood transfusion (Jahnson & Andersson, 1992; Vamvakas, 1996). Immunosuppression resulting from blood transfusion and tumor hypoxia associated with anemia are two explanations for this possible connection (Goodnough, 2005; Varlotto & Stevenson, 2005). In light of recent findings suggesting a correlation between erythropoietic therapy and decreased survival, future studies designed with primary end points of overall survival and progression-free survival are warranted.

Future research also is needed to determine the ideal time to begin IV iron supplementation during chemotherapy when an erythropoietic agent is being administered. In addition, the optimal total IV iron dose must be further explored (Henry et al., 2007). Finally, as anemia assessment and management typically have focused on objective measures (Hgb level), nursing research exploring subjective measures of anemia is needed. Monitoring the symptoms of anemic patients may help to determine patterns, potentially resulting in new strategies in the management of anemia.

Conclusion of Case Study

Recall T.C.'s case from the beginning of this chapter, and reflect on the following questions. Is T.C. at risk for anemia? If so, what are her risk factors? What concerns would the oncology nurse have, and how would the nurse monitor this patient?

T.C. has stage IIIA non-small cell lung cancer. Her baseline Hgb level reveals she is already mildly anemic. In addition, she reports experiencing symptoms of anemia, such as fatigue and dyspnea on exertion. T.C. is at significant risk for worsening anemia as her treatment begins. Risk factors include her low baseline Hgb, treatment with a platinum-based therapy, older age, and presence of symptoms. The nurse should monitor the patient's Hgb closely, assess the patient comprehensively, and advocate for early anemia treatment to enhance T.C.'s QOL and potential to tolerate treatment. The nurse's early recognition of the problem of anemia and timely intervention to manage this symptom will help T.C. to maintain her functional status and be able to continue to care for her grandchildren, which she reports is important to her.

Erythropoietic therapy can be initiated with the start of chemotherapy. Platinum-based therapy places patients at significant risk for anemia. Even with early-stage disease and aggressive treatment, lung cancer prognosis remains poor. Treatment of anemia in this population is essential to enhance QOL (Kosmidis & Krzakowski, 2005).

Conclusion

Anemia is prevalent in in oncology populations, and this symptom negatively affects patients' QOL, daily functioning, and survival. Determining the differential diagnosis of anemia may pose a challenge for the healthcare team. Oncology nurses are in an ideal position to identify symptoms of anemia and initiate treatment early to improve the Hgb level, resolve symptoms, enhance patients' QOL, and afford patients the opportunity to complete their treatment course without interruption. In light of concerns of potential serious adverse effects of erythropoietic therapies, oncology nurses must remain abreast of current research in this area and aggressively monitor the Hgb level of patients who are receiving erythropoietic therapy. Anticipating anemia, assessing the symptom comprehensively, and advocating for evidence-based treatments are the keys to providing high-quality patient care.

References

American Association of Blood Banks. (2002). *Circular of information for the use of human blood and blood components.* Bethesda, MD: Author.

Amgen Inc. (2007). Aranesp (darbepoetin alfa for injection) [Package insert]. Thousand Oaks, CA: Author.

Birgegard, G., Gascon, P., & Ludwig, H. (2006). Evaluation of anaemia in patients with multiple myeloma and lymphoma: Findings of the European Cancer Anaemia Survey. *European Journal of Haematology, 77*(5), 378–386.

Bohlius, J., Wilson, J., Seidenfeld, J., Piper, M., Schwarzer, G., Sandercock, J., et al. (2006). Recombinant human erythropoietins and cancer patients: Updated meta-analysis of 57 studies including 9353 patients. *Journal of the National Cancer Institute, 98*(10), 708–714.

Brooks, J.P. (2005). Reengineering transfusion and cellular therapy processes hospitalwide: Ensuring the safe utilization of blood products. *Transfusion, 45*(Suppl. 4), 159S–171S.

Buchsel, P.C., Murphy, B.J., & Newton, S.A. (2002). Epoetin alfa: Current and future indications and nursing implications. *Clinical Journal of Oncology Nursing, 6*(5), 261–267.

Caro, J.J., Salas, M., Ward, A., & Goss, G. (2001). Anemia as an independent prognostic factor for survival in patients with cancer: A systematic, quantitative review. *Cancer, 91*(12), 2214–2221.

Cleeland, C.S., Demetri, G.D., Glaspy, J., Cella, D.F., Portenoy, R.K., Cremieux, P., et al. (1999). Identifying hemoglobin level for optimal quality of life: Results of an incremental analysis [Abstract 2215]. *Proceedings of the American Society of Clinical Oncology, 18,* 574A.

Crawford, J., Cella, D., Cleeland, C.S., Cremieux, P.Y., Demetri, G.D., Sarokhan, B.J., et al. (2002). Relationship between changes in hemoglobin level and quality of life during chemotherapy in anemic cancer patients receiving epoetin alfa therapy. *Cancer, 95*(4), 888–895.

De Los Santos, J.F., & Thomas, G.M. (2007). Anemia correction in malignancy management: Threat or opportunity? *Gynecologic Oncology, 105*(2), 517–529.

Demetri, G.D., Kris, M., Wade, J., Degos, L., & Cella, D. (1998). Quality-of-life benefit in chemotherapy patients treated with epoetin alfa is independent of disease response or tumor type: Results from a prospective community oncology study. Procrit Study Group. *Journal of Clinical Oncology, 16*(10), 3412–3425.

Elfath, M.D. (2006). Is it time to focus on preserving the functionality of red blood cells during storage? *Transfusion, 46*(9), 1469–1470.

Foubert, J. (2006). Cancer-related anaemia and fatigue: Assessment and treatment. *Nursing Standard, 20*(36), 50–57.

Gajic, O., & Moore, S.B. (2005). Transfusion-related acute lung injury. *Mayo Clinic Proceedings, 80*(6), 766–770.

Glaspy, J. (1997). The impact of epoetin alfa on quality of life during cancer chemotherapy: A fresh look at an old problem. *Seminars in Hematology, 34*(3, Suppl. 2), 20–26.

Glaspy, J., Vadhan-Raj, S., Patel, R., Bosserman, L., Hu, E., Lloyd, R.E., et al. (2006). Randomized comparison of every-2-week darbepoetin alfa and weekly epoetin alfa for the treatment of chemotherapy-induced anemia: The 20030125 study group trial. *Journal of Clinical Oncology, 24*(15), 2290–2297.

Glaspy, J.A., Jadeja, J.S., Justice, G., Fleishman, A., Rossi, G., & Colowick, A.B. (2003). A randomized, active-control, pilot trial of front-loaded dosing regimens of darbepoetin-alfa for the treatment of patients with anemia during chemotherapy for malignant disease. *Cancer, 97*(5), 1312–1320.

Goodnough, L.T. (2005). Risks of blood transfusion. *Anesthesiology Clinics of North America, 23*(2), 241–252.

Groopman, J.E., & Itri, L.M. (1999). Chemotherapy-induced anemia in adults: Incidence and treatment. *Journal of the National Cancer Institute, 91*(19), 1616–1634.

Henke, M., Laszig, R., Rube, C., Schafer, U., Haase, K.D., Schilcher, B., et al. (2003). Erythropoietin to treat head and neck cancer patients with anaemia undergoing radiotherapy: Randomised, double-blind, placebo-controlled trial. *Lancet, 362*(9392), 1255–1260.

Henry, D.H., Dahl, N.V., Auerbach, M., Tchekmedyian, S., & Laufman, L.R. (2007). Intravenous ferric gluconate significantly improves response to epoetin alfa versus oral iron or no iron in anemic patients with cancer receiving chemotherapy. *Oncologist, 12*(2), 231–242.

Herrington, J.D., Davidson, S.L., Tomita, D.K., Green, L., Smith, R.E., & Boccia, R.V. (2005). Utilization of darbepoetin alfa and epoetin alfa for chemotherapy-induced anemia. *American Journal of Health-System Pharmacy, 62*(1), 54–62.

Hovav, T., Yedgar, S., Manny, N., & Barshtein, G. (1999). Alteration of red cell aggregability and shape during blood storage. *Transfusion, 39*(3), 277–281.

Hurter, B., & Bush, N.J. (2007). Cancer-related anemia: Clinical review and management update. *Clinical Journal of Oncology Nursing, 11*(3), 349–359.

Jahnson, S., & Andersson, M. (1992). Adverse effects of perioperative blood transfusion in patients with colorectal cancer. *European Journal of Surgery, 158*(8), 419–425.

Knight, K., Wade, S., & Balducci, L. (2004). Prevalence and outcomes of anemia in cancer: A systematic review of the literature. *American Journal of Medicine, 116*(7A), 11S–26S.

Kosmidis, P., & Krzakowski, M. (2005). Anemia profiles in patients with lung cancer: What have we learned from the European Cancer Anaemia Survey (ECAS)? *Lung Cancer, 50*(3), 401–412.

Langer, C.J., Choy, H., Glaspy, J.A., & Colowick, A. (2002). Standards of care for anemia management in oncology: Focus on lung carcinoma. *Cancer, 95*(3), 613–623.

Lappin, T.R., Maxwell, A.P., & Johnston, P.G. (2007). Warning flags for erythropoiesis-stimulating agents and cancer-associated anemia. *Oncologist, 12*(4), 362–365.

Leyland-Jones, B., Semiglazov, V., Pawlicki, M., Pienkowski, T., Tjulandin, S., Manikhas, G., et al. (2005). Maintaining normal hemoglobin levels with epoetin alfa in mainly nonanemic patients with metastatic breast cancer receiving first-line chemotherapy: A survival study. *Journal of Clinical Oncology, 23*(25), 5960–5972.

Loney, M., & Chernecky, C. (2000). Anemia. *Oncology Nursing Forum, 27*(6), 951–962.

Ludwig, H., & Strasser, K. (2001). Symptomatology of anemia. *Seminars in Oncology, 28*(Suppl. 8), 7–14.

Lyman, G.H., & Glaspy, J. (2006). Are there clinical benefits with early erythropoietic intervention for chemotherapy-induced anemia? A systematic review. *Cancer, 106*(1), 223–233.

Lynch, M.P. (2006). Overview of anemia. In D. Camp-Sorrell & R.A. Hawkins (Eds.), *Clinical manual for the oncology advanced practice nurse* (2nd ed., pp. 787–788). Pittsburgh, PA: Oncology Nursing Society.

Madjdpour, C., & Spahn, D.R. (2005). Allogeneic red blood cell transfusions: Efficacy, risks, alternatives and indications. *British Journal of Anaesthesia, 95*(1), 33–42.

Mickle, J., & Reinke, D. (2007). A review of anemia management in the oncology setting: A focus on implementing standing orders. *Clinical Journal of Oncology Nursing, 11*(4), 534–539.

Mock, V., & Olsen, M. (2003). Current management of fatigue and anemia in patients with cancer. *Seminars in Oncology Nursing, 19*(4), 36–41.

National Comprehensive Cancer Network. (2007). *NCCN Clinical Practice Guidelines in Oncology™: Cancer- and chemotherapy-induced anemia* [v.3.2007]. Retrieved July 1, 2007, from http://www.nccn.org/professionals/physician_gls/PDF/anemia.pdf

National Comprehensive Cancer Network. (2008). *NCCN Clinical Practice Guidelines in Oncology™: Cancer- and chemotherapy-induced anemia* [v.3.2009]. Retrieved October 27, 2008, from http://www.nccn.org/professionals/physician_gls/PDF/anemia.pdf

Ortho Biotech Products, L.P. (2007). Procrit (epoetin alfa for injection) [Package insert]. Raritan, NJ: Author.

Pagana, K.D., & Pagana, T.J. (2002). *Mosby's manual of diagnostic and laboratory tests* (2nd ed.). St. Louis, MO: Mosby.

Porth, C.M. (1994). *Pathophysiology: Concepts of altered health states* (4th ed.). Philadelphia: Lippincott.

Rizzo, J.D., Lichtin, A.E., Woolf, S.H., Seidenfeld, J., Bennett, C.L., Cella, D., et al. (2002). Use of epoetin in patients with cancer: Evidence-based clinical practice guidelines of the American Society of Clinical Oncology and the American Society of Hematology. *Blood, 100*(7), 2303–2320.

Ross, S.D., Allen, E., Henry, D.H., Seaman, C., Sercus, B., & Goodnough, L.T. (2006). Clinical benefits and risks associated with epoetin and darbepoetin in patients with chemotherapy-induced anemia: A systematic review of the literature. *Clinical Therapeutics, 28*(6), 801–824.

Schwartz, R.N. (2007). Anemia in patients with cancer: Incidence, causes, impact, management, and use of treatment guidelines and protocols. *American Journal of Health-System Pharmacy, 64*(Suppl. 2), S5–S13.

Shasha, D., George, M.J., & Harrison, L.B. (2003). Once-weekly dosing of epoetin-alfa increases hemoglobin and improves quality of life in anemic cancer patients receiving radiation therapy either concomitantly or sequentially with chemotherapy. *Cancer, 98*(5), 1072–1079.

U.S. Food and Drug Administration. (2007, March 9). *Information for healthcare professionals: Erythropoiesis stimulating agents (ESA)*. Retrieved September 25, 2007, from http://www.fda.gov/cder/drug/InfoSheets/HCP/RHE2007HCP.pdf

Vamvakas, E.C. (1996). Transfusion-associated cancer recurrence and postoperative infection: Meta-analysis of the randomized controlled clinical trials. *Transfusion, 36*(2), 175–186.

Varlotto, J., & Stevenson, M.A. (2005). Anemia, tumor hypoxemia, and the cancer patient. *International Journal of Radiation Oncology, Biology, Physics, 63*(1), 25–36.

Ward, N.S., & Levy, M.M. (2004). Blood transfusion practice today. *Critical Care Clinics, 20*(2), 179–186.

Weiss, G., & Goodnough, L.T. (2005). Medical progress: Anemia of chronic disease. *New England Journal of Medicine, 352*(10), 1011–1023, 1057–1060.

Wilson, B.A., Shannon, M.T., & Stang, C.L. (2006). *Nurse's drug guide 2006.* Upper Saddle River, NJ: Pearson Education.

Witzig, T.E., Silberstein, P.T., Loprinzi, C.L., Sloan, J.A., Novotny, P.J., Mailliard, J.A., et al. (2005). Phase III, randomized, double-blind study of epoetin alfa compared with placebo in anemic patients receiving chemotherapy. *Journal of Clinical Oncology, 23*(12), 2606–2617.

Worrall, L.M., Tompkins, C.A., & Rust, D.M. (1999). Recognizing and managing anemia. *Clinical Journal of Oncology Nursing, 3*(4), 153–160.

Anxiety and People With Cancer

Lisa Kennedy Sheldon, PhD, APRN, AOCNP®

Case Study

E.M. is a 47-year-old woman with a two-year history of multiple myeloma. When E.M. first came to the oncology center two years ago, she did not want her family (other than her husband) or her colleagues at work to know about her diagnosis and treatment. She had been receiving a bisphosphonate (zoledronic acid) every month to stabilize her bones and oral steroids. Now, her immunoglobulin G is climbing rapidly, and she has developed systemic symptoms, including fevers and rigors. She has failed to respond to thalidomide. The oncologist has determined that an autologous stem cell transplantation offers the best treatment option at this time. E.M. came to visit the oncology nurses after seeing the oncologist. After hearing his recommendation, she is crying. She says she does not know how to tell her college-age daughters about this, and she is scared about the transplantation and unsure of how they are going to pay for the treatment. The nurses provided her with reassurance and support, discussing her relationship with her daughters and her concerns. They also arranged for a visit from the social worker to discuss the financial arrangements and insurance coverage. To help prepare E.M. for the transplantation, the nurses offered their ongoing assistance and provided teaching materials.

One week later, E.M.'s husband called the nurses because E.M. had been very upset, and he did not know what to do to help her. She has been talking rapidly and saying that she has been so worried that she has not been able to sleep or eat all week. The nurses suggested that she come into the center to see the oncology nurse practitioner. When E.M. and her husband come into the office, E.M. is pacing around the room and talking at a quick pace. Her thoughts move from the transplantation to her daughters to her work issues in rapid sequence. Her weight is down four pounds since a week ago.

Overview

Anxiety is a common problem in patients who are coping with a cancer diagnosis. Oncology nurses often spend extended periods of time with patients with cancer, thus creating opportunities for patients to disclose their concerns. During routine care, patients may reveal their feelings about their diagnosis and treatment, allowing nurses to carefully explore and assess their concerns. How nurses respond to these patient expressions affects further assessment and the identification and treatment of anxiety in people with cancer.

Anxiety has been defined as feelings of distress or tension from known or unknown stimuli (Lehmann & Rabins, 1999). It is a subjective state characterized by emotional discomfort and apprehension that stimulates a physiologic adaptation to stress. How patients respond to stressors, such as a cancer diagnosis, depends on many factors. Patients react based on previous life experiences, prior coping strategies, age, maturity, culture, gender, and the presence of support systems, including family, friends, and spiritual sources of support. Anxiety may occur at different periods during the course of a cancer diagnosis and treatment, including around the time of diagnosis, during vulnerable points over the course of the disease, or as part of a preexisting anxiety disorder.

Patients often experience extreme levels of distress in the first few weeks after a diagnosis of cancer. High levels of anxiety are most common with a new diagnosis of cancer before patients have had an opportunity to integrate these new experiences into their frames of reality (Fedorchuk, Mendiondo, & Matar, 2003). During this initial period of shock and turmoil, patients may experience fear and worry about the future, confused and scattered thinking, and difficulty concentrating. They may have disruptions in sleep and appetite and may experience difficulty carrying out normal roles and responsibilities, such as work and family responsibilities. With the support of families and friends, attentive healthcare providers, counseling, and sometimes medications, patients usually move forward through this crisis period, make the necessary decisions, and pursue treatment for their cancer.

The presence of prolonged distress after the initial stage of crisis requires further evaluation. Many assessment strategies, including paper-and-pencil tools, are available to understand and quantify the patient's experience. Additional members of the resource team such as social workers, mental health specialists, and pastoral care providers may be recruited to assess the patient and provide the necessary interventions to decrease anxiety and improve quality of life.

During specific vulnerable periods, feelings of distress and anxiety may resurface as hopes and expectations are challenged. For example, the revelation of metastatic disease or disease progression, increasing symptoms such as pain, or the prospect of ending active treatment may stimulate anxiety and fear again. Further assessment may be needed to determine the patient's experience and need for further evaluation or intervention. The empathetic acknowledgment of patients' distress coupled with careful exploration of their concerns provides support that may be a therapeutic intervention.

Some patients may have preexisting anxiety or a generalized anxiety disorder that can be further exacerbated by a cancer diagnosis (Derogatis et al., 1983). A generalized anxiety disorder is defined by chronic, uncontrollable nervousness, fearfulness, and a sense of worry (Lantz, 2002). Patients with this disorder may have received previous treatment for anxiety, including counseling or pharmacologic agents. Determination of an underlying condition, previous treatment strategies for the disorder, and current anxiety levels helps to direct further interventions during cancer treatment.

Incidence

Anxiety is a common experience for patients with cancer. The term *distress* often is used instead of *anxiety* because it has less social stigma attached to it and may be easier for patients to discuss. Anxiety, depression, and distress often are clustered when describing the experience of patients with cancer, and some overlap exists between anxiety and depression in many patients. The actual incidence of anxiety often has been combined with depression in studies that evaluate psychiatric disorders in patients with cancer. In one of the most quoted studies, the Psychosocial Collaborative Oncology Group found that 47% of patients with cancer had psychiatric disorders (Derogatis et al., 1983). Of the group of patients with cancer who also had psychiatric diagnoses, 68% had reactive or situational anxiety and depression. Further examination revealed that 90% of these disorders were reactions to the cancer or manifestations of the cancer itself.

In other studies, 20%–40% of patients with cancer experienced distress and anxiety (Carroll, Kathol, Noyes, Wald, & Clamon, 1993; Zabora, BrintzenhofeSzoc, Curbow, Hooker, & Piantadosi, 2001). More alarming was the fact that less than 10% of patients with anxiety were identified by healthcare providers as needing psychosocial interventions. In another study, uncontrolled pain was particularly associated with adjustment disorders, including anxiety (Portenoy, Payne, & Jacobsen, 1999), making pain management a significant need for many patients with prolonged distress after an initial cancer diagnosis.

When it occurs across the cancer spectrum, anxiety is one manifestation of emotional distress that people with cancer frequently experience. The National Comprehensive Cancer Network (NCCN) has included the management of anxiety within its guidelines for distress management (NCCN, 2008). According to the NCCN guidelines, distress occurs along a continuum from normal feelings of sadness and vulnerability to problems that may become disabling, such as anxiety. The NCCN guidelines also identify specific periods of increased vulnerability (see Figure 4-1) that may put patients with cancer at risk for developing distress and anxiety. During these times, clinicians need to assess patients more carefully so that interventions to alleviate anxiety and improve quality of life are instituted in a timely manner.

Certain patients are more at risk for anxiety during the course of their cancer treatment (see Figure 4-2). Patients with a previous history of adjustment disorders with anxiety or panic attacks, sexual abuse, and other psychiatric disorders are at risk for maladjustment during the period of increased stress associated with a cancer diagnosis (Derogatis et al., 1983). Additionally, patients with depression also may have anxiety disorders and often are predisposed to more anxiety during times of stress. Further assessment of social supports and other emotional stressors may direct the frequency of future assessments and target specific interventions proved to be effective for patients with similar experiences.

FIGURE 4-1	Periods of Increased Vulnerability to Anxiety

- Upon finding a suspicious symptom
- During workup
- At the time of diagnosis
- While awaiting treatment
- During arduous treatment cycles
- With a change in treatment modality
- At the end of treatment and when encountering survivorship issues
- Upon discharge from hospital
- Before medical follow-up visits and surveillance
- When experiencing minor symptoms that could represent recurrence of disease
- After treatment failure with recurrence or progression
- With advanced cancer or worsening symptoms
- During transition to hospice or palliative care
- With awareness of the end of life

Note. Based on information from Dahlin, 2006; National Comprehensive Cancer Network, 2008.

FIGURE 4-2	Characteristics Placing Patients at Increased Risk for Anxiety

- History of psychiatric diagnosis, including depression, anxiety, and adjustment disorders
- History of alcohol or substance abuse
- Being younger
- Having young children
- Cumulative stress
- Cognitive impairment
- Communication barriers, including language and literacy issues
- Severe comorbid illnesses
- Social conditions such as inadequate social support, living alone, family conflicts, and financial problems

Note. Based on information from Dahlin, 2006; Derogatis et al., 1983; National Comprehensive Cancer Network, 2008.

Pathophysiology

Although the symptoms of anxiety may be both behavioral and physical, they often present as somatic symptoms. Feeling anxious is precipitated by stimulation of a general adaptation to stress including both the sympathetic and autonomic nervous systems. Patients with high anxiety often present with physical symptoms related to activation of the autonomic nervous system (ANS) (Dahlin, 2006). Stimulation of the ANS may produce sweating, tachycardia, cold and clammy hands, dizziness, and diarrhea. Symptoms in the musculoskeletal system include shakiness and jumpiness, trembling, inability to relax, restlessness, and fidgeting.

The most common physical symptoms of anxiety are
- Tachycardia or palpitations
- Sweating
- Perception of dyspnea or shortness of breath
- Loss of appetite
- Headaches
- Restlessness or fidgeting
- Abdominal distress.

The experience of anxiety varies among patients, and symptoms may be more subjective in nature. Both physical and psychosocial symptoms often are present in patients experiencing increased levels of anxiety.

Examples of subjective symptoms of anxiety include
- Recurrent thoughts about diagnosis and treatment
- Fears about the future and/or sense of dread
- Concerns about possible disability and pain
- Changes in body image and functioning
- Inability to sleep
- Difficulty concentrating
- Hypervigilance and scanning
- Irritability and impatience
- Worries about death.

Signs and symptoms of anxiety in patients with cancer vary by patient and circumstance. Because of the unique problems experienced by these patients, NCCN (2008) has defined the following general classifications of anxiety.
- Anxiety because of general medical condition
- Generalized anxiety disorder
- Panic disorder
- Post-traumatic stress disorder
- Phobic disorder (such as needle phobia)
- Obsessive-compulsive disorder
- Conditioned nausea/vomiting

Medical conditions and certain drugs also may cause anxiety. Hormone-secreting tumors, certain types of medications, withdrawal from alcohol and drugs, or other physical symptoms, such as pain, may produce feelings of anxiety. Clinicians must consider the possibility that physical problems are causing the feelings of anxiety in a patient and explore this carefully while instituting anxiety-reducing interventions.

Medical conditions that may cause anxiety include (Bottomley, 1998)
- Cancer with hormone-producing tumors such as pheochromocytoma
- Cardiovascular conditions such as angina, congestive heart failure, and mitral valve prolapse
- Endocrine disorders such as hyperthyroidism, diabetes, and hyper- and hypoglycemia

- Carcinoid syndrome
- Respiratory disorders such as chronic obstructive pulmonary disease, asthma, emphysema, hypoxia, and pulmonary embolus
- Neurologic conditions such as seizure disorder, cerebrovascular accident, and encephalopathy
- Withdrawal from drugs, alcohol, or benzodiazepines
- Use of steroids or stimulants
- Immune conditions such as HIV or AIDS infections.

Assessment

A thorough assessment is the cornerstone of care for patients with cancer experiencing anxiety. Determining what is appropriate anxiety and what is disabling anxiety and the etiology of these feelings may be difficult. If anxiety is affecting the patient's ability to function in normal roles, make decisions, or continue with treatment, then the anxiety may require further assessment and intervention.

Good communication skills will help nurses to assess anxiety and explore patients' experience and concerns. When a patient says "I can't stop worrying," "I am so nervous about this treatment that I can't sleep," or "I can't concentrate at work because I've been worrying about the test results," the nurse needs to hear these phrases as cues to the patient's distress. Further exploration may reveal the extent of the distress and anxiety and the impact of these feelings on the patient's ability to function and make decisions.

Specific communication skills by nurses may facilitate patient disclosure and provide psychosocial support. Active listening, open-ended questions, and effective responses can be used to assess patients' anxiety and help them to feel understood and supported. The use of these skills is not just for assessment purposes. They actually may be therapeutic interventions; allowing patients to express their concerns has been shown to diminish feelings of anxiety (Stiles, Shuster, & Harrigan, 1992). These skills also will direct the assessment of patients and identify anxiety that requires further intervention or referral to other mental health providers.

The following communication skills may facilitate patient disclosure while providing psychosocial support (Sheldon, 2005).
- Active listening—an interactive process that begins with the nurse positioned, physically and emotionally, to hear the patient's experience
- Open-ended questions—questions often beginning with *who, what, when, why,* or *how* that cannot be answered with a yes or no. These are used to explore the patient's experience.
- Responses—responses that acknowledge the patient's experience and contain messages of understanding and support
  - *Clarifying responses* use simplification and summarization to make concise statements about the patient's experience.
  - *Reflective responses* restate the patient's words with the implied emotional undertones. These are used to understand the patient's responses to the situation.
  - *Empathetic responses* convey the meaning of the patient's experience and the nurse's support and interest.

The nurse's assessment also should explore other factors that may affect the patient's anxiety level. These include current stressors, support systems, and prior coping methods that have been successful for the patient. Support systems may include significant others such as family and friends, spiritual sources of support, colleagues, and pets.

Measurement

Many tools are available to evaluate patient anxiety and distress (see Table 4-1). Nursing assessments often contain specific questions regarding patient coping and functioning but usually are limited in assessing anxiety specifically. Although traditional nursing assessments usually include questions regarding the patient's psychosocial condition, specific tools are available to rate patient anxiety and identify specific areas of concern. Mental health professionals frequently use the Structured Clinical Interview for DSM Disorders, but this tool is very lengthy, requires special training, and may be best utilized by mental health experts. Shorter tools are available to nurses, and some are brief enough to be used during routine assessment at the bedside or chairside. Some are visual scales that are appropriate for all literacy levels, whereas others use paper and pencil or handheld devices (PDAs) to capture information about the patient's experience (Cella et al., 1993; Fortner, Okon, Schwartzberg, Tauer, & Houts, 2003).

The Visual Analog Scale (VAS) is a simple tool rating distress on a scale of 0–10, with 0 being no distress and 10 being extreme distress (NCCN, 2008). The NCCN guidelines recommend incorporating this scale into every visit and referring patients with a score of four or higher for psychosocial services. The guidelines also recommend screening for medical causes of anxiety, patient safety, and decision-making ability.

Evidence-Based Interventions

Treatment of anxiety in people with cancer begins with the development of an open, trusting relationship between the patient and the oncology team. The team consists of the oncologist, oncology nurses, and people from social services and pastoral care. Addressing patient distress, especially anxiety, at the time of diagnosis sets the stage for ongoing communication between the patient and the oncology team through treatment and into a future of survivorship or palliative care.

Acknowledging that patients may need to express their concerns to their healthcare providers requires the creation of a receptive and welcoming environment. The setting needs to allow the privacy, time, and "regard" that promotes open patient-provider communication. *Regard*, or

TABLE 4-1	Tools to Measure Anxiety and Distress		
Tool	**Author**	**Items**	**Subscales**
Hospital Anxiety and Depression Scale (HADS)	Zigmond & Snaith (1983)	14	Anxiety Depression
State-Trait Anxiety Inventory (STAI)	Spielberger (1983)	20	Trait or state anxiety
Visual Analog Scale (VAS) Distress Inventory Scale (DIS)	National Comprehensive Cancer Network (2008)	1 (0–10)	Distress only Questions regarding functioning
Beck Anxiety Inventory	Beck & Steer (1993)	21 items	Anxiety
Brief Symptom Inventory (BSI®)	Derogatis & Melisaratos (1983)	53 items	3 global indices 9 symptom dimensions including anxiety

unconditional positive regard, is a term that was first used by Carl Rogers (1951) to describe the ability to accept another person's beliefs and responses regardless of one's own personal feelings. This nonjudgmental approach is important when patients are experiencing a difficult time and may be concerned as to whether their feelings of anxiety, worry, and fear are normal and understandable reactions. When nurses and other healthcare providers accept patients' experiences, they also enrich their relationship with their patients. Additionally, patients learn to trust their team and may find some relief from their anxiety after discussing their concerns.

Ongoing patient support is needed from not only the oncology team but also other sources. The team should assess patients' support systems, including family, friends, and spiritual support, and refer them to other services such as mental health services and pastoral care as necessary. Resources for additional information are available online and through community groups.

Some resources for support include
- American Cancer Society and NCCN guidelines for patients (www.nccn.org)
- American Society of Clinical Oncology's Web site for patients, Cancer.Net (www.cancer.net/portal/site/patient)
- Local branches of the American Cancer Society for scheduled support groups.

The previously mentioned NCCN (2008) treatment guidelines for distress management also provide a helpful overview of anxiety as well as pathways for evaluation, treatment, and follow-up of anxiety disorders associated with a cancer diagnosis. Because of the significant effect of symptoms such as pain on anxiety levels, interventions to address any underlying or disease-related symptoms need to be addressed in addition to initiating anxiety-specific treatment. For example, after the appropriate evaluation, diagnostic studies, and adequate treatment of symptoms and other disease-related factors, patients with anxiety should be treated with psychosocial interventions, anxiolytics medications, and/or antidepressant medications. Complementary therapies increasingly are being tried to help relieve anxiety and improve quality of life for people with cancer. Interventions include psychosocial, pharmacologic, and complementary therapies, which will be discussed in the following sections.

Psychosocial Interventions

The treatment for anxiety requires careful assessment to determine the most appropriate interventions. After eliminating medical causes of anxiety, psychosocial support is the mainstay of treatment for anxiety. Many different types of psychosocial interventions to diminish patient anxiety have been studied. Psychosocial interventions range from individual to group counseling, psychoeducational interventions, and even telephone-linked care. Two large studies showed that psychosocial interventions of cognitive behavior stress management (Antoni et al., 2006) and cognitive existential therapy (Kissane et al., 2003) decreased anxiety in patients with cancer. When patients' problems are spiritual or existential in nature, pastoral counseling may be more appropriate to address these issues and draw upon religious resources to facilitate patient coping and adaptation.

Psychosocial interventions include
- Individual therapy
- Group therapy and support groups
- Psychoeducational sessions, which provide information as well as support
- Telephone-based interventions such as telephone interpersonal counseling
- Spiritually-based psychotherapy or pastoral counseling
- Hypnosis (self and guided).

Choosing the best psychosocial intervention depends on the experience and training of the oncology nurse. Most oncology nurses have the experience to help patients in disclosing their concerns, respond empathetically, and offer psychosocial support. The NURS mnemonic often is used to describe the steps of empathetic responsiveness in patient-centered interviewing (Smith, 2002). The steps help nurses and other healthcare providers in responding to patients' emotional expressions such as anxiety and distress.

     N—Name the feeling. "I can see that you are really worried about this test."

     U—Understand the patient's experience. "Many patients feel concerned when waiting for test results."

     R—Respect the patient's coping. "You are doing the best you can to deal with this situation and help your family, too."

     S—Support the patient. "I would like to help you get through this time."

Responding empathetically allows patients to disclose their concerns in a nonjudgmental and respectful climate. By reflecting the emotional content and supporting the patient's coping strategies, the nurse empowers the patient and yet also identifies anxiety that may require further intervention to support the patient's functioning. When the nurse establishes that routine psychosocial support is not alleviating the patient's anxiety, then further pharmacologic interventions or referral may be needed for the patient.

Psychosocial interventions, such as cognitive behavioral therapy, and psychological and psychoeducational interventions have been the subject of research and systematic reviews of the literature (Andrykowski & Manne, 2006). Sufficient evidence exists to recommend psychosocial interventions (Antoni et al., 2006; Kissane et al., 2003) and psychoeducational interventions (Deshler et al., 2006; Hoff & Haaga, 2005; Jones et al., 2006) to reduce levels of anxiety in patients with cancer. The difficulty remains in identifying the specific type of intervention to benefit each patient. It may be that nurses should assess the individual patient, identifying previous strategies that have worked for the patient as a means to identify the best psychosocial interventions for the current situation. The establishment of a therapeutic and open nurse-patient relationship allows nurses to tailor the type and amount of psychosocial support to meet the needs of the individual.

Pharmacologic Interventions

If psychosocial interventions are not sufficient in treating the patient's anxiety, pharmacologic treatments may be necessary to help patients to manage their anxiety and distress. Pharmacologic agents should always be combined with psychosocial interventions. Medications may include anxiolytics (antianxiety), antidepressants, azapirones, antihistamines, and atypical neuroleptics (see Table 4-2).

Anxiolytic Medications

Anxiolytic (antianxiety) medications are used to decrease anxiety in patients with situational anxiety and generalized anxiety disorders. Patients with situational anxiety experience anxiety in relation to specific causative events in their environment. This type of anxiety usually is self-limited but may cause acute anxiety. Generalized anxiety disorder is a longer-term disorder (greater than six months) characterized by excessive worry and anxiety about numerous events (Dahlin, 2006). Although few studies have examined their effects on patients with cancer, anxiolytics have been used and studied in many patient populations and are recommended by the NCCN (2008) guidelines as one pharmacologic treatment for anxiety.

The most frequently used anxiolytics are benzodiazepines (e.g., lorazepam, diazepam), hydroxyzine, and buspirone.

Azapirones

Buspirone is an antianxiety drug used for short-term relief of anxiety and is useful in mild to moderate generalized anxiety disorders. Treatment may be needed for at least two weeks to see effectiveness. Dosages may be increased over several days to reach efficacy. Side effects include dizziness, nausea, headache, and insomnia.

Antihistamines

Hydroxyzine is an antihistamine and central nervous system depressant that may be used to treat anxiety in certain patients. It is used to treat anxiety disorders and relieve tension during stressful circumstances, such as before surgery. Side effects include drowsiness, dry mouth, and constipation.

Antidepressants

One systematic review showed that antidepressants improved symptoms of generalized anxiety disorder when used for 4–28 weeks (Rasavi et al., 1996). Studies have not shown one antidepressant to be more effective than another in treating anxiety, nor have they shown a difference in effectiveness among antidepressants, anxiolytics, or buspirone (Jackson & Lipman, 2004; Sheldon, Swanson, Dolce, Marsh, & Summers, 2008). Because each medication may have side effects, patients using these medications to treat anxiety need to be monitored by the prescriber.

Antidepressants include paroxetine, sertraline, escitalopram, venlafaxine, and mirtazapine. Nurses should monitor patients for side effects, including sedation, dizziness, nausea, falls, and sexual dysfunction, such as decreased libido (see Table 4-2).

Atypical Neuroleptics

Atypical neuroleptics are useful in treating complex patterns of anxiety and are not often used as first-line treatment in patients without preexisting mental health disorders. Examples of atypical neuroleptics are olanzapine and risperidone.

If symptoms of anxiety persist or increase, patients may need further evaluation and interventions. Patients should be reassessed every three weeks to assess their response to the medications. Depression symptoms may be seen in association with anxiety in some patients. A patient who is suicidal should immediately be referred to a mental health provider at a center or hospital. The following guidelines may indicate the need for referral to a mental health professional, social worker, or pastoral counselor.

• Score ≥ 4 on the VAS (NCCN, 2008)
• Excessive worries and fears
• Excessive sadness
• Unclear thinking
• Despair and hopelessness
• Severe family problems
• Spiritual crises
• Suicidal ideation

TABLE 4-2	Medications for the Treatment of Anxiety			
Medication	Dosage	Route	Side Effects	Contraindications
Benzodiazepines				
Lorazepam (Ativan®, Biovail Pharmaceuticals Inc.; Baxter Healthcare Corp.)	0.5–2 mg every 8–12 hours	PO/IV	Central nervous system (CNS) depression, sedation, dizziness, weakness, transient memory impairment, disorientation, sleep disturbances, agitation, and abuse potential	Contraindicated in patients with acute narrow-angle glaucoma. Use with caution with opioids and other CNS depressants, including alcohol.
Diazepam (Valium®, Roche Laboratories Inc.)	2–10 mg 2–4 times daily Increase gradually.	PO/IV	CNS depression, impaired coordination, fatigue, changes in libido and/or appetite	Contraindicated in patients with acute narrow-angle glaucoma. Use with caution with substance or alcohol abuse and depression.
Alprazolam (Xanax®, Pfizer Inc.)	Start at 0.25–0.5 mg TID. May increase every 4 days to 4 mg/day in divided doses	PO	CNS depression, fatigue, impaired coordination and memory, changes in libido and/or appetite	Contraindicated in patients with open-angle glaucoma. Use with caution in patients with suicidal ideation. Avoid abrupt cessation.
Clonazepam (Klonopin®, Roche Laboratories Inc.)	0.5–1.5 mg/day	PO	Nausea, drowsiness, impaired cognition, irritability, impaired coordination and balance	Contraindicated in older adults, those at risk for falls, and patients with schizophrenia. Not recommended for those younger than 18 years.
Azapirones				
Buspirone (BuSpar®, Bristol-Myers Squibb Co.)	7.5 mg BID initially, then may increase by 5 mg/day every 2–3 days up to 60 mg/day	PO	Dizziness, nausea, headache, nervousness, dream disturbances, insomnia	Use caution with other CNS drugs and in patients with renal and hepatic failure. Do not use with concomitant monoamine oxidase inhibitors (MAOIs). Should not be taken with grapefruit juice.
Antihistamines				
Hydroxyzine (Vistaril®, Pfizer Inc.)	25–50 mg every 4–6 hours	PO/IV	Drowsiness, dry mouth, tremor, convulsions	Use with caution in older adults.
Antidepressants				
Paroxetine (Paxil®, GlaxoSmithKline)	Start at 20 mg/day and increase by 20 mg at one-week intervals up to 60 mg/day.	PO	Asthenia, sweating, decreased appetite, dizziness, somnolence	Contraindicated in patients with seizure disorder, cardiovascular disease, and narrow-angle glaucoma.

(Continued on next page)

TABLE 4-2   Medications for the Treatment of Anxiety (Continued)

Medication	Dosage	Route	Side Effects	Contraindications
Sertraline (Zoloft®, Pfizer Inc.)	Start at 25–50 mg/day and increase at one-week intervals.	PO	Gastrointestinal (GI) upset, insomnia, sexual dysfunction	Contraindicated in patients with cardiovascular disease. Monitor for mania/hypomania and hyperglycemia. Use with caution in patients with seizure disorders.
Escitalopram (Lexapro® Forest Laboratories, Inc.)	10 mg/day May increase to 20 mg/day	PO	Nausea, insomnia, sexual dysfunction, fatigue	Do not use with concomitant MAOIs. Patients should avoid alcohol consumption.
Venlafaxine (Effexor®, Wyeth Pharmaceuticals)	75 mg/day May start at 37.5 mg/day for 4–7 days	PO	GI upset, dizziness somnolence, insomnia, headache, sexual dysfunction	Use with caution in patients with high blood pressure, heart disease, hypercholesterolemia, and seizure disorders.
Mirtazapine (Remeron®, Organon USA)	15 mg/day May increase every 7 days up to 45 mg/day	PO	Visual hallucinations, increased appetite, nightmares, drowsiness, headache	Do not use with concomitant MAOIs. Patients should avoid alcohol consumption. Use with caution with benzodiazepines.
Atypical Neuroleptics				
Olanzapine (Zyprexa®, Eli Lilly and Co.)	5–10 mg/day	PO/IM	Tardive dyskinesia, dizziness, sedation, insomnia, orthostatic hypotension, weight gain	Avoid use in older adults with dementia. Not for IV use.
Risperidone (Risperdal®, Ortho-McNeil Pharmaceutical)	1–3 mg/day Start at 0.5 mg/day in older adults.	PO	Extrapyramidal symptoms, dizziness, somnolence, nausea	Use with caution in older adults. Drug causes increased risk of cerebrovascular accident and death. Contraindicated in patients with hyperglycemia.
Other				
Propofol (Diprivan®, Abraxis BioScience, Inc.)	Titrated IV dosage for sedation and anesthesia	IV	Airway obstruction, apnea, hypoventilation	Sedative hypnotic for anesthesia

Note. Based on information from Swanson et al., 2008.

Complementary Therapies

Many different types of complementary therapies are being tried to reduce patient anxiety and thereby improve quality of life. Increasingly, patients are looking for additional therapies to improve their quality of life during their cancer treatment. Some examples of complementary therapies include

- Guided imagery
- Yoga
- Progressive relaxation and relaxation exercises
- Massage, including body and foot massage and partner-delivered massage
- Reflexology
- Self-hypnotic relaxation
- Reiki
- Aromatherapy
- Virtual reality
- Art therapy
- Stress-reducing medical devices for needle phobia
- Meditation
- Exercise.

Currently, not enough evidence exists to recommend massage, art, or exercise interventions for the reduction of anxiety in patients with cancer. However, most of the studies have had small sample sizes or were not able to detect significant changes in anxiety. A systematic review looking at homeopathy as a complementary therapy showed insufficient evidence to recommend it as an effective intervention for anxiety (Pilkington, Kirkwood, Rampes, Fisher, & Richardson, 2006). Fellowes, Barnes, and Wilkinson (2004) performed a systematic review of the effects of massage and aromatherapy on patients with cancer, using changes in anxiety as one end point. Their review did not find sufficient evidence to recommend these two therapies, but no harms appeared to be associated with either massage or aromatherapy. Future research is needed to identify complementary therapies that may reduce anxiety and improve quality of life and functioning for people living with cancer.

Expected Outcomes

Psychosocial, pharmacologic, and complementary interventions are intended to decrease anxiety levels in patients. By decreasing anxiety, patients will function better in their roles, make decisions more efficiently, and adhere to treatments without undue distress. Earlier recognition and treatment of anxiety also may decrease the number of phone calls to healthcare providers regarding unrelieved fears and worries.

Some outcomes of effective treatment of anxiety are

- Decreased distress
- Improved quality of life
- Better functioning in roles
- Increased adherence to cancer treatment recommendations
- More open and trusting relationships with healthcare providers.

Patient Teaching Points

Working with patients who are experiencing anxiety requires the nurse to assess and intervene with an individualized approach. Nurses can teach patients self-awareness regarding their physical and psychological manifestations of anxiety. Open, trusting relationships with the nurses and the oncology team allow patients to express their feelings, report changes in functioning, and provide feedback regarding effective interventions. Nurses and patients can work collaboratively to find effective coping strategies to decrease anxiety and optimize functioning. Ongoing teaching and follow-up may be necessary as patients move through vulnerable points in their care, and teaching needs to be done at appropriate times when patients are receptive. Mild anxiety may heighten awareness; however, moderate to severe anxiety may be incapacitating, thus impairing a patient's ability to focus, make decisions, and function.

Patients should be taught to

- Learn how they respond to stress and what anxiety feels like for them
- Find techniques that reduce anxiety for them, such as deep breathing, meditation, and music or art therapy, and use these techniques when the feelings appear or prophylactically before situations that patients know are anxiety-producing
- Talk with the people in their life who can provide support during difficult and stressful times
- Talk about their feelings with their oncology team so that the team can understand what patients are experiencing and plan ways to help them
- Take medications as prescribed and not discontinue them without talking with their healthcare provider
- Obtain professional help if recommended to help them to learn strategies to manage anxiety
- Join a support group, which may be effective in relieving anxiety for some people
- Keep a diary or journal as a way to put their experiences and feelings into words.

Need for Future Research

Many interventions have been used to relieve anxiety in patients with cancer, but no gold standard for care exists. Because each patient is an individual with a unique personality and history, treatment approaches need to be customized to the patient and the situation. The characteristics of patients who are at high risk for anxiety need to be identified to provide timely assessment and referral before the anxiety becomes debilitating.

Although psychosocial support is the most recommended intervention and has evidence to support its effectiveness, this treatment can be done in many different ways, including individual and group counseling and even telephone-linked care. Further research could identify effective interventions for specific population characteristics. Additionally, the training of healthcare providers, including nurses, in delivering psychosocial interventions can vary significantly and requires more clarification. The effectiveness of different methods of psychosocial interventions requires further investigation.

Further research is needed to identify the effectiveness of pharmacologic and complementary therapies for patients with cancer. Most of the research regarding medications for anxiety has not been specific to the needs of patients with cancer. Complementary therapies such as massage may be effective for some patients, but larger studies are needed to identify in which patients they are most effective.

Randomized controlled trials for anxiolytics, antidepressants, and other medications are needed to demonstrate the effectiveness of particular medications in patients with cancer.

Conclusion of Case Study

The nurse listens to the patient's concerns and responds, "E.M., this has been a tough week, and you seem very upset. You are telling me that it is hard to sleep and you don't feel like eating. You have every reason to be concerned about the transplant and how it will affect your life. But we need you to stay healthy before the transplant, and this includes sleeping and eating well. Some patients, when they are very worried, find it difficult to function or even focus on the other parts of their lives. All they can think about is what is happening to them. I would like you to talk with our nurse practitioner and social worker to find ways for you to stay healthy and talk about your concerns regarding the transplant and your finances. I want to ask your permission to have them come to talk with you."

The nurse practitioner evaluates E.M. and determines that E.M. is suffering from severe anxiety and insomnia related to her disease progression and upcoming stem cell transplantation. The nurse practitioner prescribes lorazepam for anxiety and sleep issues and refers E.M. to the oncology social worker for further evaluation and counseling. She also discusses the patient's appetite and eating issues, but E.M. does not want to see a nutritionist.

Conclusion

Anxiety is a common and pervasive issue in oncology care. Nurses are in the unique position to assess patients for symptoms of anxiety during routine care as well as at vulnerable points in their diagnosis and treatment. Formal and informal measures of anxiety may guide nurses in detecting anxiety before it affects patient functioning. Additionally, many interventions are available to prevent and alleviate anxiety and distress in patients with cancer. Psychosocial, psychoeducational, and pharmacologic interventions have evidence regarding their effectiveness, and newer treatments such as massage, Reiki, and relaxation breathing may prove useful in some patients. Oncology nurses have opportunities to prevent, detect, and treat anxiety in their patients, thereby diminishing the impact of cancer on patients' lives.

References

Andrykowski, M.A., & Manne, S.L. (2006). Are psychological interventions effective and accepted by patients with cancer? I. Standards and levels of evidence. *Annals of Behavioral Medicine, 32*(2), 93–97.

Antoni, M.H., Wimberly, S.R., Lechner, S.C., Kazi, M.S., Sifre, T., Urcuyo, M.S., et al. (2006). Reduction of cancer-specific thought intrusions and anxiety symptoms with a stress management intervention among women undergoing treatment for breast cancer. *American Journal of Psychiatry, 163*(10), 1791–1797.

Beck, A.T., & Steer, R.A. (1993). *Beck anxiety inventory manual.* San Antonio, TX: Psychological Corp.

Bottomley, A. (1998). Anxiety and the adult cancer patient. *European Journal of Cancer Care, 7*(4), 217–224.

Carroll, B.T., Kathol, R.G., Noyes, R., Jr., Wald, T.G., & Clamon, G.H. (1993). Screening for depression and anxiety in cancer patients using the Hospital Anxiety and Depression Scale. *General Hospital Psychiatry, 15*(2), 69–74.

Cella, D.F., Tulsky, D.S., Gray, G., Sarafian, B., Linn, E., Bonomi, A., et al. (1993). The Functional Assessment of Cancer Therapy scale: Development and validation of the general measure. *Journal of Clinical Oncology, 11*(3), 570–579.

Dahlin, C. (2006). Anxiety. In D. Camp-Sorrell & R.A. Hawkins (Eds.), *Clinical manual for the oncology advanced practice nurse* (2nd ed., pp. 1105–1111). Pittsburgh, PA: Oncology Nursing Society.

Derogatis, L.R., & Melisaratos, N. (1983). The Brief Symptom Inventory: An introductory report. *Psychological Medicine, 13*(3), 595–605.

Derogatis, L.R., Morrow, G.R., Fetting, J., Penman, D., Piasetsky, S., Schmale, A.M., et al. (1983). The prevalence of psychiatric disorders in patients with cancer. *JAMA, 249*(6), 751–757.

Deshler, A.M., Fee-Schroeder, K.C., Dowdy, J.L., Mettler, T.A., Novotny, P., Zhao, X., et al. (2006). A patient orientation program at a comprehensive cancer center. *Oncology Nursing Forum, 33*(3), 560–578.

Fedorchuk, M.K., Mendiondo, O.A., & Matar, J.R. (2003). Improving community cancer care: Bringing psychosocial support to private practice. *Journal of Psychosocial Oncology, 21*(2), 23–37.

Fellowes, D., Barnes, K., & Wilkinson, S. (2004). Aromatherapy and massage for symptom relief in patients with cancer. *Cochrane Database of Systematic Reviews* 2004, Issue 3. Art. No.: CD002287. DOI: 10.1002/14651858.CD002287.pub2.

Fortner, B., Okon, T., Schwartzberg, L., Tauer, K., & Houts, A.C. (2003). The Cancer Care Monitor: Psychometric content evaluation and pilot testing of a computer administered system for symptom screening and quality of life in adult cancer patients. *Journal of Pain and Symptom Management, 26*(6), 1077–1092.

Hoff, A.C., & Haaga, D.A. (2005). Effects of an education program on radiation oncology patients and families. *Journal of Psychosocial Oncology, 23*(4), 61–79.

Jackson, K.C., & Lipman, A.G. (2004). Drug therapy for anxiety in palliative care [Review]. *Cochrane Database of Systematic Reviews* 2004, Issue 1. Art. No.: CD004596. DOI: 10.1002/14651858.CD004596.

Jones, R.B., Pearson, J., Cawset, A.J., Bental, D., Barrett, A., White, J., et al. (2006). Effect of different forms of information produced for patients with cancer on their use of the information, social support, and anxiety: Randomised trial. *BMJ, 332*(7547), 942–948.

Kissane, D.W., Bloch, S., Smith, G.C., Miach, P., Clarke, D.M., Ikin, J., et al. (2003). Cognitive-existential group psychotherapy for women with primary breast cancer: A randomised controlled trial. *Psycho-Oncology, 12*(6), 532–546.

Lantz, M. (2002). Generalized anxiety in anxious times: Helping older adults cope. *Clinical Geriatrics, 10*(1), 36–38.

Lehmann, S.W., & Rabins, P.V. (1999). Clinical geropsychiatry. In J.J. Gallo, J. Busby-Whitehead, P.V. Rabins, R.A. Stillman, & J.B. Murphy (Eds.), *Reichel's care of the elderly: Clinical aspects of aging* (5th ed., pp. 179–189). Philadelphia: Lippincott Williams & Wilkins.

National Comprehensive Cancer Network. (2008). *NCCN Clinical Practice Guidelines in Oncology™: Distress management* [v.1.2008]. Retrieved March 6, 2008, from http://www.nccn.org/professionals/physician_gls/PDF/distress.pdf

Pilkington, K., Kirkwood, G., Rampes, H., Fisher, P., & Richardson, J. (2006). Homeopathy for anxiety and anxiety disorders: A systematic review of the research. *Homeopathy, 95*(3), 151–162.

Portenoy, R.K., Payne, D.K., & Jacobsen, P.B. (1999). Breakthrough pain: The characteristics and impact in patients with cancer pain. *Pain, 81*(1–2), 129–134.

Rasavi, D., Allilaire, J.F., Smith, M., Salimpour, A., Verra, M., Desclaux, B., et al. (1996). The effect of fluoxetine on anxiety and depressive symptoms in cancer patients. *Acta Psychiatrica Scandinavica, 94*(3), 205–210.

Rogers, C.R. (1951). *Client-centered therapy: Its current practice, implications, and theory.* Boston: Houghton Mifflin.

Sheldon, L.K. (2005). *Communication for nurses: Talking with patients.* Sudbury, MA: Jones and Bartlett.

Sheldon, L.K., Swanson, S., Dolce, A., Marsh, K., & Summers, J. (2008). Putting evidence into practice: Evidence-based interventions for anxiety. *Clinical Journal of Oncology Nursing, 12*(5), 217–224.

Smith, R.C. (2002). *Patient-centered interviewing: An evidence-based method* (2nd ed.). Philadelphia: Lippincott Williams & Wilkins.

Spielberger, C.D. (Ed.). (1983). *STAI: Manual for the State-Trait Anxiety Inventory* (Form Y). Palo Alto, CA: Consulting Psychologists Press.

Stiles, W.B., Shuster, P.L., & Harrigan, J.A. (1992). Disclosure and anxiety: A test of the fever model. *Journal of Personality and Social Psychology, 63*(6), 980–988.

Swanson, S., Dolce, A., Marsh, K., Summers, J., & Sheldon, L.K. (2008). *Putting evidence into practice: Anxiety.* Pittsburgh, PA: Oncology Nursing Society.

Zabora, J., BrintzenhofeSzoc, K., Curbow, B., Hooker, C., & Piantadosi, S. (2001). The prevalence of psychological distress by cancer site. *Psycho-Oncology, 10*(1), 19–28.

Zigmond, A.S., & Snaith, R.P. (1983). The Hospital Anxiety and Depression Scale. *Acta Psychiatrica Scandinavica, 67*(6), 361–370.

CHAPTER 5

Cancer Cachexia

Clara Granda-Cameron, RN, BSN, MSN, CRNP, AOCN®, ANCC,
and Mary Pat Lynch, CRNP, MSN, AOCN®

Case Study

E.B. is a 60-year-old white male plumber with a history of smoking and alcohol intake who presented with a 30-pound weight loss over six months and dysphagia. Workup revealed a mass at the base of his tongue, and biopsy was positive for squamous cell carcinoma, stage 3, with involvement of the lymph nodes in his right neck. Treatment plan included four cycles of neoadjuvant chemotherapy with cisplatin, docetaxel, and 5-fluorouracil followed by concomitant chemotherapy with weekly paclitaxel and radiotherapy. Following chemotherapy and radiotherapy, he underwent a resection of the base of his tongue and right lymph node dissection. The healthcare team is concerned that this patient is at high risk for developing cancer cachexia.

Overview

Cancer cachexia is a profound wasting syndrome usually seen in end-stage or metastatic cancer. Cachexia occurs when protein or caloric requirements are not met, either because of decreased intake, increased requirements, or inappropriate utilization of nutrients. Wasting and malnutrition have long been recognized as predictive of poor outcomes in patients with cancer. Significant weight loss at the time of diagnosis was correlated with decreased survival and impaired response to chemotherapy in 1980 by the Eastern Cooperative Oncology Group (DeWys et al., 1980). People with cancer cachexia have poor appetite and significant weight loss, leading to weakness and fatigue as well as potentially life-threatening metabolic disturbances. In addition, impaired nutritional status and protein deficiency can affect response to chemotherapy and increase toxicity from therapy, thus leading to increased morbidity and mortality (Baracos, 2006; Langer, Hoffman, & Ottery, 2001; Mattox, 2005; Slaviero, Read, Clarke, & Rivory, 2003). Patients with cancer cachexia also may have decreased quality of life (QOL), especially in physical, psychological, and social functioning (Brown, 2002).

Cancer cachexia is common; 50%–75% of patients with cancer experience some degree of cancer cachexia (Maltzman, 2004; Slaviero et al., 2003). The term *cachexia* is derived from the Greek words *kakos* ("bad") and *hexis* ("condition"). Cancer cachexia is defined as a decrease in baseline weight by 5%–10% or more in six months or 5% in one month (Bruera, 1977). Stewart, Skipworth, and Fearon (2006) stated that cancer cachexia represents a wasting syndrome involving loss of muscle and fat caused directly by tumor factors or indirectly by abnormal response to tumor presence. Baracos (2006) suggested that cachexia may be best defined as a state of depletion, synonymous with emaciation.

Weight loss in patients with cancer usually is represented by loss of muscle mass, which leads to decrease in function as measured by performance status tools such as the Karnofsky scale (Karnofsky, Abelmann, Craver, & Burchenal, 1948). Involuntary weight loss at diagnosis or as a result of treatment varies widely by tumor type and treatment modality, with the greatest risk for nutritional deficits occurring with multimodality treatments. The most common tumor types in which cachexia develops in the majority of cases are gastric (85%), pancreatic (83%), non-small cell lung (61%), small cell lung, prostate (57%), and colon (54%) (DeWys et al., 1980).

Pathophysiology

Cancer cachexia is a disorder whose etiology is very complex and fairly misunderstood. The pathophysiology of this cancer-associated syndrome has proved to be multifaceted based on current research, and its various causes can be grouped into two linked classes: primary anorexia-cachexia and secondary anorexia-cachexia (Strasser & Bruera, 2002).

Primary anorexia-cachexia is a metabolic syndrome caused directly by the cancer (see Figure 5-1). The interaction between cancer cells and the host produces immune alterations, which in turn trigger various overlapping syndromes of anorexia-cachexia. These syndromes can be divided into three categories—metabolic, neurohormonal, and anabolic al-

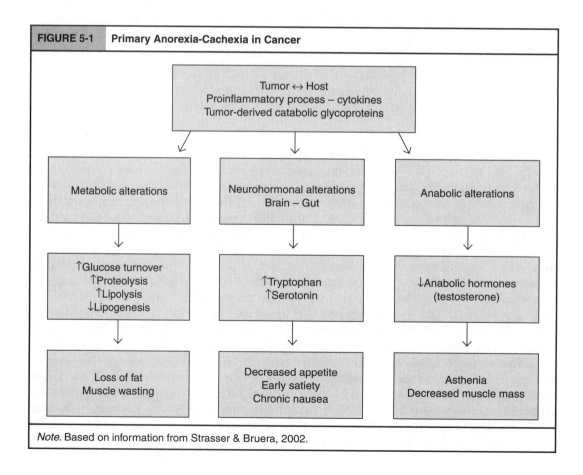

FIGURE 5-1   Primary Anorexia-Cachexia in Cancer

Tumor ↔ Host
Proinflammatory process – cytokines
Tumor-derived catabolic glycoproteins

| Metabolic alterations | Neurohormonal alterations Brain – Gut | Anabolic alterations |

| ↑Glucose turnover ↑Proteolysis ↑Lipolysis ↓Lipogenesis | ↑Tryptophan ↑Serotonin | ↓Anabolic hormones (testosterone) |

| Loss of fat Muscle wasting | Decreased appetite Early satiety Chronic nausea | Asthenia Decreased muscle mass |

Note. Based on information from Strasser & Bruera, 2002.

terations—all of which lead to loss of appetite, early satiety, asthenia, muscle wasting, and loss of fat (Strasser & Bruera, 2002).

Immune alterations between host and tumor include proinflammatory cytokines and tumor-derived catabolic glycoproteins that play a major role in all three syndromes of cancer cachexia. In response to a tumor, the body's immune system produces several proinflammatory cytokines that include interleukin (IL)-1, IL-6, tumor necrosis factor alpha (TNF-α), interferon alpha, and interferon gamma in patients with cancer (McNamara, Alexander, & Norton, 1992). Increased levels of any of these cytokines alone or in combination over time are sufficient in reproducing many of the varied features in cancer-associated cachexia (Busbridge, Dascombe, Hopkins, & Rothwell, 1989; Gelin et al., 1991; McLaughlin, Rogan, Ton, Baile, & Joy, 1992; Strassmann, Fong, Kenney, & Jacob, 1992). Also, through the use of experimental animal models, cachexia symptoms were observed to be alleviated by the use of specific cytokine antagonists, thus providing supplementary evidence to the involvement of proinflammatory cytokines in cachexia (Matthys & Billiau, 1997; Noguchi, Yoshikawa, Matsumoto, Svaninger, & Gelin, 1996; Sherry et al., 1989). These cytokines appear to be important in the metabolic processes involved in cancer cachexia and demonstrate closely interrelated activities and even synergistic effects in such patients (Argiles & Lopez-Soriano, 1999).

Circulating tumor-derived catabolic factors incite major metabolic changes that are characteristic in patients with cancer-associated cachexia. These factors derived from cancer include lipolytic as well as proteolytic factors. The former catabolic factor works directly on breaking down adipose tissue while the latter works on skeletal muscle, neither of which affect actual food intake (Beck, Mulligan, & Tisdale, 1990; Taylor, Gercel-Taylor, Jenis, & Devereux, 1992; Todorov et al., 1996).

Metabolic alterations are present in the cancer cachexia syndrome. Hypermetabolism and high rates of glucose usage are very prominent features in tumor-bearing cancers. The increased energy usage and glucose turnover through raised metabolism causes weight loss and other characteristic symptoms of cancer-associated cachexia (Lundholm, Edstrom, Karlberg, Ekman, & Schersten, 1982). Other metabolic alterations include decreased lipogenesis, increased lipolysis, and increased lysis of muscle proteins (Argiles, Meijsing, Pallares-Trujillo, Guirao, & Lopez-Soriano, 2001; Attaix, Combaret, Tilignac, & Taillandier, 1999).

Alteration of neurohormonal processes between the brain and gut plays an important role in the mechanism of cancer anorexia-cachexia. Taste sensation and neurohormonal signals from the gastrointestinal tract and neurotransmitters in the hypothalamus and other brain regions regulate food intake (Schwartz, Woods, Porte, Seeley, & Baskin, 2000). The presence of serotonin contributes to the disorder of cachexia. Abnormal use of tryptophan, the progenitor of serotonin, by tumor cells leads to excess levels of tryptophan free in blood plasma of patients with cancer (Krause, Humphrey, von Meyenfeldt, James, & Fischer, 1981). This leads to excess tryptophan in the cerebrospinal fluid, causing increased serotonin production and secretion in the ventromedial hypothalamic serotonergic system. This has a decreasing effect on appetite, and a close relationship between elevated free tryptophan levels in plasma and anorexia has been shown in patients with cancer (Cangiano et al., 1994).

Anabolic changes in cancer anorexia-cachexia comprise altered levels of anabolic hormones, including growth hormone, insulin-like growth factors, and anabolic steroids. Low levels of testosterone in patients with cancer cachexia are associated with weight loss, decreased lean body mass, and disease progression (Todd, 1988).

Secondary anorexia-cachexia represents a combination of several contributing factors (see Figure 5-2). The first factor is malnutrition caused by impaired oral intake, impaired gastrointestinal absorption, and loss of proteins through body fluids. The second factor includes catabolic states not related to cancer, such as chronic diseases or infections. The third factor is the loss of muscle mass as a result of prolonged inactivity (Strasser & Bruera, 2002).

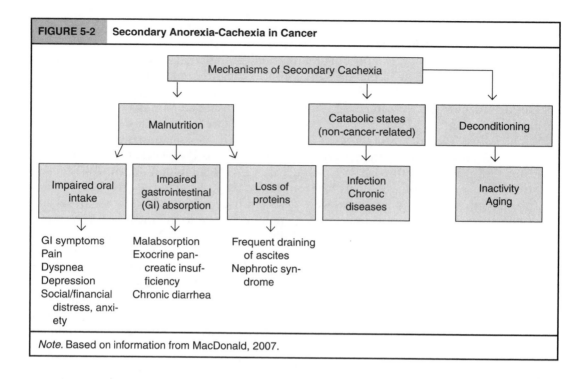

FIGURE 5-2   Secondary Anorexia-Cachexia in Cancer

Note. Based on information from MacDonald, 2007.

Impaired oral intake and gastrointestinal absorption mostly are caused by treatment- or tumor-related symptoms, including gastrointestinal symptoms (e.g., dysphagia, mucositis) and other symptoms (e.g., pain, dyspnea, delirium). Other contributing factors to impaired oral intake are emotional distress, depression, and social and financial problems.

Anorexia is the major and most prominent symptom in cancer-associated cachexia. Loss of appetite or desire to eat is one aspect of cancer-associated anorexia, as patients with cancer very often experience nausea, changes in taste, and early satiety, or the feeling that they are full before they have eaten adequately (Armes, Plant, Allbright, Silverstone, & Slevin, 1992). Abnormalities in taste and smell, causing patients to become nauseated or simply to not desire food that they may have otherwise craved, are common symptoms of cancer (DeWys & Walters, 1975; Nielsen, Theologides, & Vickers, 1980). Also, common treatments of cancer, such as chemotherapy and radiotherapy, especially to the oral cavity and esophagus, may lead to many of these same sensations and symptoms. Oral mucositis, or inflammation of the tissues of the mouth, as well as xerostomia (dry mouth) caused by damage to salivary glands often result from chemotherapy or radiation treatments to the area of the oral cavity and throat. Cancer also may affect primary or secondary organs of the alimentary tract. For example, a tumor of the esophagus or stomach that directly obstructs the passage of food prevents nutrient intake through the alimentary tract in patients with cancer. Thus, mechanical interference of the alimentary and gastrointestinal tracts exists, which leads to anorexia and malnutrition (Perez, Newcomer, Moertel, Go, & Dimagno, 1983; Ramot, 1971).

Catabolic states unrelated to cancer, such as infection, diabetes, chronic diseases (chronic heart failure, chronic renal failure), and hyperthyroidism, may contribute to the loss of skeletal muscle. Deconditioning caused by prolonged bed rest and inactivity is also associated with loss of muscle mass (Strasser & Bruera, 2002).

Cancer-associated cachexia is an incredibly complex and multifaceted manifestation in patients with cancer. The many biologic complexities of the syndrome are not fully understood.

Many factors and mechanisms contributing to its occurrence are currently being studied, but no single factor can be attributed to the cause of cachexia in patients with cancer. Rather, it is a series of many varied factors and mechanisms that, through close interaction and interrelation, formulate the intricate pathophysiology of cancer cachexia. Cancer-associated cachexia manifests itself through the interrelation of anorexia and early satiety, mechanical obstruction of the alimentary tract, and many metabolic differentiations.

Assessment

A complete history and physical examination is indicated in patients who present with signs of cancer cachexia (see Table 5-1). The history should include review of weight patterns, gain and loss cycles, and patterns of nutritional intake. A complete nutritional assessment is strongly recommended at diagnosis and periodically throughout the management of the syndrome (Ottery, 1996).

The patient's history should include the cancer diagnosis, course and treatment thus far, current medications (both prescribed and over the counter), typical 24-hour diet both cur-

TABLE 5-1	Assessment of Cancer Cachexia
Category	**Description**
General information	Cancer diagnosis and stage Cancer treatment Current medications
Symptoms	Gastrointestinal symptoms associated with cancer and/or treatment Other symptoms: Pain, dyspnea, fatigue, delirium, anxiety Edmonton Symptom Assessment Scale (symptom assessment tool)
Nutrition	Weight pattern Weight changes Dietary/caloric intake Body composition: • Skinfold thickness • Mid-arm circumference • Bioimpedance analysis • Dual energy x-ray absorptiometry Patient-Generated Subjective Global Assessment (comprehensive nutrition assessment tool)
Function	Performance status (Karnofsky, Eastern Cooperative Oncology Group) Functional Assessment of Anorexia/Cachexia Therapy (function and quality-of-life tool)
Laboratory tests	Complete blood count, renal function, liver function, electrolytes, albumin, prealbumin, transferrin, testosterone
Psychosocial	Coping with changes in self-image Emotional distress Attitudes of patient and family regarding nutrition Financial problems

Note. Based on information from Baracos, 2006; Brown, 2002; Bruera, 1977; Chang et al., 2000; Detsky et al., 1987; Karnofsky et al., 1948; Langer et al., 2001; Maltzman, 2004; Ribaudo et al., 2000; Strasser & Bruera, 2002.

rently and prior to cancer diagnosis, ability to perform activities of daily living, and any associated symptoms such as dysphagia, odynophagia, xerostomia, and altered taste. Functional status can be measured by using the Karnofsky performance status tool or a more detailed instrument such as the Functional Assessment of Anorexia/Cachexia Therapy (Karnofsky et al., 1948; Ribaudo et al., 2000). The Edmonton Symptom Assessment Scale may be used for symptom assessment (Chang, Hwang, & Feuerman, 2000).

The Patient-Generated Subjective Global Assessment (Detsky et al., 1987; see Gosselin, Gilliard, & Tinnen, 2008, pp. 783–784) can be useful in screening for cancer cachexia. This tool provides a patient- and clinician-generated score that grades the nutritional risk of patients with cancer (Bauer, Capra, & Ferguson, 2002; Brown, 2002). The Subjective Global Assessment is a validated clinician tool that measures nutritional status based on the features of a medical history (e.g., weight changes, dietary intake changes, gastrointestinal symptoms that have persisted for more than two weeks, changes in functional capacity) and physical examination (e.g., loss of subcutaneous fat, muscle wasting, ankle or sacral edema, ascites). Referral to an oncology nutritionist or other professional who is qualified to provide a comprehensive nutritional assessment is recommended if nutritional screening identifies patients with or at risk for malnutrition.

Cancer cachexia includes (a) a significant decrease in weight over the past six months, (b) a decrease in baseline weight by 5%–10% or more in six months, or (c) a decrease in weight by 5% in one month (Bruera, 1977). This includes loss of fatty tissue as well as muscle mass. Patients usually appear emaciated and report a profound loss of appetite and early satiety and possibly nausea and vomiting. Other symptoms include dry mouth, changes in smell and taste, constipation, bloating, and abdominal pain (Baracos, 2006). Patients also may report amenorrhea, polyuria, and cold intolerance (Langer et al., 2001; Rosenzweig, 2006). In addition, patients commonly report decreased mental skills, attention span, and concentration. When the cachexia is severe, alterations in metabolic functions, such as electrolyte imbalances, can occur. As a result, patients will develop loss of strength, increased fatigue and weakness, and possibly numbness, tingling, twitching, involuntary movements, and pain (Langer et al.; Maltzman, 2004). This in turn can lead to the inability to perform activities of daily living. Electrolyte imbalances also can lead to cardiac arrhythmias, which can lead to death.

The patient may present with tachycardia or tachypnea and may have dysrhythmias. Poor muscle tone and temporal wasting can indicate loss of muscle mass. A protuberant abdomen may indicate ascites. Skin will be dry with poor turgor, and the hair and nails also might be dry and brittle. An oral examination may reveal poor dentition, lesions, and dry mucous membranes.

Additionally, the physical examination should include (a) measurement of weight loss as a percentage of the patient's usual body weight, (b) current weight as it compares to ideal body weight, and (c) a history of decreased appetite or food intake. Laboratory tests such as transferrin, albumin, prealbumin, and retinol-binding protein are useful in assessing malnutrition (Brown, 2002). Quantitative measurement of body composition also is a reliable means of nutritional assessment. Body composition or anthropometrics measures the lean body mass (fat-free mass after removal of body water). Edema usually masks the detection of loss of muscle mass. Anthropometric measurements may include skinfold thickness, mid-arm circumference, bioimpedance analysis, and dual-energy x-ray absorptiometry scan (Strasser & Bruera, 2002).

Assessment of cancer cachexia should contain psychosocial and spiritual dimensions (Strasser & Bruera, 2002). Severe weight loss produces changes in body image that may generate anxiety and depression in patients and their families. A family meeting is an important tool to understand patients' and families' concerns and beliefs regarding food and nutrition, which in turn facilitates the development of an appropriate treatment plan.

Treatment

The general approach to the management of cancer cachexia is based on the understanding of its multifactorial origin. Cancer cachexia originates from a combination of factors, including reduced dietary intake, deficiency in the anabolic endocrine setting, hyperexpression of catabolic elements, lack of physical activity, and presence of comorbid conditions (Baracos, 2006).

Unfortunately, no single agent has been found to be effective in treating cancer cachexia. Implementation of a combination of modalities that requires an experienced interdisciplinary team is recommended (Ottery, Sljuka, & Hagan, 1995; Stewart et al., 2006; Strasser & Bruera, 2002). Patients with cancer cachexia should be enrolled in programs that address various aspects of care, including (a) early detection of the problem, (b) correction of secondary causes (physical and emotional symptoms), (c) inclusion of dietary counseling and other nutritional interventions, (d) exercise to maintain muscle mass, and (e) use of drug combinations that increase anabolism, reduce muscle proteolysis, and reverse the inflammatory state of cancer cachexia (see Figure 5-3) (MacDonald, 2007).

No guidelines for the management of cancer cachexia exist. However, the American Gastroenterological Association (AGA) developed guidelines for the management of cachexia associated with HIV infection that could also apply to the population of patients with cancer, given that both diseases are considered chronic life-threatening illnesses. These guidelines are summarized in Figure 5-4 (AGA, 1996).

The objectives of cancer cachexia therapy are to (a) reverse the cachexia syndrome, (b) control symptoms, (c) improve function and body image, (d) improve patients' QOL, and (e) prolong life expectancy (Strasser & Bruera, 2002). Major interventions to treat cancer cachexia include treatment of the underlying disease, nutrition, exercise, counseling, and a combination of pharmacologic therapy directed to improve symptoms and reverse the syndrome.

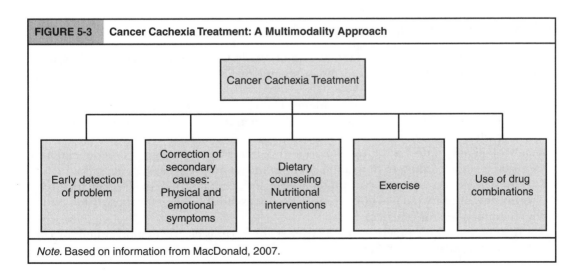

FIGURE 5-3 | Cancer Cachexia Treatment: A Multimodality Approach

Note. Based on information from MacDonald, 2007.

FIGURE 5-4	American Gastroenterological Association Guidelines for Management of Cachexia in Patients With HIV

- Evaluation of weight loss should be directed toward the systemic symptoms and signs that could indicate underlying disease. Successful treatment of the underlying disease frequently results in weight gain.
- Nutritional supplementation, when clinically indicated, represents sound clinical care.
- Therapy with appetite stimulants can improve caloric intake and result in weight gain.
- When nutritional supplementation is clinically indicated, enteral alimentation is the preferred route of administration.
- For a patient in whom enteral nutrition is contraindicated, total parenteral nutrition may be indicated under selected conditions. The use of long-term parenteral nutrition should be reserved for those patients in whom enteral nutrition is contraindicated and a meaningful life expectancy would be anticipated if nutritional therapy was given.

Note. Based on information from American Gastroenterological Association, 1996.

Cancer Treatment and Symptom Management

The best approach to treating cancer cachexia is to reverse the syndrome by eliminating cancer completely (Barber, Ross, & Fearon, 1999; Fearon & Moses, 2002). Unfortunately, this is not an option for many patients with advanced disease. Although the use of systemic antineoplastic therapy or radiation therapy may cure cancer, it also may increase the degree of treatment-related toxicities that may contribute to cancer cachexia (Couch et al., 2007). However, if cancer therapy is carefully chosen to meet patients' individual needs, treatment may provide improvement in both symptoms and QOL (Strasser & Bruera, 2002). Both early recognition of cancer cachexia and optimal symptom management are critical to improve patients' nutritional status (MacDonald, 2007; Stewart et al., 2006).

Counseling

Psychological interventions are recommended to address the severe emotional distress experienced by patients with cancer cachexia. Counseling should be directed to both the patient and the family and address concerns about body image and starvation (Del Fabbro, Dalal, & Bruera, 2006; Strasser & Bruera, 2002).

Evidence-Based Interventions

Interventions for cancer cachexia will be described in the following paragraphs based on the levels of evidence used by the Oncology Nursing Society (www.ons.org) (see Table 5-2). These levels are

- Recommended for practice (strong evidence from rigorously designed studies)
- Likely to be effective (evidence is less established than for those listed under recommended for practice)
- Benefits balanced with harms (clinicians and patients should weigh the beneficial and harmful effects according to individual circumstances and priorities)
- Effectiveness not established (current data are insufficient or are of inadequate quality)
- Effectiveness unlikely (lack of effectiveness is more established than for those listed under not recommended for practice)
- Not recommended for practice (ineffectiveness or harm is clearly demonstrated, or cost or burden exceeds potential benefit).

TABLE 5-2	Interventions for Cancer Cachexia Based on Oncology Nursing Society Levels of Evidence	
Level of Evidence	**Intervention**	**Action**
Recommended for practice	Progestational agents • Megestrol acetate • Medroxyprogesterone	Increase appetite
	Corticosteroids • Dexamethasone • Methylprednisolone • Prednisolone	Increase appetite
Likely to be effective	Nutritional support • Nutritional counseling • Enteral nutrition	Improve nutritional parameters
	Prokinetic agents • Metoclopramide	Decrease nausea Decrease early satiety
	Exercise • Repeated physical activity	Increase muscle mass Increase endurance Improve quality of life Reverse inflammatory process of cachexia*
Benefits balanced with harms	Nutritional support • Parenteral nutrition	Improve nutritional parameters Not recommended as routine intervention for cancer cachexia
Effectiveness not established	Omega-3 fatty acid supplements	Improve appetite* Decrease tumor growth*
	Anabolic agents • Growth hormone • Insulin-like growth factor • Testosterone • Testosterone analogs (oxandrolone, nandrolone)	Increase weight gain* Improve body composition* Increase strength*
	Thalidomide	Lessen weight loss* Improve functioning* Improve appetite*
	Melatonin	Stabilize weight*
	Cannabinoids	Decrease nausea Increase appetite*
Effectiveness unlikely	Cyproheptadine	Increase appetite*

(Continued on next page)

TABLE 5-2	Interventions for Cancer Cachexia Based on Oncology Nursing Society Levels of Evidence *(Continued)*	
Level of Evidence	**Intervention**	**Action**
Not recommended for practice	Hydrazine	Increase appetite*
	Pentoxifylline	Decrease muscle wasting*

* Lacks evidence

Note. Based on information from Alverdy et al., 1985; Argiles et al., 2001; Barber et al., 1999; Bauer & Capra, 2005; Bauer et al., 2005; Berenstein & Ortiz, 2005; Bozzetti et al., 1987; Brown, 2002; Bruera et al., 1999; Combaret et al., 1999; Couch et al., 2007; Davis et al., 2002; DeBoer & Marks, 2006; Del Fabbro et al., 2006; Desport et al., 2003; Dewey et al., 2007; Dezube et al., 1993; Fearon & Moses, 2002; Folador et al., 2007; Goncalves et al., 2005, 2006; Gordon et al., 2005; Graves et al., 2006; Haslett, 1998; Hryniewicz et al., 2003; Jatoi et al., 2002; Joglekar & Levin, 2004; Kardinal et al., 1990; Khan et al., 2003; Klein & Koretz, 1994; Klein et al., 1986; Kurebayashi et al., 1999; Langer et al., 2001; Lissoni et al., 1994; Lopez et al., 2004; Lundholm et al., 2004, 2007; MacDonald, 2007; Maltin et al., 1993; Maltoni et al., 2001; Mantovani et al., 1997; Martin & Wiley, 2004; McGeer et al., 1990; Mercadante, 1998; Mirhosseini et al., 2005; Muller et al., 1982; Mulligan et al., 1999; Naoi et al., 2006; Orr & Fiatarone, 2004; Ottery et al., 1995; Ovesen et al., 1993; Pawlowski, 1975; Pearlstone et al., 1995; Persson et al., 2005; Ramos et al., 2005; Rapaport & Fontaine, 1989; Ravasco et al., 2003; Smith et al., 2005; Stewart et al., 2006; Strasser & Bruera, 2002; Strasser et al., 2006; Stroud, 2005; Wilner & Arnold, 2006; Yamashita & Ogawa, 2000; Yavuzsen et al., 2005; Yeh et al., 2000; Zinna & Yarasheski, 2003.

Recommended for Practice

Orexigenic drugs are used for the treatment of cancer cachexia. These medications are appetite stimulants indicated for patients experiencing anorexia. Among all the orexigenic drugs listed in Table 5-3, the progestational agents (such as megestrol acetate [MA] and medroxyprogesterone acetate [MPA]) and corticosteroids (such as dexamethasone, methylprednisolone [MP], and prednisolone) are the only two drug types recommended for practice to improve anorexia in patients with cancer cachexia.

Progestational Agents

A systematic review of the treatment of anorexia and weight loss in cancer cachexia concluded that progestational agents were effective appetite stimulants in patients with cancer (Yavuzsen, Davis, Walsh, LeGrand, & Lagman, 2005). This review analyzed 23 randomized clinical trials evaluating MA and 6 randomized clinical trials evaluating MPA. The doses for MA ranged from 160–1,600 mg/day, and the doses for MPA ranged from 300–1,200 mg/day. The results showed that both MA and MPA improved appetite and weight, were safe with acceptable side effects, and had minimal effect on QOL. The review did not propose a final conclusion on optimal dose, time to start, or duration of treatment. A systematic review of 15 randomized clinical trials reported similar results in the evaluation of the effects of high-dose progestins for the treatment of anorexia-cachexia syndrome in patients with cancer (Maltoni et al., 2001).

Two systematic reviews on the use of MA for the treatment of anorexia-cachexia syndrome supported the benefit of this drug. A Cochrane review concluded that MA improves appetite and weight gain in anorexia-cachexia syndrome in patients with cancer, but not enough evidence existed to suggest a positive effect on QOL and the optimal dose (Berenstein & Ortiz, 2005). A review of 26 randomized controlled clinical trials reported that MA, when com-

TABLE 5-3	Interventions for Cancer Cachexia	
Intervention	**Type**	**Rationale**
Cancer treatment	Systemic and local antineoplastic treatment	Reverses primary cachexia syndrome by treating tumor
Early recognition and treatment of reversible causes associated with secondary cachexia	Symptom management (e.g., nausea, vomiting, diarrhea, constipation, mucositis, xerostomia, depression, pain)	Controls gastrointestinal symptoms, pain, and depression to improve appetite and function
Nutrition	Dietary counseling Nutritional supplements Enteral feedings Parenteral feedings	Increase caloric and protein intake
Exercise	Resistance-type activity	Maintains muscle mass
Prokinetic drugs	Metoclopramide	Improves chronic nausea and early satiety
Orexigenic drugs	Progestational agents • Megestrol acetate • Medroxyprogesterone Corticosteroids • Dexamethasone • Methylprednisolone • Prednisolone Atypical antipsychotic • Olanzapine Antidepressants • Mirtazapine Cannabinoids • Dronabinol Antihistamines • Cyproheptadine	Stimulate appetite
Anabolic agents	Testosterone derivatives • Fluoxymesterone • Nandrolone decanoate • Oxandrolone	Enhance muscle growth and strength
Metabolic inhibitor	Hydrazine sulfate	Blocks catabolic pathways
Anticytokine agents	Melatonin Pentoxifylline Thalidomide Cyclooxygenase inhibitors	Decrease tumor necrosis factor activity and effects of proinflammatory cytokines
Nutritional supplements	Omega-3 fatty acids • Eicosapentaenoic acid • Fish oils	Improve appetite and body weight

(Continued on next page)

TABLE 5-3	Interventions for Cancer Cachexia *(Continued)*	
Intervention	**Type**	**Rationale**
Nutritional supplements *(cont.)*	Beta-hydroxy-beta-methylbutyrate	Enhances the effects of weight training on muscle mass
Other	Beta-2 adrenoceptor agonists • Clenbuterol • Salbutamol	Prevent muscle protein wasting
	Beta-blocker	Improves body weight
	Adenosine 5′-triphosphate	Inhibits weight loss
	Growth hormone • Ghrelin	Increases lean body mass
Counseling	Psychosocial support to patient and family	May decrease anxiety and depression along with medical condition

Note. Based on information from Argiles et al., 2001; Baracos, 2006; Barber, 2001; Barber et al., 1999; Chlebowski et al., 1986; Couch et al., 2007; Daley & Canada, 2004; DeBoer et al., 2007; Del Fabbro et al., 2006; Fearon & Moses, 2002; Gagnon & Bruera, 1998; Jatoi, 2005; Langer et al., 2001; MacDonald, 2007; Mantovani et al., 2001; Mattox, 2005; Melstrom et al., 2007; Puccio & Nathanson, 1997; Stewart et al., 2006; Strasser & Bruera, 2002; Talukdar & Bruera, 2004; Tisdale, 2006; Wang et al., 2006.

pared to placebo, increased appetite, increased weight, and improved QOL in patients with cancer (Lopez et al., 2004). MA showed similar benefits in older adult patients with weight loss (Yeh et al., 2000).

Practice guidelines for the use of appetite stimulants in patients with cancer developed by the National Federation of French Cancer Centers (FNCLCC) recommend the use of progestins in the treatment of anorexia and weight loss. These recommendations are based on level B1 evidence, which refers to a good quality of evidence from randomized trials. These guidelines recommend a minimum dose of 160 mg/day of MA and, if no response occurs, a maximum dose of 480 mg/day. No evidence has shown that doses larger than 480 mg/day have better efficacy (Desport et al., 2003). According to the guidelines, the minimum dose of MPA shown to be effective is 200 mg/day; however, more randomized clinical trials are needed to investigate the optimal dose of this drug.

In addition to the orexigenic effect, MPA also may play a role in reducing the levels of cytokines involved in cancer cachexia. One study reported that MPA reduced the levels of IL-1-β, IL-6, TNF-α, and 5-HT (5-hydroxytryptamine) in 10 patients with advanced cancer (Mantovani et al., 1997). Other studies have shown the relationship between the effect of MPA on IL-6 in breast cancer cells in both in vitro and in vivo (Kurebayashi, Yamamoto, Otsuki, & Sonoo, 1999; Yamashita & Ogawa, 2000). In conclusion, strong evidence supports the benefits of progestational agents in increasing the appetite in patients with cancer, but more studies are necessary to confirm their impact on the inflammatory process of cancer cachexia involving cytokines.

Corticosteroids

A systematic review of the treatment of anorexia-cachexia in patients with cancer reported that corticosteroids are effective in improving appetite (Yavuzsen et al., 2005). This review involved six studies. Three studies compared oral MP or IV methylprednisolone sodium (MPSS) with placebo. MPSS and MP improved appetite and QOL. Doses of MP and MPSS ranged from 32–125 mg/day. In the same review, three studies supported the benefit of prednisolone and dexamethasone over placebo. These drugs improved appetite and well-being. Doses of prednisolone were 10 mg/day. Doses for dexamethasone ranged from 3–8 mg/day. Evidence-based research concluded that corticosteroids are effective in reversing anorexia.

The FNCLCC practice guidelines for the use of appetite stimulants in oncology recommend the use of corticosteroids in the treatment of anorexia and weight loss in patients with cancer. These recommendations are based on level B1 evidence (good-quality evidence from randomized trials). However, not enough information is available to determine the optimal dose and scheduling for their use in this indication (Desport et al., 2003).

Likely to Be Effective

Nutritional Support

Methods of nutritional administration include enteral and parenteral. Enteral nutrition (EN) can be administered either by oral intake or through the delivery of nutrients via a catheter or tube, with later absorption of nutrients by the gastrointestinal tract. The oral route is best for patients who are able to eat. EN is indicated if the gastrointestinal tract is intact but swallowing or mastication is compromised by disease, or if it is needed to pass an obstructed area. EN is used mainly in patients with cancer of the head and neck or esophagus (Mercadante, 1998). Parenteral nutrition (PN) refers to the administration of nutrients through a large IV catheter (Langer et al., 2001).

Nutritional support is provided by dietary counseling and interventions for both EN and PN. Although none of these interventions has proved to be effective in reversing the cachexia syndrome, they have improved some parameters of nutritional status. In fact, nutritional support and dietary counseling are recommended for patients with cancer cachexia who are experiencing starvation caused by gastrointestinal tumors or treatment toxicity (Del Fabbro et al., 2006).

EN is the method of choice in patients with a functioning gastrointestinal tract because it maintains the gut-mucosal barrier and immunologic function (Alverdy, Chi, & Sheldon, 1985). Both EN and PN improve some nutritional indicators, including body weight, fat mass, and nitrogen balance; however, EN is the only one that improves immune response. Other advantages of EN over PN are better tolerance, lower cost, minimal need for hospitalization, no need for frequent laboratory tests, and lower incidence of complications (Mercadante, 1998). Although EN can be administered orally in most cases, the enteral regimen requirements needed to improve lean body mass and visceral proteins are very high, which makes it impossible to achieve in patients who are unable to eat (Mercadante). The nutritional regimen recommended to improve lean body mass and visceral protein requirements is 35 kcal/kg and 1.3 g of amino acid/kg, and the recommended regimen to improve immune response is at least 42 kcal/kg and 2.3 g of amino acid/kg. These nutrition requirements are impossible to reach if the patient has impaired oral function (Mercadante).

The use of tube feeding is indicated when disease or treatment compromises swallowing or mastication (e.g., cancer of the head and neck or esophagus). The different types of tube feeding include nasogastric, gastrostomy, and jejunostomy. A nasogastric tube is easy to insert but is for short-term use because it may cause pharyngeal ulceration, sinusitis, and problems with reinsertion. Gastrostomy and jejunostomy are efficient methods of providing long-term EN and are better tolerated than the nasogastric tube. However, large volumes infused continuously may not be tolerated, causing nausea, vomiting, and diarrhea. Also, gastrostomy and jejunostomy require strict hygiene, feeding tube changes, and *Candida* prophylaxis (Mercadante, 1998).

Dietary Counseling

Some studies support the benefit of dietary counseling in patients with cancer cachexia. Ravasco, Monteiro-Grillo, and Camilo (2003) studied the impact of individualized nutritional counseling on nutritional status and QOL in 125 patients with cancer who were referred to radiation therapy. In this prospective non-control study, baseline malnutrition was prevalent. Patients reported increased nutritional intake and overall improvement in QOL after implementation of nutritional counseling. A pilot study examining the effect of nutrition intervention in seven patients receiving chemotherapy reported similar findings (Bauer & Capra, 2005).

A prospective study using an interdisciplinary team approach demonstrated benefits from nutritional counseling and symptom management. In this study, 186 patients received individualized nutritional education and aggressive symptom management. Patients were able to stop weight loss and stabilize or improve albumin or transferrin levels (Ottery et al., 1995). One multicenter randomized clinical trial by the Cancer Cachexia Study Group in Australia reported that oral nutritional supplements improved caloric intake and body composition in 200 patients with pancreatic cancer (Bauer, Capra, Battistutta, Davidson, & Ash, 2005).

On the contrary, a systematic review on symptom management of cancer-related anorexia and cachexia found no major benefit from dietary counseling (Brown, 2002). In this review, seven studies of nonpharmacologic food intake interventions were identified. All seven studies were randomized clinical trials that investigated the effects of nutritional counseling and commercial oral liquid supplements. All studies reported improved caloric intake as a result of the nutritional counseling; however, none of them reported improvement in survival, tumor response, or nutritional status (Brown). Similar findings were reported in a prospective randomized clinical trial that examined the effect of frequent nutritional counseling on oral intake, body weight, response rate, survival, and QOL in patients with lung, ovarian, and breast cancers who were undergoing chemotherapy. This study reported that dietary counseling increased daily energy intake of calories and protein with minimal gain weight, but results showed no difference in QOL between the control and experimental groups (Ovesen, Allingstrup, Hannibal, Mortensen, & Hansen, 1993). Overall, nutritional counseling increases caloric intake, and it may improve nutritional parameters and QOL.

Prokinetic Drug (Metoclopramide)

Metoclopramide has been used successfully to improve chronic nausea and early satiety associated with anorexia and cachexia in patients with cancer (Bruera et al., 1996; Nelson & Walsh, 1993). Metoclopramide is an antidopaminergic drug with effective central and antiemetic and gastric-emptying properties. It works well in the presence of autonomic failure and opioid therapy (Strasser & Bruera, 2002).

A systematic review of treatments for cancer-associated anorexia evaluated two studies using metoclopramide (Yavuzsen et al., 2005). Fifty-five patients were included. Both studies found dramatic improvement in nausea but no improvement in caloric intake or appetite. Doses ranged from 20–40 mg every 12 hours orally for controlled-release metoclopramide, and 20 mg every 6 hours orally for immediate-release metoclopramide.

Exercise

Ardies (2002) reviewed the evidence from a number of publications and concluded that repeated exercise may enhance the QOL of patients with cancer cachexia. Repeated physical activity may decrease the side effects of cancer therapy and prevent or reverse cachexia through suppression of inflammatory processes and enhancement of insulin sensitivity, protein synthesis, and antioxidant activities. Patients with cachexia who comply with a proper exercise program gain muscle protein mass, increase endurance, and improve physical function (Zinna & Yarasheski, 2003).

Benefits Balanced With Harms

This category of intervention contains the use of PN. The use of PN in patients with advanced cancer for treatment of cachexia is controversial. A review of 28 prospective randomized clinical trials evaluating the use of PN in patients with cancer reported little benefit for this patient population (Klein, Simes, & Blackburn, 1986). The authors concluded that PN may be beneficial to decrease surgical complications if used preoperatively in malnourished patients with gastrointestinal cancer. However, they also concluded that PN has no benefit in survival, treatment tolerance, treatment toxicity, or tumor response in patients treated with chemotherapy or radiotherapy. Additionally, a higher incidence of infections occurred in patients receiving chemotherapy and PN. A decade later, the same principal author reported similar findings in a review of 27 prospective randomized clinical trials that evaluated the clinical efficacy of PN and EN support in patients with cancer (Klein & Koretz, 1994).

A meta-analysis of PN in patients with cancer undergoing chemotherapy showed decreased survival and increased risk for infection (McGeer, Detsky, & O'Rourke, 1990). On the other hand, a prospective study looking at the effects of PN on the nutritional status of 12 patients with severe cancer cachexia concluded that a 20-day PN course improved some of the nutritional variables, including weight loss, body fat, and nitrogen balance (Bozzetti et al., 1987). Another study on PN showed it to be beneficial for patients with cancer, with the benefits including wound healing, reduction in sepsis, and increased responsiveness to chemotherapy (Muller, Brenner, Dienst, & Pichlmaier, 1982). A study comparing the ability of oral feeding, EN, and PN to alter plasma amino acid levels in patients with esophageal cancer concluded that PN was superior to the other two modalities (Pearlstone et al., 1995).

The use of PN is not recommended as a routine intervention in patients with cancer cachexia, but rather it should be reserved for a selected group of patients (Mantovani, Maccio, Massa, & Madeddu, 2001; Mercadante, 1998). The Capital Health Home Parenteral Nutritional Program in Edmonton in collaboration with the Regional Palliative Care Program developed clinical practice guidelines for the use of PN (see Table 5-4) (Mirhosseini, Fainsinger, & Baracos, 2005).

Effectiveness Not Established

Omega-3 Fatty Acid Supplements

Omega-3 fatty acids provided in fish oils have been investigated in patients with cancer who have anorexia and weight loss. Eicosapentaenoic acid (EPA) is the most widely investigated. Omega-3 fatty acids have a role in the treatment of anorexia by triggering the pro-

TABLE 5-4	Clinical Practice Guidelines for the Use of Parenteral Nutrition in Patients With Advanced Cancer
Category	**Criteria**
Nutrition	Potential benefit from parenteral nutrition (PN): Probable death by starvation would ensue earlier than death from disease (i.e., bowel obstruction, short bowel syndrome, malabsorption). Enteral nutrition is not an option.
Life expectancy	Patient expected to live months, and PN treatment expected to last at least six weeks.
Quality of life (QOL)	Patient is expected to improve his or her QOL with PN.
Functional status	Patient has Karnofsky score of 50 or higher.
Home environment	Patient's problems should be manageable at home or with the support of an outpatient program. Patient has a family member or other person who is willing and able to assist in care. Patient can be easily monitored for clinical follow-up and laboratory investigations. Patient and family must be cognitively and psychologically capable of administering PN at home. Home environment is safe, clean, and free of hazards.

Note. Based on information from Mirhosseini et al., 2005.

duction of orexigenic neurotransmitters in food-intake regulatory nuclei in the hypothalamus (Goncalves, Ramos, Suzuki, & Meguid, 2005). Preclinical studies in rats demonstrated that fish oil improved appetite, decreased tumor growth, and prevented body weight loss (Folador et al., 2007; Goncalves et al., 2006; Ramos et al., 2005). On the contrary, a Cochrane review directed to evaluate the effectiveness and safety of EPA in relieving symptoms associated with cachexia in patients with advanced cancer found minimal benefit (Dewey, Baughan, Dean, Higgins, & Johnson, 2007).

Anabolic Agents

Anabolic agents help to promote body composition by maintaining or enhancing lean body mass. These agents include growth hormone, insulin-like growth factor-I, testosterone, dihydrotestosterone, and the testosterone analogs oxandrolone and nandrolone decanoate (Langer et al., 2001). Anabolic steroids promote protein nitrogen accumulation; therefore, they could be used to counteract the progressive nitrogen loss associated with cancer cachexia (Argiles et al., 2001). Some of these agents have been studied in AIDS-related cachexia, but few have been evaluated in cancer cachexia (Mulligan, Tai, & Schambelan, 1999). Testosterone replacement in patients with decreased testosterone levels improves weight gain and physical activity (Langer et al., 2001). A review on the use of anabolic agents in the treatment of cancer cachexia concluded that oxandrolone is safe and effective for the treatment of AIDS-related cachexia and suggests potential benefits in patients with cancer (Langer et al.). Oxandrolone improves body composition and muscle strength (Orr & Fiatarone, 2004).

Thalidomide

Thalidomide has a number of actions, including inhibition of angiogenesis, immunomodulation, and anti-inflammatory effects (Stroud, 2005). Its clinical use is being investigated in a number of conditions, such as cancer cachexia, tuberculosis, and HIV (Joglekar & Levin, 2004). The administration of thalidomide to patients with HIV or tuberculosis-associated weight loss has resulted in weight gain (Haslett, 1998). Thalidomide has been found to attenuate weight loss, improve physical functioning, and improve appetite and nausea in patients with advanced cancer (Bruera et al., 1999; Gordon et al., 2005; Khan et al., 2003). Thalidomide for cancer cachexia should be used with caution and strictly in a research setting because of its well-known teratogenic effects (Joglekar & Levin).

Melatonin

The pineal hormone melatonin has been found to play an important role in the neuroendocrine regulation of biologic systems, inhibition of TNF secretion, and improvement of the clinical status of patients with advanced cancer (Lissoni et al., 1994). Conversely, a randomized pilot study assessing the effect of fish oil, melatonin, or their combination in patients with cancer cachexia did not demonstrate any major benefit except for stabilization in weight (Persson, Glimelius, Ronnelid, & Nygren, 2005).

Cannabinoids

Recently, the use of cannabinoids for the treatment of anorexia and cachexia has become a focus of interest. Martin and Wiley (2004) discussed the pharmacologic properties of tetrahydrocannabinol and its beneficial effect in the management of cachexia, nausea, and pain. Dronabinol is approved by the U.S. Food and Drug Administration for anorexia and weight loss in patients with AIDS. In patients with cancer, this drug may improve appetite and weight gain (Osei-Hyiama, 2007; Wilner & Arnold, 2006). On the contrary, other studies found no benefit of the cannabinoid groups over MA or placebo (Jatoi et al., 2002; Strasser et al., 2006).

Other Medications

Research has led to significant progress in understanding the pathophysiology of cancer cachexia and its associated metabolic alterations. A number of pharmacologic agents have shown promising results in normalizing some of these metabolic changes and in making a positive impact in reversing cancer cachexia. Some of these agents include cyclooxygenase inhibitors, insulin, melanocortin antagonists, beta-hydroxy-beta-methylbutyrate, adenosine 5′-triphosphate, beta antagonists and agonists, olanzapine, mirtazapine, and ghrelin (Akamizu & Kangawa, 2007; Davis, Khawam, Pozuelo, & Lagman, 2002; DeBoer & Marks, 2006; Graves, Ramsay, & McCarthy, 2006; Hryniewicz, Androne, Hudaihed, & Katz, 2003; Lundholm, Daneryd, Korner, Hyltander, & Bosaeus, 2004; Lundholm et al., 2007; Maltin et al., 1993; Naoi, Kogure, Saito, Hamazaki, & Watanabe, 2006; Rapaport & Fontaine, 1989; Smith, Mukerji, & Tisdale, 2005).

Effectiveness Unlikely

This category contains cyproheptadine, an antihistamine drug with appetite-stimulating effect. A systematic review of the treatment of cancer-associated anorexia evaluated two studies using cyproheptadine (Yavuzsen et al., 2005). One study reported major improvement in appetite and weight gain (Pawlowski, 1975), whereas the other study did not find any benefit in appetite or weight gain when compared to placebo (Kardinal et al., 1990). The most common side effect is sedation, which may limit its usefulness in patients with advanced cancer. The FNCLCC does not recommend the routine use of cyproheptadine as an appetite stimulant. This recommendation is based on level C evidence, which refers to inconsistent or weak studies (Desport et al., 2003). Not enough evidence exists to support the use of cyproheptadine to improve anorexia.

Not Recommended for Practice

Hydrazine

Hydrazine sulfate is an inhibitor of gluconeogenesis and is believed to block catabolic pathways (Strasser & Bruera, 2002). A systematic review of the treatment of cancer-associated anorexia evaluated five studies using oral hydrazine sulfate. A total of 796 patients were included. Doses ranged from 60–180 mg/day. Only one study reported improvement in appetite and weight. Four randomized clinical trials found major toxicity, significant deterioration in QOL when compared to placebo, and no body weight gain. These studies provided strong evidence against the use of hydrazine (Yavuzsen et al., 2005).

Pentoxifylline

Pentoxifylline (PTX) is a methylxanthine derivative approved for treatment of intermittent claudication. A preclinical trial in rats demonstrated that PTX suppresses the increased protein breakdown observed in cachexia by inhibiting the ubiquitin-proteasome pathway. These data suggest that PTX can prevent muscle wasting in clinical conditions where TNF production increases, such as in cancer, sepsis, and AIDS (Combaret, Ralliere, Taillandier, Tanaka, & Attaix, 1999). A pilot study involving five patients with cancer demonstrated that PTX can downregulate TNF expression and improve appetite and sense of well-being (Dezube, Sherman, Fridovich-Keil, Allen-Ryan, & Pardee, 1993). Conversely, a double-blind, placebo-controlled clinical trial including 70 patients with cancer who have a history of weight loss and anorexia who were randomized to receive 1,200 mg of PTX per day failed to show any benefit in the improvement of appetite or weight gain (Goldberg et al., 1995). PTX is not recommended for routine use as an appetite stimulant (Desport et al., 2003). This recommendation is based on level C evidence (inconsistent or weak studies).

Expected Outcomes

A realistic outcome for patients with cancer cachexia is maintenance of current weight and functional status, without reduction in either. It is unrealistic for most patients to resume their prediagnosis body weight, so the goal should be maintenance of current weight without further loss of muscle mass and maintenance of functional status without decreasing activity levels.

Patient Teaching Points

Symptom Control

Nursing care of patients with cachexia centers on the management of the symptoms related to the cancer and its treatment that may adversely affect appetite and nutritional status.

Early intervention to alleviate symptoms such as nausea, vomiting, diarrhea, pain, fatigue, and taste changes is important, especially in those diagnoses that place patients at high risk for poor nutritional outcomes, such as head and neck or gastrointestinal cancers. If early satiety is a problem, the largest proportion of required calories and protein should be provided for breakfast, when early satiety is minimal (Grant & Ropka, 1996). Frequent, small meals are helpful, but empty-calorie foods should be avoided, and each meal or snack should provide the maximum calories and protein possible.

Enlisting the help of the patient and family in symptom management of cachexia also is important. By encouraging the use of food and calorie diaries as well as the reporting of symptoms, the patient and family can partner with the healthcare team. Eliminating the symptoms will improve nutritional intake and prevent cachexia. Patients receiving EN or PN support will require additional education and support to ensure understanding and compliance.

Emotional Support

Promoting patient and family interaction and providing emotional and educational support to the family can be helpful. Encouraging family meals can help with food intake as well as family bonds. Decreasing stress and pressure at mealtimes is important. Patients often tolerate small, frequent meals better than large meals. Patients should participate in meal planning, but allowing others to cook may conserve energy and decrease the negative impact of odors on appetite. Engaging in light exercise may stimulate appetite as well, and using small amounts of seasonings can enhance taste.

The opportunity for improving outcomes in cancer cachexia exists through a standardized and proactive approach in identifying patients who are at risk for nutritional deficiencies and muscle loss. Early intervention is imperative, as deterioration caused by muscle loss frequently is irreversible. Clinicians should assess patients' nutritional status at each visit, just as with functional status. All patients should be screened at cancer diagnosis and reevaluated at regular intervals for nutritional problems. Screenings should include weight changes, dietary intake, functional status, symptoms affecting nutrition, physical examination, and projected nutritional problems (Brown, 2002).

Need for Future Research

Brown (2002) suggested that studies are needed to determine symptom clusters that predict the nutritional risk associated with various cancer diagnoses and treatments, which could lead to empirically based high-risk profiles that could be used in assessment and intervention. A number of pharmacologic agents have shown encouraging results in reversing the cancer cachexia syndrome; however, more large randomized clinical trials are needed to provide strong evidence for the agents' clinical use (Barber et al., 1999). Finally, given that cancer cachexia is a syndrome with multiple causes, a multimodal treatment approach should be the focus of future studies (Strasser & Bruera, 2002).

Conclusion of Case Study

Prior to the start of chemotherapy, E.B. was referred to the oncology nutritionist for complete assessment and evaluation of need for a feeding tube during therapy to prevent further deterioration of his nutritional status. He was found to have a low albumin and transferrin level and an additional 10-pound weight loss since surgery two weeks prior. The nutritionist recommended placement of a gastrostomy tube for enteral feedings during the two months of therapy. She also referred the patient to rehabilitation medicine for an assessment and development of a comprehensive exercise program tailored to his specific needs and abilities, with the goal of preventing or minimizing muscle loss and debilitation during the treatment. The patient was then referred to speech therapy for a swallowing evaluation and exercises for postoperative recovery while the gastrostomy tube is in place. Finally, the patient was referred to the palliative care nurse practitioner for symptom management during the treatment phase. He was determined to have symptoms consistent with reactive depression and was started on an antidepressant to help with his appetite and sleep as well as mood. He also was started on megestrol acetate for appetite stimulation and oxycodone for pain control.

The multidisciplinary team monitored the patient during the course of his chemotherapy and radiation therapy, adjusting medications as needed. As a result, the patient was able to maintain his presurgical weight without further weight loss during the concomitant therapy. He was able to avoid hospitalization for exacerbation of symptoms through the aggressive symptom management by his multidisciplinary care team.

Conclusion

Cancer cachexia is a wasting syndrome characterized by weight loss and loss of muscle and fat leading to the patient's diminished function and performance status. The pathophysiology of cancer cachexia syndrome is multifactorial; therefore, its treatment should include a combination of modalities provided by an interdisciplinary team. Oncology nurses are key members of this team. Oncology nurses need to understand the complexity of cancer cachexia to conduct a comprehensive assessment and provide appropriate treatment and care.

References

Akamizu, T., & Kangawa, K. (2007). Emerging results of anticatabolic therapy with ghrelin. *Current Opinion in Clinical Nutrition and Metabolic Care, 10*(3), 278–283.

Alverdy, J.C., Chi, H.S., & Sheldon, G.F. (1985). The effect of parenteral nutrition on gastrointestinal immunity: The importance of enteral stimulation. *Annals of Surgery, 202*(6), 681–684.

American Gastroenterological Association. (1996). American Gastroenterological Association medical position statement: Guidelines for the management of malnutrition and cachexia, chronic diarrhea, and hepatobiliary disease in patients with human immunodeficiency virus infection. *Gastroenterology, 111*(6), 1722–1752.

Ardies, C.M. (2002). Exercise, cachexia, and cancer therapy: A molecular rationale. *Nutrition and Cancer, 42*(2), 143–157.

Argiles, J., Meijsing, S.H., Pallares-Trujillo, J., Guirao, X., & Lopez-Soriano, F.J. (2001). Cancer cachexia: A therapeutic approach. *Medicinal Research Reviews, 21*(1), 83–101.

Argiles, J.M., & Lopez-Soriano, F.J. (1999). The role of cytokines in cancer cachexia. *Medicinal Research Reviews, 19*(3), 223–248.

Armes, P.J., Plant, H.J., Allbright, A., Silverstone, T., & Slevin, M.L. (1992). A study to investigate the incidence of early satiety in patients with advanced cancer. *British Journal of Cancer, 65*(3), 481–484.

Attaix, D., Combaret, L., Tilignac, T., & Taillandier, D. (1999). Adaptation of the ubiquitin-proteasome proteolytic pathway in cancer cachexia. *Molecular Biology Reports, 26*(1–2), 77–82.

Baracos, V.E. (2006). Cancer-associated cachexia and underlying biological mechanisms. *Annual Review of Nutrition, 26*, 435–461.

Barber, M.D. (2001). Cancer cachexia and its treatment with fish oil enriched nutritional supplementation. *Nutrition, 17*(9), 751–755.

Barber, M.D., Ross, J.A., & Fearon, K.C.H. (1999). Cancer cachexia. *Surgical Oncology, 8*(3), 133–141.

Bauer, J.D., & Capra, S. (2005). Nutrition intervention improves outcomes in patients with cancer cachexia receiving chemotherapy—a pilot study. *Supportive Care in Cancer, 13*(4), 270–274.

Bauer, J.D., Capra, S., Battistutta, D., Davidson, W., & Ash, S. (2005). Compliance with nutrition prescription improves outcomes in patients with unresectable pancreatic cancer. *Clinical Nutrition, 24*(6), 998–1004.

Bauer, J.D., Capra, S., & Ferguson, M. (2002). Use of the scored Patient-Generated Subjective Global Assessment (PG-SGA) as a nutritional assessment tool in patients with cancer. *European Journal of Clinical Nutrition, 56*(8), 779–785.

Beck, S.A., Mulligan, H.D., & Tisdale, M.J. (1990). Lipolytic factors associated with murine and human cancer cachexia. *Journal of the National Cancer Institute, 82*(24), 1922–1926.

Berenstein, E.G., & Ortiz, Z. (2005). Megestrol acetate for treatment of anorexia-cachexia syndrome. *Cochrane Database of Systematic Reviews* 2005, Issue 2. Art. No.: CD004310. DOI: 10.1002/14651858.CD004310.pub2.

Bozzetti, F., Ammatuna, M., Migliavaca, S., Bonalumi, M.G., Facchetti, G., Pupa, A., et al. (1987). Total parenteral nutrition prevents further nutritional deterioration in patients with cachexia. *Annals of Surgery, 205*(2), 138–143.

Brown, J. (2002). A systematic review of the evidence on symptom management of cancer-related anorexia and cachexia. *Oncology Nursing Forum, 29*(3), 517–530.

Bruera, E. (1977). ABC of palliative care: Anorexia, cachexia and nutrition. *BMJ, 315*(7117), 1219–1222.

Bruera, E., Neumann, C.M., Pituskin, E., Calder, K., Ball, G., & Hanson, J. (1999). Thalidomide in patients with cachexia due to terminal cancer: Preliminary report. *Annals of Oncology, 10*(7), 857–859.

Bruera, E., Seifert, L., Watanabe, S., Babul, N., Darke, A., Harsanyi, Z., et al. (1996). Chronic nausea in advanced cancer patients: A retrospective assessment of a metoclopramide-based antiemetic regimen. *Journal of Pain and Symptom Management, 11*(3), 147–153.

Busbridge, J., Dascombe, M.J., Hopkins, S., & Rothwell, N.J. (1989). Acute central effects of interleukin-6 on body temperature, thermogenesis and food intake in the rat [Abstract]. *Proceedings of the Nutrition Society, 48*(1), 48A.

Cangiano, C., Testa, U., Muscaritoli, M., Meguid, M.M., Mulieri, M., Laviano, A., et al. (1994). Cytokines, tryptophan and anorexia in cancer patients before and after surgical tumor ablation. *Anticancer Research, 14*(3B), 1451–1455.

Chang, V.T., Hwang, S.S., & Feuerman, M. (2000). Validation of the Edmonton Symptom Assessment Scale. *Cancer, 88*(9), 2164–2171.

Chlebowski, R.T., Herrold, J., Ali, L., Oktay, E., Chlebowski, J.S., Ponce, A.T., et al. (1986). Influence of nandrolone decanoate on weight loss in advanced non-small cell lung cancer. *Cancer, 58*(1), 183–186.

Combaret, L., Ralliere, C., Taillandier, D., Tanaka, K., & Attaix, D. (1999). Manipulation of the ubiquitin-proteasome pathway in cachexia: Pentoxifylline suppresses the activation of 20S and 26S proteasomes in muscles from tumor-bearing rats. *Molecular Biology Reports, 26*(1–2), 95–101.

Couch, M., Lai, V., Cannon, T., Guttridge, D., Zanation, A., George, J., et al. (2007). Cancer cachexia syndrome in head and neck cancer patients: Part I. Diagnosis, impact on quality of life and survival, and treatment. *Head and Neck, 29*(4), 401–411.

Daley, R., & Canada, T. (2004). Managing the cancer anorexia-cachexia syndrome: A pharmacologic review. *Oncology Nutrition Connection, 12*(4), 1–8.

Davis, M.P., Khawam, E., Pozuelo, L., & Lagman, R. (2002). Management of symptoms associated with advanced cancer: Olanzapine and mirtazapine. A World Health Organization project. *Expert Review of Anticancer Therapy, 2*(4), 365–376.

DeBoer, M.D., & Marks, D.L. (2006). Therapy insight: Use of melanocortin antagonists in the treatment of cachexia in chronic disease. *Nature Clinical Practice: Endocrinology and Metabolism, 2*(8), 459–466.

DeBoer, M.D., Zhu, X.X., Levasseur, P., Meguid, M.M., Suzuki, S., Inui, A., et al. (2007). Ghrelin treatment causes increased food intake and retention of lean body mass in a rat model of cancer cachexia. *Endocrinology, 148*(6), 3004–3012.

Del Fabbro, E., Dalal, S., & Bruera, E. (2006). Symptom control in palliative care—part II: Cachexia/anorexia and fatigue. *Journal of Palliative Medicine, 9*(2), 409–421.

Desport, J.C., Gory-Delabaere, G., Blanc-Vincent, M.P., Bachmann, P., Beal, J., Benamouzig, R., et al. (2003). Standards, options and recommendations for the use of appetite stimulants in oncology (2000). *British Journal of Cancer, 89*(Suppl. 1), S98–S100.

Detsky, A.S., McLaughlin, J.R., Baker, J.P., Johnston, N., Whittaker, S., Mendelson, R.A., et al. (1987). What is subjective global assessment of nutritional status? *Journal of Parenteral and Enteral Nutrition, 11*(1), 8–13.

Dewey, A., Baughan, C., Dean, T., Higgins, B., & Johnson, I. (2007). Eicosapentaenoic acid (EPA, an omega-3 fatty acid from fish oils) for the treatment of cancer cachexia. *Cochrane Database of Systematic Reviews* 2007, Issue 1. Art. No.: CD004597. DOI: 10.1002/14651858.CD004597.pub2.

DeWys, W.D., Begg, C., Lavin, P.T., Band, P.R., Bennett, J.M., Bertino, J.R., et al. (1980). Prognostic effect of weight loss prior to chemotherapy in cancer patients. Eastern Cooperative Oncology Group. *American Journal of Medicine, 69*(4), 491–497.

DeWys, W.D., & Walters, K. (1975). Abnormalities of taste sensation in cancer patients. *Cancer, 36*(5), 1888–1896.

Dezube, B.J., Sherman, M.L., Fridovich-Keil, J.L., Allen-Ryan, J., & Pardee, A.B. (1993). Down-regulation of tumor necrosis factor expression by pentoxifylline in cancer patients: A pilot study. *Cancer Immunology, Immunotherapy, 36*(1), 57–60.

Fearon, K.C.H., & Moses, A.G.W. (2002). Cancer cachexia. *International Journal of Cardiology, 85*(1), 73–81.

Folador, A., Hirabara, S.M., Bonatto, S.J., Aikawa, J., Yamazaki, R.K., Curi, R., et al. (2007). Effect of fish oil supplementation for 2 generations on changes in macrophage function induced by Walker 256 cancer cachexia rats. *International Journal of Cancer, 120*(2), 344–350.

Gagnon, B., & Bruera, E. (1998). A review of the drug treatment of cachexia associated with cancer. *Drugs, 55*(5), 675–688.

Gelin, J., Moldawer, L.L., Lonnroth, C., Sherry, B., Chizzonite, R., & Lundholm, K. (1991). Role of endogenous tumor necrosis factor alpha and interleukin 1 for experimental tumor growth and the development of cancer cachexia. *Cancer Research, 51*(1), 415–421.

Goldberg, R.M., Loprinzi, C.L., Mailliard, J.A., O'Fallon, J.R., Krook, J.E., Ghosh, C., et al. (1995). Pentoxifylline for treatment of cancer anorexia and cachexia? A randomized, double-blind, placebo-controlled trial. *Journal of Clinical Oncology, 13*(11), 2856–2859.

Goncalves, C.G., Ramos, E., Romanova, I., Suzuki, S., Chen, C., & Meguid, M. (2006). Omega-3 fatty acids improve appetite in cancer anorexia, but tumor resecting restores it. *Surgery, 139*(2), 202–208.

Goncalves, C.G., Ramos, E.J., Suzuki, S., & Meguid, M.M. (2005). Omega-3 fatty acids and anorexia. *Current Opinion in Clinical Nutrition and Metabolic Care, 8*(4), 403–407.

Gordon, J.N., Trebble, T.M., Ellis, R.D., Duncan, H.D., Johns, T., & Goggin, P.M. (2005). Thalidomide in the treatment of cancer cachexia: A randomised placebo controlled trial. *Gut, 54*(4), 540–545.

Gosselin, T.K., Gilliard, L., & Tinnen, R. (2008). Assessing the need for a dietitian in radiation oncology. *Clinical Journal of Oncology Nursing, 12*(5), 781–787.

Grant, M., & Ropka, M.E. (1996). Alterations in nutrition. In R. McCorkle, M. Grant, M. Frank-Stromborg, & S.B. Baird (Eds.), *Cancer nursing: A comprehensive textbook* (2nd ed., pp. 919–943). Philadelphia: Saunders.

Graves, E., Ramsay, E., & McCarthy, D.O. (2006). Inhibitors of COX activity preserve muscle mass in mice bearing the Lewis lung carcinoma, but not the B16 melanoma. *Research in Nursing and Health, 29*(2), 87–97.

Haslett, P.A. (1998). Anticytokine approaches to the treatment of anorexia and cachexia. *Seminars in Oncology, 25*(2, Suppl. 6), 53–57.

Hryniewicz, K., Androne, A.S., Hudaihed, A., & Katz, S.D. (2003). Partial reversal of cachexia by beta-adrenergic receptor blocker therapy in patients with chronic heart failure. *Journal of Cardiac Failure, 9*(6), 464–468.

Jatoi, A. (2005). Omega-3 fatty acid supplements for cancer-associated weight loss. *Nutrition in Clinical Practice, 20*(4), 394–399.

Jatoi, A., Windschitl, H.E., Loprinzi, C.L., Sloan, J.A., Dakhil, S.R., Mailliard, J.A., et al. (2002). Dronabinol versus megestrol acetate versus combination therapy for cancer-associated anorexia: A North Central Cancer Treatment Group study. *Journal of Clinical Oncology, 20*(2), 567–573.

Joglekar, S., & Levin, M. (2004). The promise of thalidomide: Evolving indications. *Drugs of Today, 40*(3), 197–204.

Kardinal, C.G., Loprinzi, C.L., Schaid, D.J., Hass, A.C., Dose, A.M., Athmann, L.M., et al. (1990). A controlled trial of cyproheptadine in cancer patients with anorexia and/or cachexia. *Cancer, 65*(12), 2657–2662.

Karnofsky, D.A., Abelman, W.H., Craver, L.F., & Burchenal, J.H. (1948, November). The use of nitrogen mustards in the palliative treatment of carcinoma. *Cancer, 1,* 634–656.

Khan, Z.H., Simpson, E.J., Cole, A.T., Holt, M., MacDonald, I., Pye, D., et al. (2003). Oesophageal cancer and cachexia: The effect of short-term treatment with thalidomide on weight loss and lean body mass. *Alimentary Pharmacology and Therapeutics, 17*(5), 677–682.

Klein, S., & Koretz, R.L. (1994). Nutrition support in patients with cancer: What do the data really show? *Nutrition in Clinical Practice, 9*(3), 91–100.

Klein, S., Simes, J., & Blackburn, G. (1986). Total parenteral nutrition and cancer clinical trials. *Cancer, 58*(6), 1378–1386.

Krause, R., Humphrey, C., von Meyenfeldt, M., James, H., & Fischer, J.E. (1981). A central mechanism for anorexia in cancer: A hypothesis. *Cancer Treatment Reports, 65*(Suppl. 5), 15–21.

Kurebayashi, J., Yamamoto, S., Otsuki, T., & Sonoo, H. (1999). Medroxyprogesterone acetate inhibits interleukin 6 secretion from KPL-4 human breast cancer cells both in vitro and in vivo: A possible mechanism of the anticachectic effect. *British Journal of Cancer, 79*(3–4), 631–636.

Langer, C., Hoffman, J.P., & Ottery, F. (2001). Clinical significance of weight loss in cancer patients: Rationale for the use of anabolic agents in the treatment of cancer-related cachexia. *Nutrition, 17*(Suppl. 1), S1–S21.

Lissoni, P., Barni, S., Tancini, G., Brivio, F., Tisi, E., Zubelewicz, B., et al. (1994). Role of the pineal gland in the control of macrophage functions and its possible implication in cancer: A study of interactions between tumor necrosis factor alpha and the pineal hormone melatonin. *Journal of Biological Regulators and Homeostatic Agents, 8*(4), 126–129.

Lopez, A.P., Figuls, M.R., Cuchi, G.U., Berenstein, E.G., Pasies, B.A., Alegre, M.B., et al. (2004). Systematic review of megestrol acetate in the treatment of anorexia-cachexia syndrome. *Journal of Pain and Symptom Management, 27*(4), 360–368.

Lundholm, K., Daneryd, P., Korner, U., Hyltander, A., & Bosaeus, I. (2004). Evidence that long-term COX-treatment improves energy homeostasis and body composition in cancer patients with progressive cachexia. *International Journal of Oncology, 24*(3), 505–512.

Lundholm, K., Edstrom, S., Karlberg, I., Ekman, L., & Schersten, T. (1982). Glucose turnover, gluconeogenesis from glycerol and estimation of net glucose cycling in cancer patients. *Cancer, 50*(6), 1142–1150.

Lundholm, K., Korner, U., Gunnebo, L., Sixt-Ammilon, P., Fouladiun, M., Daneryd, P., et al. (2007). Insulin treatment in cancer cachexia: Effects on survival, metabolism, and physical functioning. *Clinical Cancer Research, 13*(9), 2699–2705.

MacDonald, N. (2007). Cancer cachexia and targeting chronic inflammation: A unified approach to cancer treatment and palliative/supportive services. *Journal of Supportive Oncology, 5*(4), 157–162.

Maltin, C.A., Delday, M.I., Watson, J.S., Heys, S.D., Nevison, I.M., Ritchie, I.K., et al. (1993). Clenbuterol, a beta-adrenoceptor agonist, increases relative muscle strength in orthopaedic patients. *Clinical Science, 84*(6), 651–654.

Maltoni, M., Nanni, O., Scarpi, E., Rossi, D., Serra, P., & Amadori, D. (2001). High-dose progestins for the treatment of cancer anorexia-cachexia syndrome: A systematic review of randomised clinical trials. *Annals of Oncology, 12*(3), 289–300.

Maltzman, J.D. (2004, May). *Developments in the fight against cancer cachexia.* Retrieved August 20, 2007, from http://www.oncolink.org/resources/article.cfm?c=3&s=38&ss=164&id=828

Mantovani, G., Maccio, A., Esu, S., Lai, P., Santona, M.C., Massa, E., et al. (1997). Medroxyprogesterone acetate reduces the in vitro production of cytokines and serotonin involved in anorexia/cachexia and emesis by peripheral blood mononuclear cells of cancer patients. *European Journal of Cancer, 33*(4), 602–607.

Mantovani, G., Maccio, A., Massa, E., & Madeddu, C. (2001). Managing cancer-related anorexia/cachexia. *Drugs, 61*(4), 499–514.

Martin, B.R., & Wiley, J.L. (2004). Mechanism of action of cannabinoids: How it may lead to treatment of cachexia, emesis, and pain. *Journal of Supportive Oncology, 2*(4), 305–314.

Matthys, P., & Billiau, A. (1997). Cytokines and cachexia. *Nutrition, 13*(9), 763–770.

Mattox, T. (2005). Treatment of unintentional weight loss in patients with cancer. *Nutrition in Clinical Practice, 20*(4), 400–410.

McGeer, A.J., Detsky, A.S., & O'Rourke, K. (1990). Parenteral nutrition in cancer patients undergoing chemotherapy: A meta-analysis. *Nutrition, 6*(3), 233–240.

McLaughlin, C.L., Rogan, G.J., Ton, J., Baile, C.A., & Joy, W.D. (1992). Food intake and body temperature responses of rat to recombinant interleukin 1 beta and a tripeptide interleukin 1 beta antagonist. *Physiology and Behavior, 52*(6), 1155–1160.

McNamara, M.J., Alexander, H.R., & Norton, J.A. (1992). Cytokines and their role in the pathophysiology of cancer cachexia. *Journal of Parenteral and Enteral Nutrition, 16*(Suppl. 6), 50S–55S.

Melstrom, L.G., Melstrom, K.A., Jr., Ding, X.Z., & Adrian, T.E. (2007). Mechanisms of skeletal muscle degradation and its therapy in cancer cachexia. *Histology and Histopathology, 22*(7), 805–814.

Mercadante, S. (1998). Parenteral versus enteral nutrition in cancer patients: Indications and practice. *Supportive Care in Cancer, 6*(2), 85–93.

Mirhosseini, N., Fainsinger, R.L., & Baracos, V. (2005). Parenteral nutrition in advanced cancer: Indications and clinical practice guidelines. *Journal of Palliative Medicine, 8*(5), 914–918.

Muller, J.M., Brenner, U., Dienst, C., & Pichlmaier, H. (1982). Preoperative parenteral feeding in patients with gastrointestinal carcinoma. *Lancet, 1*(8263), 68–71.

Mulligan, K., Tai, V.W., & Schambelan, M. (1999). Use of growth hormone and other anabolic agents in AIDS wasting. *Journal of Parenteral and Enteral Nutrition, 23*(Suppl. 6), S202–S209.

Naoi, K., Kogure, S., Saito, M., Hamazaki, T., & Watanabe, S. (2006). Differential effects of selective cyclooxygenase (COX)-1 and COX-2 inhibitors on anorexic response and prostaglandin generation in various tissues induced by zymosan. *Biological and Pharmaceutical Bulletin, 29*(7), 1319–1324.

Nelson, K.A., & Walsh, T.D. (1993). Metoclopramide in anorexia caused by cancer-associated dyspepsia syndrome (CADS). *Journal of Palliative Care, 9*(2), 14–18.

Nielsen, S.S., Theologides, A., & Vickers, Z.M. (1980). Influence of food odors on food aversion and preference in patients with cancer. *American Journal of Clinical Nutrition, 33*(11), 2253–2261.

Noguchi, Y., Yoshikawa, T., Matsumoto, A., Svaninger, G., & Gelin, J. (1996). Are cytokines possible mediators of cancer cachexia? *Surgery Today, 26*(7), 467–475.

Orr, R., & Fiatarone, S.M. (2004). The anabolic androgenic steroid oxandrolone in the treatment of wasting and catabolic disorders: Review of efficacy and safety. *Drugs, 64*(7), 725–750.

Osei-Hyiaman, D. (2007). Endocannabinoid system in cancer cachexia. *Current Opinion in Clinical Nutrition and Metabolic Care, 10*(4), 443–448.

Ottery, F.D. (1996). Definition of standardized nutritional assessment and interventional pathways in oncology. *Nutrition, 12*(Suppl. 1), S15–S19.

Ottery, F.D., Sljuka, K., & Hagan, M. (1995, January). *Characterization of patients referred to nutrition clinic in an NCI-designated comprehensive cancer center: Baseline status and outcomes.* Presented at the 19th Clinical Congress of the American Society for Parenteral and Enteral Nutrition, Miami, FL.

Ovesen, L., Allingstrup, L., Hannibal, J., Mortensen, E.L., & Hansen, O.P. (1993). Effect of dietary counseling on food intake, body weight, response rate, survival, and quality of life in cancer patients undergoing chemotherapy: A prospective, randomized study. *Journal of Clinical Oncology, 11*(10), 2043–2049.

Pawlowski, G.J. (1975). Cyproheptadine: Weight-gain and appetite stimulation in essential anorexic adults. *Current Therapeutic Research, Clinical and Experimental, 18*(5), 673–678.

Pearlstone, D.B., Lee, J.I., Alexander, R.H., Chang, T.H., Brennan, M.F., & Burt, M. (1995). Effect of enteral and parenteral nutrition on amino acid levels in cancer patients. *Journal of Parenteral and Enteral Nutrition, 19*(3), 204–208.

Perez, M.M., Newcomer, A.D., Moertel, C.G., Go, V.L., & Dimagno, E.P. (1983). Assessment of weight loss, food intake, fat metabolism, malabsorption, and treatment of pancreatic insufficiency in pancreatic cancer. *Cancer, 52*(2), 346–352.

Persson, C., Glimelius, B., Ronnelid, J., & Nygren, P. (2005). Impact of fish oil and melatonin on cachexia in patients with advanced gastrointestinal cancer: A randomized pilot study. *Nutrition, 21*(2), 170–178.

Puccio, M., & Nathanson, L. (1997). The cancer cachexia syndrome. *Seminars in Oncology, 24*(3), 277–287.

Ramos, E.J., Romanova, I.V., Suzuki, S., Chen, C., Ugrumov, M.V., Sato, T., et al. (2005). Effects of omega-3 fatty acids on orexigenic and anorexigenic modulators at the onset of anorexia. *Brain Research, 1046*(1–2), 157–164.

Ramot, B. (1971). Malabsorption due to lymphomatous diseases. *Annual Review of Medicine, 22,* 19–24.

Rapaport, E., & Fontaine, J. (1989). Generation of extracellular ATP in blood and its mediated inhibition of host weight loss in tumor-bearing mice. *Biochemical Pharmacology, 38*(23), 4261–4266.

Ravasco, P., Monteiro-Grillo, I., & Camilo, M.E. (2003). Does nutrition influence quality of life in cancer patients undergoing radiotherapy? *Radiotherapy and Oncology, 67*(2), 213–220.

Ribaudo, J.M., Cella, D., Hahn, E.A., Lloyd, S.R., Tchekmedyian, N.S., Von Roenn, J., et al. (2000). Re-validation and shortening of the Functional Assessment of Anorexia/Cachexia Therapy (FAACT) questionnaire. *Quality of Life Research, 9*(10), 1137–1146.

Rosenzweig, M.Q. (2006). Anorexia/cachexia. In D. Camp-Sorrell & R. Hawkins (Eds.), *Clinical manual for the oncology advanced practice nurse* (2nd ed., pp. 485–490). Pittsburgh, PA: Oncology Nursing Society.

Schwartz, M.W., Woods, S.C., Porte, D., Jr., Seeley, R.J., & Baskin, D.G. (2000). Central nervous system control of food intake. *Nature, 404*(6778), 661–671.

Sherry, B.A., Gelin, J., Fong, Y., Marano, M., Wei, H., Cerami, A., et al. (1989). Anticachectin/tumor necrosis factor alpha antibodies attenuate development of cancer cachexia. *FASEB Journal, 3*(8), 1956–1962.

Slaviero, K.A., Read, J.A., Clarke, S.L., & Rivory, L.P. (2003). Baseline nutritional assessment in advanced cancer patients receiving palliative chemotherapy. *Nutrition and Cancer, 46*(2), 148–157.

Smith, H.J., Mukerji, P., & Tisdale, M.J. (2005). Attenuation of proteasome-induced proteolysis in skeletal muscle by B-hydroxy-B-methylbutyrate. *Cancer Research, 65*(1), 277–283.

Stewart, G.D., Skipworth, R., & Fearon, K. (2006). Cancer cachexia and fatigue. *Clinical Medicine, 6*(2), 140–143.

Strasser, F., & Bruera, E. (2002). Update on anorexia and cachexia. *Hematology/Oncology Clinics of North America, 16*(3), 589–617.

Strasser, F., Luftner, D., Possinger, K., Ernst, G., Ruhstaller, T., Meissner, W., et al. (2006). Comparison of orally administered cannabis extract and delta-9-tetrahydrocannabinol in treating patients with cancer-related anorexia-cachexia syndrome: A multicenter, phase III, randomized, double-blind, placebo-controlled clinical trial from the Cannabis-In-Cachexia-Study-Group. *Journal of Clinical Oncology, 24*(21), 3394–3400.

Strassmann, G., Fong, M., Kenney, J.S., & Jacob, C.O. (1992). Evidence for the involvement of interleukin 6 in experimental cancer cachexia. *Journal of Clinical Investigation, 89*(5), 1681–1684.

Stroud, M. (2005). Thalidomide and cancer cachexia: Old problem, new hope? *Gut, 54*(4), 447–448.

Talukdar, R., & Bruera, E. (2004). Cachexia. In M.D. Abeloff & J. Armitage (Eds.), *Clinical oncology* (3rd ed., pp. 749–757). Philadelphia: Elsevier Churchill Livingstone.

Taylor, D.D., Gercel-Taylor, C., Jenis, L.G., & Devereux, D.F. (1992). Identification of a human tumor-derived lipolysis-promoting factor. *Cancer Research, 52*(4), 829–834.

Tisdale, M.J. (2006). Clinical anticachexia treatments. *Nutrition in Clinical Practice, 21*(2), 168–174.

Todd, B.D. (1988). Pancreatic carcinoma and low serum testosterone; a correlation secondary to cancer cachexia? *European Journal of Surgical Oncology, 14*(3), 199–202.

Todorov, P., Cariuk, P., McDevitt, T., Coles, B., Fearon, K., & Tisdale, M.J. (1996). Characterization of a cancer cachectic factor. *Nature, 379*(6567), 739–742.

Wang, W., Andersson, M., Iresjo, B.M., Lonnroth, C., & Lundholm, K. (2006). Effects of ghrelin on anorexia in tumor-bearing mice with eicosanoid-related cachexia. *International Journal of Oncology, 28*(6), 1393–1400.

Wilner, L.S., & Arnold, R.M. (2006). Cannabinoids in the treatment of symptoms in cancer and AIDS. *Journal of Palliative Medicine, 9*(3), 802–804.

Yamashita, J.I., & Ogawa, M. (2000). Medroxyprogesterone acetate and cancer cachexia: Interleukin-6 involvement. *Breast Cancer, 7*(2), 130–135.

Yavuzsen, T., Davis, M., Walsh, D., LeGrand, S., & Lagman, R. (2005). Systematic review of the treatment of cancer-associated anorexia and weight loss. *Journal of Clinical Oncology, 23*(33), 8500–8511.

Yeh, S.S., Wu, S.Y., Lee, T.P., Olson, J.S., Stevens, M.R., Dixon, T., et al. (2000). Improvement in quality of life measures and stimulation of weight gain after treatment with megestrol acetate oral suspension in geriatric cachexia: Results of a double blind, placebo-controlled study. *Journal of the American Geriatrics Society, 48*(5), 485–492.

Zinna, E.M., & Yarasheski, K.E. (2003). Exercise treatment to counteract protein wasting of chronic diseases. *Current Opinion in Clinical Nutrition and Metabolic Care, 6*(1), 87–93.

CHAPTER 6

Chemotherapy-Induced Nausea and Vomiting

Carrie Tompkins Stricker, PhD, RN, AOCN®,
and Beth Eaby, MSN, CRNP, OCN®

Case Study

L.M. is a 43-year-old woman with stage II invasive ductal breast cancer. Her breast cancer is node positive, estrogen-receptor and progesterone-receptor negative, and negative for HER2/neu oncogene overexpression. Her oncologist plans chemotherapy with four cycles of doxorubicin and cyclophosphamide (AC) every two weeks, to be followed by four cycles of paclitaxel every two weeks. She presents to the office today for her first cycle of chemotherapy, and the nurse meets with her to discuss her antiemetic regimen. Her case will be revisited later in this chapter.

Overview

Despite significant advances in the prevention and management of nausea and vomiting over the past two decades, these symptoms remain two of the most severe and distressing for individuals undergoing chemotherapy and lead to reductions in quality of life (QOL) and daily functioning (Ballatori et al., 2007; Bloechl-Daum, Deuson, Mavros, Hansen, & Herrstedt, 2006; Cohen, de Moor, Eisenberg, Ming, & Hu, 2007; Glaus et al., 2004; Lindley et al., 1992; Osoba, Zee, Warr, et al., 1997). Fortunately, a growing arsenal of effective agents are available to prevent and treat chemotherapy-induced nausea and vomiting (CINV) and can be used together to block the multiple pathways that contribute to CINV. When used appropriately in combination, agents such as dexamethasone, serotonin-receptor antagonists, and aprepitant can prevent as much as 70%–80% of vomiting with even the most emetogenic chemotherapy treatments, although management of nausea remains a greater challenge (Ballatori et al.; Gralla, 2002; Grunberg et al., 2004).

In spite of pharmacologic advances, inconsistent prescription of and adherence to appropriate antiemetic therapy remain significant barriers to CINV prevention and management (Jordan, Sippel, & Schmoll, 2007; Roila, 2004). Oncology nurses have the potential to play a critical role in ensuring optimal management of CINV by helping to identify patients with the greatest risk and by applying national and international guidelines for CINV prevention and management (Kris et al., 2006; Multinational Association of Supportive Care in Cancer [MASCC], 2008; National Comprehensive Cancer Network [NCCN], 2008). Expert oncology nursing care is indispensable to reducing the incidence of and suffering from CINV by helping to ensure patients receive evidence-based interventions. Prevention is clearly the best management for this debilitating symptom.

CINV consists of nausea and vomiting related to chemotherapy. *Nausea* is "a subjective phenomenon of an unpleasant sensation in the epigastrium and in the back of the throat that may or may not culminate in vomiting" (Dibble, Israel, Nussey, Casey, & Luce, 2003, p. E40). *Vomiting* is "a physical protective reaction to the ingestion of toxins resulting in the expulsion of gastric contents through the mouth" (Dibble, Casey, Nussey, Israel, & Luce, 2004, p. E1). CINV typically is classified into categories of acute, delayed, anticipatory, breakthrough, or refractory CINV (see Table 6-1) (Eckert, 2001; Jordan et al., 2007; Tipton et al., 2007). Delayed CINV is more than twice as common as acute CINV in individuals receiving moderately or highly emetogenic chemotherapy regimens that include agents such as cisplatin and doxorubicin (Ballatori et al., 2007; Grunberg et al., 2004). The pattern of delayed CINV is dependent on the chemotherapy drug involved (see Figure 6-1). It may start the first day after chemotherapy and last for a few days. At other times, for example with cisplatin, after an acute peak in the first 24 hours, CINV may be delayed until the second or third day after chemotherapy administration and last for three days or longer (Martin, 1996).

TABLE 6-1	Types of Chemotherapy-Induced Nausea and Vomiting (CINV)
Type	**Definition**
Acute	Occurs within the first 24 hours of receiving chemotherapy
Delayed	Any nausea or vomiting that occurs more than 24 hours after chemotherapy administration. Typically peaks between 48 and 72 hours and may last as long as 7 days.
Anticipatory	Patient develops a conditioned response to chemotherapy based on prior CINV experience, leading to nausea and/or vomiting when exposed to stimuli associated with the chemotherapy and related nausea and vomiting.
Breakthrough	CINV that occurs despite using prophylactic medications and requires the use of "rescue" therapies
Refractory	CINV that occurs after subsequent cycles of chemotherapy after the use of prophylactic and breakthrough medications have failed

Note. Based on information from Eckert, 2001; Jordan et al., 2007; Tipton et al., 2007.

Anticipatory CINV is very difficult to manage, and prevention of acute CINV is the best strategy for avoiding this extremely challenging clinical phenomenon (Tipton et al., 2007). The trigger for anticipatory CINV may be only a thought, smell, or sight of something reminiscent of chemotherapy. As with anticipatory CINV, both breakthrough and refractory CINV often develop as a result of inadequate control of acute or delayed CINV, again highlighting the importance of preventing CINV with optimal antiemetic therapy starting with the first cycle of chemotherapy treatment.

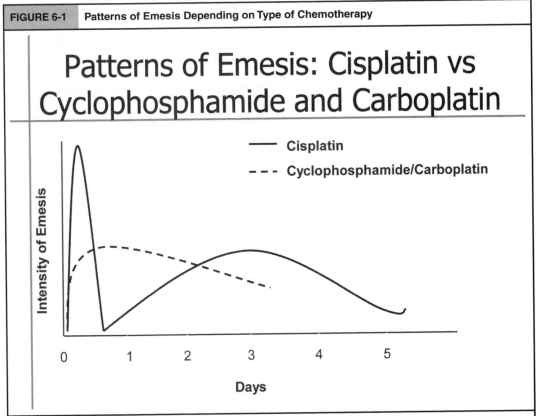

Note. From "The Severity and Pattern of Emesis Following Different Cytotoxic Agents," by M. Martin, 1996, *Oncology, 53*(Suppl. 1), p. 30. Copyright 1996 by S. Karger AG Medical and Scientific Publishers, Basel. Reprinted with permission.

Prevalence of Chemotherapy-Induced Nausea and Vomiting

Although clinical trials of antiemetic therapy report control rates for nausea and vomiting to be as high as 70%–80%, these statistics are unlikely to reflect the actual control rates in clinical practice because of both patient and provider factors (Gralla, 2002). In recent patient surveys, up to 30% of individuals receiving highly emetogenic chemotherapy reported acute-phase vomiting, and nearly half reported delayed vomiting, whereas with moderately emetogenic chemotherapy, 10%–25% of patients reported acute-phase vomiting, and 28%–40% reported delayed vomiting (Glaus et al., 2004; Grunberg et al., 2004). Rates of nausea are even higher, with up to 52% of individuals receiving moderately or highly emetogenic chemotherapy experiencing acute nausea, and 52%–82% of individuals reporting delayed nausea (Bloechl-Daum et al., 2006; Dibble et al., 2003; Glaus et al.; Grunberg et al., 2004; Stricker & Velders, 2005).

Delayed CINV clearly is a greater clinical challenge than acute CINV. Although rates of acute CINV markedly decreased in the 1990s with the introduction of the 5-hydroxytryptamine-3 (5-HT$_3$) receptor antagonists (e.g., granisetron, ondansetron), delayed nausea and vomiting remains prevalent. Nowhere is this more apparent than in the setting of adjuvant chemotherapy for women with early-stage breast cancer. A prospective, national, multisite study was undertaken with more than 300 women with early-stage breast cancer, nearly 80% of whom received anthracycline-based regimens such as AC (Dibble et al., 2003, 2004). More than half (52%) of these women experienced vomiting in the delayed setting, compared to only 18% of women who reported vomiting during the first 24 hours following chemotherapy (Dibble et al., 2004). Furthermore, 73%–82% of these women reported delayed nausea during two cycles of adjuvant chemotherapy (Dibble et al., 2003). In a more recent prospective study of 89 women receiving anthracycline-based adjuvant chemotherapy for breast cancer, the majority of whom received a 5-HT$_3$ receptor antagonist and/or dexamethasone for prevention of delayed CINV, daily rates of nausea were as high as 63% two to five days following treatment (Stricker & Velders, 2005).

Anticipatory CINV remains one of the most challenging chemotherapy-related symptoms to manage (Aapro, Molassiotis, & Olver, 2005; Eckert, 2001). Unfortunately, the incidence of anticipatory CINV did not decrease with the introduction of 5-HT$_3$ (serotonin) receptor antagonists and remains approximately 6%–7% for anticipatory vomiting and approximately 30% for anticipatory nausea (Morrow et al., 1998; Roscoe, Morrow, Hickok, & Stern, 2000; Zachariae et al., 2007). No studies have been published yet regarding the incidence or prevalence of anticipatory CINV following the introduction of the newest class of antiemetic agents, the neurokinin-1 (NK-1) receptor antagonists.

Pathophysiology

Understanding of the pathophysiology of CINV has grown over the past several decades as a result of the evolution of the science regarding neurotransmitters and pathways involved with CINV. Following the administration of chemotherapy, a number of neurotransmitters are released in both the gut and the brain, where receptors for these neurotransmitters are found, predominantly 5-HT$_3$ receptors, substance P (NK-1 receptors), and dopamine (dopamine receptors). Other neurotransmitters implicated in CINV pathogenesis are listed in Figure 6-2. These neurotransmitters may act independently or in combination to induce nausea and vomiting by binding to target receptors and initiating CINV-related neural pathways (Hesketh, Van Belle, et al., 2003). Chemotherapy-induced emesis, for example, occurs through a multistep process. First, chemotherapy and its metabolites activate receptors in the chemoreceptor trigger zone (CTZ), the gastrointestinal (GI) tract, and the cerebral cortex, which send efferent impulses to the vomiting center. In response, the vomiting center sends afferent impulses to organs such as the heart, lungs, and GI tract to slow down GI motility and speed up heart rate, often resulting in vomiting (Ettinger et al., 2007). The mechanisms underlying chemotherapy-induced vomiting are better understood than those for chemotherapy-related nausea. The sensation of nausea is controlled by a part of the central nervous system

FIGURE 6-2	Neurotransmitters/Neuropeptides Associated With Chemotherapy-Induced Nausea and Vomiting

- Acetylcholine
- Angiotensin II
- Apomorphine
- Dopamine
- Endorphins
- Gamma-aminobutyric acid
- Gastrin
- Histamine
- Neurotensin
- Norepinephrine
- Serotonin
- Substance P

Note. Based on information from Shelke et al., 2004.

(CNS) occupied with involuntary bodily functions (Shelke, Mustian, & Morrow, 2004). Two major pathways commonly are believed to be linked to CINV—the peripheral and central pathways—and their importance is thought to vary across the trajectory from acute to delayed CINV (Hesketh, Van Belle, et al.).

Peripheral Pathway

Stimulation of nausea and vomiting peripherally in the GI tract is largely related to serotonin release and binding to 5-HT_3 receptors, which predominantly is responsible for the development of nausea and vomiting in the acute setting (Cunningham, 1997; Hesketh, Van Belle, et al., 2003; Higa et al., 2006). Enterochromaffin (EC) cells line the GI tract and house most of the body's serotonin. When chemotherapy comes into contact with EC cells, either directly from oral ingestion or indirectly via the bloodstream, damage occurs and serotonin is released (see Figure 6-3). Serotonin subsequently binds to the 5-HT_3 receptors prevalent in the gut and transmits a potent signal to the vomiting center in the brain via the vagal afferent nerves. Urinary levels of 5-hydroxyindoleacetic acid (5-HIAA), the main serotonin metabolite, return to baseline within 24 hours following high-dose cisplatin chemotherapy but may remain elevated beyond 24 hours following moderate-dose cisplatin and other mod-

FIGURE 6-3   Chemotherapy-Induced Nausea and Vomiting: Serotonin Pathway

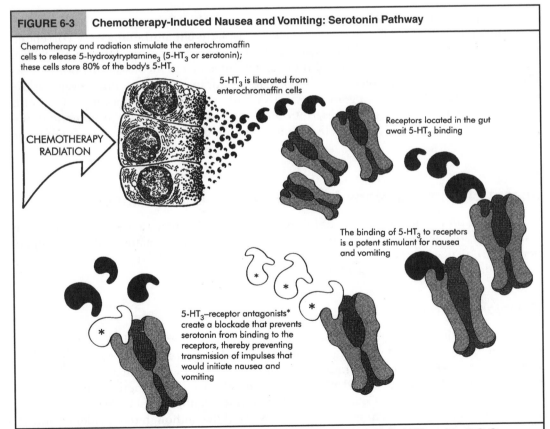

Chemotherapy and radiation stimulate the enterochromaffin cells to release 5-hydroxytryptamine$_3$ (5-HT_3 or serotonin); these cells store 80% of the body's 5-HT_3

5-HT_3 is liberated from enterochromaffin cells

CHEMOTHERAPY RADIATION

Receptors located in the gut await 5-HT_3 binding

The binding of 5-HT_3 to receptors is a potent stimulant for nausea and vomiting

5-HT_3–receptor antagonists* create a blockade that prevents serotonin from binding to the receptors, thereby preventing transmission of impulses that would initiate nausea and vomiting

Note. From "5-HT_3-Receptor Antagonists: A Review of Pharmacology and Clinical Efficacy," by R.S. Cunningham, 1997, *Oncology Nursing Forum, 24*(Suppl. 7), p. 35. Copyright 1997 by Oncology Nursing Society. Reprinted with permission.

erately emetogenic agents. These data indicate that serotonin may play a role in the causation of delayed CINV in some cases, in addition to its predominant role in the pathogenesis of acute emesis (Hesketh, Van Belle, et al.; Higa et al.). Substance P, another neurotransmitter identified as having a major role in CINV, also has been found in small amounts in the EC cells of the gut (Higa et al.), but its role in the causation of CINV via the peripheral pathway is unclear.

Central Pathway

Stimulation of central neural pathways also mediates CINV. The CTZ is located in the brain stem in an area that is not protected by the blood-brain barrier, meaning that it is accessible via the cerebrospinal fluid or blood. Located in the area postrema, part of the medulla oblongata, the CTZ receives input from neurotransmitters released because of chemotherapy (Shelke et al., 2004). Chemotherapy circulating in the bloodstream or cerebrospinal fluid also directly stimulates the CTZ (Shelke et al.). NK-1 receptors with high affinity for substance P are concentrated in the CNS and appear to be activated by chemotherapy and its metabolites (Hesketh, Van Belle, et al., 2003). Levels of substance P in the bloodstream predominantly are elevated in the delayed setting more than 24 hours following chemotherapy, although substance P may play a role in the pathogenesis of acute CINV as well (Higa et al., 2006).

Much is still unknown about the pathogenesis of CINV. Higher blood or urine levels of 5-HIAA and substance P in patients receiving cisplatin chemotherapy were correlated with greater acute and delayed CINV, supporting a clear association (Higa et al., 2006). Levels of these neurotransmitters and their metabolites varied inconsistently both across time and between patients receiving similar chemotherapy regimens, thus revealing the complex nature of CINV pathogenesis. As CINV still occurs in more than half of patients (Grunberg et al., 2004) despite prescription of optimal contemporary antiemetic therapy, additional pathways and interactions between and among them clearly remain to be elucidated.

Impact of Chemotherapy-Induced Nausea and Vomiting

Given the prevalence of CINV, careful examination of its impact is necessary. Symptom distress, physiologic consequences, and effects on QOL, functional status, and treatment adherence are all pertinent concerns. More recently, growing research is documenting the negative economic consequences of CINV.

Symptom Distress

Although patient perceptions of CINV have changed over time as antiemetic therapy has improved, both nausea and vomiting remain in the top five symptoms ranked as the most severe by heterogeneous samples of individuals with cancer. A series of similar descriptive studies was conducted in the 1980s and 1990s to determine which chemotherapy side effects patients felt were most severe (Coates et al., 1983; de Boer-Dennert et al., 1997; Griffin et al., 1996; Lindley et al., 1999). These studies demonstrated that although the incidence and severity of vomiting have decreased, control is not yet optimal, and nausea related to chemotherapy has replaced vomiting as the more distressing problem (Bloechl-Daum et al., 2006; Roila, Donati, Tamberi, & Margutti, 2002).

Physiologic Consequences

Nausea and vomiting related to chemotherapy can lead to a number of negative physiologic consequences, including impaired nutritional intake, electrolyte imbalances, dehydration, and pulmonary and GI complications (Bender et al., 2002). Impaired nutrition is a problem for as many as 40%–80% of patients with cancer (Cunningham & Huhmann, 2005), and CINV may exacerbate it as a result of decreased oral intake and inadequate caloric consumption. Impaired nutrition may result in weight loss, inadequate protein stores, and loss of muscle mass and can lead to a wasting cycle that is difficult to reverse (Brown et al., 2001). CINV results in other adverse consequences. Vomiting in particular can lead to significant electrolyte abnormalities, acid-base imbalances, and dehydration. Reduced oral intake contributes to these adverse consequences, but the primary cause is the loss of gastric fluid rich in potassium, sodium, chloride, magnesium, water, hydrochloric acid, and bicarbonate (Bender et al.). Emesis can result in metabolic acidosis because of bicarbonate loss or, in cases of severe vomiting, metabolic alkalosis because of loss of hydrogen ions. Other serious potential physiologic consequences of chemotherapy-induced vomiting include aspiration pneumonia and mucosal or submucosal tears of the lower esophagus or esophagogastric junction, known as Mallory-Weiss syndrome (Bender et al.). Although these serious adverse complications are rare, they underline the importance of CINV prevention in individuals receiving emetogenic chemotherapy.

Consequences on Quality of Life and Functional Status

Research clearly supports the negative effects of CINV on QOL and daily functioning. In the early 1990s, one of the first major studies to address this issue found that patients who experienced emesis related to chemotherapy had significant declines in QOL in the three days following chemotherapy, whereas QOL remained stable in those individuals without emesis (Lindley et al., 1992). Participants perceived that both nausea and vomiting substantially interfered with their ability to complete meals, spend time with family and friends, and maintain daily functioning, including social activities. Subsequently, a large prospective study evaluated the QOL of 832 chemotherapy-naïve patients with cancer during the first week following their initial cycle of moderately or highly emetogenic chemotherapy, using both a diary and a QOL questionnaire (Osoba, Zee, Warr, et al., 1997). Patients who experienced both nausea and vomiting had the greatest deterioration in QOL, significantly greater than for those subjects without CINV. Individuals with CINV also experienced significantly poorer physical, cognitive, and social functioning in addition to greater fatigue and other symptoms. Notably, patients with one to two emetic episodes experienced nearly the same reduction in QOL as those with three or more episodes of vomiting, thereby highlighting the importance of complete prevention of emesis.

An explosion of research in the past decade has further delineated the negative impact of CINV on QOL and functioning. In a prospective study of 119 Canadians with cancer, CINV accounted for most of the deterioration in health-related QOL scores observed over a six-day period following moderately emetogenic chemotherapy (Rusthoven et al., 1998). Furthermore, individuals experiencing CINV had greater fatigue and pain and poorer emotional functioning compared to those without CINV. A number of recent studies have used the Functional Living Index–Emesis (FLIE) instrument to examine the impact of CINV on daily functioning across diverse cancer populations residing in various countries. Greater duration, intensity, and frequency of CINV was associated with a negative impact of CINV on daily functioning in these studies, and individuals experiencing both acute and delayed CINV had the greatest declines in daily functioning (Ballatori et al., 2007; Bloechl-Daum et al., 2006; Cohen et al., 2007; Glaus et al., 2004). Even individuals who escape acute CINV are at risk for functional declines related to delayed symptoms. In one multinational sample of 298 individuals, nearly one-fourth of individuals who did not have acute CINV nonetheless reported a significant negative impact of delayed CINV on their daily lives (Bloechl-Daum et al.). Furthermore, nausea had a greater negative impact on functional status than did vomiting.

Effects on Antineoplastic Treatment Adherence

Twenty years ago, up to 20% of individuals with cancer either postponed or discontinued chemotherapy because of nausea and/or vomiting (Herrstedt, 2002). Thanks to dramatic advances in antiemetic therapy over the past two decades, CINV now affects adherence to antineoplastic therapy with much less frequency. In a study of 303 women undergoing adjuvant breast cancer chemotherapy, only 5% reported adjustment of their chemotherapy dose or schedule because of CINV (Dibble et al., 2003). In a more recent study, zero of 89 women with breast cancer had dose adjustments or treatment discontinuations because of CINV (Stricker & Velders, 2005). Recent data from more diverse populations are not available. Chemotherapy dose reductions of greater than 25% have long been known to compromise efficacy and decrease cancer survival (Bonadonna & Valagussa, 1981).

Economic Outcomes

Nausea and vomiting related to chemotherapy also may result in negative economic consequences. CINV elevates costs of care associated with cancer therapy, including both outpatient and hospital charges, as well as personal and societal economic consequences such as work loss (Grunberg, Zhang, & Zhang, 2000; Shih, Han, Zhao, & Elting, 2005). Medical costs are higher for individuals with CINV. In one study of 2,071 insurance beneficiaries with cancer, total monthly medical costs were significantly greater, by $2,619, for those with uncontrolled CINV compared to those with controlled CINV (Shih et al.). Individuals with uncontrolled CINV also lost more days from work (8.9 versus 7.2 days). Significant differences were observed in costs of inpatient care, outpatient care, and prescription medications. Other studies have documented higher hospital expenses related to CINV. An analysis of 64,000 hospital discharges found that hospital stays were two days longer and charges were approximately 30% higher for patients who developed CINV compared to those who did not (Grunberg et al., 2000).

Risk Factors

Given the significant deleterious impact of CINV on QOL, preventing nausea and vomiting is paramount. As the number, efficacy, and cost of antiemetic agents continue to increase, clinicians face a growing demand to use these agents in efficacious and cost-effective ways. The most effective antiemetic regimens must be targeted toward individuals with the highest risk for CINV. The greatest determinant of CINV risk is the emetogenicity of the chemotherapy regimen, defined as its potential for causing nausea and vomiting (Ettinger et al., 2007). National and international guidelines recommend specific antiemetic therapy based on categories of emetic risk (Kris et al., 2006; MASCC, 2008; NCCN, 2008). In the case of highly emetogenic chemotherapy, use of the most aggressive antiemetic prophylaxis clearly is indicated. In the case of moderately emetogenic chemotherapy, however, clinician judgment plays a greater role, as antiemetic guidelines offer a number of pharmacologic options for CINV prevention. Individual risk factors can help clinicians to choose the best antiemetic therapy for the individual patient.

Treatment-Related Factors

The likelihood and severity of CINV are related directly to the specific chemotherapy regimen administered because individual chemotherapeutic agents vary widely in their emetogenicity. Chemotherapy agents are assigned to categories based on their likelihood of inducing acute vomiting when prophylactic antiemetic medications are not administered (see Table 6-2). Agents are classified into four levels of emetogenic risk: high (> 90%), moderate (30%–90%), low (10%–30%), and minimal (< 10%) risk (Ettinger et al., 2007; Koeller et al., 2002; Kris et al., 2006; MASCC, 2008). A major goal of this classification system is to guide the choice of pharmacologic agents for prevention and management of CINV. Algorithms also have been proposed for calculating the emetogenicity of combined chemotherapy regimens by adding up modified scores for individual chemotherapy agents (see Figure 6-4) (Hesketh et al., 1997). Although potentially quite clinically useful, this algorithm has not been validated for routine use in clinical practice. Nonetheless, it highlights the importance of considering the potential additive effects of chemotherapy agents in increasing the likelihood of developing CINV.

TABLE 6-2	Classification of Chemotherapy Agents by Their Potential for Acute Emetogenicity	
Level of Emetogenicity	**Chemotherapy Agent**	**Rate of Emesis**
High (Level 4)	Cisplatin $\geq$ 50 mg/m^2 Dacarbazine Cyclophosphamide > 1,500 mg/m^2 Mechlorethamine Carmustine	Emesis in nearly all patients (> 90%)
Moderate (Level 3)	Oxaliplatin Carboplatin Cytarabine > 1 g/m^2 Doxorubicin, epirubicin Cyclophosphamide $\leq$ 1,500 mg/m^2 Ifosfamide Irinotecan	Emesis in > 30% (30%–90%) of patients
Low (Level 2)	Capecitabine Taxanes Gemcitabine Topotecan Methotrexate Mitoxantrone, mitomycin Etoposide Doxorubicin hydrochloride liposomal	Emesis in > 10% (10%–30%) of patients
Minimal (Level 1)	Vinca alkaloids Bleomycin Busulfan Fludarabine	Emesis in < 10% of patients

Note. Based on information from Koeller et al., 2002; Multinational Association of Supportive Care in Cancer, 2008.

FIGURE 6-4	Algorithm for Defining Emetogenicity of Combination Chemotherapy Regimens

Identify most emetogenic agent.
Increase overall rating for additional agents by:
- 1 per agent (level 3)
- 1 (level 2 agents)
- 0 (level 1 agents).

Example:
Doxorubicin + cyclophosphamide
3 + 3 = level 4 risk of emetogenicity

Note. Based on information from Hesketh et al., 1997.

One regimen combining moderately emetogenic chemotherapy agents has received particular attention for its high emetic risk, largely because of data concerning its use in women with breast cancer who have an elevated risk for developing CINV. AC historically was classified as moderately emetogenic based on the emetogenicity of its individual chemotherapy agents (Hesketh et al., 1997), but this categorization is being reconsidered. Although MASCC and the American Society of Clinical Oncology (ASCO) still classify AC as moderately emetogenic, they recognize the elevated CINV risk of this regimen (Kris et al., 2006; MASCC, 2008). In 2005, NCCN took a bolder stand by classifying AC, defined as either doxorubicin or epirubicin in combination with cyclophosphamide, as a highly emetogenic regimen in its antiemesis guidelines (NCCN, 2008).

Other treatment-related factors contributing to CINV are important to acknowledge. Experiencing acute CINV is one of the most important risk factors for delayed CINV. Individuals who have acute CINV are more likely to experience nausea and vomiting in the delayed setting (Bloechl-Daum et al., 2006; Cohen et al., 2007; Roila et al., 2002; Stricker & Velders, 2005). Furthermore, the incidence of CINV generally increases over time across cycles of chemotherapy. Fortunately, some of the newer antiemetics, such as the NK-1 receptor antagonist aprepitant, have been able to reduce the cumulative impact of treatment cycles on the CINV experience (Warr, Grunberg, et al., 2005).

Patient Characteristics

Although the emetogenicity of the chemotherapy regimen is the most important risk factor for CINV, patient experiences vary widely within these categories of risk. Identifying patients who are at higher risk for CINV at baseline before chemotherapy treatment is imperative because CINV is more difficult to manage once established. A number of individual characteristics are associated with increased risk for CINV (see Figure 6-5). These include demographic characteristics, previous experience with nausea and vomiting, and behavioral and psychological factors, such as expectations about CINV.

Demographic characteristics linked to a higher risk of CINV include female sex, younger age, and in one study, minority status (see Figure 6-5) (Alba et al., 1989; Benrubi, Norvell, Nuss, & Robinson, 1985; Dibble et al., 2004; Eckert, 2001; Hesketh et al., 2006; Liaw et al., 2003; Osoba, Zee, Pater, et al., 1997; Roila et al., 1987; Seynaeve et al., 1992; Stein et al., 1995). Behavioral and psychological factors also may help to predict the likelihood of develop-

FIGURE 6-5	Individual Risk Factors for Chemotherapy-Induced Nausea and Vomiting (CINV)

- Younger age (< 50 years old)
- Female gender
- No or low alcohol consumption (≤ 1 drink/day)
- History of nausea with stress
- History of motion sickness or hyperemesis of pregnancy
- Patient's initial expectations about developing CINV
- Pretreatment or infusion-related anxiety
- Current use of anxiolytics or antidepressants

Note. Based on information from Alba et al., 1989; Benrubi et al., 1985; Dibble et al., 2004; Eckert, 2001; Hesketh et al., 2006; Liaw et al., 2003; Osoba, Zee, Pater, et al., 1997; Roila et al., 1987; Seynaeve et al., 1992; Stein et al., 1995.

ing CINV. Pretreatment anxiety has been linked to an increased risk of anticipatory CINV (Eckert), and women on anxiolytics or antidepressants (e.g., lorazepam) prior to receiving adjuvant breast cancer chemotherapy had greater postchemotherapy CINV (Stricker & Velders, 2005). Heightened anxiety during treatment infusions is a risk factor for greater postchemotherapy nausea and vomiting (Andrykowski & Gregg, 1992; Jacobsen et al., 1988). Individuals' pretreatment expectations about CINV appear to influence their subsequent experience of nausea and vomiting following chemotherapy (Shelke et al., 2004; Stricker & Velders). In one study, individuals who thought they were "very likely" to develop CINV were much more likely (64%) to experience CINV than were individuals who thought they would be "very unlikely" to experience it (17%) (Shelke et al.). Evidence for the effect of other behavioral risk factors is less consistent, including the link between alcohol consumption and CINV risk. Regular drinkers (i.e., more than one drink/day) have a lower risk of CINV compared to individuals who drink less (Eckert), but findings are inconsistent (Osoba, Zee, Pater, et al.). A personal history of nausea and vomiting in other settings also has been linked to an increased risk of CINV (see Figure 6-5) (Dibble et al., 2003; Eckert; Leventhal, Easterling, Nerenz, & Love, 1988; Minegishi et al., 2004; Roila et al., 2002).

Continuation of Case Study

Recall L.M., the 43-year-old woman with stage II invasive ductal breast cancer who has been prescribed four cycles of AC every two weeks followed by four cycles of paclitaxel every two weeks. What risk factors does L.M. have for CINV?

L.M. is younger than 50 years old and female, both factors that put her at greater risk for developing CINV. Furthermore, NCCN (2008) recognizes AC as a highly emetogenic regimen, and her antiemetic therapy should be tailored according to these risks.

Assessment

Assessment of CINV in the clinical setting is indispensable to optimal prevention and management. Without routine assessment of nausea and vomiting experienced by individuals undergoing chemotherapy, oncology nurses will be misinformed about patient experience, as individuals with cancer tend to underreport their symptoms if not clearly prompted to do so (Johnson, Moore, & Fortner, 2007). Suboptimal management of CINV may result. Assessment of delayed CINV is especially critical given that delayed symptoms typically occur when the healthcare team no longer has the opportunity for direct observation. The phenomenon of "out of sight, out of mind" may, in part, explain why oncology nurses and physicians are able to accurately estimate the incidence of acute CINV experienced by patients receiving both highly and moderately emetogenic chemotherapy and yet significantly underestimate the incidence of delayed CINV (Grunberg et al., 2004). Provider assumptions about the efficacy of modern antiemetic regimens also may hinder assessment practices, as clinicians may have a false sense of reassurance about their effectiveness (Bender et al., 2002). The majority of oncology clinicians, including nurses, fail to integrate regular assessment of CINV and other chemotherapy-related symptoms into routine practice (Johnson et al.), thus missing a critical opportunity to optimize prevention and management.

Risk Assessment

As with any symptom, a risk assessment should first be conducted to determine the individual's likelihood of developing CINV (Ropka, Padilla, & Gillespie, 2005). Risk assessment involves an evaluation of treatment-related factors as well as patient-related characteristics that could influence CINV risk. First, the level of emetogenicity of the prescribed chemotherapy regimen should be determined, as this is central to establishing the appropriate prophylactic antiemetic regimen (NCCN, 2008). Both the NCCN antiemesis guidelines and the MASCC antiemesis guidelines provide useful tables classifying the emetic risk of chemotherapy agents. Table 6-2 provides an abbreviated summary of common chemotherapeutic agents and their corresponding emetic risk. Individuals receiving highly emetogenic regimens should be prescribed the most aggressive antiemetic prophylaxis available, consisting of agents from at least three different classes of antiemetic therapy (NCCN). For patients receiving moderately emetogenic chemotherapy regimens, however, other treatment- and patient-related characteristics play a particularly important role in determining optimal antiemetic therapy. Patients with risk factors such as younger age, female gender, prior experience with CINV, and high pretreatment expectations of developing CINV may warrant additional therapies beyond the minimum recommended antiemetic medication regimen. Risk assessments should be repeated with each new cycle of chemotherapy, as an individual's risk may change based on his or her evolving symptom experience.

Symptom Assessment

Assessment of nausea and vomiting related to chemotherapy should happen before the first day of the first cycle of chemotherapy and continue throughout the entire course of treatment. Assessment of CINV relies on both objective and subjective data and should encompass not only the symptoms of nausea and vomiting but also evaluation of potential related consequences, such as impaired nutrition and hydration (Bender et al., 2002). Because nausea is a subjective symptom, assessment relies on patient self-report data. Assessment of vomiting incorporates objective data when the clinician is able to directly observe the patient, but it typically relies heavily on self-report because most chemotherapy-related vomiting will occur in the delayed setting, when the patient typically is not clinically observable. Reliable and valid methods of assessment, such as the MASCC Antiemesis Tool (MAT) (MASCC, 2004; Molassiotis et al., 2007), are therefore essential.

Patient self-report of nausea and vomiting is the cornerstone of CINV assessment. Oncology nurses should inquire about the number, onset, duration, and severity of episodes of nausea and vomiting, as well as the use and perceived efficacy of interventions undertaken by the patient to manage CINV (Bender et al., 2002). A number of reliable and valid questionnaires are available for assessing CINV and its impact on QOL and functioning, including the Morrow Assessment of Nausea and Emesis; the Rhodes Index of Nausea, Vomiting, and Retching; the FLIE; and most recently, the Chemotherapy-Induced Nausea and Emesis QOL questionnaire (Martin, Pearson, et al., 2003; Martin, Rubenstein, Elting, Kim, & Osoba, 2003; Morrow, 1992; Rhodes & McDaniel, 1999). These instruments, however, were developed for use in research studies, and none have yet been systematically evaluated for use in clinical practice. Questionnaire length and time needed for completion and scoring are barriers to their clinical use.

In contrast, the MAT (MASCC, 2004) was designed specifically for use in clinical practice and is a reliable and valid assessment tool (Molassiotis et al., 2007). The MAT is a short self-report instrument that assesses both acute and delayed nausea and vomiting. The MAT should be filled out by the patient only twice per chemotherapy cycle—once 24 hours following chemotherapy to capture acute CINV and then again four days after chemotherapy to capture delayed nausea and vomiting. The MAT can be freely downloaded from MASCC's Web site (see www.mascc.org/content/126.html) and is recommended for the assessment of CINV in clinical practice (Molassiotis et al., 2007). Use of CINV tools such as the MAT help to facilitate discussions between clinicians and patients about the CINV experience, thereby affording opportunities to adjust a patient's antiemetic therapy on an ongoing basis throughout the entire course of chemotherapy.

Objective Assessment and Related Complications

For patients experiencing CINV, especially those with emesis, clinicians should perform a thorough objective assessment to evaluate for adverse consequences of nausea and vomiting. Nutrition assessment should include a diet history, evaluation of height and weight, a physical examination to detect signs of dehydration, sarcopenia, or muscle wasting, vital signs, and laboratory work (Bender et al., 2002). A body mass index of less than 17 is indicative of malnutrition and requires further evaluation (Bender et al.). A serum albumin less than 3.5 mg/dl and serum transferrin levels less than 200 mg/dl indicate depleted protein stores, and a prealbumin level of 15 mg/dl or less points to altered protein synthesis (Shelton & Ignatavicius, 1999). All are indicative of cachexia (see Chapter 5 for further information on cachexia) and necessitate additional evaluation and intervention. Electrolytes should be evaluated for those experiencing emesis, especially of a severe or persistent nature, because vomiting of gastric contents can lead to hypokalemia, hyponatremia, hypochloremia, and hypomagnesemia (Bender et al.). If metabolic alkalosis or acidosis is suspected, particularly in severe cases of emesis, bicarbonate levels should be checked and arterial blood gases drawn to evaluate arterial blood pH level.

Differential Diagnosis

Persistent or refractory nausea and vomiting after chemotherapy should always raise suspicion for additional abnormalities. Differential diagnoses include brain metastases, tumor infiltration of the bowel, other GI abnormalities including gastroparesis, and nausea and vomiting related to other comorbidities (Ettinger et al., 2007). In addition, chemotherapy and concomitant medications, including corticosteroids, may exacerbate gastritis or gastroesophageal reflux disease.

Evidence-Based Interventions

Overview and Goals of Management

The primary goals of managing CINV are prevention and treatment of symptoms, maintenance of QOL, and avoidance of complications, including hospitalizations. Prevention is the most important goal. The Oncology Nursing Society (ONS) Putting Evidence Into Practice (PEP) resource on CINV summarizes effective treatments for prevention and treatment of CINV (Tipton et al., 2006). When planning for CINV prevention for a patient receiving chemotherapy, the practitioner needs to identify the optimal combination of pharmacologic agents to achieve these goals and also needs to consider behavioral interventions and complementary therapies appropriate for the individual. The cornerstone of CINV management is pharmacologic antiemetic therapy. Remarkable advances in the pharmacologic management of CINV have evolved over the past 15 years. The introduction of two of the most effective classes of antiemetics, the 5-HT$_3$ receptor antagonists and NK-1 receptor antagonists, have revolutionized the control of CINV.

Pharmacologic Management

Several key principles guide pharmacologic therapy for CINV (Ettinger et al., 2007). First and foremost, prevention of both nausea and vomiting is the primary goal of antiemetic therapy, as CINV is more difficult to treat once established. The prescribed antiemetic regimen must cover the entire period of risk, which corresponds to a minimum of four days following administration of highly or moderately emetogenic chemotherapy (Ettinger et al.). The emetogenicity of the prescribed chemotherapy regimen should guide the prophylactic antiemetic therapy, which should be initiated before chemotherapy administration. Finally, combination therapy, such as concurrent dexamethasone and ondansetron (with or without aprepitant), is superior to single-agent therapy and is essential for highly and moderately emetogenic chemotherapy regimens.

Dopamine receptor antagonists, such as metoclopramide, and corticosteroids, such as methylprednisolone, were the first medications found to be helpful in treating CINV (Roila et al., 1987). High-dose metoclopramide and methylprednisolone often were combined to treat CINV associated with cisplatin-based regimens. Phenothiazines such as prochlorperazine and chlorpromazine also were a mainstay of CINV treatment in the 1980s (Wiser & Berger, 2005). These agents now are considered useful only for prevention of CINV with minimally emetogenic chemotherapy regimens or as adjunctive therapy for refractory CINV and are inappropriate for use alone with highly and moderately emetogenic chemotherapy (NCCN, 2008).

Corticosteroids are a cornerstone of antiemetic therapy. Given that a greater volume of data is available on its efficacy and tolerability compared to other corticosteroids, dexamethasone now is considered the corticosteroid of choice for combination antiemetic therapy (Kris et al., 2006). A meta-analysis of 32 studies documented the superiority of dexamethasone over placebo in both the acute and delayed settings when used with moderately and highly emetogenic regimens (Ioannidis, Hesketh, & Lau, 2000). In addition to its clear antiemetic and antinausea effects, dexamethasone also may improve CINV prevention and treatment through amelioration of anorexia and fatigue (Inoue et al., 2003).

5-Hydroxytryptamine-3 Receptor Antagonists

After being introduced in the early 1990s, 5-HT$_3$ receptor antagonists became a major advance in controlling CINV (Hesketh & Gandara, 1991). When administered immediately prior to chemotherapy, all medications in this class significantly decrease the incidence and severity of acute nausea and vomiting compared to previously available agents or placebo (Ettinger et al., 2007). Table 6-3 lists currently approved 5-HT$_3$ antagonists, all of which end in the suffix -setron, with their doses. These drugs act predominately at the peripheral level of the nervous system by binding with 5-HT$_3$ receptors in the gut to prevent transmission of signals via the vagal afferents to produce nausea and stimulate the emetic reflex (Cunningham, 1997). According to a meta-analysis of 44 studies examining oral 5-HT$_3$ antagonists for prevention of acute CINV, no significant differences in efficacy were seen between four different 5-HT$_3$ drugs when used with either cisplatin or non–cisplatin-based chemotherapy, with one exception (Jordan et al., 2007): Granisetron may be more

TABLE 6-3	Recommended Doses of Serotonin (5-HT$_3$) Receptor Antagonists for Acute Emesis	
Agent	**Route**	**Dose**
Ondansetron	IV	8 mg or 0.15 mg/kg
	Oral	16 mg*
Granisetron	IV	1 mg or 0.01 mg/kg
	Oral	2 mg (or 1 mg**)
Dolasetron	IV	100 mg or 1.8 mg/kg
	Oral	100 mg
Tropisetron	IV	5 mg
	Oral	5 mg
Palonosetron	IV	0.25 mg

* Randomized studies have tested the 8 mg twice-daily schedule.
** The 1 mg dose preferred by some panelists: small randomized study in MEC, phase II study in HEC
Ondansetron (Zofran®, GlaxoSmithKline)
Granisetron (Kytril®, Hoffman-La Roche Inc.)
Dolasetron (Anzemet®, Sanofi-Aventis)
Palonosetron (Aloxi®, MGI Pharma)
Tropisetron (used outside of the United States) (Navoban®, Novartis, Basel, Switzerland)

Note. Copyright 2007 by Multinational Association of Supportive Care in Cancer. Used with permission.

effective than tropisetron in the first 24 hours following chemotherapy. Of note, this meta-analysis did not include palonosetron.

Palonosetron is the newest 5-HT$_3$ receptor antagonist and is considered a second-generation agent in this class. It has a 100-fold higher binding affinity compared to other 5-HT$_3$ antagonists, has a half-life of about 40 hours, and is only available as an IV formulation (Aapro et al., 2006). Two separate randomized studies in individuals receiving moderately emetogenic therapy compared palonosetron to either ondansetron or dolasetron (Eisenberg et al., 2003; Gralla et al., 2003). Each drug was given only once, on day one of moderately emetogenic chemotherapy, despite differences in half-lives between the first- and second-generation 5-HT$_3$ antagonists. Palonosetron resulted in favorable control of delayed CINV compared to both ondansetron and dolasetron, but was only superior to ondansetron and not dolasetron for control of acute CINV (Eisenberg et al.; Gralla et al., 2003). When studied in patients receiving highly emetogenic chemotherapy regimens, palonosetron was equivalent to ondansetron for prevention of acute CINV (Aapro et al., 2006). None of these studies required the administration of dexamethasone on day 1 of chemotherapy. Given that 5% or less of individuals received dexamethasone in the moderately emetogenic chemotherapy trials, it is unclear whether palonosetron would maintain its superiority over ondansetron and dexamethasone if dexamethasone had been administered consistent with antiemetic guidelines. In the trial of highly emetogenic chemotherapy, however, two-thirds of participants received dexamethasone on day 1, and palonosetron maintained its superiority in preventing emesis and rescue therapy both overall (days 1–5) and during the delayed setting. Given the limitations in study design comparing palonosetron with other available 5-HT$_3$ antagonists, none of the available antiemetic guidelines support the superiority of palonosetron over other available 5-HT$_3$ antagonists (Ettinger et al., 2007; Kris et al., 2005, 2006).

Evidence supporting the use of 5-HT$_3$ antagonists as prophylaxis for delayed CINV is inconsistent. Given their superb ability to prevent acute CINV, they commonly were assumed to be effective in preventing delayed CINV as well (Hickok et al., 2005). Although individual studies have documented improved control of delayed emesis with first-generation 5-HT$_3$ antagonists compared to placebo, a recent meta-analysis found the pooled difference to be marginal—only an 8.2% reduction in the risk of vomiting with 5-HT$_3$ antagonists compared to placebo (Geling & Eichler, 2005). Furthermore, first-generation 5-HT$_3$ receptor antagonists were no better than prochlorperazine at controlling delayed CINV in a study of 691 patients receiving doxorubicin in community oncology settings (Hickok et al.). Finally, the addition of a 5-HT$_3$ receptor antagonist to dexamethasone is not superior to dexamethasone alone for prevention of delayed emesis, according to the aforementioned meta-analysis (Geling & Eichler).

Although 5-HT$_3$ antagonists are in common use thanks to their efficacy in controlling acute CINV, several potential side effects warrant attention. A small risk of electrocardiogram (ECG) changes exists, specifically a prolonged QT interval on an ECG (Schnell, 2003). A potential increased risk for ventricular arrhythmias and cardiac arrest was observed with dolasetron but not with ondansetron or granisetron (Schnell). Palonosetron used at the dose of 0.25 mg IV resulted in a lower mean post-dose change in QT interval compared to dolasetron or ondansetron (Aapro, Macciocchi, & Gridelli, 2005).

Numerous other side effects of 5-HT$_3$ antagonists can occur in up to 20% of patients. Headache is a side effect of the 5-HT$_3$ antagonists and typically is more common with ondansetron (Goodin & Cunningham, 2002), although findings are not consistent (Abali & Celik, 2007). When comparing IV palonosetron and ondansetron, headache and constipation generally were rare and occurred at almost identical rates in each drug—4.8% and 1.6%, respectively (Gralla et al., 2003). 5-HT$_3$ antagonists should be used with caution in patients with renal impairment because they could increase their risk of ECG changes (Goodin & Cunningham).

Neurokinin-1 Receptor Antagonists

The U.S. Food and Drug Administration approved the first and only NK-1 receptor antagonist, aprepitant (Emend®, Merck & Co., Inc.), in its oral form in 2003 and the IV formulation, fosaprepitant dimeglumine, in January 2008 (Merck & Co., Inc., 2008b). Aprepitant is different from and complementary to other available antiemetic agents and is approved for use in the prevention of CINV with both highly and moderately emetogenic chemotherapy in combination with dexamethasone and a 5-HT$_3$ antagonist (Merck & Co., Inc., 2008a). Aprepitant works predominately by blocking substance P within the CNS, where most NK-1 receptors are located, in contrast to 5-HT$_3$ receptor antagonists, which block serotonin receptors located predominantly in the gut. The addition of three days of aprepitant to ondansetron plus dexamethasone markedly improved the control of CINV in the first five days following administration of cisplatin-based highly emetogenic chemotherapy regimens (Hesketh, Grunberg, et al., 2003; Poli-Bigelli et al., 2003). Aprepitant particularly was effective in preventing delayed CINV, and its use in combination with dexamethasone resulted in an absolute improvement of up to 21% in complete response rates (no emesis and no rescue therapy) in the delayed setting compared to dexamethasone alone (Hesketh, Grunberg, et al., 2003; Poli-Bigelli et al.). When added to ondansetron and dexamethasone, aprepitant also improved control of CINV and reduced the impact of CINV on QOL in patients with breast cancer receiving AC chemotherapy (Warr, Hesketh, et al., 2005). The addition of aprepitant to ondansetron and dexamethasone maintained superior control of CINV across all four cycles of chemotherapy (Herrstedt et al., 2005).

Aprepitant is available in both oral and IV formulations (see Figure 6-6 for NCCN guidelines and dosing). Aprepitant generally is well tolerated, and its use did not result in a significant increase in adverse events compared to standard therapy in the AC chemotherapy tri-

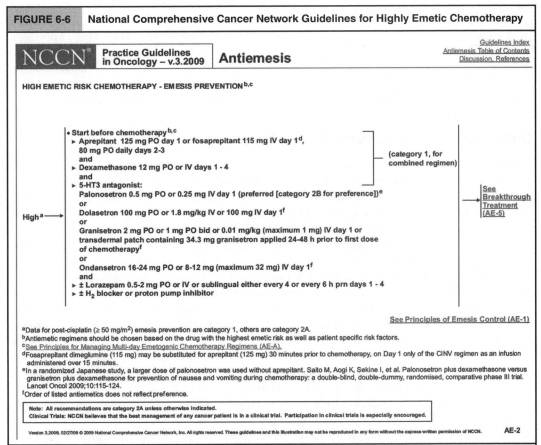

FIGURE 6-6	National Comprehensive Cancer Network Guidelines for Highly Emetic Chemotherapy

Note. Reproduced with permission from *The NCCN (3.2008) Antiemesis Clinical Practice Guidelines in Oncology.* © National Comprehensive Cancer Network, 2008. Available at http://www.nccn.org. Accessed May 5, 2008. To view the most recent and complete version of the guideline, go online to www.nccn.org. These Guidelines are a work in progress that will be refined as often as new significant data becomes available.

The NCCN Guidelines are a statement of consensus of its authors regarding their views of currently accepted approaches to treatment. Any clinician seeking to apply or consult any NCCN guideline is expected to use independent medical judgment in the context of individual clinical circumstances to determine any patient's care or treatment. The National Comprehensive Cancer Network makes no warranties of any kind whatsoever regarding their content, use or application and disclaims any responsibility for their application or use in any way.

These Guidelines are copyrighted by the National Comprehensive Cancer Network. All rights reserved. These Guidelines and illustrations herein may not be reproduced in any form for any purpose without the express written permission of the NCCN.

FIGURE 6-7	Drug-Drug Interactions With Aprepitant

Elevates Plasma Concentrations
- Pimozide*
- Terfenadine*
- Astemizole*
- Cisapride*
- Dexamethasone

Decreases Plasma Concentrations
- Phenytoin
- Warfarin

* Life threatening

Note. Based on information from Merck & Co., Inc., 2008a.

al (Warr, Hesketh, et al., 2005). Use of aprepitant resulted in a slightly increased risk of fatigue or asthenia and hiccups in the highly emetogenic chemotherapy trials (Hesketh, Grunberg, et al., 2003, Poli-Bigelli et al., 2003). More importantly, a number of potential drug-drug interactions can occur with the use of aprepitant (see Figure 6-7). Aprepitant is a substrate, moderate inducer, and moderate inhibitor of the cytochrome P450 (CYP) enzyme CYP3A4 and also induces CYP2A9 (Merck & Co., Inc., 2008a; Shadle et al., 2004). Thus, aprepitant alters the metabolism and the area under the curve of certain medications, such as dexamethasone and warfarin (Ettinger et al., 2007). Effects are more pronounced with oral forms of medications.

Other Classes of Antiemetic Medications

Cannabinoid neuromodulators have inhibitory effects on other neurotransmitters and agonist effects on cannabinoid-1 receptors found in the central and peripheral nervous systems, resulting in antinausea and antiemetic effects (Davis, Maida, Daeninck, & Pergolizzi, 2007). Pharmaceutical cannabinoids approved for use in managing CINV are nabilone (Cesamet®, Valeant Pharmaceuticals) and dronabinol (Marinol®, Solvay Pharmaceuticals, Inc.). In a meta-analysis of 30 randomized studies, cannabinoids were superior to both placebo and conventional antiemetics, such as dopamine antagonists and phenothiazines, for the control of nausea and vomiting (Tramer et al., 2001). Cannabinoids are particularly efficacious for treating refractory CINV (i.e., when patients are still experiencing CINV after standard prophylaxis and treatment) (Davis et al.). A significant barrier to the widespread use of cannabinoids in clinical practice is their side effect profile. Up to 50% of participants receiving cannabinoids in clinical trials reported dizziness, drowsiness, or somnolence; 35% had a sensation of being high; and 25% experienced hypotension (Tramer et al.). In spite of these adverse effects, twice as many patients reported a preference for cannabinoids compared to conventional antiemetics, and cannabinoids were preferred sixfold over placebo (Tramer et al.).

Anxiolytics, such as lorazepam, frequently are used as adjuncts in managing CINV but are not the drug of choice for prevention (Ettinger et al., 2007). Although they do not have direct antiemetic effects, they help to relieve anxiety symptoms that may exacerbate the CINV experience. Individuals experiencing CINV may positively perceive the sedation caused by lorazepam. This class of agents should be used carefully in older adults, given the potential for medication interactions and the propensity for adverse effects such as confusion (Wiser & Berger, 2005).

Olanzapine is another drug for which antiemetic efficacy data are emerging. Olanzapine blocks multiple neurotransmitters. Usually used to treat schizophrenia and delirium, olanzapine has shown promise for managing breakthrough, refractory, and delayed nausea and vomiting when used in combination with other antiemetics (Passik et al., 2002, 2003, 2004). A phase II study of 30 patients receiving olanzapine for four to six days in combination with granisetron on day 1 and dexamethasone on days 1–4 resulted in a 100% complete response rate (i.e., no emesis and no rescue medications) in the acute setting and complete response rates of 80%–85% for delayed CINV (Navari et al., 2005). These strong phase II data warrant additional clinical trials.

Guidelines for Antiemetic Therapy

Given the growing number and complexity of antiemetic agents available for the prevention and management of CINV, the availability of guidelines for their use has become paramount. Three major organizations have guidelines for prevention and management of CINV: NCCN, an alliance of 21 cancer centers across the United States; ASCO; and MASCC. Each of these organizations reviews and updates its guidelines with varying degrees of frequency. NCCN, for example, provides updates as often as one to three times annually depending on evolving data (NCCN, 2008). ASCO updated its guidelines in 2006 to reflect the latest clinical evidence (Kris et al., 2006), and MASCC last updated its guidelines in December 2007 (MASCC, 2008). In order to simplify and standardize antiemetic therapy, these and other national and international organizations met in Perugia, Italy, in 2004 to create unifying consensus guidelines for CINV prevention and management (Gralla et al., 2005).

In an effort to make information regarding interventions for CINV more accessible for clinical use, ONS created a PEP resource for CINV (Tipton et al., 2006, 2007) that lists interventions with varying degrees of evidence for effectiveness. Interventions that are listed under *Recommended for Practice* are supported by data either from multiple randomized clinical trials or from expert recommendations resulting from a comprehensive and critical analysis of the literature. The ONS PEP resource for CINV summarizes antiemetic guideline-based recommendations for pharmacologic therapy, all of which are listed in the category of *Recommended for Practice*.

Antiemetic Guidelines: Highly Emetogenic Chemotherapy

All three major antiemetic guidelines and the Perugia consensus guidelines offer consistent recommendations for the prevention of CINV associated with highly emetogenic chemotherapy (Ettinger et al., 2007; Kris et al., 2006; MASCC, 2008). NCCN's guidelines for highly emetogenic chemotherapy appear in Figure 6-6. All patients should receive aggressive antiemetic prophylaxis with drugs from three different classes: a corticosteroid (dexamethasone), a 5-HT$_3$ receptor antagonist, and aprepitant. NCCN recognizes AC, defined as the combination of either doxorubicin or epirubicin with cyclophosphamide, as a highly emetogenic chemotherapy regimen and therefore recommends the same triple-drug CINV prophylaxis for individuals receiving AC (Ettinger et al.). Although both ASCO and MASCC classify AC as moderately emetogenic chemotherapy, they also recommend triple therapy for women receiving this regimen because of the particularly high risk of CINV in this setting. The NCCN, MASCC, and ASCO guidelines differ slightly for antiemetic prophylaxis with AC chemotherapy (see Table 6-4).

Antiemetic Guidelines: Moderately Emetogenic Chemotherapy

With respect to antiemetic therapy for moderately emetogenic chemotherapy regimens, guidelines show greater variability. All guidelines agree that dual therapy with dexamethasone and a 5-HT$_3$ receptor antagonist on day 1 of chemotherapy should be standard therapy for the prevention of acute CINV, with the exception for AC chemotherapy as previously discussed (Ettinger et al., 2007; Kris et al., 2006; MASCC, 2008). NCCN guidelines are shown in Figure 6-8. In addition to dexamethasone and a 5-HT$_3$ receptor antagonist, NCCN recommends considering aprepitant for select patients receiving moderately emetic chemotherapy, particularly those receiving carboplatin, cisplatin, doxorubicin, ifosfamide, or similar agents (Ettinger et al.). The individual risk factors previously discussed, such as

TABLE 6-4	Summary of Antiemetic Guidelines for Doxorubicin and Cyclophosphamide Chemotherapy	
Guideline	**Acute**	**Delayed**
National Comprehensive Cancer Network (2008)	Aprepitant 125 mg PO Dexamethasone 12 mg IV/PO 5-HT$_3$ serotonin receptor antagonist*	Aprepitant 80 mg days 2 and 3 Dexamethasone 8 mg PO/IV days 2, 3, and 4
American Society of Clinical Oncology (Kris et al., 2006)	Aprepitant 125 mg PO Dexamethasone 12 mg IV/PO 5-HT$_3$ serotonin receptor antagonist*	Aprepitant 80 mg days 2 and 3 alone
Multinational Association of Supportive Care in Cancer (2008)	Aprepitant 125 mg PO Dexamethasone 8 mg 5-HT$_3$ serotonin receptor antagonist*	Aprepitant 80 mg days 2 and 3 OR Dexamethasone 8 mg/day for 2–3 days

* Dose of 5-HT$_3$ receptor antagonist depends on the particular agent used.

age, sex, and pretreatment expectations, can help to guide the selection of patients who should receive aprepitant during the first cycle of moderately emetogenic chemotherapy. For prevention of delayed CINV with moderately emetogenic chemotherapy, both NCCN and ASCO recommend either single-agent dexamethasone or a 5-HT$_3$ antagonist (Ettinger et al.; Kris et al., 2006). If palonosetron is given on day 1 of single-day chemotherapy regimens, it does not need to be repeated in the delayed setting, given its longer half-life. The MASCC guidelines differ slightly in recommending dexamethasone as the agent of choice for delayed CINV prophylaxis and recommend use of 5-HT$_3$ antagonists in the delayed setting only when dexamethasone is contraindicated (MASCC, 2008). Finally, NCCN states that aprepitant may be given alone or in combination with dexamethasone for delayed CINV prevention in those individuals who received aprepitant for acute CINV (Ettinger et al.).

Antiemetic Guidelines: Breakthrough Nausea and Vomiting

Breakthrough nausea and vomiting continues to be a significant clinical challenge. For example, even when patients receiving highly emetogenic chemotherapy are treated with the appropriate triple-drug therapy of aprepitant, dexamethasone, and a 5-HT$_3$ antagonist, 50% still experience delayed nausea or vomiting (Hesketh, Grunberg, et al., 2003; Poli-Bigelli et al., 2003). The overarching principle for managing breakthrough CINV is to give an additional agent from a different class of antiemetic medication, such as metoclopramide, prochlorperazine, or a cannabinoid (Ettinger et al., 2007). Multiple concurrent agents may be necessary. Appropriate medications and their corresponding dosages are listed in the ONS PEP resource (Tipton et al., 2006). If the chosen strategy is effective, the breakthrough medications should be continued on a scheduled rather than an as-needed basis (Ettinger et al.). If control is not achieved, then the clinician should consider changing to higher-level antiemetic prophylactic therapy with subsequent cycles of chemotherapy treatment (Ettinger et al.).

Antiemetic Guidelines: Anticipatory Nausea and Vomiting

Each of the major antiemetic guidelines recognize that the best strategy for anticipatory nausea and vomiting is to use optimal antiemetic therapy to prevent acute and delayed CINV

FIGURE 6-8   National Comprehensive Cancer Network Guidelines for Moderately Emetic Chemotherapy

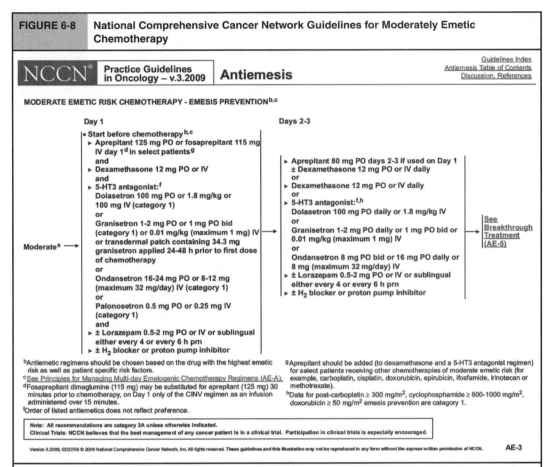

Note. Reproduced with permission from *The NCCN (3.2008) Antiemesis Clinical Practice Guidelines in Oncology.* © National Comprehensive Cancer Network, 2008. Available at http://www.nccn.org. Accessed May 5, 2008. To view the most recent and complete version of the guideline, go online to www.nccn.org. These Guidelines are a work in progress that will be refined as often as new significant data becomes available.

The NCCN Guidelines are a statement of consensus of its authors regarding their views of currently accepted approaches to treatment. Any clinician seeking to apply or consult any NCCN guideline is expected to use independent medical judgment in the context of individual clinical circumstances to determine any patient's care or treatment. The National Comprehensive Cancer Network makes no warranties of any kind whatsoever regarding their content, use or application and disclaims any responsibility for their application or use in any way.

These Guidelines are copyrighted by the National Comprehensive Cancer Network. All rights reserved. These Guidelines and illustrations herein may not be reproduced in any form for any purpose without the express written permission of the NCCN.

in all cycles of treatment (Ettinger et al., 2007; Kris et al., 2006; MASCC, 2008). Once anticipatory CINV develops, it is difficult to manage. For the treatment of anticipatory CINV, each of the three guidelines recommend behavioral and psychological strategies such as systematic desensitization, as well as the use of anxiolytics (Ettinger et al.; Kris et al., 2006; MASCC, 2008). Anxiolytic agents and doses are displayed in the ONS PEP resource (Tipton et al., 2006).

Antiemetic Guidelines: Multiday Emetogenic Chemotherapy Regimens

Patients receiving multiday chemotherapy regimens are at risk for both acute and delayed CINV of prolonged duration, depending on the drug, dose, and schedule of chemotherapy administered (Ettinger et al., 2007). Clear guidelines do not exist for specific antiemetic agents and schedules that should be prescribed for multiday chemotherapy regimens; however, each of the major guidelines provide principles for managing antiemetic therapy in this setting. NCCN and ASCO agree that antiemetics appropriate for the emetogenic risk class of chemotherapy should be administered on each day of chemotherapy and thereafter for an additional two to three days, particularly for those likely to cause delayed emesis (Ettinger et al.; Kris et al., 2006). NCCN recommends a number of additional management principles (see Figure 6-9).

Nonpharmacologic Management

A number of nonpharmacologic options for the management of CINV have been investigated, but none are supported by strong and consistent enough evidence to be classified under *Recommended for Practice* according to the ONS PEP resource for CINV. All nonpharmacologic interventions should used in conjunction with, rather than in lieu of, pharmacologic antiemetic therapy (Tipton et al., 2007). Acupuncture and acupressure, guided imagery, music therapy, progressive muscle relaxation, and the provision of psychoeducational support and information each are supported by adequate evidence and were placed in the *Likely to Be Effective* category according to PEP classification schema (Tipton et al., 2007).

Acupuncture and Acupressure

Acupuncture and acupressure have gained increasing popularity for managing various symptoms related to chemotherapy, including nausea and vomiting. Both modalities involve the stimulation of anatomic points, called acupoints, positioned along designated meridians of the body (Cohen, Menter, & Hale, 2005). Acupuncture involves the insertion of wire-thin needles into the skin at these acupoints, whereas acupressure is performed using noninvasive digital pressure or by wearing an elastic wristband with an embedded stud (Cohen et al., 2005; Ezzo et al., 2005). In Chinese medicine, acustimulation modalities are believed to help restore the body to a state of energy balance. Nausea is thought to result from a disruption in Qi, the energy flow of living beings (Gottlieb, 1995). Use of the P6 (nei guan) acupoint, an area located on the ventral aspect of the wrist approximately three fingerbreadths from the flexor crease (see Figure 6-10), is the most commonly used area for nausea and vomiting control (Ezzo et al.).

A meta-analysis of 11 randomized trials examined the effectiveness of acupuncture and acupressure for acute and delayed CINV (Ezzo et al., 2005). Most used the P6 acupoint, but a few employed the ST36 acupoint. All studies included in the meta-analysis used antiemetic medications with all participants, although not all employed modern antiemetics. Overall, acupuncture reduced the proportion of individuals experiencing acute emesis but did not reduce either acute or delayed nausea, and its efficacy for prevention of delayed emesis was not assessed. Electroacupuncture, which involves passing electric current through the acupuncture needle, was particularly effective for preventing acute emesis (Ezzo et al.). In one trial, electroacupuncture reduced emesis over a five-day period in individuals receiving myeloablative chemotherapy (Shen et al., 2000). In the meta-analysis, acupressure was effective

FIGURE 6-9	National Comprehensive Cancer Network Guidelines for Low and Minimal Emetic-Risk Chemotherapy

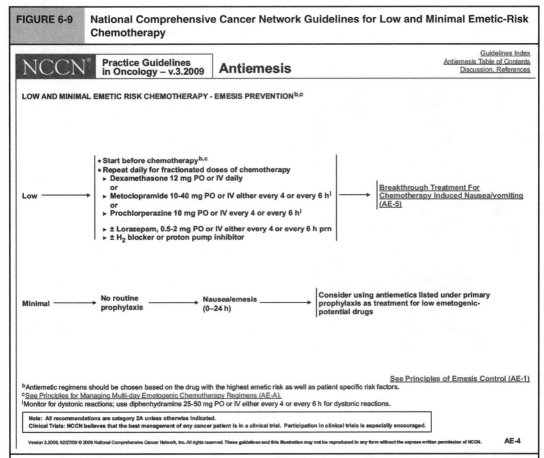

Note. Reproduced with permission from *The NCCN (3.2008) Antiemesis Clinical Practice Guidelines in On-cology.* © National Comprehensive Cancer Network, 2008. Available at http://www.nccn.org. Accessed May 5, 2008. To view the most recent and complete version of the guideline, go online to www.nccn.org.

These Guidelines are a work in progress that will be refined as often as new significant data becomes available. The NCCN Guidelines are a statement of consensus of its authors regarding their views of currently accepted approaches to treatment. Any clinician seeking to apply or consult any NCCN guideline is expected to use independent medical judgment in the context of individual clinical circumstances to determine any patient's care or treatment. The National Comprehensive Cancer Network makes no warranties of any kind whatsoever regarding their content, use or application and disclaims any responsibility for their application or use in any way.

These Guidelines are copyrighted by the National Comprehensive Cancer Network. All rights reserved. These Guidelines and illustrations herein may not be reproduced in any form for any purpose without the express written permission of the NCCN.

for control of acute nausea but not acute vomiting or delayed symptoms (Ezzo et al.). Acupressure reduced both mean acute nausea severity as well as most severe acute nausea. The efficacy of acupuncture or acupressure for controlling breakthrough or refractory CINV is not known.

Since publication of the meta-analysis, a randomized controlled trial of acupressure was undertaken in 160 women receiving moderately to highly emetogenic chemotherapy for treatment of breast cancer (Dibble et al., 2007). Digital acupressure at the P6 pressure

FIGURE 6-10	The Nei Guan P6 Acupressure Site to Control Nausea

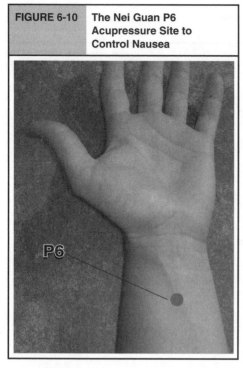

point was effective at reducing both delayed nausea and vomiting and hastening recovery from nausea (Dibble et al., 2007). The study included two control arms, one with antiemetic medication alone and a second with antiemetic medication plus placebo acupressure. Acupressure placebo was not better than the medication-alone arm, ruling out a placebo effect in this study. Based on these findings, digital acupressure can be used as an adjunct to pharmacologic therapy for the amelioration of delayed CINV in women with breast cancer.

Other Complementary Therapies

Guided imagery, music therapy, and progressive muscle relaxation have been examined as adjunctive therapies for CINV and appear particularly helpful for treating anticipatory CINV (Tipton et al., 2007). A meta-analytic review found guided imagery and progressive muscle relaxation both to be effective in reducing nausea, but no conclusion could be drawn about vomiting because of low incidence in these studies (Luebbert, Dahme, & Hasenbring, 2001). A later study, however, found progressive muscle relaxation to be effective at reducing the duration of both nausea and vomiting in 71 Chinese women with breast cancer (Molassiotis, Yung, Yam, Chan, & Mok, 2002). With guided imagery, patients are encouraged to think of a favorite or pleasant place in order to mentally block thoughts of prior experiences with chemotherapy. Self-hypnosis, distraction, massage, and aromatherapy are other methods that may be helpful for controlling CINV, but effectiveness has not yet been established by robust data (Tipton et al., 2007). With distraction, patients can watch videos or listen to music to divert attention from a situation that may cause nausea. Although further study is needed to document the effectiveness of these methods, they appear to have minimal risk and hold promise as complementary therapies for CINV.

Need for Future Research

In spite of the many advances in prevention and management of CINV in the past two decades, further research remains imperative. Research is needed to identify new agents and combinations that will best prevent delayed CINV, a persistent problem. Further research regarding pathophysiologic mechanisms underlying CINV, particularly for nausea, would go far in propelling this science forward. Future research also should seek to better individualize antiemetic management strategies using previously identified as well as yet unknown predictive factors, including potential biomarkers. The ability to tailor CINV management strategies to individuals would markedly improve not only the effectiveness but also the cost efficiency of antiemetic therapy. Finally, failure to integrate best practices for the assessment and management of CINV into individual and organizationwide clinical practice remains a major barrier to optimal prevention and management of CINV. More research is needed to examine the best strategies for promoting evidence-based practices in diverse clinical settings so that all patients can benefit from comprehensive and effective antiemetic therapy.

Conclusion of Case Study

Recall that L.M. has been prescribed the following antiemetic regimen while receiving AC chemotherapy, consistent with guidelines for highly emetogenic chemotherapy (NCCN, 2008). She received the following medications as a plan to both prevent and manage CINV.

- Day 1: Palonosetron 0.25 mg IV, dexamethasone 12 mg PO, and aprepitant 125 mg PO
- Days 2–4: Dexamethasone 8 mg PO daily plus aprepitant 80 mg PO days 2 and 3

The oncology nurse calls L.M. on day 3 to evaluate how she is tolerating AC chemotherapy. She reports that she has had no vomiting episodes and only mild nausea on the day of and day after chemotherapy. Today, however, she has had moderate nausea that is interfering with her ability to eat and which made her stay home from work today. She denies experiencing anxiety. Clearly, additional therapy is indicated. Nausea is more common and more distressing than vomiting and is particularly common in the delayed setting following anthracycline-based chemotherapy for breast cancer, where daily rates of delayed nausea are greater than 60% (Dibble et al., 2007; Stricker & Velders, 2005). Although she experienced no vomiting, L.M. is experiencing moderate nausea interfering with daily functioning despite optimal prophylactic antiemetic therapy recommended by national guidelines (NCCN, 2008). A number of options may be considered for managing her breakthrough nausea, including

- An oral 5-HT$_3$ antagonist as needed
- Metoclopramide 20 mg PO as needed
- Acupressure
- Nabilone 1–2 mg PO BID
- Prochlorperazine 10 mg PO as needed.

However, certain choices are better than others. Appropriate management of breakthrough nausea and vomiting includes the addition of an antiemetic from a different class, such as metoclopramide (a dopamine antagonist) or nabilone (a cannabinoid) (Ettinger et al., 2007). An oral 5-HT$_3$ antagonist would be the least appropriate choice at this time because L.M. received palonosetron, a 5-HT$_3$ inhibitor, on day 1, and this agent has a 40-hour half-life. Metoclopramide would likely be the best choice for L.M. given the potential for CNS and sedative side effects with the use of cannabinoids, particularly because she is trying to preserve her ability to work. A phenothiazine such as prochlorperazine would be another option. Regardless of which agent is chosen, if it is effective it should be given on a scheduled rather than an as-needed basis until nausea has dissipated and should be added to the prophylactic antiemetic regimen with future cycles of chemotherapy (Ettinger et al.). Acupressure at the P6 acupoint also would be a reasonable option for managing L.M.'s delayed nausea and has proven successful at reducing delayed CINV in women receiving chemotherapy for breast cancer (Dibble et al., 2007).

Conclusion

Despite major advances in antiemetic therapy and the availability of complementary thera-pies of varying effectiveness in managing CINV, nausea and vomiting remain two of the most distressing side effects for individuals receiving chemotherapy for cancer treatment. CINV impairs daily functioning and significantly decreases QOL. The primary goal of antiemetic therapy therefore is complete prevention of CINV, and a growing armamentarium of pharma-cologic agents is available to assist in this effort. The appropriate use of the two newest antie-metic agents, aprepitant and palonosetron, significantly improves the control of CINV com-pared to prior therapies, and these agents appear particularly promising when used togeth-er in combination with dexamethasone for regimens of the highest emetogenic risk. None-theless, CINV remains prevalent, and delayed nausea and vomiting are especially problemat-ic. Combination antiemetic therapy covering the entire period of risk is imperative, and the emetogenicity of the chemotherapy regimen as well as individual risk factors should guide the choice of antiemetic medications. National and international consensus guidelines from organizations such as ASCO, NCCN, and MASCC are based on a thorough review of the avail-able evidence regarding antiemetic therapy and should be used to guide decisions regarding optimal CINV prevention and management. Lack of routine assessment of CINV in clinical practice and poor uptake of antiemetic guidelines remain two significant barriers to optimal prevention and management of nausea and vomiting. Oncology nurses can take the lead in efforts to optimize CINV therapy by implementing standards for assessment and management of nausea and vomiting not only in their individual clinical practices but also in their institu-tional standards. Furthermore, oncology nurses should educate patients about comprehen-sive strategies for CINV, including antiemetic medications, dietary strategies, and comple-mentary therapies such as acupuncture and progressive muscle relaxation.

References

Aapro, M.S., Grunberg, S.M., Manikhas, G.M., Olivares, G., Suarez, T., Tjulandin, S.A., et al. (2006). A phase III, double-blind, randomized trial of palonosetron compared with ondansetron in preventing chemotherapy-induced nausea and vomiting following highly emetogenic chemotherapy. *Annals of Oncology, 17*(9), 1441–1449.

Aapro, M.S., Macciocchi, A., & Gridelli, C. (2005). Palonosetron improves prevention of chemotherapy-induced nausea and vomiting in elderly patients. *Journal of Supportive Oncology, 3*(5), 369–374.

Aapro, M.S., Molassiotis, A., & Olver, I. (2005). Anticipatory nausea and vomiting. *Supportive Care in Cancer, 13*(2), 117–121.

Abali, H., & Celik, I. (2007). Tropisetron, ondansetron, and granisetron for control of chemotherapy-induced emesis in Turkish cancer patients: A comparison of efficacy, side-effect profile, and cost. *Cancer Investigation, 25*(3), 135–139.

Alba, E., Bastus, R., de Andres, L., Sola, C., Paredes, A., & Lopez Lopez, J.J. (1989). Anticipatory nausea and vomiting: Prevalence and predictors in chemotherapy patients. *Oncology, 46*(1), 26–30.

Andrykowski, M.A., & Gregg, M.E. (1992). The role of psychological variables in post-chemotherapy nausea: Anxiety and expectation. *Psychosomatic Medicine, 54*(1), 48–58.

Ballatori, E., Roila, F., Ruggeri, B., Betti, M., Sarti, S., Soru, G., et al. (2007). The impact of chemotherapy-induced nausea and vomiting on health-related quality of life. *Supportive Care in Cancer, 15*(2), 179–185.

Bender, C.M., McDaniel, R.W., Murphy-Ende, K., Pickett, M., Rittenberg, C.N., Rogers, M.P., et al. (2002). Chemotherapy-induced nausea and vomiting. *Clinical Journal of Oncology Nursing, 6*(2), 94–102.

Benrubi, G.I., Norvell, M., Nuss, R.C., & Robinson, H. (1985). The use of methylprednisolone and metoclo-pramide in control of emesis in patients receiving cis-platinum. *Gynecologic Oncology, 21*(3), 306–313.

Bloechl-Daum, B., Deuson, R.R., Mavros, P., Hansen, M., & Herrstedt, J. (2006). Delayed nausea and vomiting continue to reduce patients' quality of life after highly and moderately emetogenic chemotherapy despite antiemetic treatment. *Journal of Clinical Oncology, 24*(27), 4472–4478.

Bonadonna, G., & Valagussa, P. (1981). Dose-response effect of adjuvant chemotherapy in breast cancer. *New England Journal of Medicine, 304*(1), 10–15.

Brown, J., Byers, T., Thompson, K., Eldridge, B., Doyle, C., & Williams, A.M. (2001). Nutrition during and after cancer treatment: A guide for informed choices by cancer survivors. [Erratum appears in CA Cancer J Clin 2001 Sep-Oct;51(5):320]. *CA: A Cancer Journal for Clinicians, 51*(3), 153–187.

Coates, A., Abraham, S., Kaye, S.B., Sowerbutts, T., Frewin, C., Fox, R.M., et al. (1983). On the receiving end—patient perception of the side-effects of cancer chemotherapy. *European Journal of Cancer and Clinical Oncology, 19*(2), 203–208.

Cohen, A.J., Menter, A., & Hale, L. (2005). Acupuncture: Role in comprehensive cancer care—a primer for the oncologist and review of the literature. *Integrative Cancer Therapies, 4*(2), 131–143.

Cohen, L., de Moor, C.A., Eisenberg, P., Ming, E.E., & Hu, H. (2007). Chemotherapy-induced nausea and vomiting: Incidence and impact on patient quality of life at community oncology settings. *Supportive Care in Cancer, 15*(5), 497–503.

Cunningham, R.S. (1997). 5-HT3-receptor antagonists: A review of pharmacology and clinical efficacy. *Oncology Nursing Forum, 24*(Suppl. 7), 33–40.

Cunningham, R.S., & Huhmann, M.B. (2005). Nutritional disturbances. In C.H. Yarbro, M.H. Frogge, & M. Goodman (Eds.), *Cancer nursing: Principles and practice* (6th ed., pp. 761–790). Sudbury, MA: Jones and Bartlett.

Davis, M., Maida, V., Daeninck, P., & Pergolizzi, J. (2007). The emerging role of cannabinoid neuromodulators in symptom management. *Supportive Care in Cancer, 15*(1), 63–71.

de Boer-Dennert, M., de Wit, R., Schmitz, P.I., Djontono, J., v Beurden, V., Stoter, G., et al. (1997). Patient perceptions of the side-effects of chemotherapy: The influence of 5HT3 antagonists. *British Journal of Cancer, 76*(8), 1055–1061.

Dibble, S.L., Casey, K., Nussey, B., Israel, J., & Luce, J. (2004). Chemotherapy-induced vomiting in women treated for breast cancer [Online exclusive]. *Oncology Nursing Forum, 31*(1), E1–E8. Retrieved March 8, 2008, from http://ons.metapress.com/content/j2w3070617x1r707/fulltext.pdf

Dibble, S.L., Israel, J., Nussey, B., Casey, K., & Luce, J. (2003). Delayed chemotherapy-induced nausea in women treated for breast cancer [Online exclusive]. *Oncology Nursing Forum, 30*(2), E40–E47. Retrieved March 8, 2008, from http://ons.metapress.com/content/h760703496561442/fulltext.pdf

Dibble, S.L., Luce, J., Cooper, B.A., Israel, J., Cohen, M., Nussey, B., et al. (2007). Acupressure for chemotherapy-induced nausea and vomiting: A randomized clinical trial. *Oncology Nursing Forum, 34*(4), 813–820.

Eckert, R.M. (2001). Understanding anticipatory nausea. *Oncology Nursing Forum, 28*(10), 1553–1560.

Eisenberg, P., Figueroa-Vadillo, J., Zamora, R., Charu, V., Hajdenberg, J., Cartmell, A., et al. (2003). Improved prevention of moderately emetogenic chemotherapy-induced nausea and vomiting with palonosetron, a pharmacologically novel 5-HT3 receptor antagonist: Results of a phase III, single-dose trial versus dolasetron. *Cancer, 98*(11), 2473–2482.

Ettinger, D.S., Bierman, P.J., Bradbury, B., Comish, C.C., Ellis, G., Ignoffo, R.J., et al. (2007). Antiemesis. *Journal of the National Comprehensive Cancer Network, 5*(1), 12–33.

Ezzo, J., Vickers, A., Richardson, M.A., Allen, C., Dibble, S.L., Issell, B., et al. (2005). Acupuncture-point stimulation for chemotherapy-induced nausea and vomiting. *Journal of Clinical Oncology, 23*(28), 7188–7198.

Geling, O., & Eichler, H.G. (2005). Should 5-hydroxytryptamine-3 receptor antagonists be administered beyond 24 hours after chemotherapy to prevent delayed emesis? Systematic re-evaluation of clinical evidence and drug cost implications. *Journal of Clinical Oncology, 23*(6), 1289–1294.

Glaus, A., Knipping, C., Morant, R., Bohme, C., Lebert, B., Beldermann, F., et al. (2004). Chemotherapy-induced nausea and vomiting in routine practice: A European perspective. *Supportive Care in Cancer, 12*(10), 708–715.

Goodin, S., & Cunningham, R. (2002). 5-HT(3)-receptor antagonists for the treatment of nausea and vomiting: A reappraisal of their side-effect profile. *Oncologist, 7*(5), 424–436.

Gottlieb, B. (Ed.). (1995). *New choices in natural healing: Over 1,800 of the best self-help remedies from the world of alternative medicine.* Emmaus, PA: Rodale Press.

Gralla, R., Lichinitser, M., Van Der Vegt, S., Sleeboom, H., Mezger, J., Peschel, C., et al. (2003). Palonosetron improves prevention of chemotherapy-induced nausea and vomiting following moderately emetogenic chemotherapy: Results of a double-blind randomized phase III trial comparing single doses of palonosetron with ondansetron. *Annals of Oncology, 14*(10), 1570–1577.

Gralla, R.J. (2002). New agents, new treatment, and antiemetic therapy. *Seminars in Oncology, 29*(1, Suppl. 4), 119–124.

Gralla, R.J., Roila, F., Tonato, M., Multinational Society of Supportive Care in Cancer, American Society of Clinical Oncology, Cancer Care Ontario, et al. (2005). The 2004 Perugia Antiemetic Consensus Guideline process: Methods, procedures, and participants. *Supportive Care in Cancer, 13*(2), 77–79.

Griffin, A.M., Butow, P.N., Coates, A.S., Childs, A.M., Ellis, P.M., Dunn, S.M., et al. (1996). On the receiving end. V: Patient perceptions of the side effects of cancer chemotherapy in 1993. *Annals of Oncology, 7*(2), 189–195.

Grunberg, S.M., Deuson, R.R., Mavros, P., Geling, O., Hansen, M., Cruciani, G., et al. (2004). Incidence of chemotherapy-induced nausea and emesis after modern antiemetics. *Cancer, 100*(10), 2261–2268.

Grunberg, S.M., Zhang, M., & Zhang, Q. (2000). Hospital service use associated with chemotherapy-induced emesis and nausea for patents with principal or secondary diagnosis of cancer [Abstract]. *European Journal of Cancer, 36*(Suppl.), S28.

Herrstedt, J. (2002). Nausea and emesis: Still an unsolved problem in cancer patients? *Supportive Care in Cancer, 10*(2), 85–87.

Herrstedt, J., Muss, H.B., Warr, D.G., Hesketh, P.J., Eisenberg, P.D., Raftopoulos, H., et al. (2005). Efficacy and tolerability of aprepitant for the prevention of chemotherapy-induced nausea and emesis over multiple cycles of moderately emetogenic chemotherapy. *Cancer, 104*(7), 1548–1555.

Hesketh, P.J., & Gandara, D.R. (1991). Serotonin antagonists: A new class of antiemetic agents. *Journal of the National Cancer Institute, 83*(9), 613–620.

Hesketh, P.J., Grunberg, S.M., Gralla, R.J., Warr, D.G., Roila, F., de Wit, R., et al. (2003). The oral neurokinin-1 antagonist aprepitant for the prevention of chemotherapy-induced nausea and vomiting: A multinational, randomized, double-blind, placebo-controlled trial in patients receiving high-dose cisplatin—the Aprepitant Protocol 052 Study Group. *Journal of Clinical Oncology, 21*(22), 4112–4119.

Hesketh, P.J., Grunberg, S.M., Herrstedt, J., de Wit, R., Gralla, R.J., Carides, A.D., et al. (2006). Combined data from two phase III trials of the NK1 antagonist aprepitant plus a 5HT$_3$ antagonist and a corticosteroid for prevention of chemotherapy-induced nausea and vomiting: Effect of gender on treatment response. *Supportive Care in Cancer, 14*(4), 354–360.

Hesketh, P.J., Kris, M.G., Grunberg, S.M., Beck, T., Hainsworth, J.D., Harker, G., et al. (1997). Proposal for classifying the acute emetogenicity of cancer chemotherapy. *Journal of Clinical Oncology, 15*(1), 103–109.

Hesketh, P.J., Van Belle, S., Aapro, M., Tattersall, F.D., Naylor, R.J., Hargreaves, R., et al. (2003). Differential involvement of neurotransmitters through the time course of cisplatin-induced emesis as revealed by therapy with specific receptor antagonists. *European Journal of Cancer, 39*(8), 1074–1080.

Hickok, J.T., Roscoe, J.A., Morrow, G.R., Bole, C.W., Zhao, H., Hoelzer, K.L., et al. (2005). 5-hydroxytryptamine-receptor antagonists versus prochlorperazine for control of delayed nausea caused by doxorubicin: A URCC CCOP randomised controlled trial. *Lancet Oncology, 6*(10), 765–772.

Higa, G.M., Auber, M.L., Altaha, R., Piktel, D., Kurian, S., Hobbs, G., et al. (2006). 5-hydroxyindoleacetic acid and substance P profiles in patients receiving emetogenic chemotherapy. *Journal of Oncology Pharmacy Practice, 12*(4), 201–209.

Inoue, A., Yamada, Y., Matsumura, Y., Shimada, Y., Muro, K., Gotoh, M., et al. (2003). Randomized study of dexamethasone treatment for delayed emesis, anorexia and fatigue induced by irinotecan. *Supportive Care in Cancer, 11*(8), 528–532.

Ioannidis, J.P., Hesketh, P.J., & Lau, J. (2000). Contribution of dexamethasone to control of chemotherapy-induced nausea and vomiting: A meta-analysis of randomized evidence. *Journal of Clinical Oncology, 18*(19), 3409–3422.

Jacobsen, P.B., Andrykowski, M.A., Redd, W.H., Die-Trill, M., Hakes, T.B., Kaufman, R.J., et al. (1988). Nonpharmacologic factors in the development of posttreatment nausea with adjuvant chemotherapy for breast cancer. *Cancer, 61*(2), 379–385.

Johnson, G.D., Moore, K., & Fortner, B. (2007). Baseline evaluation of the AIM Higher Initiative: Establishing the mark from which to measure. *Oncology Nursing Forum, 34*(3), 729–734.

Jordan, K., Sippel, C., & Schmoll, H.J. (2007). Guidelines for antiemetic treatment of chemotherapy-induced nausea and vomiting: Past, present, and future recommendations. *Oncologist, 12*(9), 1143–1150.

Koeller, J.M., Aapro, M.S., Gralla, R.J., Grunberg, S.M., Hesketh, P.J., Kris, M.G., et al. (2002). Antiemetic guidelines: Creating a more practical treatment approach. *Supportive Care in Cancer, 10*(7), 519–522.

Kris, M.G., Hesketh, P.J., Herrstedt, J., Rittenberg, C., Einhorn, L.H., Grunberg, S., et al. (2005). Consensus proposals for the prevention of acute and delayed vomiting and nausea following high-emetic-risk chemo-therapy. *Supportive Care in Cancer, 13*(2), 85–96.

Kris, M.G., Hesketh, P.J., Somerfield, M.R., Feyer, P., Clark-Snow, R., Koeller, J.M., et al. (2006). American Society of Clinical Oncology guideline for antiemetics in oncology: Update 2006. *Journal of Clinical Oncology, 24*(18), 2932–2947.

Leventhal, H., Easterling, D.V., Nerenz, D.R., & Love, R.R. (1988). The role of motion sickness in predicting anticipatory nausea. *Journal of Behavioral Medicine, 11*(2), 117–130.

Liaw, C.C., Chang, H.K., Liau, C.T., Huang, J.S., Lin, Y.C., & Chen, J.S. (2003). Reduced maintenance of complete protection from emesis for women during chemotherapy cycles. *American Journal of Clinical Oncology, 26*(1), 12–15.

Lindley, C., McCune, J.S., Thomason, T.E., Lauder, D., Sauls, A., Adkins, S., et al. (1999). Perception of chemotherapy side effects cancer versus noncancer patients. *Cancer Practice, 7*(2), 59–65.

Lindley, C.M., Hirsch, J.D., O'Neill, C.V., Transau, M.C., Gilbert, C.S., & Osterhaus, J.T. (1992). Quality of life consequences of chemotherapy-induced emesis. *Quality of Life Research, 1*(5), 331–340.

Luebbert, K., Dahme, B., & Hasenbring, M. (2001). The effectiveness of relaxation training in reducing treatment-related symptoms and improving emotional adjustment in acute non-surgical cancer treatment: A meta-analytical review. *Psycho-Oncology, 10*(6), 490–502.

Martin, A.R., Pearson, J.D., Cai, B., Elmer, M., Horgan, K., & Lindley, C. (2003). Assessing the impact of chemotherapy-induced nausea and vomiting on patients' daily lives: A modified version of the Functional Living Index-Emesis (FLIE) with 5-day recall. *Supportive Care in Cancer, 11*(8), 522–527.

Martin, C.G., Rubenstein, E.B., Elting, L.S., Kim, Y.J., & Osoba, D. (2003). Measuring chemotherapy-induced nausea and emesis. *Cancer, 98*(3), 645–655.

Martin, M. (1996). The severity and pattern of emesis following different cytotoxic agents. *Oncology, 53*(Suppl. 1), 26–31.

Merck & Co., Inc. (2008a, April). Emend [Package insert]. Retrieved March 8, 2008, from http://www.emend .com/aprepitant/emend/consumer/product_information/pi/index.jsp

Merck & Co., Inc. (2008b, January). *FDA approves Emend® (fosaprepitant dimeglumine) for injection, Merck's new intravenous therapy, for use in combination with other antiemetics for prevention of nausea and vomiting caused by chemotherapy.* Retrieved March 8, 2008, from http://www.merck.com/newsroom/press_releases/ product/2008_0129.html

Minegishi, Y., Ohmatsu, H., Miyamoto, T., Niho, S., Goto, K., Kubota, K., et al. (2004). Efficacy of droperidol in the prevention of cisplatin-induced delayed emesis: A double-blind, randomised parallel study. *European Journal of Cancer, 40*(8), 1188–1192.

Molassiotis, A., Coventry, P., Stricker, C., Clements, C., Eaby, B., Velders, L., et al. (2007). Validation and psychometric assessment of a short clinical scale to measure chemotherapy-induced nausea and vomiting: The MASCC Antiemesis Tool (MAT). *Journal of Pain and Symptom Management, 34*(2), 148–159.

Molassiotis, A., Yung, H.P., Yam, B.M., Chan, F.Y., & Mok, T.S. (2002). The effectiveness of progressive muscle relaxation training in managing chemotherapy-induced nausea and vomiting in Chinese breast cancer patients: A randomised controlled trial. *Supportive Care in Cancer, 10*(3), 237–246.

Morrow, G.R. (1992). A patient report measure for the quantification of chemotherapy induced nausea and emesis: Psychometric properties of the Morrow assessment of nausea and emesis (MANE). *British Journal of Cancer Supplement, 19,* S72–S74.

Morrow, G.R., Roscoe, J.A., Hynes, H.E., Flynn, P.J., Pierce, H.I., & Burish, T. (1998). Progress in reducing anticipatory nausea and vomiting: A study of community practice. *Supportive Care in Cancer, 6*(1), 46–50.

Multinational Association of Supportive Care in Cancer. (2004). *MASCC Antiemesis Tool (MAT).* Retrieved October 3, 2007, from http://www.mascc.org/content/126.html

Multinational Association of Supportive Care in Cancer. (2008, March). *MASCC consensus conference on antiemetic therapy.* Retrieved May 5, 2008, from http://www.mascc.org/media/Resource_centers/MASCC_Guidelines _Update.pdf

National Comprehensive Cancer Network. (2008). *NCCN Clinical Practice Guidelines in Oncology™: Antiemesis* [v.3.2008]. Retrieved March 7, 2008, from http://www.nccn.org/professionals/physician_gls/PDF/antiemesis .pdf

Navari, R.M., Einhorn, L.H., Passik, S.D., Loehrer, P.J., Sr., Johnson, C., Mayer, M.L., et al. (2005). A phase II trial of olanzapine for the prevention of chemotherapy-induced nausea and vomiting: A Hoosier Oncology Group study. *Supportive Care in Cancer, 13*(7), 529–534.

Osoba, D., Zee, B., Pater, J., Warr, D., Latreille, J., & Kaizer, L. (1997). Determinants of postchemotherapy nausea and vomiting in patients with cancer. Quality of Life and Symptom Control Committees of the National Cancer Institute of Canada Clinical Trials Group. *Journal of Clinical Oncology, 15*(1), 116–123.

Osoba, D., Zee, B., Warr, D., Latreille, J., Kaizer, L., & Pater, J. (1997). Effect of postchemotherapy nausea and vomiting on health-related quality of life. *Supportive Care in Cancer, 5*(4), 307–313.

Passik, S.D., Kirsh, K.L., Theobald, D.E., Dickerson, P., Trowbridge, R., Gray, D., et al. (2003). A retrospective chart review of the use of olanzapine for the prevention of delayed emesis in cancer patients. *Journal of Pain and Symptom Management, 25*(5), 485–488.

Passik, S.D., Lundberg, J., Kirsh, K.L., Theobald, D., Donaghy, K., Holtsclaw, E., et al. (2002). A pilot exploration of the antiemetic activity of olanzapine for the relief of nausea in patients with advanced cancer and pain. *Journal of Pain and Symptom Management, 23*(6), 526–532.

Passik, S.D., Navari, R.M., Jung, S.H., Nagy, C., Vinson, J., Kirsh, K.L., et al. (2004). A phase I trial of olanzapine (Zyprexa) for the prevention of delayed emesis in cancer patients: A Hoosier Oncology Group study. *Cancer Investigation, 22*(3), 383–388.

Poli-Bigelli, S., Rodrigues-Pereira, J., Carides, A.D., Julie Ma, G., Eldridge, K., Hipple, A., et al. (2003). Addition of the neurokinin 1 receptor antagonist aprepitant to standard antiemetic therapy improves control of chemotherapy-induced nausea and vomiting. Results from a randomized, double-blind, placebo-controlled trial in Latin America. *Cancer, 97*(12), 3090–3098.

Rhodes, V.A., & McDaniel, R.W. (1999). The Index of Nausea, Vomiting, and Retching: A new format of the Index of Nausea and Vomiting. *Oncology Nursing Forum, 26*(5), 889–894.

Roila, F. (2004). Transferring scientific evidence to oncological practice: A trial on the impact of three different implementation strategies on antiemetic prescriptions. *Supportive Care in Cancer, 12*(6), 446–453.

Roila, F., Donati, D., Tamberi, S., & Margutti, G. (2002). Delayed emesis: Incidence, pattern, prognostic factors and optimal treatment. *Supportive Care in Cancer, 10*(2), 88–95.

Roila, F., Tonato, M., Basurto, C., Bella, M., Passalacqua, R., Morsia, D., et al. (1987). Antiemetic activity of high doses of metoclopramide combined with methylprednisolone versus metoclopramide alone in cisplatin-treated cancer patients: A randomized double-blind trial of the Italian Oncology Group for Clinical Research. *Journal of Clinical Oncology, 5*(1), 141–149.

Ropka, M.E., Padilla, G., & Gillespie, T.W. (2005). Risk modeling: Applying evidence-based risk assessment in oncology nursing practice. *Oncology Nursing Forum, 32*(1), 49–56.

Roscoe, J.A., Morrow, G.R., Hickok, J.T., & Stern, R.M. (2000). Nausea and vomiting remain a significant clinical problem: Trends over time in controlling chemotherapy-induced nausea and vomiting in 1413 patients treated in community clinical practices. *Journal of Pain and Symptom Management, 20*(2), 113–121.

Rusthoven, J.J., Osoba, D., Butts, C.A., Yelle, L., Findlay, H., & Grenville, A. (1998). The impact of postchemotherapy nausea and vomiting on quality of life after moderately emetogenic chemotherapy. *Supportive Care in Cancer, 6*(4), 389–395.

Schnell, F.M. (2003). Chemotherapy-induced nausea and vomiting: The importance of acute antiemetic control. *Oncologist, 8*(2), 187–198.

Seynaeve, C., Schuller, J., Buser, K., Porteder, H., Van Belle, S., Sevelda, P., et al. (1992). Comparison of the anti-emetic efficacy of different doses of ondansetron, given as either a continuous infusion or a single intravenous dose, in acute cisplatin-induced emesis. A multicentre, double-blind, randomised, parallel group study. Ondansetron Study Group. *British Journal of Cancer, 66*(1), 192–197.

Shadle, C.R., Lee, Y., Majumdar, A.K., Petty, K.J., Gargano, C., Bradstreet, T.E., et al. (2004). Evaluation of potential inductive effects of aprepitant on cytochrome P450 3A4 and 2C9 activity. *Journal of Clinical Pharmacology, 44*(3), 215–223.

Shelke, A.R., Mustian, K.M., & Morrow, G.R. (2004). The pathophysiology of treatment-related nausea and vomiting in cancer patients: Current models. *Indian Journal of Physiology and Pharmacology, 48*(3), 256–268.

Shelton, S.N., & Ignatavicius, D.D. (1999). Intervention for clients with malnutrition and obesity. In D.D. Ignatavicius, M.L. Workman, & M.A. Mishler (Eds.), *Medical-surgical nursing across the health care continuum* (3rd ed., pp. 1543–1569). Philadelphia: Saunders.

Shen, J., Wenger, N., Glaspy, J., Hays, R.D., Albert, P.S., Choi, C., et al. (2000). Electroacupuncture for control of myeloablative chemotherapy-induced emesis: A randomized controlled trial. *JAMA, 284*(21), 2755–2761.

Shih, Y.T., Han, S., Zhao, L., & Elting, L.S. (2005). Economic burden of uncontrolled chemotherapy-induced nausea and vomiting among working-age cancer patients [Abstract]. *Journal of Clinical Oncology, 23*(Suppl. 16), 541S.

Stein, B.N., Petrelli, N.J., Douglass, H.O., Driscoll, D.L., Arcangeli, G., & Meropol, N.J. (1995). Age and sex are independent predictors of 5-fluorouracil toxicity. Analysis of a large scale phase III trial. *Cancer, 75*(1), 11–17.

Stricker, C.T., & Velders, L. (2005). Predictors of chemotherapy-induced nausea and vomiting in women with early stage breast cancer [Abstract]. *Supportive Care in Cancer, 13*(6), 422.

Tipton, J., McDaniel, R., Barbour, L., Johnston, M.P., LeRoy, P., Kayne, M., et al. (2006). *Putting evidence into practice: Chemotherapy-induced nausea and vomiting*. Pittsburgh, PA: Oncology Nursing Society.

Tipton, J.M., McDaniel, R.W., Barbour, L., Johnston, M.P., Kayne, M., LeRoy, P., et al. (2007). Putting evidence into practice: Evidence-based interventions to prevent, manage, and treat chemotherapy-induced nausea and vomiting. *Clinical Journal of Oncology Nursing, 11*(1), 69–78.

Tramer, M.R., Carroll, D., Campbell, F.A., Reynolds, D.J., Moore, R.A., & McQuay, H.J. (2001). Cannabinoids for control of chemotherapy induced nausea and vomiting: Quantitative systematic review. *BMJ, 323*(7303), 16–21.

Warr, D.G., Grunberg, S.M., Gralla, R.J., Hesketh, P.J., Roila, F., Wit, R., et al. (2005). The oral NK(1) antagonist aprepitant for the prevention of acute and delayed chemotherapy-induced nausea and vomiting: Pooled data from 2 randomised, double-blind, placebo controlled trials. *European Journal of Cancer, 41*(9), 1278–1285.

Warr, D.G., Hesketh, P.J., Gralla, R.J., Muss, H.B., Herrstedt, J., Eisenberg, P.D., et al. (2005). Efficacy and tolerability of aprepitant for the prevention of chemotherapy-induced nausea and vomiting in patients with breast cancer after moderately emetogenic chemotherapy. *Journal of Clinical Oncology, 23*(12), 2822–2830.

Wiser, W., & Berger, A. (2005). Practical management of chemotherapy-induced nausea and vomiting. *Oncology, 19*(5), 637–645.

Zachariae, R., Paulsen, K., Mehlsen, M., Jensen, A.B., Johansson, A., & von der Maase, H. (2007). Anticipatory nausea: The role of individual differences related to sensory perception and autonomic reactivity. *Annals of Behavioral Medicine, 33*(1), 69–79.

CHAPTER 7

Cognitive Impairment

Tamsin Mulrooney, ARNP, PhD, OCN®, CBCN

Case Study

A.M. is a 48-year-old RN who was diagnosed with breast cancer 18 months ago. She received four cycles of doxorubicin and cyclophosphamide every two weeks followed by four cycles of paclitaxel every two weeks. She started daily tamoxifen after her chemotherapy finished. Her menstrual cycle has been irregular since receiving chemotherapy, and she reports that she does not feel as mentally sharp as she did prior to her chemotherapy treatments. She has been forgetting names of people she knows well and has trouble coming up with words she wants to use in conversation. She also finds it difficult to multitask on the busy inpatient surgical unit where she works, and she is very concerned that her performance at work has declined. She is afraid that she may forget something important that could negatively affect one of her patients. A.M. notices she is frequently misplacing items, such as her car keys and her purse. She also is having a difficult time keeping track of the activities of her husband and two school-age children. This is a big change for her, as she always has been able to juggle the demands of home and work life. She finds this very upsetting and asks if anything can be done to help her with these issues.

Overview

Nurses play an important role in helping patients with cancer to cope with the short- and long-term effects of cancer therapy. This chapter will review the literature regarding cognitive impairment (CI) in patients with cancer. The mechanisms thought to play a role in the development of CI will be presented. The pathophysiology of the normal mechanisms of cognition and methods that are used in cognitive testing will be discussed. Treatments for CI will be provided, including interventions with medication, cognitive behavioral therapy (CBT), and helpful tips from patients with cancer who have experienced CI. Finally, suggestions for future research will be discussed.

A growing body of literature is examining CI experienced by patients with cancer (Tannock, Ahles, Ganz, & van Dam, 2004; Wefel, Lenzi, Theriault, Davis, & Meyers, 2004). This CI tends to manifest as a decline in memory, concentration, and multitasking functions and can occur during or after treatment for cancer. Patients with cancer have commonly referred to this experience as *chemo brain* or *chemo fog*, although patients with cancer who have not received chemotherapy have reported the symptom as well. Experts in the field have suggested that the experience be referred to as *cancer or cancer therapy–associated cog-*

nitive change (Hurria, Somlo, & Ahles, 2007), as many other factors could be implicated in the development of this impairment. For the purpose of this chapter, the phenomenon will be referred to as CI.

Early research examining CI focused on children treated for childhood cancers. As a result of such research, cancer treatments for children were adjusted to lessen the damage on cognitive function (Duffner, 2006). The challenges facing children are much different than those facing adult patients with cancer and will not be addressed in this chapter. Instead, the focus will be solely on CI in adult patients with cancer.

Most of the research evaluating CI in adult patients with cancer focuses on women with breast cancer. In more recent years, this field of study has widened and includes research of CI in patients with prostate cancer, brain tumors, and lung cancer, as well as those with hematologic malignancies. Methodologic challenges in this area of research have made it difficult to generalize results to a broader group of patients with cancer. Some of these challenges include small sample sizes and differing methods of testing cognitive function. In addition, statistical analyses have not been standardized across studies, thereby making it difficult to compare and draw definitive conclusions about CI in patients with cancer (Shilling, Jenkins, & Trapala, 2006). Despite these methodologic problems and lack of consistent measurement tools, patients with cancer are reporting that CI is problematic for them. It thus is important to better understand this experience, as it can negatively affect quality of life and potentially interfere with work, educational, and personal goals (Ahles et al., 2002; Mulrooney, 2007).

CI has been found across groups of patients with varying cancer diagnoses. In hematology patients treated with bone marrow transplantation after high-dose chemotherapy or total body irradiation, about 60% (n = 24 out of 40) of the sample were found to have mild to moderate impairment in attention, information processing speed, verbal learning, and memory. Predictors for CI in this sample included fatigue, overall health status, and higher level of education (Harder et al., 2002). In patients with breast cancer treated with chemotherapy, the incidence of CI has been broad, with estimates of 17%–75% of participants having measureable CI on neuropsychological testing (van Dam et al., 1998; Wieneke & Dienst, 1995).

Descriptions and Consequences of Cognitive Impairment

The vast majority of the research on CI in patients with cancer has focused on neuropsychological test results and very little on clinical significance or the impact of CI on the day-to-day life of patients with cancer. In a recent qualitative study that described the lived experiences of patients with breast cancer and CI, 10 women who had been treated with chemotherapy gave vivid descriptions about what it felt like to experience this problem (Mulrooney, 2007). The participants of this study described problems with short-term memory, attention, concentration, word retrieval, and multitasking. These incidents of cognitive failures were unpredictable and could happen several times a day one week and just once or twice in another week. Participants often described CI as being part of a "vicious cycle." For example, they could be in the middle of a conversation and have trouble coming up with a particular word. This would cause a feeling of dread followed by anxiety that would then make word retrieval nearly impossible. Anxiety was described as a component of the experience of CI not only when it was occurring but also when thinking about important things that could potentially be forgotten. CI often resulted in negative consequences both at home and at work. Some of the participants described altered relationships with their families. Family members often would get frustrated and angry with the memory loss experienced by the participants. Changes in employment status also were noted. Out of 10 participants, 2 retired earlier than they had planned, 3 had reduced their workloads, and 2 others had lost their jobs as a result of CI (Mulrooney). This small study provided preliminary evidence that CI can negatively affect quality of life throughout many dimensions of a cancer survivor's life.

Pathophysiology

CI occurring in patients with cancer is believed to be multifactorial. A panel of experts convened in 2003 to discuss the research on CI in patients with cancer. One of the goals of this meeting was to identify the factors that potentially could affect cognitive function in this population. The factors then were incorporated into a model and included endogenous hormones, genetic predisposition, depression, anxiety, fatigue, cytokines, cancer treatment, and clotting in small blood vessels (Tannock et al., 2004). This model provides a useful framework to better understand the complexities of CI experienced by patients with cancer. Each of the factors in the model will now be discussed in greater detail.

Endogenous Hormones: Androgens, Estrogen, and Cognition

The hippocampus is the area of the brain most responsible for memory and learning. It is the area that registers new memories that then are stored elsewhere in the brain (Lezak, Howieson, & Loring, 2004). Because many estrogen receptors are present in the hippocampus, estrogen is believed to play an important role in its function. Estrogen also is believed to affect cognition by preventing cerebral ischemia, enhancing neurotransmitter activity, and promoting favorable lipoprotein alterations (Yaffe, Sawaya, Lieberburg, & Grady, 1998). As the aging process occurs and as women enter menopause either naturally or prematurely because of cancer treatment, estrogen levels drop. As a result of these lowered estrogen levels, cognitive function, in particular memory and learning functions, can decline (Yaffe et al.).

The relationship between testosterone and cognitive ability is not well understood. Patients with lower levels of testosterone are hypothesized to have lower levels of cognition, but the mechanism by which this occurs is unclear. In a literature review, Beauchet (2006) found several studies providing evidence that older men with low testosterone levels scored lower on some tests of cognitive function.

Genetic Predisposition

Some believe the development of CI may be related to a genetic predisposition. Ahles et al. (2003) examined a group of long-term survivors of breast cancer and lymphoma who had been treated with chemotherapy to see if the presence of the epsilon 4 allele of the apolipoprotein E (APOE) gene was associated with a higher degree of CI compared with survivors who did not carry this allele. The presence of this allele has been linked with a higher risk of developing Alzheimer disease as well as CI following head injuries (both single traumatic brain injuries and those injuries sustained with repeated trauma from sports such as boxing or football). Ahles et al. (2003) found that the participants with the epsilon 4 allele scored significantly lower in neuropsychological measures of visual memory ($p < 0.03$) and spatial ability domains ($p < 0.05$) compared with the participants who did not have the epsilon 4 allele. No group differences were found on fatigue, depression, or anxiety. This study provided preliminary data to support that chemotherapy-related CI may, in part, be related to the presence of the epsilon 4 allele of the APOE gene, and research in this area is ongoing.

Depression, Anxiety, and Fatigue

The symptoms of depression, anxiety, and fatigue commonly are found in women with breast cancer before, during, and after cancer treatment (Ferrell, Grant, Funk, Otis-Green, & Garcia, 1998; Ganz et al., 2002; Gelinas & Fillion, 2004; Schreier & Williams, 2004). Bender et al. (2006) found that self-report of CI was associated with depression. Castellon et al. (2004) found that women who reported higher levels of anxiety, depression, or fatigue reported more cognitive complaints than women who did not have anxiety, depression, or fatigue. Some studies assessing cognitive function after chemotherapy found CI even when depression, anxiety, and fatigue were controlled (Ahles et al., 2002; Schagen et al., 2002; van Dam et al., 1998).

Lehto and Cimprich (1999) found that higher levels of anxiety were significantly correlated with poor ratings on a self-report measurement of attentional function (the Attentional Function Index) in women with newly diagnosed breast cancer who were about to undergo surgery. However, anxiety did not correlate significantly with standard neuropsychological measurement of attentional function. In another study, Cimprich (1999) found that the most common symptoms experienced and reported by women with newly diagnosed breast cancer prior to any treatment were insomnia, mood disturbance, fatigue, and inability to concentrate. Greater numbers of symptoms were significantly correlated with lower cognitive function (subjectively rated) and mood disturbance (as measured by the Profile of Mood States). In contrast, Tchen et al. (2003) found no significant correlation between higher levels of fatigue, menopausal symptoms, or poorer quality of life with CI.

Some of the research supports that anxiety, fatigue, and mood disturbance, including depression and insomnia, may have an effect on cognitive function. However, other studies have found no association between CI and these common symptoms that patients with cancer may experience. Insufficient data exist on the relationship between the aforementioned symptoms and the effect on cognitive function and whether better control of these symptoms will lead to improved cognitive function.

Cytokines

Research supports that cytokines may play a role in the development of CI in patients with cancer. Cytokines are proteins secreted by cells of the immune system that help to regulate immunity, the inflammatory process, and hematopoiesis. Interleukins (ILs) and interferons are examples of cytokines that occur naturally and yet can be administered as a type of biotherapy to treat certain types of cancer. Although the naturally occurring cytokines are released peripherally, they can act upon the central nervous system (CNS). The exact mechanism is unclear, but various pathways appear to allow cytokines to cross the blood-brain barrier, travel to the brain, and induce behavioral changes. Dantzer (2001) discussed the term *sickness behavior*, whereby the release of proinflammatory cytokines can induce a decrease in general activity, exploratory behavior, oral intake, and brain stimulation, as well as impair memory and learning. In patients with cancer, cytokines have been associated with the development of many symptoms, including anorexia-cachexia, asthenia, pain, sleep disturbances, mood disturbances, and fatigue (Dunlop & Campbell, 2000).

mor histology, and treatment regimen may play a part in the presence of CI in patients with brain tumors. As with other patients with cancer, age, fatigue, sleep disturbance, depression, and anxiety can influence the degree of CI.

Location of the brain tumor can affect cognition. Patients with frontal tumors scored lower overall on cognitive testing (Kaleita et al., 2004), whereas patients with tumors of the left hemisphere had more depressive symptoms and memory impairment (Hahn et al., 2003). Histology of the brain tumor may or may not affect cognition. Hahn et al. found that patients with GBMs scored lower on tests of psychomotor function and visual scanning compared to patients who did not have a GBM histology. However, Kayl and Meyers (2003) found no differences on neuropsychological testing between patients with GBMs and those with anaplastic astrocytomas.

In patients with brain tumors, treatments with surgery or radiation did not appear to be significant predictors of cognitive function (Kaleita et al., 2004). When evaluating differences between whole brain radiation with or without radiosurgery, researchers found control of disease to be the most important factor in maintaining cognitive function (Aoyama et al., 2007) and that the tumor itself was more detrimental to cognitive function than the treatment.

As with other patients with cancer, certain factors play a role in CI in patients with brain tumors. Neuropsychological testing in these patients showed that younger patients scored better than middle-aged or older patients (Kaleita et al., 2004). Depression, fatigue, sleep disturbance, CI, and pain have been found to be a symptom cluster in patients with high-grade gliomas (Fox, Lyon, & Farace, 2007). Long-term survivors of GBM were found to have significant CI, anxiety, depression, and a decrease in social functioning and ability to work. However, the quality-of-life scores of this group of GBM survivors generally were reported to be good (Steinbach et al., 2006).

Assessment

Domains of Cognition and Standard Neuropsychological Testing

Cognition involves complex thought processes, which can be classified in various ways. The four broad components of general cognitive function include (a) receptive functions, (b) memory and learning, (c) thought processes, and (d) expressive functions (Lezak et al., 2004). *Receptive abilities* are the ways in which individuals receive, classify, and integrate information. *Memory and learning* include the storage and retrieval of information. *Thought processes* include the ability to form concepts and organize information. *Expressive functions* refer to the ability to communicate information. Many steps are necessary for these cognitive functions to be operational. Within each of these classifications are components that can be verbalized and those that cannot, such as visual or sound patterns. The ability to direct attention is necessary for each of these four classes of cognitive functioning to operate efficiently. Neuropsychological testing generally is performed to test levels of functioning in all aspects of cognition.

A typical battery of neuropsychological testing can take up to eight hours to complete, with many of the measures used assessing more than one cognitive domain. Table 7-1 provides an overview of the domains of cognition, the functions associated with each domain, and examples of neuropsychological tests that are used to assess each domain. Global assessment measures are tools that look at many areas of cognitive function and often are used to quickly screen for abnormalities. One such global assessment tool, the High Sensitivity Cognitive Screen (HSCS), can predict (but not measure) how cognitively intact a person will be

TABLE 7-1	Domains of Cognitive Functioning and Neuropsychological Measures	
Domain of Cognition	**Definition**	**Examples of Neuropsychological Tests of This Domain**
Abstract reasoning	The ability to solve complex problems by generating a hypothesis and incorporating feedback that may then modify the problem-solving effort.	D-KEFS Card Sorting Test
Attention and concentration	The ability to not only focus on direct attention to a particular problem, but to ignore extraneous stimuli not required to solve the problem. This domain also includes the ability to multitask, or concentrate on more than one task at a time.	PASAT CPT D-KEFS subtests (Trail Making, Color-Word Interference, Verbal Fluency)
Information processing speed	Refers to how quickly one can internalize and assess information.	PASAT D-KEFS Trail Making Tests Digit Symbol-Coding (WAIS-III)
Language and verbal skills	Refers to both receptive and expressive skills. Enables one to comprehend directions and correctly respond using verbal abilities.	D-KEFS Verbal Fluency Tests WASI Vocabulary subtest WRAT-3 Reading subtest
Learning and memory	The ability to commit new information to memory so that it may be retrieved. Tests assessing this domain will assess both long- and short-term memory function as well as verbal and nonverbal learning and memory.	Logical Memory I and II (WMS-III) Faces I and II (WMS-III) CVLT and CVLT-II
Visuospatial and visuoconstructional	Visuospatial and visuoconstructional abilities include the capacity to process visual features of a stimulus and to coordinate motor output to construct or reproduce visual stimuli.	WASI Block Design subtest
Motor skills	Tests of motor skill assess the speed and dexterity of motor functioning, as well as how quickly the brain can signal the body to perform tasks that vary in complexity.	Grooved pegboard Digit Symbol-Coding (WAIS-III) D-KEFS Trail Making Tests

CPT—Continuous Performance Test; CVLT—California Verbal Learning Test; D-KEFS—Delis-Kaplan Executive Function System; PASAT—Paced Auditory Serial Addition Test; WAIS-III—Wechsler Adult Intelligence Scale, Third Edition; WASI—Wechsler Abbreviated Scale of Intelligence; WMS-III—Wechsler Memory Scale, Third Edition; WRAT-3—Wide Range Achievement Test, Revision 3

Note. Based on information from Lezak et al., 2004.

in six domains of cognition (Fogel, 1991). The HSCS takes approximately 25 minutes to administer and initially was developed to screen for mild delirious states. As it was not developed to detect the changes in cognitive function in patients with cancer, it may not be the most accurate tool to use in this setting.

One of the problems with using standard neuropsychological testing in patients with cancer is that these tests were not developed specifically for the CI reported by this population. Patients with cancer who were functioning at a high level prior to their diagnosis may still test in the normal range, despite experiencing what they would consider a decline in cognitive function. Therefore, such tests may not fully identify subtle changes that an individual finds very meaningful. In a study assessing cognitive function in patients with ovarian cancer who were receiving chemotherapy, researchers found that women with more education perceived memory and concentration declines despite the fact that they tested in normal rang-es on neuropsychological testing (Hensley et al., 2006).

Self-report of CI in the face of normal neuropsychological measures has been associated with depression (Bender et al., 2006; Castellon et al., 2004), anxiety (Castellon et al.; Scha-gen et al., 1999), fatigue (Castellon et al.; Downie, Mar Fan, Houede-Tchen, Yi, & Tannock, 2006), menopausal symptoms (Downie et al.), distress (Schagen et al., 1999; Shilling & Jen-kins, 2007), and self-report of poor quality of life (Shilling & Jenkins). At present, accurate measurement may not be possible for changes in cognition reported by patients with cancer that takes into consideration both objective measurement and self-report. In other studies, patients were found to have CI prior to the start of cancer therapy (Grosshans et al., 2008; Hermelink et al., 2007; Wefel et al., 2004). These results raise more questions about how best to measure this experience in patients with cancer. Until an appropriate tool is developed, the best method for nurses to use when evaluating patients with reports of CI may be to ask them to describe details of their experience.

Radiologic Findings

Aside from patients with brain tumors or as a metastatic workup for acute cognitive chang-es in patients with cancer, use of radiologic studies of the brain is not the standard of care as part of the workup for CI. However, a growing body of research is using such radiologic studies to assess for changes in the brains of patients with cancer. Magnetic resonance imaging (MRI) studies were used to assess the brains of patients with lung cancer who had completed chemo-therapy. The MRIs indicated areas of neuronal loss and demyelination (Ciszkowska-Lyson et al., 2003). Similar abnormal findings of the brain also have been found in patients with breast cancer. Functional positron-emission tomography scans evaluated the brains of women with breast cancer treated 5–10 years prior with chemotherapy with or without tamoxifen and com-pared them with healthy controls. The researchers found significant alterations in the activity of the frontal cortex, cerebellum, and basal ganglia in the breast cancer group (Silverman et al., 2007). Studies using functional MRIs to document for changes in neural activity patterns over time in women being treated with chemotherapy for breast cancer are ongoing.

Interventions

The study of CI in patients with cancer is relatively new. Research to date has focused on documenting the existence of CI and related factors. At this time, very few evidence-based interventions are available to help with the changes in cognition experienced by patients with cancer. Most of the research assessing interventions for CI has focused on patients with breast cancer. Research using pharmacologic interventions to treat CI is limited to poster presentations using medications that have been approved for other uses. Many other inter-ventions are common-sense tips that patients with cancer themselves have identified to help them in coping with this experience. Although they are not yet based on scientific evidence, these tips can be of assistance to those challenged by CI.

Pharmacologic Interventions

Small studies have examined the use of pharmacologic interventions for CI in patients with cancer. However, these studies have not yet been published in peer-reviewed journals and have used medications that are not approved for CI in patients with cancer. One study found significant improvement in memory speed and attention in fatigued patients with breast cancer with the use of modafinil (Provigil®, Cephalon, Inc.), a medication approved to improve wakefulness (Kohli, Fisher, Tra, Wesnes, & Morrow, 2007). Another study found that dexmethylphenidate (Focalin®, Novartis Pharmaceuticals), a medication approved for attention-deficit/hyperactivity disorder (ADHD), improved fatigue levels and memory in patients with breast and ovarian cancer (Lower et al., 2005). However, improvement in cognitive function or fatigue was not found when d-threo-methylphenidate HCl (Concerta®, Alza Corp.), also approved for ADHD, was used in patients with metastatic and primary brain tumors who were undergoing radiation therapy (Butler et al., 2007). Again, these agents currently are not approved to treat CI associated with cancer.

Cognitive Behavioral Therapy

CBT is a form of psychotherapy that is based on the idea that perceptions and beliefs held by an individual affect how the individual feels emotionally about a particular situation. CBT tends to be goal oriented and can be completed in a relatively short amount of time (i.e., over several weeks to months). A form of CBT was found to improve cognitive function in patients with breast cancer who reported CI following chemotherapy (Ferguson et al., 2007). Ferguson et al. developed a CBT-based program titled "Memory and Attention Adaptation Training." This program was delivered to 29 patients with breast cancer who reported CI and were an average of eight years after therapy. Treatment consisted of the use of a workbook, a series of office visits, and telephone contacts to teach participants compensatory strategies to cope with the CI they had been experiencing. The participants were highly satisfied with the treatment, and significant improvement occurred in neuropsychological testing, self-reported cognitive function, and quality of life. This study suggests that intervening with a form of CBT aimed at teaching coping strategies may be helpful to women treated for breast cancer who are experiencing CI.

Patient Teaching Points

Many patients with cancer trying to deal with CI have developed their own coping strategies. The following tips have been provided by patients with breast cancer who participated in a small study evaluating the lived experience of breast cancer (Mulrooney, 2007). Although these tips are not based in scientific evidence, they may be useful to patients with cancer who are experiencing CI.

Common strategies to cope with CI include writing down important information, keeping calendars, using lists and notes to jog the memory, and participating in relaxation activities such as listening to music. Doing "brain exercises" such as crossword and Sudoku puzzles is believed to improve concentration, but again this has not been formally studied. The breast cancer survivors interviewed for this study reported that greater efforts must go into planning certain activities so that memory lapses do not impede the task at hand. Some concrete examples include using lists to go grocery shopping and placing items next to the door if the item would be needed on an outing. Frequently used items such as car keys, pocketbooks, and calendars should be kept in the same place so that they are not lost. The individuals found that keeping detailed notes about work-related activities helped to preserve their competency at work (Mulrooney, 2007).

Self-talk can be an important strategy when anxiety occurs during an incident of CI. Many of the breast cancer survivors in the study stated that if they were experiencing a memory lapse or difficulty finding words, they would talk to themselves, take deep breaths, and tell themselves that everything was all right and that they were doing fine. This would help them to calm down and reduce the anxiety they experienced with an occurrence of CI. Once calm, they could sometimes (but not always) do what they needed to do, whether it be recalling a word or remembering how to drive to a familiar place (Mulrooney, 2007).

A relationship between social support, either through family, friends, or coworkers, and the ability to cope with CI was found (Mulrooney, 2007). Those with little support seemed to keep their struggles a secret. With no one to talk to, they kept their experiences and frustrations with CI to themselves and thus felt they did not cope well with CI. Those who reported having strong support were more apt to divulge to those around them that they were having problems and enlist the assistance of family and friends, and they reported much better coping. Ensuring that patients with cancer have a social support network, either through family, friends, or a support group, may be a helpful strategy for helping them to cope with CI.

In conclusion, research examining interventions for CI experienced by patients with cancer is just beginning. Until more evidence-based interventions are developed, patients can easily implement the tips in Figure 7-1 to improve function. Evidence supports the use of CBT to learn strategies for coping with CI. Patients who experience CI report social support to be helpful as well. Nurses can play an important role in evaluating a patient's support network and can ensure that patients are referred to outside networks, such as support groups, as necessary. Caution should be used when prescribing medications for CI, as some of the studies presented in this chapter have not yet been published in peer-reviewed journals and the medications mentioned have not been approved for use in the setting of CI.

FIGURE 7-1	Strategies for Coping With Cognitive Impairment

- "A place for everything and everything in its place"
  - Make sure you put frequently used items back in the same place all the time. For example, hang car keys in the same place, and keep your purse or wallet on the kitchen counter.
  - If you are going to need to bring something out of the house with you, place it close to the door. For example, if movies need to be returned to the video store, place them in a bag on the doorknob.
- Get organized.
  - Keep to-do lists, and start to rely on grocery lists.
  - Use a day planner or calendar to write things down.
  - Sticky notes may be helpful reminders.
  - Keep detailed notes.
- Keep a journal.
  - Track to see if patterns exist of when cognitive impairment occurs. This may help you to plan accordingly.
  - Monitor the frequency and characteristics of your symptoms, and share them with your healthcare provider.
- Enlist your coworkers, friends, and family to help.
  - Read your journal so that you can identify where you need help.
  - Try to offload some responsibilities, both at home and at work.
  - Have friends call and remind you of plans you have made together.
  - Share your experience with those around you so that they can understand how you feel and what is happening to you.
- Work your mind.
  - Crossword and Sudoku puzzles may help with concentration and word-finding skills.
  - Try to do math problems in your head, like multiplication tables or figuring out the change you will receive when paying for a purchase.

(Continued on next page)

FIGURE 7-1	Strategies for Coping With Cognitive Impairment *(Continued)*

- Work your body.
  - Exercise helps to fight fatigue, which has been associated with cognitive impairment.
  - Exercise can help you to sleep better, which in turn may help with cognitive impairment.
- Take good care of yourself.
  - Use a pill box to organize your medications.
  - Ask your healthcare provider if you can tape record conversations so you do not forget important information.
  - Take notes at healthcare visits.
- Try to fix any underlying problems.
  - Report any depression, anxiety, fatigue, or sleep problems to your healthcare provider to receive the appropriate treatment.
  - Have your blood tested for anemia or thyroid problems.
- Try self-talk.
  - If an episode of cognitive impairment occurs, rather than feeling anxious and upset about it, try to talk to yourself and calm yourself down. Some survivors of cancer have found this helpful, as the anxiety only makes the impairment worse.
- De-stress.
  - Try yoga, exercise, reading, meditation, listening to calming music, and other quiet activities.
  - Laugh!

Note. Based on information from Mulrooney, 2007.

Need for Future Research

The research on CI in patients with cancer is in its infancy with many avenues left to explore. Neuropsychological testing and screening tools such as the HSCS may not be the most accurate tools for measuring CI in patients with cancer. Therefore, measurement tools specifically for CI in this population need to be developed. The relationship between common symptoms experienced by patients with cancer (e.g., depression, anxiety, fatigue, insomnia) and CI warrants further investigation. Better control of the aforementioned symptoms may improve cognitive function, but this has not yet been formally studied. More interventions must be developed to help patients with cancer to cope with this experience. To accomplish this, more descriptive research evaluating the experience of CI is necessary.

Conclusion of Case Study

Recall that A.M. was a patient with breast cancer who, following treatment, has experienced significant levels of CI. The oncology nurse provides a list of helpful tips (see Figure 7-1) that A.M. can use in coping with this change in her cognition. The nurse also refers A.M. to the cancer center psychologist who specializes in CBT to see if learning additional coping strategies may be helpful. The oncologist is notified of the cognitive changes the patient is experiencing and also is informed of A.M.'s hot flashes and sleep disturbances.

A.M. returns to the clinic in four months for follow-up. She has implemented some of the strategies she learned from the oncology nurse and the psychologist and finds she is coping better with CI. She always places her keys and her purse by the door when she arrives home so as not to misplace these items. She has a large calendar on her kitchen wall where she keeps track of her children's extracurricular activities and her husband's travel schedule. She is using lists at work to remember tasks she must accomplish. Her hot flashes are under better control, and she is sleeping better. She thinks that her improved sleep has helped her to concentrate better. Although she does not feel as though she is back to her baseline, she does feel more in control of her life and less fearful of making mistakes at work.

Conclusion

The presence of CI has been found across patients with varied cancer diagnoses. CI tends to manifest as a change in attention, concentration, memory, and multitasking abilities. It can negatively affect many dimensions of a cancer survivor's life. Multiple factors are thought to play a role in the development of CI. These include endogenous hormones, genetic predisposition, depression, anxiety, fatigue, cytokines, clotting in small blood vessels, and cancer therapy, as well as the cancer itself. Debate is ongoing about how best to evaluate patients who report CI, and research examining interventions is sparse. Future directions in this field of research must address how best to evaluate CI, examine the relationships between CI and other associated factors, and develop more treatment options. Nurses can play an important role in identifying patients with CI as well as providing helpful tips and support to patients reporting this experience.

References

Ahles, T.A., Saykin, A.J., Furstenberg, C.T., Cole, B., Mott, L.A., Skalla, K., et al. (2002). Neuropsychologic impact of standard-dose systemic chemotherapy in long-term survivors of breast cancer and lymphoma. *Journal of Clinical Oncology, 20*(2), 485–493.

Ahles, T.A., Saykin, A.J., Noll, W.W., Furstenberg, C.T., Guerin, S., Cole, B., et al. (2003). The relationship of APOE genotype to neuropsychological performance in long-term cancer survivors treated with standard dose chemotherapy. *Psycho-Oncology, 12*(6), 612–619.

Aoyama, H., Tago, M., Kato, N., Toyoda, T., Kenjyo, M., Hirota, S., et al. (2007). Neurocognitive function of patients with brain metastasis who received either whole brain radiotherapy plus stereotactic radiosurgery or radiosurgery alone. *International Journal of Radiation Oncology, Biology, Physics, 68*(5), 1388–1395.

Beauchet, O. (2006). Testosterone and cognitive function: Current clinical evidence of a relationship. *European Journal of Endocrinology, 155*(6), 773–781.

Bender, C., Sereika, S., Brufsky, A., Ryan, C., Vogel, V., Rastogi, P., et al. (2007). Memory impairments with adjuvant anastrozole versus tamoxifen in women with early-stage breast cancer. *Menopause, 14*(6), 995–998.

Bender, C.M., Sereika, S.M., Berga, S.L., Vogel, V.G., Brufsky, A.M., Paraska, K.K., et al. (2006). Cognitive impairment associated with adjuvant therapy in breast cancer. *Psycho-Oncology, 15*(5), 422–430.

Butler, J., Case, L., Atkins, J., Frizzell, B., Sanders, G., Griffin, P., et al. (2007). A phase III, double-blind, placebo-controlled prospective randomized clinical trial of d-threo-methylphenidate HCl in brain tumor patients receiving radiation therapy. *International Journal of Radiation Oncology, Biology, Physics, 69*(5), 1496–1501.

Caraceni, A., Martini, C., Belli, F., Mascheroni, L., Rivoltini, L., Arienti, F., et al. (1993). Neuropsychological and neurophysiological assessment of the central effects of interleukin-2 administration. *European Journal of Cancer, 29A*(9), 1266–1269.

Castellon, S.A., Ganz, P.A., Bower, J.E., Petersen, L., Abraham, L., & Greendale, G.A. (2004). Neurocognitive performance in breast cancer survivors exposed to adjuvant chemotherapy and tamoxifen. *Journal of Clinical and Experimental Neuropsychology, 26*(7), 955–969.

Choi, S.M., Lee, S.H., Yang, Y.S., Kim, B.C., Kim, M.K., & Cho, K.H. (2001). 5-fluorouracil-induced leukoencephalopathy in patients with breast cancer. *Journal of Korean Medical Science, 16*(3), 328–334.

Cimprich, B. (1999). Pretreatment symptom distress in women newly diagnosed with breast cancer. *Cancer Nursing, 22*(3), 185–194.

Ciszkowska-Lyson, B., Krolicki, L., Teska, A., Janowicz-Zebrowska, A., Krzakowski, M., & Tacikowska, M. (2003). [Brain metabolic disorders after chemotherapy in the study by magnetic resonance spectroscopy]. *Neurologia i Neurochirurgia Polska, 37*(4), 783–798.

Dantzer, R. (2001). Cytokine-induced sickness behavior: Where do we stand? *Brain, Behavior, and Immunity, 15*(1), 7–24.

Downie, F.P., Mar Fan, H.G., Houede-Tchen, N., Yi, Q., & Tannock, I.F. (2006). Cognitive function, fatigue, and menopausal symptoms in breast cancer patients receiving adjuvant chemotherapy: Evaluation with patient interview after formal assessment. *Psycho-Oncology, 15*(10), 921–930.

Duffner, P.K. (2006). The long term effects of chemotherapy on the central nervous system. *Journal of Biology, 5*(7), 21.

Dunlop, R.J., & Campbell, C.W. (2000). Cytokines and advanced cancer. *Journal of Pain and Symptom Management, 20*(3), 214–232.

Ferguson, R.J., Ahles, T.A., Saykin, A.J., McDonald, B.C., Furstenberg, C.T., Cole, B.F., et al. (2007). Cognitive-behavioral management of chemotherapy-related cognitive change. *Psycho-Oncology, 16*(8), 772–777.

Ferrell, B.R., Grant, M., Funk, B., Otis-Green, S., & Garcia, N. (1998). Quality of life in breast cancer. Part II: Psychological and spiritual well-being. *Cancer Nursing, 21*(1), 1–9.

Fogel, B.S. (1991). The high sensitivity cognitive screen. *International Psychogeriatrics, 3*(2), 273–288.

Fox, S., Lyon, D., & Farace, E. (2007). Symptom clusters in patients with high-grade glioma. *Journal of Nursing Scholarship, 39*(1), 61–67.

Ganz, P.A., Desmond, K.A., Leedham, B., Rowland, J.H., Meyerowitz, B.E., & Belin, T.R. (2002). Quality of life in long-term, disease-free survivors of breast cancer: A follow-up study. *Journal of the National Cancer Institute, 94*(1), 39–49.

Gelinas, C., & Fillion, L. (2004). Factors related to persistent fatigue following completion of breast cancer treatment. *Oncology Nursing Forum, 31*(2), 269–278.

Green, H.J., Pakenham, K.I., Headley, B.C., Yaxley, J., Nicol, D.L., Mactaggart, P.N., et al. (2002). Altered cognitive function in men treated for prostate cancer with luteinizing hormone-releasing hormone analogues and cyproterone acetate: A randomized controlled trial. *BJU International, 90*(4), 427–432.

Grosshans, D., Meyers, C., Allen, P., Davenport, S., & Komaki, R. (2008). Neurocognitive function in patients with small cell lung cancer: Effect of prophylactic cranial irradiation. *Cancer, 112*(3), 589–595.

Hahn, C., Dunn, R., Logue, P., King, J., Edwards, C., & Halperin, E. (2003). Prospective study of neuropsychologic testing and quality-of-life assessment of adults with primary malignant brain tumors. *International Journal of Radiation Oncology, Biology, Physics, 55*(4), 992–999.

Harder, H., Cornelissen, J.J., Van Gool, A.R., Duivenvoorden, H.J., Eijkenboom, W.M., & van den Bent, M.J. (2002). Cognitive functioning and quality of life in long-term adult survivors of bone marrow transplantation. *Cancer, 95*(1), 183–192.

Harder, H., Holtel, H., Broomberg, J., Poortmans, P., Haaxma-Reiche, H., Kluin-Nelemans, H., et al. (2004). Cognitive status and quality of life after treatment for primary CNS lymphoma. *Neurology, 62*(4), 544–547.

Hensley, M., Correa, D., Thaler, H., Wilton, A., Venkatraman, E., Sabbatini, P., et al. (2006). Phase I/II study of weekly paclitaxel plus carboplatin and gemcitabine as first-line treatment of advanced-stage ovarian cancer: Pathologic complete response and longitudinal assessment of impact on cognitive functioning. *Gynecologic Oncology, 102*(2), 270–277.

Hermelink, K., Untch, M., Lux, M., Kreienberg, R., Beck, T., Bauerfiend, I., et al. (2007). Cognitive function during neoadjuvant chemotherapy for breast cancer: Results of a prospective, multicenter, longitudinal study. *Cancer, 109*(9), 1905–1913.

Hurria, A., Somlo, G., & Ahles, T. (2007). Renaming "chemobrain." *Cancer Investigation, 25*(6), 373–377.

Joly, F., Alibhai, S.M., Galica, J., Park, A., Yi, Q.L., Wagner, L., et al. (2006). Impact of androgen deprivation therapy on physical and cognitive function, as well as quality of life of patients with nonmetastatic prostate cancer. *Journal of Urology, 176*(6, Pt. 1), 2443–2447.

Kaleita, T., Wellisch, D., Cloughesy, T., Ford, J., Freeman, D., Belin, T., et al. (2004). Prediction of neurocognitive outcome in adult brain tumor patients. *Journal of Neuro-Oncology, 67*(1–2), 245–253.

Kayl, A., & Meyers, C. (2003). Does brain tumor histology influence cognitive function? *Neuro-Oncology, 5*(4), 255–260.

Keime-Guibert, F., Chinot, O., Taillandier, L., Cartalat-Carel, S., Frenay, M., Kantor, G., et al. (2007). Radiotherapy for glioblastoma in the elderly. *New England Journal of Medicine, 356*(15), 1527–1535.

Keime-Guibert, F., Napolitano, M., & Delattre, J.Y. (1998). Neurological complications of radiotherapy and chemotherapy. *Journal of Neurology, 245*(11), 695–708.

Knobf, M.T. (2001). The menopausal symptom experience in young mid-life women with breast cancer. *Cancer Nursing, 24*(3), 201–210.

Kohli, S., Fisher, S.G., Tra, Y., Wesnes, K., & Morrow, G.R. (2007). The cognitive effects of modafinil in breast cancer survivors: A randomized clinical trial [Abstract 9004]. *Journal of Clinical Oncology, 25*(Suppl. 18), 494s. Retrieved November 1, 2008, from http://meeting.ascopubs.org/cgi/content/abstract/25/18_suppl/9004

Lezak, M.D., Howieson, D.B., & Loring, D.W. (2004). *Neuropsychological assessment* (4th ed.). New York: Oxford University Press.

Lehto, R., & Cimprich, B. (1999). Anxiety and directed attention in women awaiting breast cancer surgery. *Oncology Nursing Forum, 26*(4), 767–772.

Lower, E., Fleishman, S., Cooper, A., Zeldis, J., Faleck, H., & Manning, D. (2005). A phase III, randomized placebo-controlled trial of the safety and efficacy of d-MPH as new treatment of fatigue and "chemobrain" in adult cancer patients [Abstract 8000]. *Journal of Clinical Oncology, 23*(Suppl. 16), 729s. Retrieved November 1, 2008, from http://meeting.ascopubs.org/cgi/content/abstract/23/16_suppl/8000

Mulrooney, T. (2007). *The lived experience of cognitive impairment in women treated with chemotherapy for breast cancer.* Unpublished doctoral dissertation, University of Utah. Retrieved March 31, 2008, from http://content.lib.utah.edu/cdm4/item_viewer.php?CISOROOT=/us-etd2&CISOPTR=150&CISOBOX=1&REC=9

National Comprehensive Cancer Network. (2008a). *NCCN Clinical Practice Guidelines in Oncology™: Breast cancer* [v.1.2009]. Retrieved November 2, 2008, from http://www.nccn.org/professionals/physician_gls/PDF/breast.pdf

National Comprehensive Cancer Network. (2008b). *NCCN Clinical Practice Guidelines in Oncology™: Ovarian cancer* [v.1.2008]. Retrieved November 2, 2008, from http://www.nccn.org/professionals/physician_gls/PDF/ovarian.pdf

National Comprehensive Cancer Network. (2008c). *NCCN Clinical Practice Guidelines in Oncology™: Prostate cancer* [v.1.2009]. Retrieved November 2, 2008, from http://www.nccn.org/professionals/physician_gls/PDF/prostate.pdf

Reichenberg, A., Yirmiya, R., Schuld, A., Kraus, T., Haack, M., Morag, A., et al. (2001). Cytokine-associated emotional and cognitive disturbances in humans. *Archives of General Psychiatry, 58*(5), 445–452.

Rugo, H., & Ahles, T. (2003). The impact of adjuvant therapy for breast cancer on cognitive function: Current evidence and directions for research. *Seminars in Oncology, 30*(6), 749–762.

Schagen, S.B., Muller, M.J., Boogerd, W., Rosenbrand, R.M., van Rhijn, D., Rodenhuis, S., et al. (2002). Late effects of adjuvant chemotherapy on cognitive function: A follow-up study in breast cancer patients. *Annals of Oncology, 13*(9), 1387–1397.

Schagen, S.B., van Dam, F.S., Muller, M.J., Boogerd, W., Lindeboom, J., & Bruning, P.F. (1999). Cognitive deficits after postoperative adjuvant chemotherapy for breast carcinoma. *Cancer, 85*(3), 640–650.

Schreier, A.M., & Williams, S.A. (2004). Anxiety and quality of life of women who receive radiation or chemotherapy for breast cancer. *Oncology Nursing Forum, 31*(1), 127–130.

Shilling, V., & Jenkins, V. (2007). Self-reported cognitive problems in women receiving adjuvant therapy for breast cancer. *European Journal of Oncology Nursing, 11*(1), 6–15.

Shilling, V., Jenkins, V., & Trapala, I. (2006). The (mis)classification of chemo-fog-methodological inconsistencies in the investigation of cognitive impairment after chemotherapy. *Breast Cancer Research and Treatment, 95*(2), 125–129.

Silverman, D., Dy, C., Castellon, S., Lai, J., Pio, B., Abraham, L., et al. (2007). Altered frontocortical, cerebellar, and basal ganglia activity in adjuvant-treated breast cancer survivors 5-10 years after chemotherapy. *Breast Cancer Research and Treatment, 103*(3), 303–311.

Steinbach, J.P., Blaicher, H.P., Herrlinger, U., Wick, W., Nagele, T., Meyermann, R., et al. (2006). Surviving glioblastoma for more than 5 years: The patient's perspective. *Neurology, 66*(2), 239–242.

Tannock, I.F., Ahles, T.A., Ganz, P.A., & van Dam, F.S. (2004). Cognitive impairment associated with chemotherapy for cancer: Report of a workshop. *Journal of Clinical Oncology, 22*(11), 2233–2239.

Tchen, N., Juffs, H.G., Downie, F.P., Yi, Q.-L., Hu, H., Chemerynsky, I., et al. (2003). Cognitive function, fatigue, and menopausal symptoms in women treated with adjuvant chemotherapy for breast cancer. *Journal of Clinical Oncology, 21*(22), 4175–4183.

van Dam, F.S., Schagen, S.B., Muller, M.J., Boogerd, W., Wall, E., Droogleever Fortuyn, M.E., et al. (1998). Impairment of cognitive function in women receiving adjuvant treatment for high-risk breast cancer: High-dose versus standard-dose chemotherapy. *Journal of the National Cancer Institute, 90*(3), 210–218.

Wefel, J.S., Lenzi, R., Theriault, R.L., Davis, R.N., & Meyers, C.A. (2004). The cognitive sequelae of standard-dose adjuvant chemotherapy in women with breast carcinoma: Results of a prospective, randomized, longitudinal trial. *Cancer, 100*(11), 2292–2299.

Wieneke, M.H., & Dienst, E.R. (1995). Neuropsychological assessment of cognitive functioning following chemotherapy for breast cancer. *Psycho-Oncology, 4*(1), 61–66.

Yaffe, K., Sawaya, G., Lieburg, I., & Grady, D. (1998). Estrogen therapy in postmenopausal women: Effects on cognitive function and dementia. *JAMA, 279*(9), 688–695.

CHAPTER 8

Constipation

Cathy Fortenbaugh, RN, MSN, AOCN®

Case Study

M.L. is a 43-year-old woman who was diagnosed six months ago with stage IV ovarian epithelial cancer. She had a total abdominal hysterectomy bilateral salpingo-oophorectomy (TAHBSO) and received three cycles of paclitaxel and paraplatin. Her last cycle was three weeks ago. M.L. is recovering from a second surgery done one week ago to evaluate her response to chemotherapy treatment. She has been home from the hospital for three days. She has no other medical conditions and has had no other surgeries. Current medications include ferrous sulfate one tablet PO daily, ibuprofen 600 mg PO PRN for headache, and oxycodone and acetaminophen 5/325 mg, two tablets PO PRN for pain. She is experiencing moderate incisional pain at a rating of 6 on a 0–10 pain scale.

She reports taking two tablets of oxycodone and acetaminophen 5/325 mg approximately four to five times a day with adequate relief. M.L. returns to her gynecologic (GYN) oncologist for her first postoperative visit. During the assessment, the oncology nurse sees that M.L. appears to be uncomfortable. Upon further questioning, the nurse learns that M.L. has not had a bowel movement in three days, and her last bowel movement occurred just before discharge from the hospital. M.L. currently is experiencing abdominal cramping. She reports that she is passing flatus at least hourly. M.L. reports that the constipation started postoperatively and that she had a similar problem after the TAHBSO surgery while taking pain medications.

Overview

Definition

Constipation is a common symptom in patients with cancer that causes physical, emotional, and psychosocial distress and has a significant impact on quality of life. Oncology nurses are in an ideal position to proactively and effectively anticipate and manage constipation because they frequently are on the front lines of cancer symptom management.

The definition of constipation is difficult to quantify because the perception of what a normal bowel movement is varies from person to person (Massey, Haylock, & Curtiss, 2003). For example, one patient may not have a bowel movement in two days and perceive this to be constipation, whereas that same pattern may be another patient's usual bowel elimination. In general, constipation can be defined as the difficult, infrequent passage of hard stool associated with abdominal cramping and rectal pain or discomfort (Kuck & Ricciardi, 2005). Using this definition, constipation has four main characteristics: (a) infrequent timing of bowel movements, (b) hard stool, (c) sensation of abdominal bloating or cramping, and (d) straining with bowel movements causing rectal pain.

Feeling of incomplete evacuation after a bowel movement is another common component of constipation (Massey et al., 2003). If fecal impaction is present, liquid stool sometimes will ooze around the impaction, causing incontinence (Kuck & Ricciardi, 2005). A normal bowel pattern is defined as at least three stools per week and no more than three stools per day (National Cancer Institute [NCI], 2007).

Incidence

The incidence of constipation in patients with cancer also is difficult to quantify because this symptom is subjective. In one study, 40% of adult patients with cancer from 15 community oncology clinics participating in the AIM (Assessment, Information, Management) Higher Initiative reported experiencing constipation during their most recent chemotherapy cycle. The AIM Higher Initiative was a quality improvement program intended to improve symptom assessment, information distribution, and management of five chemotherapy-related symptom areas: anemia, neutropenia, nausea and vomiting, diarrhea and constipation, and anxiety and depression (Johnson, Moore, & Fortner, 2007). In another study, researchers estimated that 70%–100% of hospitalized patients with cancer had a problem with constipation (McMillan, 2002).

Patients with cancer in other settings also experience a high incidence of constipation. Studies using hospice patients with cancer have reported varying incidences of constipation at 24%–84% (McMillan, 2002). The incidence of constipation is as high as 40%–50% in studies using patients who were referred for palliative care (Plaisance & Ellis, 2002; Vanegas, Ripamonti, Sbanotto, & De Conno, 1998).

Risk Factors and Etiology

One of the best approaches to management of constipation is to anticipate and prevent it before it occurs, whenever possible. Oncology nurses should have a good understanding of the risk factors related to constipation in individuals with cancer in order to identify patients who are at risk and to initiate measures to prevent or lessen constipation effects. Patient and caregiver education is an essential component of this process.

Formal risk assessment evaluates patients who are at risk for developing a symptom prior to treatment (Ropka, Padilla, & Gillespie, 2005). Documenting risk factors in patients will likely increase the oncology team's awareness and provide a rationale for interventions (Johnson et al., 2007). Common factors that contribute to constipation in the general population include altered bowel habits, inadequate fluid intake, inadequate fiber in the diet, lack of exercise, lack of privacy, older age, and comorbidities causing debilitation (Kuck & Ricciardi, 2005; NCI, 2007). Many of the factors likely to cause constipation in the general population have a similar effect on the development of constipation in patients with cancer. The most common risk factors in patients with cancer are inadequate fluid intake and opioid analgesics (Polovich, White, & Kelleher, 2005). In addition, other specific risks for constipation in patients with cancer fit into the following five different categories.

- A symptom of the cancer itself: Tumor or malignant ascites fluid can press on and partially or totally occlude the bowel. For example, this is common in patients with ovarian cancer who develop peritoneal metastasis. In patients with small cell lung cancer, altered nervous system function, such as paraneoplastic autonomic neuropathy, can occur. Patients with advanced breast or prostate cancer or other cancers may develop spinal cord compression, and if spinal cord injury is present, it leads to bowel atony. Constipation can occur as a result of this oncologic emergency (Kuck & Ricciardi, 2005; NCI, 2007).

- Cancer-related immobility, dehydration, and paralysis could decrease peristalsis, which leads to constipation (Kuck & Ricciardi, 2005; NCI, 2007).
- A side effect or complication of cancer therapy: Being treated for cancer with surgery, chemotherapy, or radiation is a risk factor for developing constipation (Kuck & Ricciardi, 2005; NCI, 2007). For example, radiation to the anorectal area can lead to fibrosis, change innervation to the rectum or anal sphincter, and result in constipation (Massey et al., 2003). Depression and anxiety from the cancer treatment can lead to immobility, which can cause constipation because of decreased peristalsis (Polovich et al., 2005).
- Medications used to manage cancer-related symptoms, such as opioid analgesics, antiemetics, antihistamines, tricyclic antidepressants, and aluminum antacids, can lead to constipation (Kuck & Ricciardi, 2005; NCI, 2007).
- Preexisting issues such as hemorrhoids, laxative abuse, and other comorbidities are additional risk factors (Kuck & Ricciardi, 2005; NCI, 2007).

Pathophysiology

To understand the pathophysiology of constipation, an understanding of normal bowel function is important. Basically, the body is designed to take in fuel in the form of food and discharge it in the form of stool. The intestines are divided into the small intestine (the duodenum, jejunum, and ileum), which absorbs nutrients from food, and the large intestine (the ascending, transverse, and descending colon and the rectum), which absorbs water from digested food and forms stool. Figure 8-1 illustrates the anatomy of the small and large intestines. Gastric contents spend two to four hours in the small intestine and 24–48

| FIGURE 8-1 | The Human Digestive System |

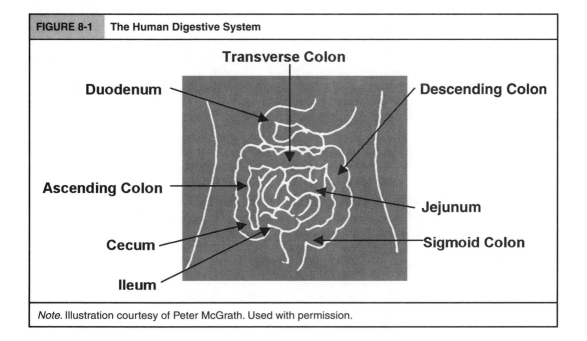

Note. Illustration courtesy of Peter McGrath. Used with permission.

hours traveling through the colon. Approximately seven liters of fluid is secreted into the intestines each day, and about 1.5 liters of dietary fluid passes through each day. The jejunum and the rest of the small bowel absorb most of the fluid. Only about one liter of fluid enters the colon. The average water content in the stool is about 200 ml. The colon plays a crucial role in fine-tuning fluid absorption. Nerves and muscles in the rectum and anus help to facilitate normal bowel movements. In addition, rhythmic contractions of the colon and abdominal muscles play a part in moving stools toward the rectum. When stool enters the rectum, nerves relay the signal that the bowels can be emptied. Usually, this action can be delayed until the appropriate privacy can be maintained (Sykes, 2006).

Decreased motility of the large intestine largely contributes to constipation. For example, as innervation to the colon decreases, the motility in the colon also decreases, slowing the movement of stool through the colon and increasing the absorption of fluid. Other physical factors include altered strength of contractions within the intestines, poor muscle tone within the colon, and sensory changes within the rectum and anus (Polovich et al., 2005).

Many causes of constipation exist in patients with cancer, and each one affects different portions of normal bowel function. Major causes include diet, decreased activity, medications, scarring from cancer treatments, compression from tumor or ascites, bowel disorders, neuromuscular disorders, metabolic disorders, distress, and environmental factors (NCI, 2007). Having adequate fluid and fiber in the diet is essential to normal bowel function. Many reasons can account for decreased fluid or fiber intake, ranging from side effects of treatments such as chemotherapy and radiation (e.g., nausea and vomiting, taste changes, anorexia, fatigue, mucositis) to baseline inadequate diet. These factors frequently are interrelated in patients with cancer. Decreased oral intake slows down peristalsis because less fluid-absorbing bulk will be moving through the intestines (NCI, 2007). With decreased intake, fewer stools occur, the transit time increases, and the stool is hard and difficult to eliminate (Polovich et al., 2005).

As previously mentioned, decreased activity adversely affects constipation. For example, decreased activity can be caused by cancer or treatment-related effects and other comorbidities, such as diabetes, which actually causes fatigue, peripheral neuropathy, and spinal cord compression or injury to T8-L3, which are physical causes of immobility (Kuck & Ricciardi, 2005).

Many different classes of medications cause constipation, including chemotherapy. For example, vinca alkaloids such as vincristine, vinblastine, and vinorelbine cause autonomic nerve dysfunction. Rectal emptying is affected because afferent and efferent pathways from the sacral cord are affected. In addition, vincristine and vinblastine cause neurotoxicity to the gastrointestinal tract causing decreased colonic transit time, which leads to decreased peristalsis or paralytic ileus (Polovich et al., 2005). The next most common chemotherapeutic agents that cause constipation are the taxanes, including paclitaxel, docetaxel, oxaliplatin, and thalidomide (Polovich et al.).

Opioid analgesics, sedatives, antiemetics, phenothiazines, calcium and aluminum antacids, diuretics, iron, calcium, and antidepressants are all medications commonly taken by patients with cancer. Opioid analgesics act directly on mu receptor sites in the intestine and the central nervous system to delay gastric emptying and decrease peristalsis. The severity of constipation is dose dependent. The higher the opioid dose, the greater the severity of constipation will be if it is not adequately prevented or managed (Massey et al., 2003; Woolery et al., 2008). General anesthesia and pudendal blocks contribute to constipation (NCI, 2007). Figure 8-2 is a list of medications that can cause constipation.

Treatments causing scarring to the bowel, such as radiation therapy or surgical anastomosis, can be expected to contribute to constipation because of narrowing of the bowel lumen

(Kuck & Ricciardi, 2005; NCI, 2007). Compression to the bowel comes from a tumor either inside or outside the bowel lumen or from ascites fluid (Kuck & Ricciardi; NCI). Bowel disorders generally are preexisting conditions, such as irritable colon or diverticulitis. Neuromuscular disorders interrupting bowel innervation leading to bowel atony can be the result of spinal cord injury or compression and stroke. Weak abdominal muscles also can lead to bowel atony (Kuck & Ricciardi; NCI).

Metabolic disorders leading to constipation include hypothyroidism, lead poisoning, uremia, dehydration, hypercalcemia, hypokalemia, and hyponatremia (Kuck & Ricciardi, 2005; NCI, 2007). Depression and anxiety are contributing factors in constipation, as are other forms of distress, because they can lead to inactivity, which decreases peristalsis and leads to constipation (Kuck & Ricciardi; NCI). Environmental factors include the proximity of the patient to the bathroom, the patient's need for assistance in getting to the bathroom, an unfamiliar environment, inadequate lighting, change in bathroom habits such as use of the commode or bedpan, lack of privacy in the bathroom, and excessive temperatures (Kuck & Ricciardi; NCI).

FIGURE 8-2	Classes of Medications That Cause Constipation

- Chemotherapeutic agents
  - Vincristine
  - Vinblastine
  - Vinorelbine
  - Paclitaxel
  - Docetaxel
  - Oxaliplatin
- Opioid analgesics
- Sedatives
- Antiemetics
- Phenothiazines
- Calcium and aluminum antacids
- Diuretics
- Iron
- Calcium
- Antidepressants

Note. Based on information from Kuck & Ricciardi, 2005.

Assessment

Although constipation is a common problem for patients with cancer, the symptom is underassessed and underreported by the healthcare team (McMillan, 2002). Underassessment of constipation can lead to the development of or increase in severity of a largely preventable symptom. Oncology nurses need to be skilled in assessment of constipation to effectively manage this troublesome symptom.

Assessment of constipation is achieved through a thorough history and physical examination. The first step in the assessment of a patient with constipation is for the nurse to take a thorough constipation history. To obtain a complete history, the nurse asks questions such as whether risk factors are present. Next, if constipation is present, determining what has changed from the usual bowel pattern is important. Has the frequency of stool changed? Is the stool hard or soft? Is abdominal cramping present? Is there an increased use of laxatives? Does the patient have rectal fissures, abscesses, or hemorrhoids? If any of these are present, are they painful?

Next, the oncology nurse inquires about factors that might contribute to constipation, such as fluid and fiber intake and activity level of the patient, because each one of these changes can be easily modified. In addition, the nurse must assess the patient's perception of the experience. Is the patient tense or anxious? Does the patient appear depressed? Does he or she perceive incomplete evacuation specifically of stool following a bowel movement? Is rectal pain present? What impact has constipation had on the individual's activities of daily living? What other symptoms are present, such as anorexia or nausea and vomiting?

Pain assessment can serve as a template for constipation assessment. Just as with pain assessment, clinicians must note the characteristics of constipation, such as onset, frequency, and severity and precipitating, aggravating, and relieving factors. What interventions worked in the past when the patient was constipated? If diarrhea is present, the patient should be assessed for fecal impaction (Kuck & Ricciardi, 2005). A three-day dietary history is helpful in assessing the patient's current diet. Consultation with a dietitian can be a helpful addition to the assessment process of a patient with constipation (Bisanz et al., 2007). Figure 8-3 presents questions that nurses can ask patients to assess for constipation.

FIGURE 8-3	Constipation Patient Assessment Questions

- What is the usual frequency, amount, and timing of your bowel movements?
- When was your last bowel movement?
- Are you experiencing any abdominal pain or discomfort, cramping, nausea or vomiting, excessive gas, or rectal fullness?
- Do you normally use any laxatives, stool softeners, or enemas?
- What do you usually do for constipation?
- What type of diet do you follow?
- What type and how much fluid do you take each day?
- What are your usual activities?
- What are the doses and frequency of your medications?

Note. Based on information from National Cancer Institute, 2007.

Once a history has been taken, the nurse should perform a patient examination. The typical physical examination related to constipation includes inspection, auscultation, palpation, percussion, and examination. Inspection of the abdomen includes checking for symmetry, contour, distention, bulges, and peristaltic waves. Auscultation of bowel sounds includes noting the character, frequency, and presence or absence of bowel sounds in all four quadrants of the abdomen. Hypoactive bowel sounds include a reduction in the loudness, tone, or regularity of the sounds and can indicate a slowing of intestinal activity. Hypoactive bowel sounds are normal during sleep and also occur normally for a short time after abdominal surgery. Decreased bowel sounds often indicate constipation. Absent bowel sounds can indicate paralytic ileus, which is a potentially life-threatening problem for patients.

Hyperactive bowel sounds reflect an increase in intestinal activity. This sometimes can occur with diarrhea and after the patient has eaten. Palpation of the abdomen includes noting any masses or stool in the colon or any areas of increased tenderness or resistance. If resistance is present, the abdomen would feel firm instead of pliable. Abdominal tenderness and muscular resistance can be associated with chronic constipation. Deep palpation can be used to detect abdominal masses, including sausage-shaped fecal material in the left colon. A feces-filled colon can indicate the presence of constipation. Percussion involves checking for dullness in an otherwise tympanic area of the abdomen, as dullness is heard over areas with abdominal fluid or stool present. Rectal examination can be performed with caution to check for fecal impaction, hemorrhoids, or fissures in patients with adequate neutrophil counts of $1,500/mm^3$ and platelet counts of $150,000/mm^3$. Report changes such as abdominal distention, fecal impaction, bleeding, and absent bowel sounds (Fortenbaugh & Rummel, 2007; Kuck & Ricciardi, 2005). The tool in Table 8-1 (NCI Cancer Therapy Evaluation Program Common Terminology Criteria for Adverse Events for constipation) provides clinicians with assessment criteria to grade constipation severity and common language for de-

TABLE 8-1	Common Terminology Criteria for Adverse Events for Constipation				
Adverse Event	**Grade**				
	1	**2**	**3**	**4**	**5**
Constipation	Occasional or intermittent symptoms; occasional use of stool softeners, laxatives, dietary modification, or enema	Persistent symptoms with regular use of laxatives or enemas; limiting instrumental ADL	Obstipation with manual evacuation indicated; limiting self care ADL	Life-threatening consequences; urgent intervention indicated	Death

Definition: A disorder characterized by irregular and infrequent or difficult evacuation of the bowels. ADL—activities of daily living

Note. From *Common Toxicity Criteria for Adverse Events* (Version 4.0), by National Cancer Institute Cancer Therapy Evaluation Program, 2009. Retrieved July 24, 2009, from http://ctep.cancer.gov/protocolDevelopment/electronic_applications/docs/ctcaev4.pdf.

scribing symptoms. This tool can help nurses to determine types of interventions that are needed based on the severity of the toxicity. For example, level one indicates the preventive need for a stool softener and dietary interventions; level two indicates that constipation is possible or present requiring a laxative; level three indicates a serious event, such as obstipation, requiring intervention such as manual evacuation; and level four is a serious life-threatening event requiring immediate attention (Massey et al., 2003). Figure 8-4 lists expected patient outcomes related to the management of constipation.

FIGURE 8-4	Expected Outcomes

- The patient will report a normal pattern of bowel functioning, such as no less than three stools a week and no more than three stools a day.
- The patient and significant others will identify the need to contact the healthcare provider when self-care measures are ineffective.
- The patient is able to manage and titrate medications for constipation as instructed.
- The patient and significant others will identify and manage risk factors that affect constipation, such as diet, stress, lack of privacy, physical activity, and neurogenic conditions.
- The patient will not experience any adverse effects or complications of constipation.
- The patient will engage in usual activities.

Note. Based on information from Kuck & Ricciardi, 2005.

Management and Evidence-Based Interventions

The Oncology Nursing Society (ONS) published a scientific review for constipation in its Putting Evidence Into Practice (PEP) resources (Bisanz et al., 2007) (see www.ons.org/outcomes/volume2/constipation.shtml). Interventions for constipation were grouped into categories: *Recommended for Practice* (for which no interventions existed at the time of the PEP literature search), *Likely to Be Effective, Benefits Balanced With Harms, Effectiveness Not Established, Not Recommended for Practice,* and *Expert Opinion.* Figure 8-5 is a summary of the interventions in the *Likely to Be Effective* and *Expert Opinion* categories.

FIGURE 8-5	Management of Constipation

Likely to Be Effective

Interventions for which effectiveness has been demonstrated by supportive evidence from a single rigorously conducted controlled trial, consistent supportive evidence from well-designed controlled trials using small samples, or guidelines developed from evidence and supported by expert opinion

• Opioid-Induced Constipation: Prophylactic Regimen

   A proactive approach, including initiation of a prophylactic regimen, is needed to prevent constipation when taking opioids. However, not enough evidence exists to identify the most effective regimen (see *Expert Opinion* section).

• Opioid-Induced Constipation: Opioid Rotation

   Research has demonstrated that some opioids have less constipating effect than others, and rotating opioids would decrease the associated side effects.

   – Switching opioids from sustained-release oral morphine to transdermal fentanyl patches may decrease constipation.

   – Switching opioids to methadone may result in a reduction in laxative use.

• Refractory Constipation in Adults

   The National Comprehensive Cancer Network recommends the use of polyethylene glycol (PEG) as a treatment alternative for patients with cancer with persistent constipation. Standard-dose PEG with electrolytes in the United States is known as Golytely® (Braintree Laboratories) and Colyte® (Schwarz Pharma). Low-dose PEG, referred to as PEG 3350, is available without electrolytes in the United States and is marketed as Miralax® (Schering-Plough). Stimulant or osmotic laxatives are effective in improving bowel function in patients with cancer with persistent constipation and/or at the end of life, and some patients may need both types of laxatives to achieve optimal results.

Expert Opinion

Low-risk interventions that are (1) consistent with sound clinical practice, (2) suggested by an expert in a peer-reviewed publication (journal or book chapter), and (3) for which limited evidence exists. An expert is an individual who has authored articles published in a peer-reviewed journal in the domain of interest.

Special Note: Myelosuppressed Patients

Avoid rectal agents and/or manipulation (i.e., rectal examinations, suppositories, and enemas) in myelosuppressed patients. These actions can lead to development of bleeding, anal fissures, or abscesses. In addition, avoid manipulation of the stoma of neutropenic patients.

General Constipation (Both Adult and Pediatric)

• Prevention

   – Take preventive measures in anticipation for patients receiving medications such as vincristine, vinblastine, vinorelbine, or other chemotherapies that slow colonic transit times.

• Interventions

   – Teach the patient about bowel function.

   – Provide a comfortable, quiet, private environment for defecating.

   – Provide a toilet, bedside commode, and any necessary assistive devices. Avoid the use of a bedpan when possible.

   – Minimize use of constipating medications whenever possible.

   – Involve the patient in development of a bowel regimen.

   – Encourage the intake of warm or hot fluids.

Opioid-Induced Constipation

• Stimulant Laxatives Plus Stool Softener

   This combination is recommended when initiating opioid therapy. A useful bowel regimen includes docusate sodium (100–300 mg/day) along with senna (two to six tablets twice a day). Bulk laxatives are not recommended for opioid-induced constipation because of the risk of bowel impaction in poorly hydrated patients.

   – The laxative dose should be individually titrated for effectiveness according to bowel functions, not opioid dosing.

(Continued on next page)

FIGURE 8-5 | **Management of Constipation** *(Continued)*

Constipation in Adults
- Pharmacologic Interventions
  - Prokinetic medication (i.e., metoclopramide) should be reserved for use in individuals with severe constipation and those resistant to bowel programs. Caution: Avoid in patients with large abdominal tumors or bowel obstruction.
  - Oral mineral oil is effective for hard stool but should not be used for routine prevention of constipation because it may interfere with absorption of some nutrients.
  - Expert opinion supports the use of a stimulant laxative plus a stool softener in preventing and managing constipation in patients at the end of life.
- Nonpharmacologic Interventions
  - Recommended fluid intake per day is eight 8-oz servings in adults.
  - Treat high and low impactions differently.
  - High impactions: These are comfortably relieved with low-volume (< 300 ml) milk and molasses enemas up to four times per day along with an oral laxative. For enema recipe, see definition table at www.ons .org/outcomes.
  - Low impactions: Oil-retention enemas soften hard stool. In nonmyelosuppressed patients, stool can be manually disimpacted followed by enemas of choice.
- Individualized Bowel Management Program
  - After the patient has gone three days without a bowel movement, initiate a bowel management program.
  - A good program includes fluids, fiber, and a decrease in constipating medications or provision of medications to offset constipating side effects of medications.

Constipation in Pediatric Patients
- Pharmacologic Interventions
  - Disimpaction can be achieved with either oral or rectal medications, including enemas in age-appropriate children.
- Nonpharmacologic Interventions
  - A balanced diet containing whole grains, fruits, and vegetables is recommended as part of the treatment of constipation.

Note. From *Putting Evidence Into Practice: Constipation,* by A. Bisanz, M. Woolery, H.F. Lyons, L. Gaido, M.C. Yenulevich, and S. Fulton, 2007, Pittsburgh, PA: Oncology Nursing Society. Copyright 2007 by Oncology Nursing Society. Adapted with permission.

Prevention

A preventive approach to constipation should take place whenever possible. If the patient is found to have one or more risk factors during assessment, a prevention program should begin immediately. This program should consist of increased consumption of dietary fiber, including whole grains and vegetables; fluid intake to include eight 8-ounce servings a day; and consumption of warm or hot liquids to stimulate the bowel. The use of constipating medications, such as chemotherapeutic agents, opioid analgesics, sedatives, and antiemetics, should be reduced if possible. A program of active and passive exercise should be initiated based on the patient's tolerance level. The patient will need a comfortable, quiet, private environment to have a bowel movement. Avoid the use of a bedpan when possible, and encourage the patient to use any assistive devices necessary, such as a raised toilet seat (Bisanz et al., 2007; Massey et al., 2003).

If constipation occurs despite a preventive approach or if the patient risk factors include opioid analgesics or chemotherapeutic agents such as vinca alkaloids, oxaliplatin, or thalidomide, which are known to cause constipation, a more aggressive approach is necessary. A stool softener plus a stimulating laxative is recommended when initiating opioid therapy. One recommended regimen is docusate sodium 100–300 mg/day along with senna two to six tablets a day (Bisanz et al., 2007). The laxative dose should be titrated to achieve results, not based on the opioid dose. Bulk-forming laxatives are not recommended for opioid-induced constipation. In addition, research has shown that some opioids are less constipating than others. For example, switching from long-acting oral morphine to transdermal fentanyl may decrease constipation, and switching to methadone may result in decreased laxative use (Bisanz et al.).

Laxatives

The goal of laxative therapy is to promote regular bowel elimination function without side effects such as abdominal cramping or diarrhea. Laxative therapy is not indicated in patients with suspected bowel obstruction caused by fecal obstipation (also known as impaction), tumor, or other factors because of the risk of bowel perforation. The seven categories of laxatives are
- Bulk-forming laxatives
- Lubricants
- Saline laxatives
- Osmotic laxatives
- Detergent laxatives
- Stimulating laxatives
- Polyethylene glycol.

These drugs are available in the form of oral agents, suppositories, and enemas, depending on the agent selected (Massey et al., 2003).

Bulk-forming laxatives include fiber, bran, psyllium, methylcellulose, mucilloids, malt soup extracts, and carboxymethylcellulose. Bulk-forming laxatives increase peristalsis by absorbing water and allowing the stool to retain water, which in turn increases both the bulk and weight of the stool and distends the bowel. Fluid intake must be increased to three liters a day with bulk-forming laxatives (Bisanz et al., 2007). Bulk-forming laxatives are not indicated for patients who require fluid restrictions or who cannot tolerate drinking an increased volume of fluid, nor are they recommended for opioid-induced constipation or patients who are unable to drink adequate amounts of fluids because of the risk of bowel impaction (Bisanz et al.; Massey et al., 2003).

Lubricants are used to coat and soften the stool, which allows it to move through the intestine without difficulty. Examples include mineral oil and liquid petrolatum. The onset of their action is between 24–48 hours. Long-term use of lubricants can lead to malabsorption of fat-soluble vitamins, making them not useful as a prophylactic bowel regimen. Mineral oil alters the availability of vitamin K, therefore altering coagulation. Excess doses of lubricant can lead to rectal seepage and perianal irritation (Massey et al., 2003).

Saline or osmotic laxatives increase peristalsis by pulling water into the intestine and the stool to add to the weight of the stool. Saline laxatives include magnesium citrate, sodium biphosphate, and magnesium hydroxide. They are not indicated for the prevention of constipation but instead are used for acute constipation management. High doses produce watery stool within one to two hours. Lower doses work within 6–12 hours. Patients should be instructed not to take aluminum-containing antacids with magnesium-containing laxatives. Sodium salts are contraindicated in patients with cardiac or renal disease, hypertension, and edema (Massey et al., 2003).

Osmotic laxatives increase peristalsis by working through colonic bacteria that metabolize them, causing an increased osmotic pressure gradient, which pulls water into the intestines and then into the stool. Examples of osmotic laxatives include glycerin, lactulose, and sorbitol. Glycerin is available in suppository form. Both lactulose and sorbitol have a very sweet taste and may be difficult for some patients to tolerate. Increased doses of this type of laxative can result in watery diarrhea (Massey et al., 2003).

Detergent laxatives also are known as emollient laxatives or stool softeners and include docusate, docusate sodium, and docusate potassium. They act on the colon to reduce surface tension, which allows water and fat to enter the stool and reduce water and electrolyte absorption from the colon. Onset of action is 12–24 hours for oral preparations and 2–15 minutes with rectal preparations. These laxatives are best used for short periods of time when straining with stool is to be avoided. They are not appropriate when used alone in a prophylactic bowel management program for long-term constipation. Enteric-coated detergent laxatives must be taken whole and not altered in any way in order to be effective (Massey et al., 2003).

The two classes of stimulant laxatives are diphenylmethanes and anthraquinones. The diphenylmethanes include phenolphthalein and bisacodyl, which act directly on the colon by local irritation and stimulation of the intramural nerve plexus to stimulate intestinal motility. The diphenylmethanes take 6–10 hours to work when taken orally and 15–60 minutes when taken rectally. They are not effective when biliary obstruction is present because they must be excreted in the bile to be effective. Bisacodyl should not be used within one hour of taking antacids, cimetidine, or milk. Bisacodyl should be avoided when ulcerative lesions of the colon are suspected. The anthraquinones include senna products, casanthrol, cascara, and danthron and work by activating bacterial degradation in the intestine. Onset of action usually is 6–12 hours but can act as long as 24 hours for oral preparations and 15–60 minutes rectally. Both classes of stimulant laxatives can cause dependence, and normal bowel function may be lost with use (Massey et al., 2003).

The National Comprehensive Cancer Network recommends the use of polyethylene glycol as a treatment alternative for patients with cancer who have persistent constipation. Polyethylene glycol is available as standard dose with electrolytes and low dose without electrolytes. Polyethylene glycol should not be administered to patients with compromised kidney function (Bisanz et al., 2007).

Suppositories come from several different laxative classes and include glycerin, bisacodyl, senna, and phenolphthalein. Their onset of action is from 15–60 minutes. They are useful as a second step to oral laxatives that have not been effective. Suppositories should not be placed within the stool; they should be placed between the rectal mucosa and the stool in order to be effective. Tolerance can develop, and suppositories are not recommended for long-term use. Rectal irritation can occur with repeated use of suppositories. Furthermore, no type of rectal manipulation, including administering a suppository, should be attempted in the presence of rectal fissures or when the patient's neutrophil count is below $1,500/mm^3$ or if the platelet count is below $150,000/mm^3$ (Massey et al., 2003).

Enemas

Enemas are used to cleanse the distal colon after removal of impaction and are not useful for long-term constipation management. The type of enema fluid used determines the mechanism of action. Vegetable oil and lubricants soften and lubricate the stool and are useful for relieving low impactions. Tap water and normal saline work by increasing the fluid volume in the colon. Soap is an irritant that stimulates peristalsis (Massey et al., 2003). Milk and molasses enemas are useful for removing high impactions because the high sugar content in the molasses brings water into the bowel and helps to soften the stool (Bisanz et al., 2007).

Nonpharmacologic Interventions

The effectiveness of nonpharmacologic interventions in adult patients has not been established. Dietary fiber often is recommended for the prevention and management of constipation, but the research evidence is inconclusive (Woolery et al., 2008). Fiber should not be used in patients with advanced disease or those with inadequate fluid intake (Woolery et al.). Increased activity and exercise increase blood flow to the digestive organs, thereby improving motility, and are thought to be useful in preventing and managing constipation. However, few research studies exist, and they are conflicting (Woolery et al.). Other nonpharmacologic interventions, such as aromatherapy, massage therapy, and biofeedback, have been examined but lack conclusive research evidence on their effectiveness (Woolery et al.).

Obstipation

Fecal obstipation also is known as impaction. It occurs when constipation has not been adequately managed. Large amounts of dry hard stool sit in the rectum and cannot be properly eliminated. The patient may experience leakage of liquid stool around the obstipated area, which can be perceived as diarrhea. Other symptoms include rectal discomfort, tenesmus, lower abdominal pain, lower back pain, urinary retention, and urinary incontinence.

If obstipation progresses, late symptoms may include nausea, vomiting, altered mental status, hypotension, respiratory and circulatory compromise, and, in some instances, death. Rectal examination reveals large amounts of dry, hard stool in the rectum, unless the obstipation is located higher than the rectum in the sigmoid colon. Other obstipation assessment criteria are similar to the assessment of constipation. Additionally, an abdominal x-ray may be performed. Once obstipation has been identified, the goal of treatment is to lubricate the bowel and soften the stool so that it can be successfully removed. A nonstimulating laxative, glycerin suppository, oil retention enema, or hypertonic phosphate enema may be used (Massey et al., 2003). The goal is to prevent damage, such as fissures or hemorrhoids, to rectal tissues. If manual removal of obstipation is necessary, the patient could receive premedication with an antianxiety agent or short-acting opioid to reduce the physical and psychological discomfort related to the procedure. A topical anesthetic and a water-soluble lubricant is applied to the rectal area below the obstipation.

Next, a rectal examination is performed using a gloved finger lubricated with lidocaine ointment. Once the anal sphincter has relaxed, a second finger can be inserted, and the two fingers break apart the stool. When most of the stool has been removed, a cleansing enema and an aggressive bowel program should follow the procedure. This procedure should be avoided in neutropenic and/or thrombocytopenic patients (Massey et al., 2003).

Patient Teaching Points

Patients and families need to be active participants in the patients' care to effectively prevent and manage constipation. Nurses can teach patients to control constipation through fluid intake, dietary modification, medications, and activity level. The teaching should take place at a time when the patient is feeling well. Ideally, the patient should not be actively suf-

fering from a symptom such as constipation during the teaching session.
Teaching begins as soon as a risk factor for constipation is identified and
continues through treatment. Figure
8-6 includes points to cover related
to constipation in a teaching session
with patients and families.

Need for Future Research

More research is needed in almost every aspect of describing, preventing, and managing constipation.
Because constipation is a well-estab-

FIGURE 8-6	Patient Teaching Points

- Instruct patients to avoid laxative abuse.
- If necessary, encourage a combination of a laxative and stool softener.
- Teach patients about selecting high-fiber foods, such as fresh fruits and vegetables, whole-grain breads and cereals, and bran.
- Encourage a daily fluid intake of at least 3,000 ml unless patients are on fluid restriction.
- Instruct patients to plan a daily schedule for having a bowel movement after meals, when the gastrocolic reflexes are active.
- Discuss the need to plan for privacy.
- Encourage patients to exercise regularly.

Note. Based on information from Kuck & Ricciardi, 2005.

lished problem for patients with cancer, continuation of nursing research in this area is important. The true incidence of constipation in patients with cancer needs to be validated.
Much research still is needed to determine what interventions are most effective for preventing and treating constipation in people with cancer. As of September 2006, no interventions were available for which effectiveness has been demonstrated by strong evidence
from rigorously conducted studies, meta-analyses, or systematic reviews (Bisanz et al., 2007).
Pharmacologic interventions currently are based on high-level evidence in the non-oncol-
ogy population and need to be studied in the oncology population. Oncology nurses are
on the front lines of cancer symptom management, and the challenge is to now be on the
forefront of symptom management research.

Conclusion of Case Study

After discharge, M.L. has been gradually advancing her diet and beginning to ambulate
around her home. She has not resumed her usual activities. M.L. reports feeling extremely
fatigued. She has not resumed her usual fluid intake because she reports she is too tired
to eat or drink. M.L. also reports feeling extremely anxious about the outcome of the sec-
ond-look surgery. M.L. is experiencing no nausea, vomiting, or diarrhea.

The oncology nurse performs a physical examination and notes that M.L.'s abdomen is
symmetrical, slightly firm, and distended but not tender. M.L. has decreased bowel sounds
in all four quadrants.

Recall that M.L. has a history of ovarian cancer. Because she is having bowel sounds in
all four quadrants, passing gas, and had a bowel movement three days ago, M.L. does not
appear to be having obstruction from the ovarian cancer itself at this time. She received
paclitaxel chemotherapy; however, she has received only three cycles, and the last dose
was three weeks ago. M.L. is experiencing decreased mobility and change in diet as well as
decreased fluid intake since her recent surgery. M.L. has undergone two abdominal surgeries in the past six months. She currently is taking a narcotic analgesic and reports that
the narcotic was a factor in developing constipation following her first surgery.

The nurse shares the findings with M.L.'s GYN physician, who orders docusate sodium
100 mg and senna. M.L. is to take one tablet of each in the morning and again in the evening and may increase both medications to two tablets as needed for the period of time

that she will be taking the narcotic analgesic. The oncology nurse reviews foods that are high in fiber, such as bran, fruit, beans, and vegetables, and instructs M.L. to gradually increase the fiber in her diet and drink at least three liters of fluids a day. Fluids also can be in the form of gelatin and broth. The oncology nurse describes energy conservation techniques, as fatigue is a component of M.L.'s decreased fluid intake. They discuss that mild exercise can help to relieve constipation, and M.L. describes activities that she can tolerate, such as taking a short walk each day. M.L. states that if she experiences constipation that is not relieved in three days, blood in her stool, or nausea and vomiting, she will call the office for further instructions. Two weeks later, M.L. returns for her next cycle of chemotherapy and reports that the constipation has resolved.

Conclusion

Oncology nurses can make a significant impact on the management of constipation. This symptom continues to be underreported and therefore underaddressed and has a great impact on quality of life. The end result to the patient can be uncomfortable at the least, and life threatening at the worst, such as with bowel perforation. By using the ONS PEP resource on constipation, oncology nurses can identify patients who are at risk and implement evidence-based guidelines. Management of constipation should center on prevention through patient and family caregiver education and proactive interventions. Further research still is needed to determine the best intervention to prevent and manage constipation.

References

Bisanz, A., Woolery, M., Lyons, H.F., Gaido, L., Yenulevich, M.C., & Fulton, S. (2007). *Putting evidence into practice: Constipation.* Pittsburgh, PA: Oncology Nursing Society.

Fortenbaugh, C.C., & Rummel, M.A. (2007). *Case studies in oncology nursing: Text and review.* Sudbury, MA: Jones and Bartlett.

Johnson, G.D., Moore, K., & Fortner, B. (2007). *Baseline evaluation of the AIM higher initiative: Establishing the mark from which to measure.* Retrieved July 2, 2007, from http://www.ons.org/publications/journals/ONF/Volume34/Issue3/3403729.asp

Kuck, A.W., & Ricciardi, L. (2005). Alterations in elimination. In J.K. Itano & K.N. Taoka (Eds.), *Core curriculum for oncology nursing* (4th ed., pp. 318–344). St. Louis, MO: Elsevier Saunders.

Massey, R.I., Haylock, P.J., & Curtiss, C. (2003). Constipation. In C.H. Yarbro, M.H. Frogge, & M. Goodman (Eds.), *Cancer symptom management* (3rd ed., pp. 512–523). Sudbury, MA: Jones and Bartlett.

McMillan, S.C. (2002). Presence and severity of constipation in hospice patients with advanced cancer. *American Journal of Hospice and Palliative Care, 19*(6), 426–430.

National Cancer Institute. (2007). *Gastrointestinal complications (PDQ®).* Retrieved July 2, 2007, from http://www.cancer.gov/cancertopics/pdq/supportivecare/gastrointestinalcomplications/HealthProfessional/page2

Plaisance, L., & Ellis, J.A. (2002). Opioid-induced constipation: Management is necessary but prevention is better. *American Journal of Nursing, 102*(3), 72–73.

Polovich, M., White, J.M., & Kelleher, L.O. (Eds.). (2005). *Chemotherapy and biotherapy guidelines and recommendations for practice* (2nd ed.). Pittsburgh, PA: Oncology Nursing Society.

Ropka, M.E., Padilla, G., & Gillespie, T.W. (2005). Risk modeling: Applying evidence-based risk assessment in oncology nursing practice. *Oncology Nursing Forum, 32*(1), 49–56.

Sykes, N.P. (2006). The pathogenesis of constipation. *Journal of Supportive Oncology, 4*(5), 213–218.

Vanegas, G., Ripamonti, C., Sbanotto, A., & De Conno, F. (1998). Side effects of morphine administration in cancer patients. *Cancer Nursing, 21*(4), 289–297.

Woolery, M., Bisanz, A., Lyons, H.F., Gaido, L., Yenulevich, M., Fulton, S., et al. (2008). Putting evidence into practice: Evidence-based intervention for the prevention and management of constipation in patients with cancer. *Clinical Journal of Oncology Nursing, 12*(2), 317–337.

CHAPTER 9

Depression

Kathy Sharp, MSN, FNP-BC, AOCNP®

Case Study

Z.S. is a 44-year-old woman who found a lump in her right breast during her monthly breast self-examination. A biopsy revealed infiltrating ductal carcinoma, and she received a right modified radical mastectomy and right axillary node dissection. She currently is receiving the sixth dose of every-two-week dose-dense ACT (doxorubicin, cyclophosphamide, and paclitaxel). The same nurse has administered each of Z.S.'s chemotherapy regimens and has established a good rapport with the patient. During the infusion, the nurse asks Z.S. how she is tolerating the treatments and how she has been feeling during the time since her last treatment. Z.S. replies that she is tired of being tired and wonders when she will get her energy back. She also states that her hormones are "out of whack" because she is having mood swings and crying spells.

Overview

Although this chapter specifically addresses depression in patients with cancer, depression must be recognized as being one part of a much larger picture. The National Comprehensive Cancer Network (NCCN, 2008) regards depression as part of the continuum of distress. NCCN's definition of distress is

> A multifactorial unpleasant emotional experience of a psychological (cognitive, behavioral, emotional), social, and/or spiritual nature that may interfere with the ability to cope effectively with cancer, its physical symptoms and its treatment. Distress extends along a continuum, ranging from common normal feelings of vulnerability, sadness, and fears to problems that can become disabling, such as depression, anxiety, panic, social isolation, and existential and spiritual crisis. (p. DIS-2)

In this context, an important consideration is that not all symptoms may be caused by depression. Other problems, such as spiritual distress or crisis, existential crisis, and anxiety, may overlap and should be carefully explored separately from depression. Also important is to try to discern the cause of physical symptoms that may accompany depression. NCCN has published standards of care for distress management, which are applicable but not specific to depression (see Figure 9-1). The complete distress management guideline for depression is available from the NCCN Web site at www.nccn.org/professionals/physician_gls/PDF/distress .pdf (NCCN, 2008).

Depression is a serious health problem that will affect 1 in 4 women and 1 in 10 men during their lifetime (Mental Health America, 2007c). According to the World Health Organization (WHO, 2008), depression is the leading cause of disability as measured by years lived with disability. The lifetime risk for depression in women is 20%–25% versus 7%–12% in men (Schwenk, Terrell, Harrison, Shadigan, & Valenstein, 2005). In any given year, approximately 6.7% of the U.S. population aged 18 and older suffers from major depressive disorder (Kessler, Chiu, Demler, Merikangas, & Walters, 2005).

The rates of depression in people with cancer have not been studied in a large population. However, the National Institute of Mental Health (NIMH) and Mental Health America (formerly known as the National Mental Health Association) both reported that one in four people with cancer also suffers from clinical depression (Mental Health America, 2007a; NIMH, 2007). Depression symptoms in patients with cancer often are attributed to cancer or to the side effects of cancer treatment. For example, fatigue, a common side effect of cancer treatment, also is a common presenting symptom of depression. Patients with cancer frequently have other comorbid conditions that may be blamed for depression symptoms and result in depression continuing to be undetected and untreated (Mental Health America, 2007a). One example would be the patient who has comorbid hypothyroidism, which, if not properly controlled, results in fatigue, lack of energy, sleepiness, and weight gain, all of which can be symptoms of depression.

The impact of depression on individuals and society is enormous. WHO collected data from more than 240,000 people in 60 countries and found that depression impairs health status to a greater degree than four other major chronic conditions—asthma, angina, arthritis, and diabetes. WHO researchers found that depression rates varied from 9%–23%, and depression often was paired with other illnesses. The most disabling combination of diagnoses was depression with diabetes (Kahn, 2007). People with depression were more likely to develop diabetes and to suffer death from comorbid heart disease two years sooner than those without depression. Depression complicates and lengthens the recovery period from medical illnesses (Mental Health America, 2007a). Absenteeism from work increased by 50% in people with depression and resulted in approximately 5.6 hours a week of lost productivity, costing the United States $105 billion in lost productivity. Up to 9% of adults are estimated to have depression, but less than half of these have been diagnosed. The majority of those who are diagnosed with depression are treated in family practice, with less than 3% receiving specialized mental health services (Mental Health America, 2007a).

Depression is common in patients with advanced cancer, with overall occurrence rates for all types of cancer estimated to be 5%–25%. The highest rates were found in those with breast (1.5%–46%), pancreatic (33%–50%), lung (11%–44%), and oropharyngeal cancer (22%–57%). Shorter survival, reduction in treatment adherence, lengthened hospitalization, and diminished quality of life are all associated with depression in patients with cancer (Massie, 2004; Nelson, 2007; NIMH, 2007; Zabora, BrintzenhofeSzoc, Curbow, Hooker, & Piantadosi, 2001). NCCN (2008) reported that 20%–40% of patients with cancer have some level of distress; however, less than 10% are identified and referred for psychological help. Less than half of palliative care patients who exhibit symptoms of moderate to severe depression are on antidepressants (Nelson). These facts and figures may seem startling to some, but they highlight the need for improved education, additional screening, and increased intervention for depression. All of these improvements can begin with the oncology nurse, whose presence at the chairside or bedside is ideal for establishing the patient rapport necessary for effective intervention to begin. Interventions, including medications to alleviate depression, will be discussed later in this chapter.

FIGURE 9-1	Standards of Care for Distress Management

- Distress should be recognized, monitored, documented, and treated promptly at all stages.
- All patients should be screened for distress at their initial visit, at appropriate intervals, and as clinically indicated, especially with changes in disease status.
- Screening should identify the level and nature of the distress.
- Distress should be assessed and managed according to clinical practice guidelines.
- Multidisciplinary institutional committees should be formed to implement standards for distress management.
- Educational and training programs should be developed to ensure that healthcare professionals and pastoral caregivers have knowledge and skills in the assessment and management of distress.
- Licensed mental health professionals and certified pastoral caregivers experienced in psychosocial aspects of cancer should be readily available as staff members or by referral.
- Medical care contracts should include reimbursement for services provided by mental health professionals.
- Clinical health outcomes measurement should include assessment of psychosocial domain (e.g., quality of life, patient and family satisfaction).
- Patients, families, and treatment teams should be informed that management of distress is an integral part of total medical care and provided with appropriate information about psychosocial services in the treatment center and the community.
- Quality of distress management should be included in institutional continuous quality improvement projects.

Note. Reproduced with permission from *The NCCN (1.2008) Distress Management Clinical Practice Guidelines in Oncology.* © National Comprehensive Cancer Network, 2008. Available at http://www.nccn.org. Accessed December 4, 2008. To view the most recent and complete version of the guideline, go online to www.nccn.org.

These Guidelines are a work in progress that will be refined as often as new significant data becomes available.

The NCCN Guidelines are a statement of consensus of its authors regarding their views of currently accepted approaches to treatment. Any clinician seeking to apply or consult any NCCN guideline is expected to use independent medical judgment in the context of individual clinical circumstances to determine any patient's care or treatment. The National Comprehensive Cancer Network makes no warranties of any kind whatsoever regarding their content, use or application and disclaims any responsibility for their application or use in any way.

These Guidelines are copyrighted by the National Comprehensive Cancer Network. All rights reserved. These Guidelines and illustrations herein may not be reproduced in any form for any purpose without the express written permission of the NCCN.

Pathophysiology

Historically, depression was thought of in stigmatized terms and looked upon as a personal weakness (To, Zepf, & Woods, 2005). A survey by Mental Health America (2007c) showed that societal attitudes about depression are changing. Currently, 72% of Americans view depression as a health problem, versus 38% just 10 years ago (Mental Health America, 2007b). Depression is recognized, both by society and the medical community, as a biologic/chemical problem, with alterations in the neurotransmitters serotonin, norepinephrine, and dopamine implicated as the culprit behind the illness (To et al.). This theory originated in the 1950s from the observation that the antimicrobial agent iproniazid was associated with mood alterations. Later, the antihypertensive agent reserpine was found to correlate with depleted brain neurochemicals. Research has not been conducted that conclusively proves this assertion, although intensive research has been conducted for decades to elucidate the neurobiologic base of depression. Epidemiologic studies revealed that genetic and environmental factors contribute to the risk of depression, noting that adverse experiences early in life have a role in the pathogenesis of depression. Although the exact mechanisms are still being determined, theories postulate that the functional capacity of neurocircuits are essentially overloaded and dysfunctional as a result of an increased stress load early in life. Scientists have discovered two different alleles on the genes that are associated with the occurrence and types of depression and are altered in response to stress (Heim, Plotsky, & Nemeroff, 2004; Robertson, 2007). Studies have demonstrated improvement in depression symptoms with the administration of these neurotransmitters, and enhanced vulnerability to depression is shown when the quantity of these neurochemicals has been decreased (Sullivan, Neale, & Kendler, 2000; To et al.). Caspi et al. (2003) reported a link between genetic abnormalities in the serotonin transporter gene and the development of pathologic reactions to stressful life events.

Many medications have been implicated as the cause of depression symptoms, including chemotherapy agents, especially vinca alkaloids, oncologics such as thalidomide, biologics such as interferon, and steroids, all of which are part of cancer treatment. Other medications include but are not limited to antihypertensives, anticonvulsants, antiarrhythmics, beta-blockers, histamine-2 receptor blockers, digoxin, antiparkinsonian drugs, antihistamines, nonsteroidal anti-inflammatory drugs (NSAIDs), and psychoactive drugs (Goolsby, 2002; Kramer, 2004; Newport, 2005; Schwenk et al., 2005). The estrogen blocker tamoxifen also has been associated with an increased rate of depression in women with breast cancer (Spollen & Gutman, 2003).

Tamoxifen, widely used in patients with estrogen receptor–positive breast cancer, was retrospectively studied in 2,439 female patients (Spollen & Gutman, 2003). An electronic database was used to identify patients who had the onset of depression diagnosed within one year of breast cancer according to *International Classification of Diseases, Ninth Revision* codes, or who had antidepressant medication initiated with or without tamoxifen. The rate of new-onset depression was marginally higher in the tamoxifen group (n = 1,930, 17.82%) versus the control group (n = 509, 14.34%, p = 0.0641). A subset analysis using a variable follow-up period showed a 27.3% rate of depression in the tamoxifen group versus 21.99% in the non-tamoxifen group (p = 0.0076). Although this study was relatively small, it suggested that patients with breast cancer who are receiving tamoxifen may be at increased risk for depression (Spollen & Gutman).

Assessment

Depression is categorized as major, minor, or as a dysthymic disorder with chronic depression lasting more than two years. Major depressive disorder is described as a despairing mood with loss of interest in nearly all activities previously considered pleasurable. In addition to a despairing mood, the person must experience at least four other symptoms, such as change in appetite or weight (gain or loss), changes in sleep (disturbed, interrupted, early morning awakening, or insomnia), difficulty concentrating or making decisions, or agitation, fatigue, and recurrent thoughts of suicide. Symptoms must persist for at least two consecutive weeks. These symptoms can be remembered easily using one of two mnemonics: A SAD FACES or SIG E CAPS (see Figures 9-2 and 9-3) (Schwenk et al., 2005; Valdivia & Rossy, 2004).

Some healthcare providers may take for granted that depression is a normal response to cancer, and depression therefore is often ignored or overlooked. All healthcare providers, particularly those in oncology, should remember to screen for depression because research suggests that the best improvement in health status is when depression and other comorbid conditions are optimally treated (Kahn, 2007). Many depression questionnaires, inventories, screening tools, and self-reporting questions have been used to discover, rate, or categorize depression. In 2006, the Oncology Nursing Society (ONS) reviewed the available screening tools for depression. An extensive table listing the screening tool, the author, a description of the scaling and scoring method, and each tool's psychometric properties is available in the Outcomes Resource Area of the ONS Web site (www.ons.org/outcomes/measures/depression.shtml). Depression evaluation tools are numerous, but some of the most common are by Beck, Zung, and Hamilton. Although each one of these tools has been validated and widely used, they can be too lengthy for easy use by the bedside nurse. Figure 9-4 contains online screening tools, some of which may be printed for patient evaluation.

Although nurses may not be specifically trained in the use of a structured clinical interview tool, they are the most likely to have excellent rapport with the patient and may be the first healthcare provider to uncover clues or symptoms suggesting depression. In 2004, the U.S. Preventive Services Task Force (USPSTF) recommended routine screening for depression by simply asking the patient two questions: first, "Over the last two weeks, have you felt down, depressed, or hopeless?" and second, "Over the last two weeks, have

FIGURE 9-2	**A SAD FACES Mnemonic**
A	Appetite
S	Sleep (insomnia or hypersomnia)
A	Anhedonia (loss of interest or pleasure in usual activities)
D	Depressed mood
F	Fatigue
A	Agitation
C	Concentration
E	Esteem (sense of worthlessness or diminished/lost self-esteem)
S	Suicidal

Note. Based on information from Montano, 1994.

FIGURE 9-3	**SIG E CAPS Mnemonic**
S	Sleep (insomnia or hypersomnia)
I	Interests (diminished interest or pleasure in usual activities)
G	Guilt (feelings of worthlessness, excessive or inappropriate guilt)
E	Energy (loss of energy or fatigue)
C	Concentration (indecisiveness or diminished concentration)
A	Appetite (decreased or increased)
P	Psychomotor retardation or agitation
S	Suicidal

Note. Based on information from American Psychiatric Association, 2000; Remick, 2002.

you felt little interest or pleasure in doing usual activities?" A positive answer to either question should result in a more in-depth discussion with the patient (USPSTF, 2002). Although this two-question screening was designed for the general population and is not specific to cancer, it can easily be included in conversations with patients and may serve to cultivate a more in-depth evaluation and involvement of other members of the healthcare team. Specifically, the bedside nurse can use this simple screening tool to identify the potential for depression. If a patient responds yes to either of the questions in the screening tool, an assess-

FIGURE 9-4	**Links for Depression Screening Tools**

Beck Depression Inventory (BDI) and Beck Depression Inventory–Short Form (BDI-SF): Available online for purchase only, see www.pearsonassess.com
Center for Epidemiologic Studies Depression Scale (CES-D): http://counsellingresource.com/quizzes/cesd/index.html
Hamilton Rating Scale for Depression: http://healthnet.umassmed.edu/mhealth/HAMD.pdf
Patient Health Questionnaire (PHQ)-2: www.cmwf.org/usr_doc/phq2.pdf
PHQ-9: www.phqscreeners.com
Zung Self-Rating Depression Scale (ZSDS): http://healthnet.umassmed.edu/mhealth/ZungSelfRated DepressionScale.pdf

ment for symptoms of depression is warranted. The bedside nurse may perform an assessment but should report both the screening and assessment findings to the nurse practitioner, physician assistant, or physician who is responsible for the patient's oncology care.

When assessing patients for depression, nurses must look at physical symptoms as well as emotional, psychological, or behavioral clues. Psychological and physical symptoms may include fatigue, lack of energy, inability to concentrate, insomnia or drowsiness, subjectively described restlessness, a sense of hopelessness, decreased interest in usual activities, irritability, or appetite changes (either loss of appetite or carbohydrate craving). Emotional symptoms include depressed mood, pessimism, loss of self-esteem, crying, social withdrawal, anhedonia, or pathologic guilt (Hentz, 2005). Physical symptoms often are present in depressed patients with cancer both during and after treatment. Gielissen, Verhagen, Witjes, and Bleijenberg (2006) reported that "persistent fatigue is a long-term adverse effect experienced by 30% to 40% of patients cured of cancer" (p. 4882). Fatigue and other physical symptoms without an identifiable source should be triggers that cause the nurse to consider depression as the origin. Fulcher (2006) reported that patients with pain, disability, and the perceived absence of social support have higher rates of depression. The phenomenon of symptom clustering has been identified in patients with cancer and may include combinations of depression, fatigue, insomnia, anxiety, and pain. Kim, McGuire, Tulman, and Barsevick (2005) identified the symptom cluster of depression and fatigue. This symptom cluster also was associated with a diminished quality of life. Other research by Beck, Dudley, and Barsevick (2005) explored the relationship among pain, fatigue, and sleep disturbance. Their analysis indicated that pain influenced fatigue both directly and indirectly, and the combination indirectly affected sleep. Both of these studies suggest that symptom intervention may improve patients' quality of life.

Newport and Nemeroff (1998) and Trask (2004) described four approaches to assessing depression in patients with cancer: (a) inclusive, (b) etiologic, (c) substitutive, and (d) exclusive. Each approach reflects how depression is both defined and measured. The inclusive approach, as the name implies, includes all the symptoms of depression, regardless of whether they may be caused by medical illness. Etiologic approaches include only symptoms that are not the result of physical illness. The substitutive approach substitutes physical symptoms, such as fatigue, and adds additional psychological symptoms, such as crying. The exclusive approach eliminates the most common symptoms of weight changes and fatigue, allowing more focus on the psychological symptoms. Each approach has pros and cons and variable sensitivity; however, the inclusive approach is recommended because it is the most sensitive (see Zung, 1965, for the Zung Self-Rating Depression Scale).

Evidence-Based Interventions

What does all this mean to the oncology nurse? How can the oncology nurse make a difference in the life of a patient with cancer who is depressed? What interventions are supported by evidence-based research? A team of dedicated individuals from ONS reviewed the available literature regarding treatments for depression that were evidence-based and divided these into three categories: (1) *Recommended for Practice*, (2) *Likely to Be Effective*, and (3) *Effectiveness Not Established*. Interventions supported as beneficial and thus recommended for practice were psychoeducational/psychosocial interventions and pharmacologic interventions. See Table 9-1 for a summary of interventions (Fulcher, Badger, Gunter, Marrs, & Reese, 2008).

Recommended for Practice

Evidence at the highest level supports psychoeducational and psychosocial interventions during and following cancer treatment. Although data on the frequency and duration of these therapies are widely variable, the majority of research reports improvement in depression symptoms. Psychoeducational and psychosocial interventions include cognitive behavioral therapy (CBT), patient education, counseling and psychotherapy, behavioral therapy, and social support. The strongest evidence supports CBT as being the most beneficial (Fulcher et al., 2008). Most psychoeducational and psychosocial interventions generally require advanced education and training and usually are performed by professionals other than nurses. The professionals who provide these therapies may not always be readily available for consult by the bedside nurse.

TABLE 9-1	Interventions by Level of Evidence
Level of Evidence	**Interventions**
Recommended for practice	Psychoeducational/psychosocial • Patient education • Cognitive behavioral therapy • Counseling/psychotherapy • Behavioral therapy • Social support Pharmacologic—antidepressants • Selective serotonin reuptake inhibitors • Tricyclic antidepressants • Serotonin-norepinephrine reuptake inhibitors • Other antidepressants
Likely to be effective	Methylphenidate (Ritalin®, Novartis Pharmaceuticals Corp.) Relaxation therapy
Effectiveness not established	Massage therapy Hypnotherapy

Note. Based on information from Badger et al., 2007.

CBT is used to help patients to recognize and change thought distortions or perceptions that cause or exacerbate psychological distress. CBT is guided by a therapist who works collaboratively with patients to uncover how thoughts, emotions, and behavior interrelate and how experiences or other external stimuli influence perceptions. A therapist challenges patients to evaluate their perceptions against reality to overcome (in the case of depression) distortions about self-worth. CBT is goal oriented, based on learning principles of behavior change, and directed toward a specific result. This intervention works best with patients who have some ability for introspection (i.e., the ability to look inward) (Mulhauser, 2007; Osborn, Demoncada, & Feuerstein, 2006; Schwenk et al., 2005). For instance, a female patient may be told that she will lose her hair from chemotherapy. Her long flowing hair and frequent compliments about its beauty are part of her perception of self-worth. Her husband's past comments about not liking short hair represent external stimuli and serve to increase the perception that her hair and her appeal are tied together. She feels ugly, begins to worry about losing her husband, and becomes depressed about the loss of her hair and the potential loss of her husband. CBT with a therapist would serve to redirect her thinking about her self-value, acknowledge the reality of her husband's reassurances, and correct her thought distortions.

Gielissen et al. (2006) studied CBT in disease-free cancer survivors compared with those awaiting therapy. Although the randomized controlled trial included only 112 cancer survivors, it showed that CBT was effective in reducing the severity of fatigue. Cancer survivors with persistent fatigue were randomized to immediate CBT or assigned to a waiting list. Evaluations of functional impairment and fatigue severity were assessed at baseline and six months later. Patients who received immediate therapy (n = 50) had significant improvement compared to those who were on the waiting list (n = 48), with a 50% improvement in fatigue scores in the treatment group versus 18% in the waiting list control group. Functional impairment improved in 54% of the treatment group versus 4% in the waiting list control group.

Although CBT is available only from a trained therapist, patient education is an intervention available to every nurse, and its importance cannot be overemphasized. Philosopher Sir Francis Bacon stated, "Knowledge is power" (BrainyQuote.com, n.d.). For patients with cancer, knowledge begins with education regarding their specific diagnosis and the treatment or treatments that are recommended. Patients with cancer who have depression also need education about the diagnosis of depression and specific medications they may be taking that are known to cause depression. Patients experiencing depression need reassurance and education about the biologic causes of depression. Providing reading material to patients is a way of extending acceptance to those who may be struggling with a new diagnosis of depression and also arms them with an understanding of the cause of their symptoms. The "power" gleaned from patient education should not be underestimated, for it is one more weapon for patients to use in their secondary battle with depression.

Counseling, psychotherapy, and behavioral therapy are interventions that require special training and education to administer; however, the primary nurse is in a unique position to recognize the need for these interventions and to make recommendations to the patient's primary healthcare provider. Miovic and Block (2007) reported empathetic listening to be the most important communication skill oncologists can use with patients, but nurses may employ empathetic listening as well. This simply involves listening and giving patients time and encouragement to express their thoughts, fears, and concerns. Historically, listening to their patients is a task at which nurses have been exceptionally skillful. Consider this example: Mrs. Jones has recently been diagnosed with metastatic colon cancer with lesions in the liver and lung. She is on her second cycle of FOLFIRI (folinic acid, fluorouracil, and irinotecan) and is scheduled for a total of 12 cycles. She struggled through multiple side effects, particularly fatigue, with her adjuvant FOLFOX (fluorouracil, leucovorin, and oxaliplatin) treatment just two years ago. She states to the nurse that she is not sure she can go through this treatment and wonders if she should just go home, forget about it, and die. The nurse understands that Mrs. Jones is likely frustrated and possibly depressed but senses that she needs to express some of those emotions. The nurse says, "Mrs. Jones, I know you must be frustrated over having a recurrence so soon, and may dread the treatment. Why don't you tell me about the things that worry and bother you the most." The nurse then sits with the patient, maintains eye contact, and is attentive to what Mrs. Jones has to say. The nurse should not interrupt or offer opinions but rather should simply listen.

Although many other factors are recognized to be involved in depression, treatment has focused largely on medications. The first pharmacologic therapies were the monoamine oxidase inhibitors (MAOIs), introduced in the 1950s. The monoamine neurotransmitter hypothesis began with the use of the antihypertensive agent reserpine, which depletes the brain of the neurotransmitters norepinephrine, serotonin, and dopamine. Study of this phenomenon ultimately led to the development of the many antidepressants on the market today. MAOIs inhibit monoamine oxidase, an enzyme that breaks down the neurotransmitter at the synapse. The effect is to increase neurotransmitter binding at postsynaptic receptors, thereby increasing levels of available neurotransmitters. MAOIs have been linked with potential dangers because of the many side effects and food/drug interactions, for instance, the dangerous interaction with foods containing tyramine such as aged cheese, wine, and pickled fish. This interaction can cause the release of norepinephrine from nerve endings, resulting in severe hypertension (Khouzam, 2007; To et al., 2005).

Pharmacologic interventions have frequently been written about and are recommended for patients with depression and cancer, but few studies have specifically addressed their effectiveness using randomized controlled trials. Studies of patients with cancer and depression generally support the use of tricyclic antidepressants (TCAs), selective serotonin reuptake inhibitors (SSRIs), and others, but only four reviews were found that upheld the benefits (Goodnick & Hernandez, 2000; Ly, Chidgey, Addington-Hall, & Hotopf, 2002; Pirl, 2004; Schwartz, Lander, & Chochinov, 2002). No differences in effectiveness were noted between TCAs and SSRIs; however, SSRIs are preferable because of a lower incidence of side effects. Although the serotonin-norepinephrine receptor inhibitor (SNRI) venlafaxine has been studied repeatedly for its usefulness in managing hot flashes associated with estrogen blockade, no studies were found that evaluated its effectiveness in treating patients with cancer who had depression. Likewise, duloxetine has not been specifically studied in the cancer population. Refer to Table 9-2 for information on medications.

TABLE 9-2	Antidepressant Medications Used in Patients With Cancer		
Medication	**Trade Name/ Manufacturer**	**Comments/ Positive Effects**	**Common Side Effects/Concerns**
Selective Serotonin Reuptake Inhibitors (SSRIs)			
Fluoxetine	Prozac® (Eli Lilly & Co.)	Activating, good for patients with lack of energy, long half-life, good for forgetful or poorly compliant patients	Very long half-life, potent inhibitor of CYP2D6 isoenzymes, not good for patients on multiple medications or medications that are anticipated to require frequent titration, sexual side effects
Sertraline	Zoloft® (Pfizer Inc.)	Low drug-drug interaction, good for patients with psychomotor retardation	Increased alertness, insomnia, weak inhibitor of CYP2D6 isoenzymes, diarrhea, sexual side effects
Paroxetine	Paxil® (Glaxo-SmithKline)	Good for patients with comorbid anxiety disorder	Nausea, anticholinergic effects, dizziness, headache, may occasionally increase anxiety, increased half-life in older adults, weight gain, potent inhibitor of CYP2D6 isoenzymes, sexual side effects
Citalopram	Celexa® (Forest Laboratories, Inc.)	Low drug-drug interaction potential, few gastrointestinal (GI) side effects; good for older adults, those with agitated depression, and those with GI sensitivity	Hypersomnia, sexual side effects Use with caution in patients with renal impairment.
Escitalopram	Lexapro® (Forest Laboratories, Inc.)	Low drug-drug interaction potential, few GI side effects, good for older adults and those with agitated depression	Hypersomnia, sexual side effects Use with caution in patients with renal impairment.
Serotonin-Norepinephrine Reuptake Inhibitors (SNRIs)			
Venlafaxine	Effexor® (Wyeth Pharmaceuticals)	Good for comorbid depression and pain	Hypertension at higher doses, constipation, vivid dreams, significant withdrawal syndrome requires slow taper, nausea and vomiting, headache, sexual side effects

(Continued on next page)

TABLE 9-2	Antidepressant Medications Used in Patients With Cancer *(Continued)*		
Medication	**Trade Name/ Manufacturer**	**Comments/ Positive Effects**	**Common Side Effects/Concerns**
Duloxetine	Cymbalta® (Eli Lilly & Co.)	Good for comorbid depression and pain	Nausea, constipation, major CYP1A2 and CYP2D6 inhibitor, sexual side effects Use with extreme caution in patients with heavy alcohol use or chronic liver disease.
Desvenlafaxine	Pristiq™ (Wyeth Pharmaceuticals)	Does not interfere with most medications (except ketoconazole, desipramine, monoamine oxidase inhibitors, and midazolam), so is good for patients with polypharmacy	May worsen hypertension Increased risk of bleeding May activate mania
Tricyclic Antidepressants			
Amitriptyline (tertiary amines)	Elavil® (AstraZeneca Pharmaceuticals)	Good for patients with peripheral neuropathy and insomnia	Sedating, dry mouth, constipation, dizziness, weight gain
Imipramine (tertiary amine)	Tofranil® (Tyco Healthcare)	Good for patients with chronic pain and comorbid depression Long-term use may be associated with an increased risk of breast cancer in women.	Hypotension, QT prolongation, drowsiness, dry mouth, dizziness, low blood pressure, thrombocytopenia, leukopenia, nausea, vomiting, weakness, blurred vision, constipation, urinary retention, may increase suicidality Adjust dose for older adults and patients with hepatic impairment and glaucoma.
Desipramine (secondary amine)	Norpramin® (Sanofi-Aventis)	Long-term use may be associated with an increased risk of breast cancer in women.	Dry mouth, drowsiness, urinary retention, constipation, dizziness
Nortriptyline (secondary amine)	Pamelor® (Tyco Healthcare)	–	Orthostatic hypotension, urinary retention, constipation, dry mouth, drowsiness
Protriptyline (secondary amine)	Vivactil® (Barr Laboratories, Inc.)	Used also for panic disorder	Long-term use may be associated with an increased risk of breast cancer in women. Dry mouth, drowsiness, urinary retention, constipation, dizziness
Doxepin (dibenzoxazepine derivative)	Sinequan® (Pfizer Inc.)	Good for anxious, depressed patients	Long-term used may be associated with an increased risk of breast cancer in women. Dry mouth, drowsiness, urinary retention, constipation, dizziness

(Continued on next page)

TABLE 9-2	Antidepressant Medications Used in Patients With Cancer *(Continued)*		
Medication	**Trade Name/ Manufacturer**	**Comments/ Positive Effects**	**Common Side Effects/Concerns**
Other Antidepressants			
Mirtazapine (sero-tonin and alpha-2 receptor blocker)	Remeron® (Organon USA)	Good for patients with an-orexia, insomnia, nausea, low drug-drug interaction	Weight gain, very sedating Reduce dose by 50% for hepatic impairment and 25% for renal impairment.
Bupropion (nor-epinephrine/do-pamine reuptake inhibitor)	Wellbutrin® (Glaxo-SmithKline)	Good for apathetic, low-energy depression, no sexual side effects, may be used in combination with SSRIs and SNRIs	May increase heart rate and lower seizure threshold Do not use if patient has history of seizure, substance abuse, bulimia, anorexia, or electrolyte disturbance.
Trazodone (triazol-opyridine)	Desyrel® (Bristol-Myers Squibb Co.)	Good for insomnia	Used as adjunct for sleep but rarely used for depression because dose needed to treat causes over-sedation
Nefazodone (sero-tonin-2 antagonist/ reuptake inhibitor, triazolopyridine)	Brand name (Ser-zone) discontinued in the United States; only avail-able as a generic.	Good for anxious patients with insomnia	Fatigue, dizziness, sedation, weight gain, interactions with many com-mon medications **Black box warning: may cause hepatic damage/failure.** Contraindicated with most statins, sildenafil (Viagra®, Pfizer Inc.), and pimozide; increases digoxin level; inhibits CYP3A3/4
Monoamine Oxidase Inhibitors			
Phenelzine	Nardil® (Pfizer Inc.)	Also used for bulimia	Avoid aged cheese, wine, and pick-led meats, which can interact and cause severe hypertension.
Tranylcypromine	Parnate® (Glaxo-SmithKline)	Same	Same as above
Isocarboxazid	Marplan® (Validus Pharmaceuticals, Inc.)	Same	Same as above

Note. Based on information from Agency for Healthcare Research and Quality, 2007; American Psychiatric Association, 2000; *Epocrates Online*, 2008; Gutman & Nemeroff, 2002; Hentz, 2005; Khouzam, 2007; Newport, 2005; Oncology Nursing Society, 2007; Oquendo & Liebowitz, 2006; Schwenk et al., 2005; Sharpe et al., 2002; Valdivia & Rossy, 2004.

The medications used in patients with cancer who have depression should be selected and dosed based on a number of factors, including comorbid conditions, current treatments and medications, side effect profile, potential toxicities, hepatic and renal function, and published indications (Gutman & Nemeroff, 2002; Schwenk et al., 2005; Valdivia & Rossy, 2004). For example, antidepressants with short half-lives (i.e., sertraline and paroxetine) are preferred for those patients who have impaired hepatic or renal function. Because of potential of in-teraction, caution should be used when any patient on pain medication starts an antidepressant. Because of their sedating effects, TCAs in particular may potentiate the effect of opioid analgesia; however, clinical practice guidelines state that patients with cancer may respond to lower doses of TCAs (American Psychiatric Association, 2000).

Major depression is a well-known side effect of interferon-alfa, which is used to treat malignant melanoma. One small study by Musselman et al. (2001) found that prophylactic treatment with paroxetine two weeks before starting interferon significantly reduced the likelihood that interferon would have to be discontinued because of depression. The associated depression is a phenomenon that also occurs in acute trauma and infections and is referred to as *cytokine-mediated sickness*. It is thought to result because of a normal illness adaptive behavior, manifested as increased sleep, decreased appetite, and decreased sex drive that cannot be turned off. The repetitive administration of interferon continues this process, and continual stimulation is thought to cause stimulation of the adrenocorticotropic hormone/ cortisol axis. Stimulation of the hypothalamic-pituitary-adrenal axis is consistently observed in patients with depression (Chen, 2003).

Likely to Be Effective

Methylphenidate and relaxation therapy are the only two interventions that were supported as likely to be effective. These interventions did not have the rigorous supporting data to allow classification in the *Recommended for Practice* category.

Methylphenidate (Ritalin®, Novartis Pharmaceuticals Corp.), a central nervous system stimulant, most often has been used for its mood elevating properties, to negate the effect of opioid-induced somnolence, and to improve cognitive functioning. Ritalin, often used in children with attention-deficit disorder and attention-deficit/hyperactivity disorder, has an extrapyramidal effect in adults. In a review of nine studies, methylphenidate was found to be useful in treating depression, with 80% of the patients having a favorable response. Less than 20% reported side effects, which included nausea, headache, anxiety, and tachycardia (Rozans, Dreisbach, Lertora, & Kahn, 2002). Although favorable, the studies were small, with only one well-designed controlled trial by Homsi et al. (2001).

Complementary and alternative therapies consist of relaxation therapy, massage therapy, hypnotherapy, and herbal preparations. Relaxation therapy is a technique that focuses on inducing a relaxed physical and mental state using guided imagery, hypnosis, and autogenic training. A meta-analysis of 15 studies by Leubbert, Dahme, and Hasenbring (2001) found relaxation therapy to have a significant effect on reducing cancer treatment–related side effects, including depression. Studies of other complementary therapies did not meet criteria for recommendation. It is important to point out that these interventions may be useful, but it also is important to recognize that randomized clinical trials have not been conducted to prove the level of effectiveness.

Effectiveness Not Established

Several other kinds of intervention were evaluated. However, studies lacked sufficient evidence of effectiveness. One of these, hypnotherapy, is a behavior therapy using hypnosis to induce heightened concentration, receptivity, and relaxation. Hypnotherapy is only performed by a trained hypnotherapist, usually a psychologist or psychiatrist, who uses various methods to induce a tranquil state during which the patient can focus on positive behavior changes. A review of 27 studies using hypnotherapy for symptom relief in terminally ill patients with cancer revealed only one study that was a randomized controlled trial. Although one trial did show improvement in depression with hypnosis, the small sample size was not adequate to suggest hypnotherapy as a reliable intervention (Rajasekaran, Edmonds, & Higginson, 2005). The only randomized controlled trial conducted was by Liossi and White (2001). Although statistically significant reductions in depression and anxiety occurred for the group treated with hypnotherapy, the study only included 50 patients.

Other complementary interventions noted in the literature include St. John's wort, S-adenosylmethionine (known as SAMe), dehydroepiandrosterone (known as DHEA), folate and other herbal supplements, yoga, acupuncture, aromatherapy, exercise, and meditation (Fredman & Rosenbaum, 2004; Kramer, 2004). These therapies have not been sufficiently studied, so no evidence exists to recommend them for regular practice. Nurses must ask about the use of complementary therapies when evaluating patients. Although many therapies will not interfere with standard treatment, herbal preparations may interact with prescription medications and chemotherapy. It is imperative for the nurse to ask specifically about herbal preparations, because some people may be unlikely to think of vitamins or supplements as harmful. Example questions to ask include, "Are you taking any type of medicine, vitamins, or herbs that are not prescription? Do you use any over-the-counter medicines such as laxatives, vitamins, or other supplements such as garlic or ginseng? Do you see an herbalist or mountain healer for suggestions or herbal mixtures?"

Although not included in the ONS categorization of depression interventions, electroconvulsive therapy has been shown to be effective in a select group of patients who are profoundly depressed and suicidal. The decision to utilize this therapy is made by professionals trained in its use (i.e., psychiatrists) (Brody & Serby, 2004).

Experiential Suggestions From the Author

During the past 30 years, a common theme that this author has heard from others is the frustration or awkwardness of opening a conversation with patients about depression. Although depression is becoming more accepted as a medical illness in our society, significant stigma still exists in some populations, particularly in older adults. The following are several examples of ways to open a dialogue with patients when their body language, the nurse's observations and assessment, or a "sixth sense" indicates that depression is a possibility but may be difficult for the patient to discuss.

Each of these scenarios should lead fairly easily into asking the two survey questions recommended by the USPSTF (2002).

- Mrs. S, you look sad today. Would you like to talk about how you are feeling?
- Mr. M, I know you have been feeling fatigued lately. I was reading an article on fatigue last evening that said fatigue is caused by many things, including anemia, chemotherapy, and other medications. It also says that depression may be a cause of fatigue. Do you think that depression could be part of the reason you have been fatigued for several weeks?
- Mrs. M, I was recently surprised to read that more than 50% of patients with cancer suffer from depression that is never diagnosed. Do you think that number is accurate? Have you ever felt depressed?
- How are you coping with your cancer and chemotherapy?
- How is your stress level?
- I know that being in the hospital away from your family must be difficult. How are you doing? How are you coping with that?
- Mrs. C, you have had to deal with a lot of side effects (substitute bad news, stress, or other problem). How are you coping emotionally?

Keep the following pointers in mind: If the patient says "fine" or "OK" in response to your question and you have a high suspicion of depression, press the issue by saying "Really?" or "Are you sure?" Some patients need encouragement to open up. One key to obtaining information is asking the question and then **being quiet long enough** for the patient to formulate a response. Remember that if you do not look for it, you cannot find it.

Patient Teaching Points

Multiple resources and Web sites are available for patient information about depression and its treatment, but important to note is that not all Web sites contain factual or appropriate information. Advise patients to only follow recommendations from well-known sites, such as the American Cancer Society or the National Institutes of Health. Figure 9-5 lists a few helpful and informational Web sites. Nurses must have an adequate understanding of the information presented in this chapter and be able to guide patients to information they can retrieve themselves. Nurses play the primary role in patient education, and the nurse/patient relationship is an important part of treatment adherence. When patients feel comfortable and sense that the nurse is interested in their health and well-being, positive outcomes ensue. Nurses should recognize the role they play in the patient's self-esteem. Teaching should be done in a nonjudgmental manner with an accepting attitude, particularly for those patients who still associate depression with some social or personal stigma (Harper-Jones, 2004; Vanderhoef, 2006). For patients who may be resistant to taking antidepressants, the analogy of taking insulin for diabetes or chemotherapy for cancer often is effective in helping them to grasp the understanding of depression as a biologic/medical illness.

Example of what to say to a patient: "You admit that you are depressed, and the symptoms you are experiencing would indicate you are correct. Depression is a physical illness, resulting in part because of the lack of adequate chemicals in the brain. Taking medication for depression is just like taking insulin for diabetes. If the pancreas does not produce enough insulin, you take insulin in the form of an injection. Treatment for depression is in the form of a pill, taken daily to replace the chemicals in the brain. Just like you should not skip a day's insulin dosage, you must not skip a day of your depression medicine."

FIGURE 9-5	**Online Depression Information, Guidelines, and Standards**

American Academy of Family Physicians, "Practice Guidelines: Clinical Review of Recent Findings on the Awareness, Diagnosis and Treatment of Depression," by M. Preboth, *American Family Physician* (May 15, 2000): www.aafp.org/afp/20000515/practice.html

American Psychiatric Association, *Treatment of Patients With Major Depressive Disorder* (2nd ed.): www.psychiatryonline.com/pracGuide/pracGuideChapTOC_7.aspx

American Psychological Association: www.apa.org/topics/topicdepress.html

Medscape Depression Resource Center (requires free registration on Medscape.com): www.medscape.com/resource/depression

National Cancer Institute Physician Data Query (PDQ®) Summary (health professional version): www.cancer.gov/cancertopics/pdq/supportivecare/depression/healthprofessional

National Cancer Institute Depression PDQ® Summary (patient version): www.cancer.gov/cancertopics/pdq/supportivecare/depression/patient

National Guidelines Clearinghouse, Depression Clinical Practice Guidelines: www.guidelines.gov/summary/summary.aspx?doc_id=9632&nbr=

National Institutes of Mental Health: www.nimh.nih.gov/health/topics/depression/index.shtml

Need for Future Research

What does the future hold for patients with depression? What changes in health care must be made to improve treatment? A random sample of palliative care nurses who belong to ONS were mailed a survey using a case study for feedback. Interestingly, respondents rated depression as the most important clinical issue, and 98% of nurses reported feeling adequate to assess and treat depression. Surprisingly, only 54% indicated they would notify the patient's physician. The majority also reported little familiarity with self-rating depression scales. These findings indicate the urgent need for education regarding depression screening and evaluation tools, the need for further study of nurses' knowledge, and more emphasis on assessment of patients with cancer for depression (Little, Dionne, & Eaton, 2005).

A cognitive marker of clinical depression is a reduced ability to be specific in recalling personal memories, a phenomenon known as *overgeneral memory*. A 2007 study by McBride, Segal, Kennedy, and Gemar showed that both CBT and pharmacotherapy resulted in improved specific memory and a decrease in overgeneral memory. Many patients with cancer have cognitive impairment after treatment with chemotherapy (see Chapter 7 for more information on cognitive impairment). This new research, although not focused on cognitive impairment, offers insight into possible connections between depression and cognitive memory and promises hope toward future research in this area. Another study of 840 patients at the Mayo Clinic demonstrated a synergistic interaction between depression and the apolipoprotein E genotype, and concluded that healthy older adult individuals who develop depression are at increased risk for subsequent mild cognitive impairment (Geda et al., 2006).

In the future, research may provide information about genetic variations that will predict how different patients will respond to specific serotonin-norepinephrine medications. Current studies are looking at acupuncture, high- and low-intensity exercise, vagal nerve stimulation, and rapid transmagnetic stimulation, as well as alternative therapies. Other research is looking at various combinations of medications and combining psychotherapy with medications (Saenger, 2005). NIMH has numerous ongoing studies regarding a variety of depression treatments. Many of these studies are specifically designed to investigate depression in patients with cancer. For a complete list of available clinical trials, go to www .nimh.nih.gov/health/trials/depression.shtml (NIMH, 2008).

Ford and Erlinger (2004) found that major depression is strongly associated with increased levels of C-reactive protein among men, which could help to explain the association between cardiovascular disease and depression. Findings presented at the 2006 meeting of the American Society of Clinical Oncology revealed that increased levels of proinflammatory cytokines have been linked to depression in patients with cancer (Medscape Medical News, 2006). A 2007 report by Reuters found that the presence of depression may slow healing. A total of 183 subjects received a circular wound on the roof of the mouth under local anesthesia. The average healing time was seven days in nondepressed participants and almost four times that in the depressed individuals. More research is needed to illuminate these associations and to identify the exact nature of the correlation between inflammatory markers and cancer.

Although performed on a small sample size of 17, imaging studies on patients with major depression showed response-specific regional changes when scanned with positron-emission tomography after receiving CBT. Changes included increases in hippocampus and dorsal cingulate and decreases in dorsal and medial frontal cortex. When patients were treated with paroxetine, increases were seen in prefrontal areas, and decreases occurred in hippocampal and subgenual cingulate (Goldapple et al., 2004). This preliminary research needs to be continued to explore the relationship between certain areas of the brain and specific therapies.

Since SSRIs were introduced in the 1980s, controversy has existed about the increased risk of suicide ideation. This led to more research about the relationship between suicide ideation and antidepressants, and ultimately a black box warning ensued in the early 2000s. New findings from the Sequenced Treatment Alternatives to Relieve Depression (STAR*D) trial (Laje, 2007) revealed the presence of two genetic markers in patients with suicide ideation. Both of the genetic markers encode nerve cell receptors for glutamate, a chemical messenger, and their presence suggests a genetic basis underlying suicide ideation. This groundbreaking news underscores the need for continued research into potential genetic connections and depression.

The American Psychiatric Association (2000) reviewed trials that combined psychotherapy with pharmacotherapy in patients with mild to moderate depression and those with major or recurrent depression. They concluded that combination therapy was useful for those suffering from major or recurrent depression but not for those with mild depression. All the studies reviewed were in the general population and not specific to patients with cancer, which suggests an area for future research.

Conclusion of Case Study

The nurse asks Z.S. if she believes her mood swings are really hormonal or if she is feeling depressed. Z.S. replies that she does not know for sure but admits she probably is depressed. The nurse asks Z.S. about her activities over the past two weeks. Z.S. states she has been at home and does not care if she ever goes out again. The nurse asks Z.S. if she would be willing to fill out a depression screening questionnaire to help clarify how she is feeling. Z.S. agrees, and the nurse provides her with a copy of the Zung Self-Rating Depression Scale. The nurse completes the scoring and recognizes that Z.S. has a score equivalent with significant depression. She confirms to Z.S. that the screening tool suggests depression and asks if she can schedule an appointment for her to discuss this further with the oncology nurse practitioner or physician. The nurse also takes the opportunity to reassure Z.S. that depression is a medical illness that occurs in up to half of patients with cancer. The nurse provides Z.S. with some reading material about depression to review before the next office visit and also reassuringly explains depression, the causes, and the treatment. At the next chemotherapy appointment, the nurse asks Z.S. about her visit with the oncology nurse practitioner. Z.S. reports that the oncology nurse practitioner discussed depression and the symptoms Z.S. was experiencing, along with the available treatment options. Z.S. and the nurse practitioner jointly agreed to a trial of escitalopram (Lexapro®, Forest Laboratories, Inc.), based on her other medications and health problems. The nurse practitioner also arranged an appointment with a counselor and suggested that Z.S. might benefit from attending a support group meeting for breast cancer survivors. Although it has been only three weeks since Lexapro was added, Z.S. believes that she is already sleeping better and feeling more hopeful.

The oncology nurse is in a unique position to be a catalyst for significant change in the recognition, screening, diagnosis, and treatment of depression in patients with cancer. The opportunities are ripe for dramatic improvement in patient education by the informed oncology nurse. Educated patients, in turn, can be advocates for more research into the causes and treatment of depression.

Conclusion

Oncology nurses are often the first healthcare professionals to recognize the signs and symptoms of depression. Their skills and unique one-on-one interaction with patients with cancer enhance the opportunity to initiate intervention for depression. Excellent care is one of the hallmarks of oncology nurses, and active listening is one of the most important, most caring, and most appreciated interventions nurses can provide for depressed patients with cancer. Even if they do nothing else, nurses should listen well—patients will usually tell them what they need to do.

References

Agency for Healthcare Research and Quality. (2007, September 26). *Comparative effectiveness of second-generation antidepressants in the pharmacologic treatment of adult depression: AHRQ executive summary.* Retrieved February 9, 2008, from http://www.medscape.com/viewprogram/7793

American Psychiatric Association. (2000). *Diagnostic and statistical manual of mental disorders* (4th ed., text revision). Washington, DC: Author.

Badger, T.A., Fulcher, C.D., Gunter, A.K., Marrs, J.A., & Reese, J.M. (2007). *Putting evidence into practice: Depression.* Pittsburgh, PA: Oncology Nursing Society.

Beck, S.L., Dudley, W.N., & Barsevick, A. (2005). Pain, sleep disturbance, and fatigue in patients with cancer: Using a mediation model to test a symptom cluster. *Oncology Nursing Forum, 32*(3), 48–55.

BrainyQuote.com. (n.d.). *Francis Bacon quotes.* Retrieved February 15, 2008, from http://www.brainyquote.com/quotes/authors/f/francis_bacon.html

Brody, D.W., & Serby, M. (2004, September). What you should know about adult depression. *Clinical Advisor,* pp. 19–25.

Caspi, A., Sugden, K., Moffitt, T.E., Taylor, A., Craig, I.W., Harrington, H., et al. (2003). Influence of life stress on depression: Moderation by a polymorphism in the 5-HTT gene. *Science, 301*(5631), 386–389.

Chen, J.J. (2003). *Neuroimmunology of mood disorders and multiple sclerosis.* Retrieved February 18, 2008, from http://www.medscape.com/viewarticle/448447

Epocrates Online. (2008). Retrieved December 4, 2008, from http://www.epocrates.com

Ford, D.E., & Erlinger, T.P. (2004). Depression and C-reactive protein in US adults: Data from the Third National Health and Nutrition Examination Survey. *Archives of Internal Medicine, 164*(9), 1010–1014.

Fredman, S.J., & Rosenbaum, J.F. (2004). *The application of nutrition to psychiatric illness.* Retrieved March 4, 2005, from http://www.medscape.com/viewarticle/480926

Fulcher, C.D. (2006). Clinical challenges: Depression management during cancer treatment. *Oncology Nursing Forum, 33*(1), 33–35.

Fulcher, C.D., Badger, T., Gunter, A.K., Marrs, J.A., & Reese, J.M. (2008). Putting evidence into practice: Interventions for depression. *Clinical Journal of Oncology, 12*(1), 131–140.

Geda, Y.E., Knopman, D.S., Mrazek, D.A., Jicha, G.A., Smith, G.E., Negash, S., et al. (2006). Depression, apolipoprotein E genotype, and the incidence of mild cognitive impairment: A prospective cohort study. *Archives of Neurology, 63*(3), 435–440.

Gielissen, M.F., Verhagen, S., Witjes, F., & Bleijenberg, G. (2006). Effects of cognitive behavior therapy in severely fatigued disease-free cancer patients compared with patients waiting for cognitive behavior therapy: A randomized controlled trial. *Journal of Clinical Oncology, 24*(30), 4882–4887.

Goldapple, K., Segal, Z., Garson, C., Lau, M., Bieling, P., Kennedy, S., et al. (2004). Modulation of cortical-limbic pathways in major depression: Treatment-specific effects of cognitive behavior therapy. *Archives of General Psychiatry, 61*(1), 34–41.

Goodnick, P.J., & Hernandez, M. (2000). Treatment of depression in comorbid medical illness. *Expert Opinion on Pharmacotherapy, 1*(7), 1367–1384.

Goolsby, M.J. (2002). Screening, diagnosis, and clinical care for depression. *Journal of the American Academy of Nurse Practitioners, 14*(7), 286–288.

Gutman, D., & Nemeroff, C.B. (2002). *The neurobiology of depression: Unmet needs.* Retrieved December 4, 2008, from http://www.medscape.com/viewprogram/2123

Harper-Jones, S. (2004). Diabetes and depression. *American Journal of Nursing, 104*(9), 55–59.

Heim, C., Plotsky, P.M., & Nemeroff, C.B. (2004). Importance of studying the contribution of early adverse experience to neurobiological findings in depression. *Neuropsychopharmacology, 29*(4), 641–648.

Hentz, P.B. (2005, June). Effective management strategies for depression. *Clinical Advisor Supplement,* pp. 15–20.

Homsi, J., Nelson, K.A., Sarhill, N., Rybicki, L., LeGrand, S.B., Davis, M.P., et al. (2001). A phase II study of methylphenidate for depression in advanced cancer. *American Journal of Hospice and Palliative Care, 18*(6), 403–407.

Kahn, M. (2007, September 7). *Depression more damaging than some chronic illnesses.* Retrieved September 9, 2007, from http://www.reuters.com/article/healthNews/idUSL0683687520070907

Kessler, R.C., Chiu, W.T., Demler, O., Merikangas, K.R., & Walters, E.E. (2005). Prevalence, severity, and comorbidity of twelve-month DSM-IV disorders in the national comorbidity survey replication. *Archives of General Psychiatry, 62*(6), 617–627.

Khouzam, H.R. (2007). Depression: Guidelines for effective primary care, part 2, treatment. *Consultant, 47*(9), 841–847.

Kim, H.J., McGuire, D.B., Tulman, L., & Barsevick, A.M. (2005). Symptom clusters: Concept analysis and clinical implications for cancer nursing. *Cancer Nursing, 28*(4), 270–282.

Kramer, T.A.M. (2004). *The relationship between depression and physical symptoms.* Retrieved September 30, 2007, from http://www.medscape.com/viewarticle/480898

Laje, G. (2007). Genetic markers of suicide ideation emerging during citalopram treatment of major depression. *American Journal of Psychiatry, 164*(10), 1530–1538.

Leubbert, K., Dahme, B., & Hasenbring, M. (2001). The effectiveness of relaxation training in reducing treatment-related symptoms and improving emotional adjustment in acute non-surgical cancer treatment: A meta-analytic review. *Psycho-Oncology, 10*(6), 490–502.

Liossi, C., & White, P. (2001). Efficacy of clinical hypnosis in the enhancement of quality of life of terminally ill cancer patients. *Contemporary Hypnosis, 18*(3), 145–160.

Little, L., Dionne, B., & Eaton, J. (2005). Nursing assessment of depression among palliative care cancer patients. *Journal of Hospice and Palliative Nursing, 7*(2), 98–106. Retrieved September 23, 2007, from http://www.medscape.com/viewarticle/501961

Ly, K.L., Chidgey, J., Addington-Hall, J., & Hotopf, M. (2002). Depression in palliative care: A systematic review. Part 2: Treatment. *Palliative Medicine, 16*(4), 279–284.

Massie, M.J. (2004). Prevalence of depression in patients with cancer. *Journal of the National Cancer Institute Monographs, 2004*(32), 57–71.

McBride, C., Segal, Z., Kennedy, S., & Gemar, M. (2007). Changes in autobiographical memory specificity following cognitive behavior therapy and pharmacotherapy for major depression. *Psychopathology, 40*(3), 147–152.

Medscape Medical News. (2006). *Cancer patients typically have increased interleukin-6 levels.* Retrieved February 5, 2008, from http://www.medscape.com/viewarticle/537309

Mental Health America. (2007a). *Mental Health America.* Retrieved September 17, 2007, from http://www.mentalhealthamerica.net/go/information/get-info/depression/depression-what-you-need-to-know/depression-what-you-need-to-know

Mental Health America. (2007b). *Mental Health America attitudinal survey. Part IV: Understanding of and attitudes towards mental illness.* Retrieved October 1, 2007, from http://www.mentalhealthamerica.net/go/surveys

Mental Health America. (2007c). *National depression screening day.* Retrieved February 14, 2008, from http://www.mentalhealthamerica.net/index.cfm?objectid=DDAD50B5-1372-4D20-C869143B77A53916

Miovic, M., & Block, S. (2007). Psychiatric disorders in advanced cancer. *Cancer, 110*(8), 1665–1676.

Montano, C.B. (1994). Recognition and treatment of depression in a primary care setting. *Journal of Clinical Psychiatry, 55*(Suppl. 12), 18–34.

Mulhauser, G. (2007). *An introduction to cognitive therapy and cognitive behavioural approaches.* Retrieved September 9, 2007, from http://counsellingresource.com/types/cognitive-therapy/index.html

Musselman, D.L., Lawson, D.H., Gumnick, J.F., Manatunga, A.K., Penna, S., Goodkin, R.S., et al. (2001). Paroxetine for the prevention of depression induced by high-dose interferon alfa. *New England Journal of Medicine, 344*(13), 961–966.

National Comprehensive Cancer Network. (2008). *NCCN Clinical Practice Guidelines in Oncology™: Distress management* [v.1.2008]. Retrieved December 4, 2008, from http://www.nccn.org/professionals/physician_gls/PDF/distress.pdf

National Institute of Mental Health. (2007). *Depression.* Retrieved September 20, 2007, from http://www.nimh.nih.gov/health/topics/depression/index.shtml

National Institute of Mental Health. (2008). *Depression clinical trials.* Retrieved February 14, 2008, from http://www.nimh.nih.gov/health/trials/depression.shtml

Nelson, R. (2007, September 19). *Psychiatric disorders common in patients with advanced cancer.* Retrieved September 27, 2007, from http://www.medscape.com/viewarticle/563028

Newport, D.J. (2005). *Family medicine and primary care: Working toward the 3 "Rs" for managing depression.* Retrieved September 30, 2007, from http://www.medscape.com/viewprogram/3795

Newport, D.J., & Nemeroff, C.B. (1998). Assessment and treatment of depression in the cancer patient. *Journal of Psychosomatic Research, 45*(3), 215–237.

Oncology Nursing Society. (2007). *Depression.* Retrieved February 15, 2008, from http://www.ons.org/outcomes/measures/summaries.shtml#dep

Oquendo, M., & Liebowitz, M. (2006). *The diagnosis and treatment of depression in primary care: An evidence-based approach.* Retrieved August 13, 2007, from http://www.medscape.com/viewprogram/4571

Osborn, R.L., Demoncada, A.C., & Feuerstein, M. (2006). Psychosocial interventions for depression, anxiety, and quality of life in cancer survivors: Meta-analyses. *International Journal of Psychiatry in Medicine, 36*(1), 13–34.

Pirl, W.F. (2004). Evidence report on the occurrence, assessment, and treatment of depression in cancer patients. *Journal of the National Cancer Institute Monographs, 2004*(32), 32–39.

Rajasekaran, M., Edmonds, P.M., & Higginson, I.L. (2005). Systematic review of hypnotherapy for treating symptoms in terminally ill adult cancer patients. *Palliative Medicine, 19*(5), 418–426.

Remick, R.A. (2002). Diagnosis and management of depression in primary care: A clinical update and review. *Canadian Medical Association Journal, 167*(11), 1253–1260.

Reuters. (2007). *Depression may slow healing of mouth sores.* Retrieved February 5, 2008, from http://www.reuters.com/article/healthNews/idUSSAT10157120071031

Robertson, B. (2007). *Progress in discerning endophenotypes in depression.* Retrieved September 23, 2007, from http://www.medscape.com/infosite/nsi/content/article-0805-endophenotypes

Rozans, M., Dreisbach, A., Lertora, J.J., & Kahn, M.J. (2002). Palliative use of methylphenidate in patients with cancer: A review. *Journal of Clinical Oncology, 20*(1), 335–339.

Saenger, E. (2005). Evidence-based approaches to treating and predicting success in the long-term management of depression: An expert interview with Alan Schatzberg, MD. *Medscape Psychiatry and Mental Health, 10*(1). Retrieved September 26, 2007, from http://www.medscape.com/viewarticle/506598

Schwartz, L., Lander, M., & Chochinov, H.M. (2002). Current management of depression in cancer patients. *Oncology, 16*(8), 1102–1115.

Schwenk, T.L., Terrell, L.B., Harrison, R.V., Shadigan, E.M., & Valenstein, M.A. (2005). *Guidelines for clinical care: Depression.* Retrieved September 30, 2007, from http://www.cme.med.umich.edu/pdf/guideline/depression04.pdf

Sharpe, C.R., Collet, J.P., Belzile, E., Hanley, J.A., & Boivin, J.F. (2002). The effects of tricyclic antidepressants on breast cancer risk. *British Journal of Cancer, 86*(1), 92–97.

Spollen, J.J., & Gutman, D.A. (2003). *New research in depression.* Retrieved February 5, 2008, from http://www.medscape.com/viewarticle/457166

Sullivan, P.F., Neale, M.C., & Kendler, K.S. (2000). Genetic epidemiology of major depression: Review and meta-analysis. *American Journal of Psychiatry, 157*(10), 1552–1562.

To, S.E., Zepf, R.A., & Woods, A.G. (2005). The symptoms, neurobiology, and current pharmacological treatments of depression. *Journal of Neuroscience Nursing, 37*(2), 102–107.

Trask, P.C. (2004). Assessment of depression in cancer patients. *Journal of the National Cancer Institute Monographs, 2004*(32), 80–92.

U.S. Preventive Services Task Force. (2002). *Screening for depression: Recommendations and rationale.* Rockville, MD: Agency for Healthcare Research and Quality. Retrieved September 28, 2007, from http://www.ahrq.gov/clinic/3rduspstf/depression/depressrr.htm

Valdivia, I., & Rossy, N. (2004, February 2). *Brief treatment strategies for major depressive disorder: Advice for the primary care clinician.* Retrieved September 30, 2007, from http://www.medscape.com/viewarticle/467185

Vanderhoef, D. (2006, February). Nurse practitioner commentary. In In M.S. Keene, L. Pesko, D.L. Roberts, D. Sheehan, & D. Vanderhoef, *Depression and anxiety disorders: The value of compliance for improved clinical outcomes* (p. 13). Englishtown, NJ: Princeton Media Associates, LLC.

World Health Organization. (2008). *Depression.* Retrieved February 14, 2008, from http://www.who.int/mental_health/management/depression/definition/en

Zabora, J., BrintzenhofeSzoc, K., Curbow, B., Hooker, C., & Piantadosi, S. (2001). The prevalence of psychological distress by cancer site. *Psycho-Oncology, 10*(1), 19–28.

Zung, W.W. (1965). A self-rating depression scale. *Archives of General Psychiatry, 12,* 63–70.

CHAPTER 10

Diarrhea

JoAnn Coleman, RN, MS, AOCN®, ACNP

Case Study

C.B. is a 68-year-old man with a history of small cell lung cancer with bony metastases who reports to the clinic complaining of four to six bouts of explosive diarrhea over the past 12 hours. The patient had completed chemotherapy one week earlier with cisplatin and etoposide along with radiation therapy and irinotecan. He states that the diarrhea started within the past couple of days and has gotten progressively worse. Sometimes he eliminates just a small amount, but the urge to go to the bathroom comes on quickly and strongly.

Overview

Diarrhea is one of the most common symptoms that may complicate the treatment of a patient with cancer. Etiologies of diarrhea may arise from many factors with more than one causative agent or condition, including a single treatment or combination of cancer treatments, which presents a challenge to both assessment and treatment of diarrhea in a patient receiving cancer therapy. Any condition that causes increased intestinal secretions, decreased mucosal absorption, or altered motility can produce diarrhea (Sabol & Carlson, 2007).

Definition

Diarrhea is a physical sign of a gastrointestinal disturbance. The definition of diarrhea is often subjective, with both patients and healthcare providers having different views as to what constitutes diarrhea. The patient may consider one episode of loose stool as diarrhea, whereas the nurse would want a more detailed account of the patient's regular bowel habits to assess for any significant change in bowel movements (Sabol & Carlson, 2007).

Although formal definitions vary, diarrhea usually is defined as an abnormal increase in stool liquidity (altered consistency or looseness of stool), stool frequency (more than three times per day), and stool weight of more than 200 g/day. Diarrhea often occurs when the fecal contents move so rapidly through the small intestine and colon that there is not enough time for the gastrointestinal secretions and oral contents to be absorbed (Camilleri & Murray, 2008).

Small bowel diarrhea is suggested by the passage of large volumes of stool. The stool tends to be light in color, watery or soupy, and generally non-bloody. Foul-smelling, greasy stools that are difficult to flush suggest steatorrhea (foul-smelling, oily, or frothy stools). When pain accompanies large volume diarrhea, it is likely to be periumbilical or in the right lower quadrant, often intermittent and crampy.

Diarrhea from large bowel disease may be smaller in volume, usually is dark in color, and rarely is foul-smelling. The stools are soft, jelly-like, and often mixed with mucus or blood. Abdominal pain associated with large bowel ailments usually is hypogastric, left or right lower quadrant, or sacral. The pain often is continuous and may be associated with tenesmus (a feeling of incomplete defecation) if anorectal disease also is present (Sabol & Carlson, 2007). Stool consistency and the number of episodes are the more common indicators of diarrhea because the consensus among healthcare providers is that loose or watery stools are abnormal, and any other measurements are not practical in a clinical setting (Engelking, 2004).

Diarrhea may or may not be associated with discomfort, and the stool may contain abnormal constituents such as blood, pus, or mucus. Symptoms associated with diarrhea include abdominal pain, cramping and tenderness, urge to defecate, perineal discomfort, and fecal incontinence. Diarrhea can range from mild and self-limiting to severe and life-threatening when uncontrolled diarrhea leads to volume depletion (dehydration), electrolyte imbalance, renal insufficiency, and cardiovascular compromise. These symptoms can occur rapidly in patients receiving cancer-related therapy, alone or in any combination, and whose diarrhea is not adequately managed (Engelking, 2004).

Diarrhea may be characterized as acute or chronic in accordance with onset and duration. See Figure 10-1 for differential diagnosis of acute and chronic diarrhea. Diarrhea is considered acute when it occurs within 2–48 hours of the onset of the causative factor and lasts 7–14 days or less with appropriate intervention. Acute diarrhea most often is associated with infection and usually is self-limiting (Engelking, 2004). Causative factors of acute diarrhea include infectious agents such as viruses, bacteria, and parasites. Other important causes include food poisoning, medications, inflammatory or ischemic bowel disease, fecal impaction, and recent ingestion of poorly absorbable sugars such as lactulose (Marcos & DuPont, 2007). Chronic diarrhea may have a very late onset depending on the cause, persists for more than two to three weeks, and often results from an unidentified causative agent, disease, or response to treatment-related tissue damage that interferes with normal physiologic functioning (Engelking, 2004). Nosocomial diarrhea begins more than 72 hours after admission to the hospital and often is caused by medications, enteral feedings, or superinfection from broad-spectrum antibiotic therapy, either during the course of antibiotic therapy or up to eight weeks after the commencement of treatment (Camilleri & Murray, 2008).

Incidence

Diarrhea related to cancer and its treatment is recognized as a cause of symptom distress and may have severe consequences in a variety of patient populations. The incidence of patients who may experience diarrhea following chemotherapy and/or radiation therapy may be up to 90% (Tuchmann & Engelking, 2001). Patients with cancer-related diarrhea include those with carcinoid tumors, carcinoid syndrome (Kulke, 2007), endocrine hormone-producing tumors (vasoactive intestinal peptide tumor [VIPoma], gastrinoma, insulinoma, glucagonoma) (Jani, Moser, & Khalid, 2007; Maser, Toset, & Roman, 2006; Singh, Teller, Esrasin, & Abbas, 2007), and medullary thyroid tumor (Traugott & Moley, 2005).

Patients undergoing high-dose chemotherapy, as in bone marrow transplantation (Saltz, 2003), and patients receiving radiation therapy to the abdominal and pelvic area are more susceptible to diarrhea (Bismar & Sinicrope, 2002). Patients treated with certain chemotherapeutic

---

| FIGURE 10-1 | Differential Diagnosis of Diarrhea |

Acute Diarrhea
- Infectious
  - Bacterial
    * Salmonella
    * Shigella
    * Campylobacter
    * *Escherichia coli* O157:H7
    * *Staphylococcus aureus*
    * *Clostridium perfingens*
    * *Bacillus cereus*
    * *Yersina enterocolitica*
  - Viral
    * Norwalk virus
    * Vibrio species
  - Protozoal
    * Ova and parasites
    * *Giardia lamblia*
    * *Entamoeba histolytica*
    * Cryptosporidium
- Medications
  - Broad-spectrum antibiotics
  - Sorbitol-containing elixirs
  - Magnesium or phosphate-containing antacids
  - Antiarrhythmics
  - Antineoplastics
  - Antihypertensives
  - Osmotically active agents
  - Prokinetic agents
- Enteral feeding tube nutrition
  - Infusion rate
  - Position of feeding tube
  - Tonicity of formula
  - Formula contamination
- Gastrointestinal disorders
  - Partial bowel obstruction
  - Ischemic bowel
  - Initial attack of ulcerative colitis and Crohn's disease
  - Diverticulitis
  - Pseudomembranous colitis
- Other
  - Excessive alcohol ingestion
  - Dietary indiscretion
    * Mushrooms
    * Unripened fruit
    * Bran
    * Fiber
    * Fructose
  - Heavy metal poisoning

Chronic Diarrhea
- Osmotic diarrhea
  - Malabsorption syndromes
  - Maldigestion syndromes
- Secretory diarrhea
  - Zollinger-Ellison syndrome (gastrinoma)
  - Pancreatic cholera (VIPoma)
  - Neoplasm (colon and villous adenoma)
  - Stimulant or laxative abuse
  - Bile salt malabsorption
- Mucosal inflammation
  - Crohn's disease
  - Ulcerative colitis
  - Lymphocytic colitis
  - Collangenous colitis
  - Radiation enteritis
- Motor disorders
  - Irritable bowel syndrome
  - Endocrine disorders
    * Diabetic diarrhea
    * Adrenal insufficiency
    * Hyperthyroidism
    * Hypothyroidism
    * Addison's disease
  - Surgical procedures
    * Obstruction
    * Gastrectomy
    * Pyloroplasty
    * Vagotomy
    * Antrectomy
    * Small-bowel resection
  - Infiltrative disorders
    * Lymphoma
    * Scleroderma

Note. From "Diarrhea," by V.K. Sabol and F.K. Friedenberg, 1997, *AACN Clinical Issues, 8*(3), p. 427. Copyright 1997 by Lippincott Williams & Wilkins. Reprinted with permission.

FIGURE 10-2	**Cancer Treatment Agents Causing Diarrhea**

Chemotherapy	**Targeted Molecules**
• Dacarbazine	• Bortezomib
• Dactinomycin	• Erlotinib
• Docetaxel	• Gefitinib
• 5-fluorouracil	• Gemtuzumab
• Irinotecan	• Imatinib
• Paclitaxel	• Lapatinib
• Topoisomerase inhibitors	• Sorafenib
• Topotecan	• Sunitinib
	• Vandetanib
Biologic Agents	
• Interferons	**Other**
• Interleukin-2	• Cytarabine
	• Fludarabine
Monoclonal Antibodies	• Mitotane
• Bevacizumab	• Sargramostim
• Cetuximab	• Vidarabine
• Panitumumab	
• Trastuzumab	

Note. Based on information from Polovich et al., 2005.

agents, such as fluoropyrimidines and irinotecan, have a high occurrence of diarrhea (Rosenoff et al., 2006). Diarrhea also has occurred as a side effect of some supportive care pharmaceutical agents such as epoetin alfa and newer antineoplastic agents such as epidermal growth factor receptor inhibitors (Bennett & Engelking, 2002). High-risk agents and regimens, which more likely cause diarrhea, are found in Figure 10-2. Diarrhea also may be the primary manifestation in a cluster of symptoms.

As more aggressive cancer therapy regimens and new therapies are developed and integrated into clinical practice, the scope of the problem of diarrhea in patients with cancer is likely to expand. Oncology nurses need to be vigilant in providing thorough assessment and proactive management in patients undergoing cancer-related therapy that may lead to diarrhea. Severe diarrhea may affect treatment outcomes by having to reduce the antineoplastic drug dosage, delay administration, or discontinue antineoplastic or radiation therapy altogether in response to physical indicators of toxicity (Sonis et al., 2004). Diarrhea often is reported as a dose-limiting toxicity in clinical trials and is a common cause of oncology treatment modification (Engelking, 2004). Although drug or radiation dose reduction, delay, or elimination may temporarily ameliorate diarrhea, it also reduces the desired antineoplastic dose, which in turn limits the optimal levels for treatment with a potentially negative effect on tumor response (Arbuckle, Huber, & Zacker, 2000).

Patients with severe diarrhea can consume costly healthcare resources, including treatment in an emergency department or hospitalization for IV hydration and electrolyte supplementation (Dranitsaris, Maroun, & Shah, 2005). Immunocompromised patients who are hospitalized for diarrhea management incur the added risk of developing secondary complications such as nosocomial infection, which can interfere with achieving positive treatment outcomes (Engelking, 2004). Diarrhea from cancer and cancer treatment also may cause impairment to the quality of a patient's life (O'Brien, Kaklamani, & Benson, 2005).

Risk Factors

Diarrhea resulting from the administration of chemotherapy or specific biologic agents is a frequent problem. If diarrhea is not treated, consequences can lead to severe dehydration, hospitalizations, cancer treatment delays, dose reductions, and even death (Arbuckle et al., 2000). The specific agent, dose, schedule, and combination of anticancer therapies all influence the severity of chemotherapy-induced diarrhea.

Radiation therapy to the pelvis, abdomen, or lower thoracic and lumbar spine can lead to destruction of the cells of the lumen of the bowel, which can lead to severe and life-threatening diarrhea. Minimizing the severity of diarrhea from radiation therapy may increase the probability of completing the planned treatment without interruption and improve the outcome (Bismar & Sinicrope, 2002).

Pathophysiology

Approximately 8–9 liters of fluid enter the intestines daily; 1–2 liters represent food and liquid intake, and the rest is from endogenous sources such as salivary, gastric, pancreatic, biliary, and intestinal secretions. Most of the fluid, about 6–7 liters, is absorbed in the small intestine, and only about 1–2 liters are presented to the colon. Most of this fluid is absorbed as it passes through the colon, leaving a stool output of about 100–200 g daily (Sellin, 1998).

Water is absorbed passively in the gut, dependent on the osmotic gradient. Thus, diarrhea results from excess osmotically active substances in the stool, the result of either decreased absorption of nutrients and electrolytes, excess secretion of electrolytes, or both (Field, 2003).

Causes

A number of etiologies cause cancer-related diarrhea, which results from an imbalance between absorptive and secretive processes produced by an array of causative factors. A list of common causes of diarrhea related to cancer or its treatment can be found in Figure 10-3. Identifying the etiology of the diarrhea aids in the appropriate selection of interventions. Mechanisms of diarrhea that may be seen in patients with cancer are categorized as (1) osmotic, (2) malabsorptive, (3) secretory, (4) infectious/exudative, (5) dysmotility-associated,

---

FIGURE 10-3	Causative Factors in Cancer-Related Diarrhea

Disease-Related Etiologies
- Neuroendocrine tumors
  - VIPomas
  - Gastrinomas
  - Insulinomas
  - Medullary thyroid tumor
  - Carcinoid
- Neoplasia
  - Colorectal tumors
  - Lymphoma
- Partial small bowel obstruction
- Enterocolonic fistula
- Ischemic colitis
- Enzyme deficiency
- Pancreatic cancer
- Reduced luminal bile acid
- Infectious processes
  - Invasive bacterial infection (*Clostridium difficile, Escherichia coli*)
  - Ulcerating viral infection (cytomegalovirus, Herpes simplex)
  - Invasive parasites (amebiasis)

Treatment-Related Etiologies
- Surgical procedures
  - Pancreatectomy
  - Ileal resection
  - Colon resection
  - Anorectal surgery
  - Gastrectomy
  - Vagotomy
  - Sympathectomy
- Chemotherapeutic agents
  - Fluoropyrimidines
  - Topoisomerase inhibitors
  - Cisplatin
- Radiation therapy effects
  - Abdominal
  - Pelvic
- Supportive care therapies
  - Supplemental feeding formulas
  - Anti-infective agents
  - Cytoprotective agents (e.g., metoclopramide)
  - Narcotic withdrawal

Note. From "Diarrhea," by C. Engelking in C.H. Yarbro, M.H. Frogge, and M. Goodman (Eds.), *Cancer Symptom Management* (3rd ed., p. 531), 2004, Sudbury, MA: Jones and Bartlett. Copyright 2004 by Jones and Bartlett. Adapted with permission.

and (6) cancer treatment–related diarrhea from chemotherapy or radiation treatments (Engelking, 2004). These mechanisms may overlap with more than one mechanism occurring in a patient. Figure 10-3 presents an overview of cancer-related diarrhea.

Osmotic Diarrhea

Osmotic diarrhea is related to the ingestion of poorly absorbable substances, dietary factors, or problems with digestion leading to malabsorptive function of the bowel. Water is pulled into the bowel lumen by the osmotic pressure of unabsorbed particles, increasing the water content of the gastrointestinal tract. There is a rapid fluid shift and dilution and poor mixing of bile and pancreatic juices, thereby slowing the reabsorption of water (Gibson & Keefe, 2006). Common causes of osmotic diarrhea can result from ingestion of poorly absorbed hyperosmolar substances such as sorbitol, magnesium-based antacids, citrates, lactulose, enteral feeding solutions, and carbohydrates. Pancreatic insufficiency can also trigger osmotic diarrhea when the release of pancreatic enzymes is slowed or prevented. Incomplete digestion of fat in the small intestine occurs secondary to biliary or pancreatic obstruction or surgery, leading to osmotic diarrhea. Blood in the bowel from intestinal hemorrhage, which is common in patients with esophageal, gastric, and intestinal malignancies, creates an osmotic pull of water into the lumen, leading to osmotic diarrhea (Schiller, 2007; Sellin, 1998).

Malabsorptive Diarrhea

Malabsorptive diarrhea is a combination of mechanical and biochemical mechanisms that prevent effective absorptive processes. Malabsorption of fluid occurs when the lumen or mucosal integrity or other gut wall characteristics are altered. Enzyme deficiencies may occur after gastrectomy or pancreatectomy, which inhibits complete digestion such as with lactose intolerance and pancreatic insufficiency, or surgical resection may reduce the mucosal surface for the process of absorption (Mackay, Hayes, & Yeo, 2006; Savaiano, Boushey, & McCabe, 2006; Zgodzinski, Dekoj, & Espat, 2005). The degree of malabsorption depends on the length and portion of bowel resected. Ileal resection causes diarrhea through disruption of the enterohepatic circulation of bile salts allowing nonabsorbed, osmotically active substances to enter the colon, exerting a stimulant effect on the bowel. The amount of colon resected also can result in decreased fluid reabsorption by reducing the intestinal mucosal contact and transit time, thus resulting in a decrease in the absorption of electrolytes and/or bile salts. This is called short bowel or short gut syndrome and occurs when more than 200 cm of bowel is resected (Misialos, Macheras, Lapetanakis, & Liakatos, 2007). A primary feature of malabsorptive diarrhea is large-volume steatorrhea.

Patients with hypoalbuminemia (serum albumin < 2.5 mg/dl) may exhibit malabsorptive diarrhea. The low albumin leads to a decrease in oncotic pressure and results in edema of the intestinal mucosa. The fluid in the intestines cannot be reabsorbed and ultimately is eliminated as liquid stool (Camilleri & Murray, 2008).

Secretory Diarrhea

Secretory diarrhea results from overstimulation of the intestinal tract's secretory capacity. The small intestines and large bowel mucosas secrete more fluids and electrolytes than can be absorbed by the bowel. Secretory diarrhea is characterized by large stool volume, which can exceed 1 L/hr in a well-hydrated person. Usually, red or white blood cells are not present in the stool and the patient lacks a fever or other systemic symptoms. Secretory diarrhea persists when a patient fasts because the secretory process is independent of ingested substances (McMahan & DuPont, 2007).

Common causes of secretory diarrhea include (a) bacterial enterotoxins resulting in inflammation and infection of the gut (Bartlett, 2002), (b) damage from chemotherapy or radiation (Gwede, 2003), (c) graft-versus-host disease (GVHD) (Ross & Couriel, 2005), (d) endocrine hormone-secreting tumors (e.g., carcinoid tumors, VIPomas, gastrinoma, insulinoma, glucagonoma, medullary thyroid cancer) (Jani et al., 2007; Maser et al., 2006; Singh et al., 2007) and medullary thyroid tumor (Traugott & Moley, 2005), (e) inflammatory bowel disease such as Crohn disease (Ruthruff, 2007), and (f) bile salt malabsorption seen in distal small bowel resection (> 100 cm resected) (Westergaard, 2007).

Bacterial enterotoxins can produce secretory diarrhea as certain pathogens (e.g., *Clostridium [C.] difficile* and *Escherichia coli*) produce infections that irritate the bowel wall, leading to intestinal stimulation and oversecretion. Large bowel irritation from bacterial enterotoxins leads to secretion of large amounts of water, electrolytes, and mucus as a protective mechanism, causing dilution of the irritating enterotoxins and rapid movement through the colon (Gore & Surawicz, 2003). Antibiotic therapy also may cause secretory diarrhea in up to 20% of patients, which usually is benign and self-limiting (Engelking, 2004). Pseudomembranous enterocolitis can develop from an overgrowth of toxic strains of *C. difficile* following administration of antibiotic therapy in both immunocompromised and healthy people. If left untreated, *C. difficile* infection can lead to severe diarrhea, hypovolemia, toxic megacolon with dilation and possible perforation of the colon, hemorrhage, and even death (Bartlett, 2002). Patients receiving chemotherapy are at the highest risk for pseudomembranous enterocolitis (Engelking, 2004).

In chemotherapy-induced diarrhea, an imbalance between absorption and secretion leads to the production of a large volume of fluid and electrolytes in the small bowel. This fluid overwhelms the absorptive capacity of the colon, leading to large volumes of diarrhea. This type of diarrhea usually does not resolve with fasting (Stringer et al., 2007).

Radiation enteritis is a complication of abdominal and pelvic radiation. Radiation therapy interacts with cells to cause cellular death, which leads to diarrhea, especially when the cells are most vulnerable to the killing effect of radiation therapy during the G_2 and M phases. Rapidly proliferating tissues, such as small intestine crypt cells, are particularly sensitive to radiation. They undergo apoptosis (programmed cell death), and the crypt cells are shed from the intestinal villi. Acute diarrhea from radiation enteritis is seen during this phase. Concurrent administration of chemotherapy may enhance apoptosis and exacerbate the diarrhea. Late or chronic radiation enteritis is secondary to mucosal atrophy with vasculitis and fibrosis progressing over time, resulting in narrowing of the intestinal lumen with dilation of the bowel proximal to the stricture. The affected segments of intestine become thickened. Ulceration, necrosis, and occasional perforation of the bowel wall may occur (Nguyen, Antoine, Dutta, Karlsson, & Sallah, 2002; Toomey, Cahill, Geraghty, & Thirion, 2006).

Secretory diarrhea is a major feature of acute intestinal GVHD. Patients undergoing allogeneic hematopoietic stem cell transplantation have an autoimmune response to donor T lymphocytes in specific target tissues including the epithelial lining of the intestinal wall. This response generally occurs within 20–30 days after receiving the donor cell infusion. A cascade of events cause the proliferation of inflammatory cells that ultimately produce mucosal tissue damage and may even completely denude the entire gastrointestinal tract. Damage to intestinal tract tissue is manifested by large-volume, greenish-colored liquid diarrhea in amounts that correlate with the extent of tissue damage. Patients may produce as much as eight liters within 24 hours (Ross & Couriel, 2005).

Hormones produced by endocrine tumors, such as vasoactive intestinal peptide in VIPomas, affect the intestinal transport of water and electrolytes, causing an accumulation of intestinal fluids. The patient has a large volume of watery stool (> 1,000 ml/day) and may have severe loss of electrolytes, which can lead to severe dehydration and arrhythmias (Maser et al., 2006).

Diarrhea associated with inflammatory bowel disease may result from a number of causative factors, including location, extent, and severity of inflammation. The result of inflammatory bowel disease is now thought to be the result of an exaggerated or insufficiently suppressed immune response to some unknown antigen probably derived from the normal bowel microbial flora. This inflammatory process leads to mucosal damage and a disturbance of the epithelial barrier function, resulting in an increased influx of bacteria into the intestinal wall causing intestinal overstimulation and secretion of fluid (Scaldaferri & Fiocchi, 2007).

A patient with bile acid malabsorption typically presents with chronic, watery diarrhea. Bile acids recirculate between the liver and small intestine. They reabsorb in the distal small intestine, and normally only a small fraction of the bile acids goes into the colon during each cycle. In a patient with bile acid malabsorption, a larger amount of bile acids stimulate electrolyte and water secretion, which results in loose to watery stools. The most common cause of bile acid malabsorption is ileal resection (Westergaard, 2007).

Infectious Diarrhea

Infectious diarrhea is characterized by a systemic fever, pus, blood, or mucus in the stool. The diarrhea is caused by an infectious agent invading the intestinal mucosa. Within the intestinal wall, the hydrostatic pressure in the blood vessels and lymphatics cause water and electrolytes, mucus, protein, and cells to accumulate in the lumen of the bowel. The destruction of enzymes essential to carbohydrate and protein digestion combines to produce moderate to severe amounts of diarrhea. Fecal leukocytes are often found in fecal smears. The sudden onset of loose or watery stools in a previously healthy individual usually is of infectious origin (bacterial, viral, or parasitic). The majority of causative microbial agents may never be identified (Gadewar & Fasano, 2005). *C. difficile* is the most commonly (up to about 50%) identified microbial causative agent in antibiotic-associated diarrhea in the hospital. Causes of infectious diarrhea include the use of excessive antibiotics (penicillin, clindamycin, cephalosporins, and quinolones) (Bartlett & Gerding, 2008), contaminated enteral feedings (Eisenberg, 2002), or the ingestion of contaminated foods (DuPont, 1997).

Anemia and hypoalbuminemia caused by cumulative blood and protein loss through the intestinal wall also are associated with infectious diarrhea. Albumin levels of less than 2 g/dl, which is common in patients with various types and stages of cancer, cause intestinal wall edema, which further disrupts absorptive processes of the bowel. The volume of diarrhea is usually less than 1,000 ml/day with high-frequency stools (> 6/day) (Engelking, 2000).

Dysmotility-Associated Diarrhea

Dysmotility-associated diarrhea occurs when intestinal motility becomes altered in response to changes in mechanical stretch receptors and neural stimuli that determine peristaltic activity. This results in the rapid transit of stool through the colon, limiting the exposure time for absorption. Small semiliquid to liquid high-weight stools in variable volume and frequency are characteristic of diarrhea associated with bowel motility problems.

Many causative factors may be responsible for dysmotility-associated diarrhea, including (a) fecal impaction from drug therapy (e.g., narcotics) that results in overflow diarrhea around the impaction (Abraham & Sellin, 2007); (b) obstructive processes that distend the bowel beyond its normal size (e.g., tumor, adhesions from surgery, radiation therapy); (c) the over-ingestion of peristaltic stimulants (e.g., laxatives) (Camilleri & Murray, 2008); (d) opioid withdrawal syndrome (Gowing, Ali, & White, 2006); or (e) the psychoneuroimmunologic effects of stress and fear (Hertig, Cain, Jarrett, Burr, & Heitkemper, 2007).

Chemotherapy-Induced Diarrhea

The pathophysiology of chemotherapy-induced diarrhea is not well understood and is probably the result of a combination of mechanisms. Cytotoxic agents damage the mucosal lining of the intestine, altering water absorption. Within the colon, water follows chloride, and in normal tissue, both are absorbed readily from the lumen of the bowel. When the crypts of the colon are damaged from chemotherapy, chloride absorption is reduced and water is released into the lumen, resulting in diarrhea. Gut motility also is altered, with reduced transit time for bowel contents, again resulting in a decrease in water absorption. Chemotherapy-induced diarrhea may be classified as osmotic or secretory (Engelking, 2004).

Many antineoplastic agents cause mucosal damage characterized by sloughing of surface epithelial cells without basement membrane replacement, resulting in superficial ulceration and extensive bowel wall inflammation. Epithelial cell necrosis and inflammation trigger a cascade of events that stimulate intestinal wall secretion of large quantities of fluid and electrolytes producing diarrhea. These mucosal reactions contribute to the destruction of brush border enzymes needed for carbohydrate and protein digestion, thus producing a malabsorptive effect. In neutropenic patients, endotoxin released by opportunistic pathogens exaggerates the mucosal inflammation and intensifies the severity of the diarrhea. These responses combine to produce moderate to severe diarrhea immediately following and up to 10–14 days after chemotherapy (Engelking, 2000).

The severity of chemotherapy-induced diarrhea depends upon the particular agent or combination of agents, dosage schedule, route of administration, and multimodality regimens including both chemotherapy and radiation (Richardson & Dobish, 2007). Diarrhea is a dose-limiting toxicity for certain chemotherapeutic agents, particularly the fluoropyrimidines (e.g., 5-fluorouracil, floxuridine) and the topoisomerase inhibitors (e.g., irinotecan), although the mechanisms and manifestations differ. Diarrhea associated with fluoropyrimidine therapy is characterized by a unique syndrome and may be either acute (within 24 hours after therapy) or late (2–10 days after therapy). The acute form of diarrhea is sudden, and the patient may exhibit other symptoms such as diaphoresis, flushing, abdominal cramping, salivation, and nasal congestion. This reaction resolves rapidly following atropine administration (Engelking, 2000). Late-onset diarrhea related to irinotecan occurs in up to 80% of patients and can be attributed to an intestinal accumulation of the drug's active metabolite SN-38. Late-onset diarrhea can occur as early as two days after therapy but most commonly presents within one to two weeks following irinotecan administration. Incidence of diarrhea is higher in patients receiving concomitant fluorouracil. The median duration of late-onset diarrhea is about three days with appropriate management (Richardson & Dobish).

Radiation-Induced Diarrhea

The pathology of radiation-induced diarrhea is not well understood. Radiation-induced mucosal damage results in decreased absorption of water and electrolytes, causing diarrhea. Another possible mechanism is decreased bile acid absorption in the ileum caused by mucosal damage. When passing through the bowel, the excess bile acid irritates and damages the protective mucosa of the intestine. This results in the passage of fluid and electrolytes into the lumen and causes diarrhea. Acute and chronic diarrhea can result from radiation therapy directed to the abdominal, pelvic, and lumbosacral area of the body. Severity of the diarrhea depends on the total dose of radiation, anatomic location, and amount of bowel included in the field. The production of replacement crypt stem cells is arrested following radiation. This results in denudement and atrophy of the villi in the small intestine and flattening of the epithelial surface in the large bowel. These changes cause protein and fibrin formations, leukocyte infiltration, and edema of the bowel wall, producing loss of epithelial function and giving rise to the loss of water, electrolytes, and protein. Conjugated bile salts, which normally are reabsorbed in the small intestine, enter the colon instead and are deconjugated by colonic bacterial flora, resulting in water retention and diarrhea. A reduction in brush border lactase interferes with enzyme degradation of lactose. This allows lactose to accumulate in the gut where it ferments, thus producing flatulence, distention, and diarrhea (Bismar & Sinicrope, 2002).

Acute radiation enteritis develops in 30%–49% of patients receiving a total radiation dose in the range of 15–30 gray and may be seen in up to 70% of patients, depending on treatment and predisposing factors. Late-onset effects of abdominal radiotherapy may occur 8–12 months or as late as 15 years after radiation and are manifested as chronic radiation enteritis (Nguyen et al., 2002).

Chronic radiation enteritis results from vascular insufficiency, which develops gradually over time and is secondary to damaged epithelial cells in blood vessels and connective tissues found in the bowel wall. Ischemic changes may lead to fistula formation, ulceration, obstruction, abscess formation, stricture, perforation, and chronic bleeding. Functional changes include malabsorption, narrowing of the bowel lumen predisposing to obstruction, and changes that may result in intestinal fibrosis and ischemia. Late effects have been documented in 5%–15% of patients treated with abdominal, pelvic, and lumbosacral radiation (Otterson, 2007).

Assessment

A complete assessment of the patient's medical, social, and family history in addition to the patient's present physical examination and laboratory studies is needed to determine the etiology of diarrhea. This information is necessary, as all possible causes of diarrhea need to be considered for appropriate treatment interventions. Figure 10-4 discusses the assessment of risk factors for diarrhea.

In patients with cancer, nurses must anticipate the risk of occurrence, potential severity of diarrhea from the patients' particular cancer, and its treatment, as well as evaluate the onset and clinical course of the diarrhea. Through assessment of diarrhea in a patient with cancer, nurses need to sort through the disease, its treatment, and supportive care interventions to help to identify the primary cause (Polovich, White, & Kelleher, 2005).

FIGURE 10-4	Assessment of Risk Factors for Diarrhea

- Normal bowel habits
- Diet history and any recent changes
  - Fluids
  - Fat
  - Fiber
  - Fruit
  - Caffeine
  - Lactose intolerance
  - Alcohol
  - Spicy foods
- Familial diseases
  - Crohn disease or ulcerative colitis
  - Celiac disease
  - Cystic fibrosis
  - Hyperthyroidism
  - Diabetes mellitus
- Medical history
  - Inflammatory condition
    * Diverticulitis
    * Irritable bowel syndrome
    * Crohn disease or ulcerative colitis
    * Intestinal infection secondary to mucositis and neutropenia
    * Graft-versus-host disease
  - Cancer diagnosis and stage
  - Cancer treatment
    * Surgery
    * Chemotherapy
    * Radiation therapy

- Medications
  - Antacids, especially magnesium-containing compounds
  - Antiarrhythmics
  - Antihypertensives
  - Antibiotics
  - Diuretics
  - Nonsteroidal anti-inflammatory drugs
  - Laxatives or stool softeners
  - Magnesium oxide
  - Theophylline
  - Antidiarrheals
  - Immunosuppression
  - Opioid withdrawal
- Activity level
  - Exercise—heavy exercise may induce diarrhea.
- Previous surgery
  - Small intestine or large bowel resection
  - Gastrectomy
  - Manipulation of bowel during surgery may cause diarrhea or ileus.
- Travel history
- Anxiety and stress
- Alternative therapies such as herbal remedies
- Other
  - Sorbitol-based gum
  - Hyperosmotic dietary supplements

Patient Report

A patient's complaint of diarrhea initiates a complete bowel elimination profile to assess normal bowel habits and any alterations related to the cancer and its treatment, as well as any comorbid conditions associated with impaired bowel function. Current bowel function pattern assessment should include descriptions of stool color, consistency, odor, daily amount, and number of episodes per day. Ascertaining the patient's definition of diarrhea is important, as stool frequency may have increased rather than loose or liquid stool occurring. Determining the relationship of stools to administration of antineoplastic agents or treatments, eating, or stressful events allows one to place the timing of the onset of the event. Visual inspection of the stool is important to confirm patient report of stool character and to identify the presence of any blood or pus. The patient also may complain of abdominal cramps, distention, intestinal rumbling (i.e., borborygmus), anorexia, and thirst. Painful, spasmodic contractions of the anus and ineffective straining (i.e., tenesmus) may occur with defecation (Schiller, 2007).

The National Cancer Institute (NCI) Cancer Therapy Evaluation Program's (2009) Common Terminology Criteria for Adverse Events is a useful tool for assessing patients' complaints of diarrhea and is presented in Table 10-1. It is a five-point Likert-type scale for rating the severity of diarrhea. Other grading scales include the Eastern Cooperative Oncology Group (2007) Common Toxicity Criteria for diarrhea and the World Health Organization (n.d.) Toxicity Criteria by Grade for diarrhea (see Figure 10-5).

TABLE 10-1	National Cancer Institute Common Terminology Criteria for Diarrhea				
Adverse Event	**Grade**				
	1	**2**	**3**	**4**	**5**
Diarrhea	Increase of < 4 stools per day over baseline; mild increase in ostomy output compared to baseline	Increase of 4–6 stools per day over baseline; moderate increase in ostomy output compared to baseline	Increase of ≥ 7 stools per day over baseline; incontinence; hospitalization indicated; severe increase in ostomy output compared to baseline; limiting self care ADL	Life-threatening consequences; urgent intervention indicated	Death

Definition: A disorder characterized by frequent and watery bowel movements.
ADL—activities of daily living

Note. From *Common Terminology Criteria for Adverse Events* (Version 4.0), by National Cancer Institute Cancer Therapy Evaluation Program, 2009. Retrieved July 24, 2009, from http://ctep.cancer.gov/protocol Development/electronic_applications/docs/ctcaev4.pdf.

FIGURE 10-5	Common Toxicity Criteria for Diarrhea*
Eastern Cooperative Oncology Group Common Toxicity Criteria for Diarrhea 0 = none 1 = increase of 2–3 stools/day over pre-Rx 2 = increase of 4–6 stools/day, or nocturnal stools, or moderate cramping 3 = increase of 7–9 stools/day, or incontinence or, severe cramping 4 = increase of ≥ 10 stools/day, or grossly bloody diarrhea, or need for parenteral support	

*The World Health Organization's Toxicity Criteria by Grade for Diarrhoea are the same as presented here.

Note. From *ECOG Common Toxicity Criteria*, by Eastern Cooperative Oncology Group, 2007. Retrieved December 19, 2007, from http://www.ecog.org/general/ctc.pdf.

The patient's use of complementary and alternative therapies needs to be elicited because patients may self-administer herbal supplements and teas without the knowledge of healthcare providers. It is important for nurses to query patients about the use of complementary and alternative therapies. A number of herbals that may cause diarrhea can be found in Figure 10-6.

Urine output needs to be assessed to assist in delineating the amount of fluid depletion. Ascertaining the frequency of stool, consistency of stool, and associated symptoms may help to identify the etiology or the interventions that may be effective. Figure 10-7 depicts points of evaluation of patients' bowel patterns.

Physical Findings

Physical assessment of the patient with a complaint of diarrhea is necessary to assist in determining dehydration and electrolyte imbalance, infectious processes, and impaired perianal or peristomal skin integrity. To determine whether a patient is dehydrated, assessment of the following signs and symptoms is performed: Assess for dry mucosal surfaces, poor skin turgor, sunken eyes, tachycardia, orthostatic blood pressure changes, fluctuations in mental status, and urine that is dark in color with a high specific gravity. Weight loss of 1%–2% in a week may be related and a significant problem by itself (Engelking, 2004).

FIGURE 10-6	Herbs and Supplements That Can Cause Diarrhea
• High-dose vitamin C • Magnesium • Potassium • Aloe • Bromelain • Buckhorn • Cascara • Cat's claw • Creatine • "Dieter's" teas • Eucalyptus oil	• Fish oil • Flaxseed and flaxseed oil • Garlic • Guggulipid • Lecithin • Milk thistle • Rhubarb • Rose hips • Sarsaparilla • Senna

Physical examination includes auscultation of bowel sounds and abdominal palpation to assess for abdominal bruits, masses, ascites, hepatosplenomegaly, and perianal irritation or fistulas. Findings on physical examination may give a clue in identifying the location in the bowel where the problem is originating. Absent or hyperactive bowel sounds may indicate that the patient is experiencing an obstructive process. Fecal impaction may be determined by a rectal examination. Examination of the perianal or peristomal area for impaired skin integrity from repetitive cleansing or wiping is required.

The presence of fever, blood in the stool, abdominal pain, weakness, or dizziness warrants medical attention to rule out infection, bowel obstruction, or dehydration (Benson et al., 2004). Following the order of the abdominal assessment (inspection, auscultation for bowel sounds, percussion, and then palpation) is important to obtain critical information without causing discomfort to the patient.

FIGURE 10-7	Evaluation of a Patient's Bowel Pattern

Frequency of Stool
• Increase from baseline
• Timing
  – Onset
  – Duration
  – Early morning bowel is most active; after eating; not in relation to intake

Consistency of Stool
• Formed or liquid
• Color—light color may indicate lack of bile salts.
• Odor—possible indication of infection or inadequate fat metabolism
• Presence of other constituents
  – Blood increases bowel contents transit time.
  – Pus may indicate infection or inflammation.
  – Stool mixed with blood, pus, or exudates points toward an inflammatory process, ischemia, infection, or neoplastic disease.

Associated Symptoms
• Nausea
• Flushing, feeling hot
• Diaphoresis
• Sense of incontinence
• Abdominal cramping, bloating, or gaseous feeling

The presence of fecal impaction must be considered, as diarrhea may occur because of impaired absorption at the site of obstruction, allowing only fluid to pass through the obstructed area. This may be suspected if a patient complains of acute and severe cramping that occurs before small amounts of diarrhea occur in the absence of any other risk factors. Patients with thrombocytopenia and/or neutropenia must be considered before any digital rectal examination or disimpaction. A patient's diet history and medication intake also need to be assessed.

Patient assessment is of the utmost importance to determine if the clinical manifestations are severe in a patient receiving treatment for cancer, as consideration for ongoing treatment may be affected (Viele, 2003). Administration of an antineoplastic agent or agents may need to be held or modified, or a radiation treatment may need to be held.

Patients may be reluctant to tell the nurse about any toxicity because they may believe that it might lead to dose reduction, which will cause treatment to be less effective. It is important to inform the patient that side effects and adjustments in doses of chemotherapy and radiation are common. The nurse should stress to the patient the importance of relaying any symptoms accurately and in a timely manner, as failure to adjust doses early may lead to severe, life-threatening toxicities, treatment delay, and possibly a greater dose reduction.

Critical clinical manifestations related to diarrhea include
- Dehydration
- Life-threatening hypokalemia, metabolic acidosis, hypercalcemia, and malnutrition
- Cardiovascular compromise
- Impaired immune function following frequent episodes of chemotherapy-induced diarrhea
- Reduced absorption of oral medications
- Pain
- Anxiety
- Exhaustion
- Decreased quality of life.

Laboratory Results

No specific diagnostic tests validate diarrhea, but several tests may help to clarify the etiology. Stool analysis may be performed for bacteria, fungus, ova and parasites, specific bacterial toxins (specifically *C. difficile*), blood, and fecal leukocytes. Laboratory data are essential to determine electrolyte imbalance, particularly potassium level and hypoalbuminemia to check for protein-calorie malnutrition. A complete blood count is checked to determine the presence of infection. Any invasive radiographic imaging with contrast or endoscopic evaluation with biopsy should be reserved for patients with persistent diarrhea refractory to antidiarrheal interventions, particularly in immunocompromised individuals. Patients suspected of having an endocrine hormone-producing tumor may need a 24-hour urine collection for 5-hydroxyindoleacetic acid or serum analysis for chromogranin A, C-peptide, gastrin, glucagon, insulin growth factor, pancreatic polypeptide, vasoactive intestinal peptide–binding protein, and calcitonin (Warner, 2005). Chronic diarrhea of unknown origin investigations can include breath tests to evaluate lactose, bile acid, and carbohydrate absorption, small intestine biopsy, intestinal angiograms, and vitamin B_{12} analysis (Sellin, 1998).

Evidence-Based Interventions

The Oncology Nursing Society (ONS) developed a Putting Evidence Into Practice (PEP) resource for diarrhea (Muehlbauer et al., 2008). This resource provides evidence-based oncology nursing interventions for diarrhea that can be used in the clinical setting. Recommendations for the treatment of chemotherapy-induced and radiation-induced diarrhea are presented along with levels of evidence used in the nursing interventions. Treatment of diarrhea entails the use of targeted pharmacotherapy and adjunctive supportive care, such as dietary modification, bowel rest, fluid and electrolyte replacement, and skin care, as well as delay or discontinuation of the causative agent. Patients and caregivers need to be educated about which symptoms require immediate attention and how to monitor and document symptoms effectively. To accomplish these goals, interventions must match the identified cause and the specific needs of the patient by incorporating both nonpharmacologic and pharmacologic strategies (Stern & Ippoliti, 2003).

Nonpharmacologic Interventions

Anticipation and prompt management of diarrhea related to cancer and its treatment may be more realistic to minimize toxicity and associated side effects than any prevention strategies. Patients with diarrhea should discontinue foods, beverages, and medications known to produce or aggravate diarrhea. Dietary modification as a pretreatment prophylaxis for both chemotherapy and radiation therapy has evolved from expert opinion. A diet low in fiber and residue may minimize the severity of cancer treatment–related diarrhea. Initiating a low-lactose diet in individuals with temporary lactose intolerance may prevent, reduce, or control diarrhea in some patients. The use of a lactase enzyme supplement such as Lactaid® (McNeil Nutritionals, LLC) may be a helpful adjunct (Engelking, 2000). Initiating a nutrition consult with a dietitian can be beneficial to assist the patient in assessing and choosing foods and to customize a diet to maintain adequate nutrition and hydration. Dietary recommendations to alleviate or eliminate diarrhea are presented in Table 10-2.

TABLE 10-2	Dietary Recommendations	
Recommendation for Homeostasis	**Consume**	**Avoid**
Hydration	8–10 large glasses of clear liquids, which may include weak, tepid tea and gelatin Sports drinks Juice* Fluids with glucose, as glucose absorption drives sodium and water back into the body Clear broth/bouillon	Alcohol Coffee and tea with caffeine Very hot or cold beverages Milk Carbonated drinks Prune and orange juice
Nutrition	Small amounts of soft, bland food Consider BRAT diet: **B**ananas, **R**ice, **A**pplesauce, **T**oast Foods high in protein (beef, chicken, turkey, eggs) Potassium-rich food (bananas, fruit juices*, potatoes without the skin, avocados, asparagus tips) Foods containing pectin (beets, unspiced applesauce, peeled apples, ginger tea) Low-fiber foods (white bread, white rice) Eat food at room temperature.	Milk and dairy products Spicy, greasy, or fried foods High-fiber foods (whole-grain products, beans, raw vegetables, seeds, popcorn, pickles, fruit) Hyperosmotic supplements (Ensure® [Abbott Laboratories])

* Do not eat or drink grapefruit products until cleared by your doctor.

Note. Based on information from Engelking, 2004.

The addition of soluble fiber supplements for the prevention of diarrhea related to radiation therapy has been established by clinical practice guidelines and is likely to be effective (Muehlbauer et al., 2008). Patients requiring tube feedings may have psyllium or pectin added to their formula to prevent diarrhea. Using lactose-free and fiber-containing products, minimizing risk of bacterial contamination of formulas during preparation, diluting medications with water, and altering the feeding infusion rate to infuse over time rather than bolus administration are other considerations to prevent diarrhea (Eisenberg, 2002). More research is needed on psyllium fiber supplementation to identify the type and dose that will effectively treat and/or prevent diarrhea for any patient having chemotherapy or radiation therapy (Muehlbauer et al.).

Nonpharmacologic interventions considered likely to be effective include probiotic oral supplementation used for the prevention of diarrhea from radiation to the pelvis. Supplementation with *Lactobacillus acidophilus* NDC0 1748, *Lactobacillus rhamnosus*, and VSL#3 have been studied and may be effective (Bowen et al., 2007; Marteau, de Vrese, Cellier, & Schrezenmeir, 2001). Further research is needed to determine the probiotic strain, dosage, and timing of administration needed to prevent or treat diarrhea from radiation therapy (Muehlbauer et al., 2008).

Careful monitoring of the use and frequency of laxatives and stool softeners may help to avoid diarrhea. A healthy bowel regimen with adequate exercise, fluid intake, and dietary fiber should be encouraged. Incorporation of a bowel regimen in patients who require narcotics for pain management needs to be assessed and monitored to see if it reduces the incidence of fecal impaction.

Perianal, perineal, and any peristomal skin must be assessed in a patient experiencing diarrhea. Liquid stool contains acids and can be very caustic to bare skin, causing excoriation and skin breakdown depending on the length of exposure and recurring episodes of stooling. The affected area should be cleansed after each episode to limit exposure time of stool on the skin. Mild soap and water or baby wipes are the cleansing products of choice. The skin should be patted dry, rather than rubbed, and if possible, allowed to air dry. Sitz baths of tepid water several times a day may minimize discomfort. A skin barrier product such as petroleum jelly, Desitin® (Johnson & Johnson) ointment, or other moisture-barrier products may be used but must be removed carefully, as skin damage from rubbing may cause additional damage.

Rectal pouches may be used in hospitalized patients to promote skin integrity in cases of severe diarrhea or persistent fecal incontinence. Nurses must remind patients receiving radiation therapy to be careful to not wash off treatment field markings and check with the radiation therapy team before application of any skin products (Engelking, 2004).

Diarrhea is usually high in sodium, potassium, and bicarbonate. The use of oral rehydration formulas (commercial products are Pedialyte® [Abbott Laboratories], Ricelyte® [Mead Johnson], and Gatorade® [Quaker Oats Co.]) is based on the principle that carbohydrate absorption, especially glucose, in the small bowel facilitates sodium and water reabsorption from the intestinal lumen into the intravascular compartment. The effectiveness of these products has not been established. Sports drinks that claim to replenish fluid and electrolyte loss during exercise may be used for fluid replenishment but have little effect on increasing stool consistency and may actually increase diarrhea in some people because of the high osmolality of the drinks (Rao et al., 2006).

Early nutrition interventions are crucial to avoid poor outcomes including malnutrition, persistent diarrhea, and death. Controversy exists as to what type of foods are best indicated during an acute episode of diarrhea, as well as which foods may provide sufficient calories and easily absorbable nutrients and are palatable. Because of water and electrolyte loss during diarrhea, any dietary plan should always include oral rehydration to effectively treat and prevent dehydration in patients with diarrhea. Other foods recommended for the treatment of diarrhea include avocados, asparagus tips, beets, unspiced applesauce, and peeled apples as well as ginger tea (Viele, 2003). Table 10-3 provides dietary guidelines developed from expert opinion.

Complications of diarrhea include the potential for cardiac dysrhythmias because of significant fluid and electrolyte loss, especially the loss of potassium (< 3.5 mEq/L). Urinary output of less than 30 ml/hr for two to three consecutive hours, muscle weakness, paresthesias, hypotension, anorexia, and drowsiness must be reported.

Proactive assessment and management of diarrhea by nurses and patients to effectively manage the symptom and its consequences are essential to have a positive effect on the treatment outcome and well-being of patients. Oncology nurses are in a unique position to identify patients who are at high risk for potentially life-threatening symptoms (Arnold et al., 2005).

TABLE 10-3	Low-Residue Dietary Guidelines by Food Group	
Food Group	**Foods Allowed**	**Foods to Avoid**
Breads and cereals	Breads: enriched white, Vienna, French, light rye without seeds, melba toast, zwieback, corn Muffins: plain muffins, corn muffins, plain pancakes, waffles	Breads: whole grains such as whole wheat, sprouted wheat, bran breads with seeds or nuts such as poppy, sesame, rye, nut breads Muffins: made with nuts or seeds, fruit skins, or whole grains such as whole wheat or bran
	Cereals: refined cereals such as oatmeal, buckwheat, cream of wheat or rice, corn flakes, Rice Krispies®, Rice Chex®, Cheerios®, etc.	Cereals: bran cereals, whole grain, fiber, cereals with nuts
Potato and potato substitutes	White rice, brown rice, most pastas, potatoes, sweet potatoes	Pasta/rice: wild rice, whole-wheat noodles
Fresh/frozen fruit	Banana	All except banana
Canned fruit	Applesauce, apricots, cherries, peaches, pears, pineapple, mandarin oranges, orange/grapefruit sections, jellies, fruit cocktail	Berries, grapes, berry pie filling, jams and preserves
Dried fruits	None	AVOID ALL.
Fruit/vegetable juices	Fruit juices without pulp (except prune), vegetable juices without pulp, citrus juices in moderation	Prune juice, large quantities of citrus juices
Fresh vegetables/ frozen vegetables	NO UNCOOKED VEGETABLES; well-cooked green beans, beets, squash, pumpkin, white/red potatoes without skin, sweet potatoes without skin, carrots, spinach, asparagus, strained tomatoes, celery, mushrooms	ALL FRESH RAW VEGETABLES, cooked onions, cabbage, Brussels sprouts, broccoli, green peppers, corn, cauliflower, dried beans/peas/lentils, turnips, rutabagas, vegetables cooked in cream sauce, potato skins, French fries, eggplant

(Continued on next page)

TABLE 10-3	Low-Residue Dietary Guidelines by Food Group *(Continued)*	
Food Group	**Foods Allowed**	**Foods to Avoid**
Canned vegetables	Green beans, peas, beets, squash, pumpkin, tomato sauce, tomato paste, tomato puree, carrots, asparagus, strained tomatoes, mushrooms	Onions, cabbage, Brussels sprouts, dried beans/peas/lentils, olives, pickles
Fats	Margarine, sour cream, butter, gravy, mayonnaise, dressing, and bacon	Large amounts of added mayonnaise, margarine, gravies, and dressings
Beverages/Liquids	Water, weak or decaffeinated tea, ginger ale, 7UP® or clear soft drinks, decaffeinated colas, Gatorade®, sports drinks	Regular coffee and tea, decaffeinated sodas, alcohol (beer, wine, liquor, mixed drinks)
Miscellaneous	All herbs and spices, such as parsley, oregano, salt, catsup, soy sauce, and vinegar	Hot pepper, black or white pepper used in large quantities, popcorn, potato chips
Meat/Other Protein	Stewed, boiled, baked, barbecued, well-trimmed, low-fat meats Nonfried eggs Low-fat cottage cheese, cream cheese, processed skim-milk cheese, part-skim mozzarella and ricotta, farmer cheese, string cheese, parmesan, and any other cheese with 5 g of fat or less per serving (read the label)	Fried meats, fatty meats, cured meats, cold cuts, poultry skin Fried eggs High-fat cheeses (natural cheese) Lima beans, peas, all dried legumes
Soups	Broth-based soups with allowed foods, cream-based soups made with low-fat milk with allowed foods (e.g., chicken noodle, cream of asparagus soup made with low-fat milk)	Broth-based soups made with foods to avoid, cream-based soups made with whole milk or made with foods to avoid (e.g., French onion, cream of broccoli)
Desserts	Popsicles, sherbet, water ice, gelatin, angel food cake, vanilla wafers, ginger snaps, plain cake, hard candy, jelly beans, pudding made with low-fat milk, arrowroot cookies, frozen yogurt, ice milk, low-fat desserts, honey, jelly, syrup	Rich desserts, pies, frostings made with fat and whole milk, coconut, candied fruits
Milk	2 cups or the equivalent per day of skim milk, low-fat milk, powdered milk, buttermilk, evaporated milk, skim-milk or low-fat yogurt, low-fat chocolate milk, ice milk, frozen yogurt, low-fat frozen desserts	All other milk beverages or products

Note. From "Diarrhea," by C. Engelking in C.H. Yarbro, M.H. Frogge, and M. Goodman (Eds.), *Cancer Symptom Management* (3rd ed., pp. 540–541), 2004, Sudbury, MA: Jones and Bartlett. Copyright 2004 by Jones and Bartlett. Reprinted with permission.

Pharmacologic Interventions

Many agents are being investigated for the management of diarrhea, but none have been shown to be effective at this time. Innovative strategies to minimize diarrhea secondary to radiation therapy also are being evaluated, such as pretreatment with cholestyramine to bind bile acids, and glutathione to bind free radicals released by tissues being radiated (Barasch, Elad,

Altman, Damato, & Epstein, 2006). Probiotic preparations, which usually are made from lactic acid–producing bacteria such as *Lactobacillus* species found in fermented foods and cultured milk products, are being evaluated as agents in the prevention of chemotherapy-induced diarrhea (Bowen et al., 2007; Jenkins, Holsten, Bengmark, & Martindale, 2005).

The following evidence-based interventions for the management of chemotherapy- and radiation therapy–induced diarrhea are found in the ONS PEP resource by Muehlbauer et al. (2008) (see Table 10-4 for definitions of the levels of evidence).

TABLE 10-4	Levels of Evidence
Level	**Description**
Recommended for practice	Interventions for which effectiveness has been demonstrated by strong evidence from rigorously conducted studies, meta-analyses, or systematic reviews and for which expectation of harm is small compared with the benefits
Likely to be effective	Interventions for which effectiveness has been demonstrated by supportive evidence from a single rigorously conducted controlled trial, consistent supportive evidence from well-designed controlled trials using small samples, or guidelines developed from evidence and supported by expert opinion
Benefits balanced with harms	Interventions for which clinicians and patients should weigh the beneficial and harmful effects according to individual circumstances and priorities
Effectiveness not established	Interventions for which insufficient or conflicting data or data of inadequate quality currently exist, with no clear indication of harm
Effectiveness unlikely	Interventions for which lack of effectiveness has been demonstrated by negative evidence from a single rigorously conducted controlled trial, consistent negative evidence from well-designed controlled trials using small samples, or guidelines developed from evidence and supported by expert opinion
Not recommended for practice	Interventions for which lack of effectiveness or harmfulness has been demonstrated by strong evidence from rigorously conducted studies, meta-analyses, or systematic reviews, or interventions for which the costs, burdens, or harms associated with the intervention exceed anticipated benefit
Expert opinion	Low-risk interventions that are (1) consistent with sound clinical practice, (2) suggested by an expert in a peer-reviewed publication (journal or book chapter), and (3) for which limited evidence exists. An expert is an individual who has published articles in a peer-reviewed journal in the domain of interest.

Note. From "PEP Up Your Practice" (p. 6), by B.H. Gobel and J.M. Tipton in L.H. Eaton and J.M. Tipton (Eds.), *Putting Evidence Into Practice: Improving Oncology Patient Outcomes,* 2009, Pittsburgh, PA: Oncology Nursing Society. Copyright 2009 by Oncology Nursing Society. Reprinted with permission.

Recommended for Practice

The interventions that have been found to be effective and are recommended for practice for the treatment of diarrhea as a result of chemotherapy are loperamide and octreotide acetate. Loperamide is an oral opiate, and the recommended dosage is 4 mg as the initial dose followed 2 mg every four hours (Benson et al., 2004). High-dose loperamide (2 mg every four hours and 4 mg every four hours at night) has also been shown to be moderately effective in controlling chemotherapy-induced diarrhea. Octreotide acetate is a somatostatin analog that is recommended for second-line treatment of chemotherapy-induced diarrhea that does not respond to loperamide. The standard dose is 100–150 mcg three times a day given subcutaneously (Benson et al.; Zidan et al., 2001).

Loperamide and diphenoxylate are recommended for the treatment of radiation-induced diarrhea. For mild diarrhea, an initial dose of 4 mg of loperamide followed by 2 mg every 4 hours or after every unformed stool is recommended. For persistent diarrhea lasting more than 24 hours, the dose can be increased to 2 mg every two hours (Benson et al., 2004). The recommended dose of diphenoxylate is 2 tablets four times a day, which may be necessary until control of diarrhea has been achieved, and then the dose can be reduced to meet the individual's requirements (Pfizer Inc., 2005).

Likely to Be Effective

The treatment of chemotherapy-induced diarrhea with octreotide acetate injection (Sandostatin LAR® Depot [Novartis Pharmaceuticals Corp.]) is given as a 20–30 mg once-monthly intramuscular injection as secondary prophylaxis after an individual fails loperamide with or without diphenoxylate hydrochloride with atropine sulfate (Lomotil®, Pfizer Inc.) (Rosenoff, 2004; Rosenoff et al., 2006). Octreotide acetate 100 mcg given three times a day by subcutaneous injection has been found to be more effective than diphenoxylate 10 mg by mouth in individuals with grade 2 or 3 diarrhea from radiation (Benson et al., 2004; Yavuz, Yavuz, Aydin, Can, & Kavgaci, 2002).

Benefits Balanced With Harms

The administration of neomycin for the prevention of irinotecan-induced diarrhea requires careful consideration of the risks and benefits as well as any harmful effects regarding an individual's circumstances (Muehlbauer et al., 2008). Likewise, the administration of amifostine for the treatment of diarrhea from chemotherapy other than irinotecan needs the same consideration (Muehlbauer et al.).

Effectiveness Not Established

Oral alkalization (Maeda et al., 2004; Moreno et al., 2006; Takeda et al., 2001), budesonide (a glucocorticoid steroid) (Karthaus et al., 2005), and charcoal (Maeda et al.; Michael et al., 2004) are agents that have been investigated for prevention of irinotecan-induced diarrhea in a few studies. These interventions had insufficient, conflicting, or inadequate quality data to recommend their use. The agents did not appear to pose any harm to individuals. Studies looking at probiotics and glutamine for the prevention of diarrhea from chemotherapy other than irinotecan have not shown them to be effective.

Glutamine and the antioxidant vitamins E and C have been studied for their potential benefit in the prevention and treatment of radiation-induced diarrhea, but no benefit was found (Kennedy et al., 2001; Kozelsky et al., 2003; Savarese, Savy, Vahdat, Wischmeyer, & Corey, 2003).

Effectiveness Unlikely

Lack of effectiveness was demonstrated for the use of sulfasalazine for the prevention of radiation-induced diarrhea (Benson et al., 2004) as well as pentosan polysulfate for the treatment of radiation-induced diarrhea (Pilepich et al., 2006).

Not Recommended for Practice

Evidence has shown lack of effectiveness of sucralfate for the prevention of radiation-induced diarrhea, and it is not recommended for practice (Benson et al., 2004; Martenson et al., 2000). No evidence supports the use of selenium supplementation as a protective mechanism against diarrhea from chemotherapy or radiation therapy (Dennert & Horneber, 2006).

Expert Opinion

The administration of atropine (0.25–1 mg IV or subcutaneous) may prevent early diarrhea resulting from irinotecan (Pharmacia & Upjohn, 1998). Late diarrhea from irinotecan can be life-threatening and should be treated promptly with loperamide. Tincture of opium may be a second-line therapy for diarrhea from chemotherapy-induced diarrhea. Deodorized tincture of opium is the preferred preparation as it more concentrated (10 mg/ml morphine). The recommended dose is 10–15 drops in water every three to four hours (Benson et al., 2004). Camphorated tincture of opium (paregoric) is less concentrated (0.4 mg/ml morphine) and the recommended dose is 1 tsp (5 ml) in water every three to four hours (Benson et al.).

Care of the patient with diarrhea should be guided by the evidence and best known practices available. Treatment varies and is driven by the etiology and pathophysiologic mechanism. A telephone triage algorithm that incorporates subjective and objective assessment findings and employs NCI severity grading of diarrhea may direct treatment recommendations.

Expected Outcomes

The goals of managing diarrhea in patients with cancer should be to
- Prevent diarrhea.
- Enhance recovery of intestinal mucosa from the effects of chemotherapy or radiation therapy.
- Restore normal bowel function.
- Eliminate causative factors.
- Maintain nutrition and fluid and electrolyte balance through hydration and supplementation.
- Minimize the risk of complications.
- Eliminate or reduce diarrhea-associated morbidity and mortality.
- Prevent cancer treatment delays or regimen modifications.
- Improve cancer treatment outcomes.
- Protect skin integrity.
- Optimize patients' quality of life.

Measurable outcomes are needed to assess the effectiveness of the management of diarrhea. Reduction in the number of daily stool episodes with a concomitant decrease in stool liquidity are objective parameters. Tools need to be developed and tested for use in a variety of settings to measure the effectiveness of interventions.

Emergency management of diarrhea-associated complications such as hypotension or acidosis may be an initial priority. Monitoring the number, amount, and consistency of bowel movements is critical. Fluid and electrolyte replacement is necessary. Antidiarrheal medication should be administered as appropriate to reduce stool frequency, volume, and peristalsis. The severity of diarrhea must be reassessed at an appropriate interval after administering antidiarrheal medication.

Patient and Family Teaching Points

- Instruct patients to report any signs of diarrhea.
- Educate patients who are at high risk for developing diarrhea about measures to prevent or ameliorate the severity of diarrhea.
- Assist patients in understanding when diarrhea can be self-managed and when to seek help.
- Educate patients about when to start antidiarrheal medications (e.g., with certain chemotherapeutic agents, antidiarrheal medication should be provided so that patients can self-administer at the onset of diarrhea).
- Educate patients regarding appropriate hydration and nutrition.
- Instruct patients to clean their rectal area with mild soap and water after each bowel movement, rinse well, and pat dry with a soft towel. Additional protection may be provided by applying a moisture-barrier ointment.
- Inform patients to take warm sitz baths to relieve pain related to perianal inflammation.
- Educate patients about symptoms that may be life-threatening, including excessive thirst, fever, dizziness or lightheadedness, palpitations, rectal spasms, excessive abdominal cramping, watery or bloody stools, and continued diarrhea while on antidiarrheal treatment. Stress that these symptoms require patients to immediately contact their healthcare provider.
- Provide written materials with specific healthcare provider contact numbers, and review information at each visit. Consider visual and cognitive impairments.
- Stress the importance of reporting the occurrence and character of diarrhea and any self-care measures employed at home.
- Customize patient self-care sheets to assist in the control of diarrhea.
- Provide a self-care behavior log for the patient to relate side effects of cancer treatment and rate the severity of the side effect and its resultant distress using a visual analog scale or some other measurement scale.
- Provide information that is culturally sensitive and understandable to patients whose first language is not English.

Need for Future Research

All oncology nurses have a responsibility to use available evidence as they assess and manage diarrhea and its associated fluid, electrolyte, and metabolic disturbances. Significant questions remain about the most effective way to assess and manage cancer treatment–induced diarrhea. Identification of those patients who are at risk for diarrhea and how to prevent and treat the symptom will continue to evolve as new antineoplastic agents and novel treatments are employed.

Effective treatment must be a continuous process based on an initial comprehensive and accurate clinical assessment, subsequent targeted reassessment, and the administration of appropriate pharmacologic and nonpharmacologic therapies at the optimal time. Initial assessment should consider the onset and duration of diarrhea and the potential for dehydration and sepsis. Standardized, globally accepted guidelines for the management of cancer treatment–related diarrhea and validated, evidence-based measures of diarrhea need to be implemented and studied in clinical trials as part of quality cancer care. Further investigation into the pathophysiology of cancer treatment–related diarrhea may allow for more directed approaches in the prophylaxis and treatment of this symptom. The study of individual genotype to predict the toxicity and efficacy of chemotherapeutic agents may be important for better application of these agents (Yang et al., 2005).

Conclusion of Case Study

The nurse carefully assesses C.B.'s report of diarrhea, which he relates as liquid stools occurring four to six times a day and noticeably changed from his normal stool consistency and bowel regimen. Upon consideration of the type of chemotherapeutic agents received, particularly irinotecan, the recommended initial pharmacologic intervention for diarrhea is to start the patient on loperamide at an initial dose of 4 mg orally followed by 2 mg every four hours (Muehlbauer et al., 2008). Review of general diet strategies with the patient includes consuming five to six small, frequent meals and consuming at least 8–10 servings (8 oz. each) of room-temperature liquid per day. Close monitoring of the patient for continued or increasing frequency of diarrhea is emphasized. The patient is encouraged to report any of these changes immediately. This late diarrhea may lead to dehydration and electrolyte imbalance, which, if not treated early and promptly, could lead to life-threatening consequences.

Conclusion

Nursing assessment of diarrhea related to cancer and its treatment is essential to appropriate management that influences patient outcomes. Early intervention for the symptom of diarrhea using evidence-based practice provides quality cancer care. The impact of the morbidity of diarrhea may be decreased by employing guidelines and stressing the aggressive management of diarrhea. Education of healthcare providers and patients regarding the importance of assessing and managing diarrhea is essential to improve the control of diarrhea and, in turn, positively affect patients' quality of life.

References

Abraham, B., & Sellin, J.H. (2007). Drug-induced diarrhea. *Current Gastroenterology Reports, 9*(5), 365–372.

Arbuckle, R.B., Huber, S.L., & Zacker, C. (2000). The consequences of diarrhea occurring during chemotherapy for colorectal cancer: A retrospective study. *Oncologist, 5*(3), 250–259.

Arnold, R.J., Gabrail, N., Raut, M., Kim, R., Sung, J.C., & Zhou, Y. (2005). Clinical implications of chemotherapy-induced diarrhea in patients with cancer. *Journal of Supportive Oncology, 3*(3), 227–232.

Barasch, A., Elad, S., Altman, A., Damato, K., & Epstein, J. (2006). Antimicrobials, mucosal coating agents, anesthetics, analgesics, and nutritional supplements for alimentary tract mucositis. *Supportive Care in Cancer, 14*(6), 528–532.

Bartlett, J.G. (2002). Antibiotic-associated diarrhea. *New England Journal of Medicine, 346*(5), 334–339.

Bartlett, J.G., & Gerding, D.N. (2008). Clinical recognition and diagnosis of Clostridium difficile infection. *Clinical Infectious Diseases, 46*(Suppl. 1), S12–S18.

Bennett, V., & Engelking, C. (2002). *Current perspectives on cancer treatment-induced diarrhea (CTID)* (pp. 1–22). Tampa, FL: Moffitt Cancer Center.

Benson, A.B., Ajani, J.A., Catalano, R.B., Engelking, C., Kornblau, S.M., Martenson, J.A., et al. (2004). Recommended guidelines for the treatment of cancer treatment-induced diarrhea. *Journal of Clinical Oncology, 22*(14), 2918–2926.

Bismar, M.M., & Sinicrope, F.A. (2002). Radiation enteritis. *Current Gastroenterology Reports, 4*(5), 361–365.

Bowen, J.M., Stringer, A.M., Gibson, R.J., Yeoh, A.S.J., Hannam, S., & Keefe, D.M.K. (2007). VSL#3 probiotic treatment reduces chemotherapy-induced diarrhea and weight loss. *Cancer Biology and Therapy, 6*(9), 1–6.

Camilleri, M., & Murray, J.A. (2008). Diarrhea and constipation. In A.S. Fauci, E. Braunwald, D.L. Kasper, S.L. Hauser, D.L. Longo, J.L. Jameson, et al. (Eds.), *Harrison's principles of internal medicine* (17th ed., pp. 245–252). New York: McGraw-Hill.

Dennert, G., & Horneber, M. (2006). Selenium for alleviating the side effects of chemotherapy, radiotherapy and surgery in cancer patients. *Cochrane Database of Systematic Reviews* 2006, Issue 3. Art. No.: CD005037. DOI: 10.1002/14651858.CD005037.pub2.

Dranitsaris, G., Maroun, J., & Shah, A. (2005). Estimating the cost of illness in colorectal cancer patients who were hospitalized for severe chemotherapy-induced diarrhea. *Canadian Journal of Gastroenterology, 19*(2), 83–87.

DuPont, H.L. (1997). Guidelines on acute infectious diarrhea in adults. The Practice Parameters Committee of the American College of Gastroenterology. *American Journal of Gastroenterology, 92*(11), 1962–1975.

Eastern Cooperative Oncology Group. (2007). *ECOG common toxicity criteria.* Retrieved April 20, 2008, from http://www.ecog.org/general/ctc.pdf

Eisenberg, P. (2002). An overview of diarrhea in the patients receiving enteral nutrition. *Gastroenterology Nursing, 25*(3), 95–104.

Engelking, C. (2000). Cancer treatment-related diarrhea: Challenges and barriers to clinical practice. *American Journal of Nursing, 100*(Suppl. 4), 1–16.

Engelking, C. (2004). Diarrhea. In C.H. Yarbro, M.H. Frogge, & M. Goodman (Eds.), *Cancer symptom management* (3rd ed., pp. 528–557). Sudbury, MA: Jones and Bartlett.

Field, M. (2003). Intestinal ion transport and the pathophysiology of diarrhea. *Journal of Clinical Investigation, 111*(7), 931–943.

Gadewar, S., & Fasano, A. (2005). Current concepts in the evaluation, diagnosis and management of acute infectious diarrhea. *Current Opinion in Pharmacology, 5*(6), 559–565.

Gibson, R.J., & Keefe, D.M.K. (2006). Cancer chemotherapy-induced diarrhea and constipation: Mechanisms of damage and prevention strategies. *Supportive Care in Cancer, 14*(9), 890–900.

Gore, J.I., & Surawicz, C. (2003). Severe acute diarrhea. *Gastroenterology Clinics of North America, 32*(4), 1249–1267.

Gowing, L., Ali, R., & White, J. (2006). Buprenorphine for the management of opioid withdrawal. *Cochrane Database of Systematic Reviews* 2006, Issue 2. Art. No.: CD002025. DOI: 10.1002/14651858.CD002025.pub3.

Gwede, C.K. (2003). Overview of radiation- and chemoradiation-induced diarrhea. *Seminars in Oncology Nursing, 19*(4, Suppl. 3), 6–10.

Hertig, V.L., Cain, K.C., Jarrett, M.E., Burr, R.L., & Heitkemper, M.M. (2007). Daily stress and gastrointestinal symptoms in women with irritable bowel syndrome. *Nursing Research, 56*(6), 399–406.

Jani, N., Moser, A.J., & Khalid, A. (2007). Pancreatic endocrine tumors. *Gastroenterology Clinics of North America, 36*(2), 431–439.

Jenkins, B., Holsten, S., Bengmark, S., & Martindale, R. (2005). Probiotics: A practical review of their role in specific clinical scenarios. *Nutrition in Clinical Practice, 20*(2), 262–270.

Karthaus, M., Ballo, H., Abenhardt, W., Steinmetz, T., Geer, T., Schimke, J., et al. (2005). Prospective, double-blind, placebo-controlled, multicenter, randomized phase III study with orally administered budesonide for prevention of irinotecan (CPT-11)-induced diarrhea in patients with advanced colorectal cancer. *Oncology, 68*(4–6), 326–332.

Kennedy, M., Bruninga, K., Mutlu, E.A., Losurdo, J., Choudhary, S., & Keshavarzian, A. (2001). Successful and sustained treatment of chronic radiation proctitis with antioxidant vitamins E and C. *American Journal of Gastroenterology, 96*(4), 1080–1084.

Kozelsky, T.F., Meyers, G.E., Sloan, J.A., Shanahan, T.G., Dick, S.J., Moore, R.L., et al. (2003). Phase III double-blind study of glutamine versus placebo for the prevention of acute diarrhea in patients receiving pelvic radiation therapy. *Journal of Clinical Oncology, 21*(9), 1669–1674.

Kulke, M.H. (2007). Clinical presentation and management of carcinoid tumors. *Hematology/Oncology Clinics of North America, 21*(3), 433–455.

Mackay, S., Hayes, T., & Yeo, A. (2006). Management of gastric cancer. *Australian Family Physician, 35*(4), 208–211.

Maeda, Y., Ohune, T., Nakamura, M., Yamasaki, M., Kiribayashi, Y., & Murakami, T. (2004). Prevention of irinotecan-induced diarrhoea by oral carbonaceous adsorbent (Kremezin) in cancer patients. *Oncology Reports, 12*(3), 581–585.

Marcos, L.A., & DuPont, H.L. (2007). Advances in defining etiology and new therapeutic approaches in acute diarrhea. *Journal of Infection, 55*(5), 385–393.

Marteau, P.R., de Vrese, M., Cellier, C.J., & Schrezenmeir, J. (2001). Protection from gastrointestinal diseases with the use of probiotics. *American Journal of Clinical Nutrition, 72*(Suppl. 2), 430S–436S.

Martenson, J.A., Bollinger, J.W., Sloan, J.A., Novotny, P.J., Urias, R.E., Michalak, J.C., et al. (2000). Sucralfate in the prevention of treatment-induced diarrhea in patients receiving pelvic radiation therapy: A North Central Cancer Treatment Group phase III double-blind placebo-controlled trial. *Journal of Clinical Oncology, 18*(6), 1239–1245.

Maser, C., Toset, A., & Roman, S. (2006). Gastrointestinal manifestations of endocrine disease. *World Journal of Gastroenterology, 12*(20), 3174–3179.

McMahan, Z.H., & DuPont, H.L. (2007). Review article: The history of acute infectious diarrhoea management—from poorly focused empiricism to fluid therapy and modern pharmacotherapy. *Alimentary Pharmacology and Therapeutics, 25*(7), 759–769.

Michael, M., Brittain, M., Nagai, J., Feld, R., Hedley, D., Oza, A., et al. (2004). Phase II study of activated charcoal to prevent irinotecan-induced diarrhea. *Journal of Clinical Oncology, 22*(21), 4410–4417.

Misialos, E.P., Macheras, A., Lapetanakis, T., & Liakatos, T. (2007). Short bowel syndrome: Current medical and surgical trends. *Journal of Clinical Gastroenterology, 41*(1), 5–18.

Moreno, V.V., Vidal, J.B., Alemany, H.M., Salvia, A.S., Serentill, M.L., Montero, I.C., et al. (2006). Prevention of irinotecan associated diarrhea by intestinal alkalization. A pilot study in gastrointestinal cancer patients. *Clinical and Translational Oncology, 8*(3), 208–212.

Muehlbauer, P., Thorpe, D.M., Davis, A., Drabot, R.C., Kiker, E.S., & Rawlings, B.L. (2008). *Putting evidence into practice: Diarrhea.* Pittsburgh, PA: Oncology Nursing Society.

National Cancer Institute Cancer Therapy Evaluation Program. (2009). *Common terminology criteria for adverse events* (version 4.0). Retrieved July 24, 2009, from http://ctep.cancer.gov/protocolDevelopment/electronic_applications/docs/ctcaev4.pdf

Nguyen, N.P., Antoine, J.E., Dutta, S., Karlsson, U., & Sallah, S. (2002). Current concepts in radiation enteritis and implications for future clinical trials. *Cancer, 95*(5), 1151–1163.

O'Brien, B.E., Kaklamani, V.G., & Benson, A.B. (2005). The assessment and management of cancer treatment-related diarrhea. *Clinical Colorectal Cancer, 4*(6), 375–381.

Otterson, M.F. (2007). Effects of radiation upon gastrointestinal motility. *World Journal of Gastroenterology, 13*(19), 2684–2692.

Pfizer Inc. (2005). Lomotil (diphenoxylate hydrochloride and atropine sulfate tablets, USP) [Package insert]. New York: Author.

Pharmacia & Upjohn. (1998). Camptosar (irinotecan hydrochloride injection) [Package insert]. Kalamazoo, MI: Author.

Pilepich, M.V., Paulus, R., St. Clair, W., Barasacchio, R.A., Rostock, R., & Miller, R.C. (2006). Phase III study of pentosanpolysulfate (PPS) in treatment of gastrointestinal tract sequelae of radiotherapy. *American Journal of Clinical Oncology, 29*(2), 132–137.

Polovich, M., White, J., & Kelleher, L.O. (Eds.). (2005). *Chemotherapy and biotherapy guidelines and recommendations for practice* (2nd ed.). Pittsburgh, PA: Oncology Nursing Society.

Rao, S.S., Summers, R.W., Rao, G.R., Ramana, S., Devi, U., Zimmerman, B., et al. (2006). Oral rehydration for viral gastroenteritis in adults: A randomized, controlled trial of 3 solutions. *Journal of Parenteral and Enteral Nutrition, 30*(5), 433–439.

Richardson, G., & Dobish, R. (2007). Chemotherapy induced diarrhea. *Journal of Oncology Pharmacy Practice, 13*(4), 181–198.

Rosenoff, S. (2004). Resolution of refractory chemotherapy-induced diarrhea (CID) with octreotide long-acting formulation in cancer patients: 11 case studies. *Supportive Care in Cancer, 12*(8), 561–570.

Rosenoff, S.H., Gabrail, N.Y., Conklin, R., Hohneker, J.A., Berg, W.J., Ghulam, W., et al. (2006). A multicenter, randomized trial of long-acting octreotide for the optimum prevention of chemotherapy-induced diarrhea: Results of the STOP trial. *Journal of Supportive Oncology, 4*(6), 289–294.

Ross, W.A., & Couriel, D. (2005). Colonic graft-versus-host disease. *Current Opinion in Gastroenterology, 21*(1), 64–69.

Ruthruff, B. (2007). Clinical review of Crohn's disease. *Journal of the American Academy of Nurse Practitioners, 19*(8), 392–397.

Sabol, V.K., & Carlson, K.K. (2007). Diarrhea: Applying research to bedside practice. *AACN Advanced Critical Care, 18*(1), 32–44.

Saltz, L.B. (2003). Understanding and managing chemotherapy induced diarrhea. *Journal of Supportive Oncology, 1*(1), 35–46.

Savaiano, D.A., Boushey, C.J., & McCabe, G.P. (2006). Lactose intolerance symptoms assessed by meta-analysis: A grain of truth that leads to exaggeration. *Journal of Nutrition, 136*(4), 1107–1113.

Savarese, D.M., Savy, G., Vahdat, L., Wischmeyer, P.E., & Corey, B. (2003). Prevention of chemotherapy and radiation toxicity with glutamine. *Cancer Treatment Reviews, 29*(6), 501–513.

Scaldaferri, F., & Fiocchi, C. (2007). Inflammatory bowel disease: Progress and current concepts of etiopathogenesis. *Journal of Digestive Diseases, 8*(4), 171–178.

Schiller, L.R. (2007). Management of diarrhea in clinical practice: Strategies for primary care physicians. *Reviews in Gastroenterological Disorders, 7*(Suppl. 3), S27–S38.

Sellin, J.H. (1998). Intestinal electrolyte absorption and secretion. In M. Feldman, B.F. Scharschmidt, M.H. Sleisinger, & J.S. Fordtran (Eds.), *Sleisinger & Fordtran's gastrointestinal and liver disease: Pathophysiology, diagnosis, management* (pp. 1451–1471). Philadelphia: Saunders.

Singh, H.M., Teller, T., Esrasin, K.T., & Abbas, M.A. (2007). VIPoma: A rare cause of acute diarrhea. *Surgical Rounds, 30*(9), 414–418.

Sonis, S.T., Elting, L.S., Keefe, D.M., Peterson, D.E., Schubert, M.M., Hauer-Jenson, M., et al. (2004). Perspectives on cancer therapy-induced mucosal injury: Pathogenesis, measurement, epidemiology, and consequences for patients. *Cancer, 100*(Suppl. 9), 1995–2025.

Stern, J., & Ippoliti, C. (2003). Management of acute cancer treatment-induced diarrhea. *Seminars in Oncology Nursing, 19*(4, Suppl. 3), 11–16.

Stringer, A.M., Gibson, R.J., Bowen, J.M., Logan, R.M., Yeoh, A.S., & Keefe, D.M. (2007). Chemotherapy-induced mucositis: The role of gastrointestinal microflora and mucins in the luminal environment. *Journal of Supportive Oncology, 5*(6), 259–267.

Takeda, Y., Kobayashi, K., Akivama, Y., Soma, T., Handa, S., Kudoh, S., et al. (2001). Prevention of irinotecan (CPT-11)-induced diarrhea by oral alkalization combined with control of defecation in cancer patients. *International Journal of Cancer, 92*(2), 269–275.

Toomey, D.P., Cahill, R.A., Geraghty, J., & Thirion, P. (2006). Radiation enteropathy. *Irish Medical Journal, 99*(7), 215–217.

Traugott, A., & Moley, J.F. (2005). Medullary thyroid cancer: Medical management and follow-up. *Current Treatment Options in Oncology, 6*(4), 339–346.

Tuchmann, L., & Engelking, C. (2001). Cancer-related diarrhea. In R.A. Gates & R.M. Fink (Eds.), *Oncology nursing secrets* (2nd ed., pp. 310–322). Philadelphia: Hanley & Belfus.

Viele, C.S. (2003). Overview of chemotherapy-induced diarrhea. *Seminars in Oncology Nursing, 19*(4, Suppl. 3), 2–5.

Warner, R.R. (2005). Enteroendocrine tumors other than carcinoid: A review of clinically significant advances. *Gastroenterology, 128*(6), 1668–1684.

Westergaard, H. (2007). Bile acid malabsorption. *Current Treatment Options in Gastroenterology, 10*(1), 28–33.

World Health Organization. (n.d.). *WHO toxicity criteria by grade for diarrhoea.* Retrieved April 20, 2008, from http://www.fda.gov/cder/cancer/toxicityframe.htm

Yang, X., Hu, Z., Chan, S., Chan, E., Goh, B., Wei, D., et al. (2005). Novel agents that potentially inhibit irinotecan-induced diarrhea. *Current Medicinal Chemistry, 12*(11), 1343–1358.

Yavuz, M.N., Yavuz, A.A., Aydin, F., Can, G., & Kavgaci, H. (2002). The efficacy of octreotide in the therapy of acute radiation-induced diarrhea: A randomized controlled study. *International Journal of Radiation Oncology, Biology, Physics, 54*(1), 195–202.

Zgodzinski, W., Dekoj, T., & Espat, N.J. (2005). Understanding clinical issues in postoperative nutrition after pancreaticoduodenectomy. *Nutrition in Clinical Practice, 20*(6), 654–661.

Zidan, J., Haim, N., Beny, A., Stein, M., Gez, E., & Kuten, A. (2001). Octreotide in the treatment of severe chemotherapy-induced diarrhea. *Annals of Oncology, 12*(2), 227–229.

CHAPTER 11

Dyspnea

Margaret M. Joyce, PhD(c), RN, AOCN®

Case Study

B.L. is a 62-year-old Caucasian man with a diagnosis of stage IV non-small cell lung cancer diagnosed three months ago. His medical history is significant for chronic obstructive pulmonary disease (COPD). He quit smoking cigarettes more than six months ago after smoking a pack per day for 40 years. Currently, he is being treated with systemic chemotherapy. The ambulatory care nurse is evaluating him today before administering his second cycle of chemotherapy. He tells the nurse that he has become increasingly short of breath with walking short distances and has decreased his activities accordingly. He is considering getting one of those scooters that he saw advertised on television so that he can get around better. He is a widower who lives alone but has two supportive daughters who check in on him. In addition to the dyspnea, he reports occasional dry cough, increasing fatigue, and anorexia. His weight has decreased three pounds since his first cycle of chemotherapy three weeks ago. He denies anxiety or depression but admits to feeling panic during one of his "difficult breathing" episodes. In addition to an antinausea regimen, B.L.'s current medications include sustained-release morphine sulfate 30 mg every 12 hours for posterior thorax pain and two puffs four times a day of albuterol/ipratropium metered dose inhaler. The nurse assesses his lung sounds and notes, in general, that the breath sounds are distant bilaterally and that there are absent breath sounds one-third the way up at the base of the left lower lung field. His vital signs include: 97.8°F (36.6°C) oral temperature, 92 regular heart rate, respiratory rate of 20, and blood pressure of 128/77. He denies pain and reports a fatigue rating of 4 and a dyspnea rating of 6. His oxygen percent saturation at rest on room air is 94%; however, his percent oxygen desaturates to 88% with exertion on room air.

Overview

Definition

The clinical term *dyspnea* describes difficult or labored breathing and generally is applied to the sensation that individuals experience as unpleasant or uncomfortable respiration (Bruera & Ripamonti, 1998). The word *breathlessness* often is used synonymously with dyspnea, although someone who is breathless may or may not be in distress. The American Thoracic Society (ATS) (1999) in a consensus statement broadly defined dyspnea as "a term used to characterize a subjective experience of breathing discomfort that consists of qualitatively distinct sensations that vary in intensity. The experience derives from interactions among multiple physiological, psychological, social, and environmental factors and may induce secondary physiological and behavioral responses" (p. 322). Thus, dyspnea is a complex subjective symptom that can be difficult to manage effectively because it has more than one dimension, can vary in time, and can have multiple causes.

Acute dyspnea refers to "the onset of breathlessness that may occur with explosive rapidity and lead to a feeling of impending doom" (Mahler, 1990, p. 127). This form of dyspnea frequently causes a person to seek emergency care. Common etiologies of acute dyspnea are airway obstruction, hyperventilation syndrome, pneumothorax (traumatic or spontaneous), pneumonia, pulmonary embolism, or hemorrhage (Mahler).

On the other hand, the usual onset of chronic dyspnea is slow or gradual. The nature of chronic dyspnea is that it is persistent and can vary in intensity with a baseline that gradually increases over time (McCarley, 1999). Some people initially attribute dyspnea to "getting old" or "being out of shape." However, chronic dyspnea prompts an individual to seek health care when the breathlessness interferes with activities of daily living despite insidious but substantial reduction in exertion or activity level (Ries & Mahler, 1990). This chapter primarily focuses on chronic cancer-related dyspnea. Information and evidence about dyspnea related to non-cancer etiologies also is presented to facilitate further understanding. However, important to note is that the theory or intervention for dyspnea as a general symptom may not have been tested in patients with cancer, and the outcome may be different in cancer-related dyspnea.

Incidence

In the general cancer population, the prevalence of dyspnea varies according to the setting and time measured during the illness trajectory. Ripamonti and Fusco (2002) reported dyspnea prevalence to be 15%–55.5% at referral to palliative care services with increases as high as 79% during the last week of life. Reuben and Mor (1986) examined data from a National Hospice Study collected during the last six weeks of life and determined the incidence of dyspnea in terminal patients with cancer was 70%. In one study of 923 general outpatients with cancer, 46% of the participants reported some shortness of breath (Dudgeon, Kristjanson, Sloan, Lertzman, & Clement, 2001).

Risk and Associated Factors

Dyspnea is particularly common in patients with cancer who have primary or metastatic lung tumors or pleural involvement; however, many patients with cancer without direct lung involvement also report it. Vainio and Auvinen (1996) measured the prevalence of symptoms by primary cancer site among patients from seven hospice programs in the United States, Europe, and Australia and found the prevalence of dyspnea to be highest in people with lung cancer (46%) and most common among patients with malignancies in the chest, such as in the breast (24%) and esophagus (19%), but remained below 20% in other primary sites.

The symptom of dyspnea can be a primary complaint in a large and varied number of medical conditions, including cardiac, pulmonary, neurologic, vascular, and psychogenic disturbances (Harver & Mahler, 1990). Underlying pulmonary or cardiac disease and low Karnofsky performance status were factors significantly associated with dyspnea in one study of terminally ill patients with cancer (Reuben & Mor, 1986). Significant predictors of breathlessness in another study were anxiety, history of smoking, and partial pressure of carbon dioxide level (Dudgeon et al., 2001). Dudgeon and Lertzman (1998) described a median of at least five abnormalities associated with reported shortness of breath in a study involving 100 terminally ill patients with cancer. Findings included abnormal chest radiographs (91%), abnormal pulmonary function tests (93%) including decreased pulmonary maximum inspiratory pressure (MIP), hypoxia (40%), history of cardiac disease (21%), and anemia (20%). An interesting pulmonary function finding was the study's median MIP measured at -16 cm H_2O (normal is -50 cm H_2O), indicating severely decreased respiratory muscle function. Respiratory muscle dysfunction can be caused in part by the malnutrition of cancer cachexia, electrolyte abnormalities, and other disorders of chronic cancer and thus may explain the high prevalence of dyspnea in people with advanced cancer (Dudgeon & Lertzman). Figure 11-1 summarizes cancer-related dyspnea risk factors and correlates.

FIGURE 11-1   **Risk Factors and Correlates for Moderate to Severe Dyspnea in Patients With Cancer**

- Smoking—past or present
- Chronic obstructive pulmonary disease
- Cardiac disease, especially congestive heart disease
- Asthma
- Environmental exposures (asbestos, coal dust, cotton dust, grain dust)
- Lung radiation
- Lung cancer—primary or metastatic
- Anxiety—either as cause or effect of dyspnea
- Fatigue/tiredness
- Maximal inspiratory pressure < 80% predicted
- Vital capacity < 80%
- Low Karnofsky performance score

Note. From "Dyspnea," by C.M. Williams, 2006, *Cancer Journal, 12*(5), p. 365. Copyright 2006 by Jones and Bartlett. Reprinted with permission.

Additional potential contributors to the prevalence of cancer-related dyspnea include cardiac or pulmonary toxicity of certain cancer therapies such as surgery, radiotherapy, or chemotherapy (Ripamonti, Fulfaro, & Bruera, 1998). Surgical procedures such as pneumonectomy or lobectomy can reduce pulmonary function (Brunelli et al., 2007) and thus may result in chronic dyspnea. Radiotherapy where the beam includes a portion of the lung may result in pneumonitis or fibrosis. Dyspnea is a primary presenting symptom of pneumonitis or pulmonary fibrosis. Chemotherapy agents associated with acute pneumonitis include bleomycin, carmustine, gemcitabine, methotrexate, mitomycin, procarbazine, and the vinca alkaloids, and those known to cause pulmonary fibrosis include bleomycin, carmustine, cyclophosphamide, methotrexate, and mitomycin (Fischer, Knobf, Durivage, & Beaulieu, 2003). Additionally, anthracycline chemotherapy agents are associated with cardiac toxicity, most commonly cardiomyopathy, which may progress to heart failure that produces dyspnea.

Mechanisms of Dyspnea

Normally, a person has no awareness of breathing (Thomas & von Gunten, 2003). Three possible derangements underlie uncomfortable breathing sensations: disorder of (a) the respiratory controller, (b) the ventilatory pump, and (c) the gas exchanger (ATS, 1999). The goal of the respiratory controller is to satisfy the metabolic requirements of the body. One theory is that dyspnea results from a mismatch between outgoing central respiratory motor activity and incoming information from both central and peripheral chemoreceptors and mechanoreceptors in the airways, lungs, and chest wall structures. This mismatch between the motor command and the mechanical response is what produces a sensation of respiratory discomfort.

ATS (1999) classified four physiologic mechanisms underlying dyspnea and possible targets for intervention. They are

- Heightened ventilatory demand as demonstrated by increased dyspnea with exertion. This is attributable to an increase in respiratory motor output and corresponding increase in sense of effort.
- Respiratory muscle abnormalities as seen with muscle weakness or mechanical inefficiency limiting maximum ventilation. The pressure-generating capacity of respiratory muscles is decreased, thereby limiting the ability to meet the respiratory control center demands.
- Abnormal ventilatory impedance as noted when central respiratory motor output increases to overcome ventilatory resistance. Asthma and COPD can narrow airways, increasing resistance to ventilation.
- Abnormal blood gas parameters such as hypoxia or hypercapnia, which stimulate respiratory drive through central perception of dyspnea.

Similar to pain, dyspnea has an affective component. The affective component is an emotional or behavioral response to the physiologic stimulus of respiratory compromise. This component can vary greatly among people to modulate the intensity of the symptom so that the "just noticeable difference" for shortness of breath among patients with similar lung pathology can vary greatly as a result of the affective response (Carrieri-Kohlman, Gormley, Douglas, Paul, & Stulbarg, 1996). Hence, the threshold perception of dyspnea and intensity of breathing discomfort varies widely among individuals and is related only moderately to the degree of pulmonary dysfunction (ATS, 1999). Psychological factors, behavioral style, and social and environmental factors are thought to contribute to the affective dimension of dyspnea.

Assessment

Dyspnea assessment is a challenge because of the symptom's subjective nature, complicated by the fact that the sensation often arises from multiple sources or pathophysiologic mechanisms (ATS, 1999). In addition, assessment of the quality and intensity of dyspnea can vary with time. Therefore, measuring the patient's perception of dyspnea is important. Regular and consistent assessment of dyspnea is facilitated by the use of a form or tool that will document the patient's rating of the symptom and change over time.

Assessment Tools

Dyspnea usually is classified as to the context in which it occurs, such as on exertion, at rest, or nocturnally. The most common method of screening for dyspnea is self-report of the activity level that causes awareness of the symptom.

The Medical Research Council (MRC) dyspnea scale (MRC's Committee on the Aetiology of Chronic Bronchitis, 1960) has been used for many years to grade the effect of dyspnea or breathlessness on daily activities. The dyspnea grading is part of a standardized interview guide and respiratory epidemiologic questionnaire. The MRC dyspnea scale is very similar to the Grades of Breathlessness Scale developed and published in 1978 by the ATS Division of Lung Disease. The scale measures perceived respiratory disability as it allows patients to indicate with a yes or no response the extent to which their breathlessness impairs their mobility (Bestall et al., 1999). The tool has established content validity and reliability (Farncombe, 1997; Mahler et al., 1987; Mahler & Wells, 1988). The MRC scale is easy to administer and useful for general screening and categorizing of individuals (Meek, 2004).

The MRC is an incremental grading scale that asks questions about activities that precipitate shortness of breath (see Figure 11-2). The grade or level of dyspnea is assigned based on the number of the last question answered with a "yes" indicating the most disability experienced by the respondent. These or similar questions help providers in clinical practice to determine and label the extent that dyspnea interferes with function.

FIGURE 11-2	Medical Research Council Dyspnea Scale

1. "Are you ever troubled by shortness of breath when hurrying on level ground or walking up a slight hill?"
2. "Do you get short of breath walking with other people at ordinary pace on level ground?"
3. "Do you have to stop for breath when walking at your own pace on level ground?"
4. "Are you short of breath on washing or dressing?" Another version is "Are you too breathless to leave the house or on dressing or undressing?"

Note. Based on information from Medical Research Council's Committee on the Aetiology of Chronic Bronchitis, 1960.

Instruments to Measure Dyspnea

Many tools or instruments are available to measure a person's subjective perception of dyspnea. A disciplined assessment of dyspnea includes measurement and documentation terms that allow longitudinal appraisal of the symptom, as well as response to interventions. A description of various dyspnea measuring tools is presented in Table 11-1. The table excludes physiologic parameters, such as pulmonary function studies or measures of oxygen saturation that assess respiratory compromise, and does not include items or dyspnea subscales from other multidimensional symptom or quality-of-life instruments.

Of these instruments, only the visual analog scale (VAS) and the Cancer Dyspnoea Scale (CDS) have evidence of either reliability or validity in patients with cancer (Joyce & Beck, 2005). The CDS measures three dimensions of dyspnea (sense of effort, sense of anxiety, and sense of discomfort) and has been tested and used primarily in Asian populations (Tanaka, Akechi, Okuyama, Nishiwaki, & Uchitomi, 2000). The VAS measures only one dimension of dyspnea (intensity or severity). Figure 11-3 demonstrates an example of a VAS. A common problem in administering the VAS is difficulty seeing the line or understanding the orientation of the anchors. Although not tested directly in people with cancer, numerical rating scale (NRS) scores (e.g., 0–100) have been shown to correlate highly with dyspnea VAS scores, and when compared for "present dyspnea," the NRS and VAS scores were not significantly different, thus supporting construct validity for the NRS (Gift & Narsavage, 1998). The choice of instrument or tool to measure dyspnea depends on one's purpose or reason for measuring dyspnea, such as to obtain a clinical baseline, to determine the effect of treatment, or as part of a protocol answering a specific research question. The feasibility of using one tool versus another also depends on the clinical or research situation.

History and Physical Examination

Evaluation of dyspnea includes a complete history and a focused review surrounding the symptom, such as dyspnea intensity and descriptors, temporal onset and duration, precipi-

TABLE 11-1	Description of Dyspnea Assessment Tools				
Name of Tool	Author/Year	Domains or Factors	Number of Items	Scaling	Scoring	Language
Baseline Dyspnea Index (BDI) or Transition Dyspnea Index (TDI)	Mahler et al., 1984	Severity of dyspnea in three different categories: functional impairment, magnitude of task, and magnitude of effort	3 categorical items assessed by observer interviewer then dyspnea graded from severe to unimpaired	BDI – 5 grade rating from 0 (severe) to 4 (unimpaired) TDI – change in dyspnea rated by seven grades ranging from –3 (major deterioration) to +3 (major improvement)	BDI has baseline focal score range from 0 to 12. TDI has a transition focal score range from –9 to +9.	English
British Medical Research Council (BMRC) or Medical Research Council (MRC) Dyspnea Scale and Modified MRC scale	Bestall et al., 1999 Mahler et al., 1987, 1988, 1989 (secondary source)	Grades of breathlessness experienced with physical activities (e.g., walking, hurrying on level ground, walking up hill)	5-point scale self-administered or by an interviewer	Categorical scale quantifying breathlessness in grades: 1 (I only get breathless with strenuous exercise) to 5 (I am too breathless to leave the house).	Grades 1–5	English
Cancer Dyspnoea Scale (CDS)*	Tanaka et al., 2000	Multidimensional nature of dyspnea (sense of effort, sense of anxiety, sense of discomfort)	12 items	5 point scale from 1 (not at all) to 5 (very much)	The maximum total score is 48: 20 points for sense of effort, 16 for sense of anxiety, and 12 for sense of discomfort. The higher the score, the more severe the dyspnea.	English Japanese

(Continued on next page)

TABLE 11-1 **Description of Dyspnea Assessment Tools** *(Continued)*

Name of Tool	Author/Year	Domains or Factors	Number of Items	Scaling	Scoring	Language
Chronic Respiratory Disease Questionnaire (CRQ)	Guyatt et al., 1987	Dyspnea, fatigue, emotional function, mastery (the feeling of control over disease)	20 items administered by interviewer	1 (extreme) to 7 (none or not at all) Likert categorical scale	Overall score can be reported for all four components. Author recommends scoring dyspnea separately and not including in overall score.	English
Modified Borg Scale (MBS)	Borg, 1982	Exertional dyspnea. Rating of perceived exertion "suitable for determining other subjective symptoms such as breathing difficulties, aches and pains" (Borg, 1982, p. 380).	Vertical 0–10+ item scale with words describing degrees of perceived exertion anchored to numbers	Categorical scale with ratio properties	One point in time value indicated by subject	English French German Japanese Hebrew Russian
Oxygen-cost diagram (OCD)	McGavin et al., 1978	Daily activities corresponding to perceived increasing oxygen demand	100 mm vertical visual analog scale with 13 activities listed at various points along the line	Patients place a mark on the line corresponding to point above which they think their breathlessness would not let them go.	Score is the distance of the mark in millimeters above zero.	English

(Continued on next page)

TABLE 11-1	Description of Dyspnea Assessment Tools *(Continued)*					
Name of Tool	Author/Year	Domains or Factors	Number of Items	Scaling	Scoring	Language
Pulmonary Function Status and Dyspnea Questionnaire (PFSDQ)	Lareau et al., 1994	Dyspnea intensity with activities and the effect of dyspnea on activities of daily life (ADL)	164-item paper and pencil self-administered questionnaire	Dyspnea component: 0 to 10 numerical rating scale with the words none, mild, moderate, and very severe at numbers 0, 3, 5, and 10 to rate dyspnea with each of 79 activities. Functional ability component: a Likert scale from 1 (as active as I've ever been) to 7 (have omitted entirely) to rate the degree to which activities have been modified at the present time compared with before the onset of COPD	Dyspnea index is obtained by summing the dyspnea scores rated 7 or greater, and an activity index is obtained by adding activity ratings 6 or greater.	English
University of California, San Diego Shortness of Breath Questionnaire (SOBQ)	Eakin et al., 1998	ADL-related shortness of breath	24 items	6-point Likert categorical scaling (0 = not at all to 5 = maximal or unable to do) to indicate severity of shortness of breath during 21 ADLs	Scored by summing responses across all 24 items to form total score (range 0–120)	English
Visual Analog Scale (VAS)*	—	Symptom intensity	1 item	100 mm line (either vertical or horizontal) with anchors at either end to indicate extremes of the sensation	Measuring the distance from the bottom of the scale (or left if it is horizontal) to the level indicated by the subject	

*This tool has evidence of either reliability or validity in patients with cancer. Most of the included tools report measurement of dyspnea in various respiratory diagnoses. When possible, the table indicates if the tools measure dyspnea or exertional dyspnea.

Note. From *Measuring Oncology Nursing-Sensitive Patient Outcomes: Evidence-Based Summary,* by M. Joyce and S. Beck, March 2005. Retrieved September 6, 2007, from http://www.ons.org/outcomes/measures/pdf/DyspneaTools.pdf. Copyright 2005 by Oncology Nursing Society. Reprinted with permission.

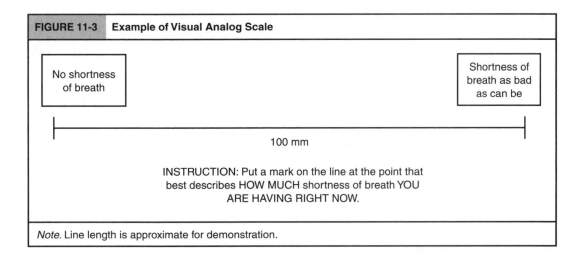

FIGURE 11-3   **Example of Visual Analog Scale**

No shortness
of breath

Shortness of
breath as bad
as can be

100 mm

INSTRUCTION: Put a mark on the line at the point that
best describes HOW MUCH shortness of breath YOU
ARE HAVING RIGHT NOW.

Note. Line length is approximate for demonstration.

tating or relieving events, and response to medication or behavioral approaches (Ripamonti & Fusco, 2002). The stability and the circumstances of the patient's condition will guide the urgency of this evaluation. A rapid initial assessment of airway, breathing, and circulation is appropriate when confronted with acute dyspnea.

Aspects of the medical history pertinent to dyspnea evaluation include assessment of co-existing diagnoses such as cardiac or pulmonary disease, history of current or past tobacco use or exposure to secondhand or environmental tobacco smoke, relevant work history that provides information about toxin exposure (e.g., asbestos), and current medications and cancer therapy, as well as prior radiotherapy or chemotherapy.

A dyspnea-focused physical examination centers on three primary areas: ventilation mechanics, cardiovascular function, and tissue oxygenation (Shepherd & Geraci, 1999). Initial evaluation includes all vital signs (blood pressure, pulse, respiratory rate, and temperature). Evaluation of ventilatory mechanics includes (a) observation of the use of accessory respiratory muscles or pursed-lip breathing, (b) stethoscope auscultation for absent breath sounds or the presence of adventitious sounds such as rales, rhonchi, wheezing, or friction rub, (c) lung field percussion to assess for dullness indicating atelectasis, consolidation, or effusion, and (d) chest palpation for respiratory excursion and fremitus. Cardiovascular assessment focuses on heart sounds, palpation of central pulses, and observation of jugular venous distention. Deficient tissue oxygenation findings are listed in Figure 11-4.

FIGURE 11-4   **Physical Signs of Deficient Tissue Oxygenation**

- Pallor (relative absence of oxyhemoglobin with its characteristic red color)
- Cyanosis of fingernails, lips, and mucous membranes
- Clubbing of the digits (indicating chronic hypoxia)
- Mental status changes (indicating cerebral hypoxia) such as restlessness, anxiety, disorientation, and confusion

Note. Based on information from Shepherd & Geraci, 1999.

Diagnostic Testing

The choice of appropriate diagnostic tests is guided by the stage of disease, usefulness of the information for possible therapeutic intervention, and patient choice. Basic dyspnea diagnostic testing includes noninvasive pulse oximetry at rest and with exertion and a complete blood count (CBC). Pulse oximetry results that show oxygen saturation equal to or greater than 92% reflect normal oxygen levels in blood and tissue (Mack & Altman, 2004). A CBC may show any decrease in hemoglobin concentration from one's usual baseline hemoglobin that is attended by a corresponding decline in the oxygen-carrying capacity of the blood.

A chest radiograph may be indicated to evaluate acute problems, such as pneumothorax, pneumonia, or pleural effusion. Computed tomography may provide information such as tumor outline or tumor progression if sequential scans are performed for comparison. Ventilation-perfusion scan can indicate the probability of pulmonary emboli as one potential cause of dyspnea. Pulmonary function tests that measure lung volumes and gas diffusion may be helpful to diagnose a reversible airway obstruction or hypoxemia, which can be improved with therapy. Extensive diagnostic testing is appropriate only to determine pathophysiologic causes of dyspnea that are potentially reversible with therapy. Patient clinical status and wishes should guide testing efforts.

Goal of Assessment

Considering the complex nature of dyspnea, an important goal of assessment is to differentiate an acute and possibly reversible cause of dyspnea from a condition that requires supportive or palliative intervention. The best intervention for dyspnea is treatment of the underlying cause. Although dyspnea may be a progressive complication of the underlying cancer, sometimes patients present with a sudden onset or an acute exacerbation of shortness of breath that could be considered a medical emergency depending on the presenting context and broad differential possibilities (Houlihan, Inzeo, Joyce, & Tyson, 2004).

Evidence-Based Interventions

The overall goals in treating dyspnea are to promote patient comfort, increase exercise tolerance, and promote physical and social well-being (Carrieri-Kohlman & Janson-Bjerklie, 1986). Modest alterations in a number of physiologic and psychological variables as a result of therapy can result in a clinically meaningful reduction in symptoms (ATS, 1999). For example, one physiologic mechanism of dyspnea may be inspiratory muscle deconditioning. A therapeutic intervention, such as inspiratory muscle training or body positioning to alter or improve inspiratory muscle function, is one approach to lessen the symptom (ATS).

Management of dyspnea can be divided into two categories: therapeutic and palliative. The optimal treatment of dyspnea is to treat reversible causes with specific therapies (therapeutic) and to treat irreversible causes with nonspecific or palliative therapies. Dudgeon et al. (2001) organized cancer-related dyspnea into categories related to cause, including directly caused by tumor, indirectly caused by tumor, caused by cancer therapy, and unrelated to cancer (see Figure 11-5). Dyspnea treatment options can be organized accordingly.

Therapeutic Treatment of Dyspnea

Dyspnea Caused by Tumor

If the etiology of a patient's dyspnea is the tumor itself, appropriate therapy to treat the underlying cause with surgery, radiotherapy, or chemotherapy could reduce dyspnea. Even a minor response to cancer treatment can reduce breathlessness. Relief of airway obstruction

---

FIGURE 11-5	**Causes of Dyspnea in Patients With Cancer**

Dyspnea Directly Due to Cancer
- Pulmonary parenchymal involvement (primary or metastatic)
- Lymphangitic carcinomatosis
- Intrinsic or extrinsic airway obstruction by tumour
- Pleural tumour
- Pleural effusion
- Pericardial effusion
- Ascites
- Hepatomegaly
- Phrenic nerve paralysis
- Multiple tumour microemboli
- Pulmonary leukostasis
- Superior vena cava syndrome

Dyspnea Indirectly Due to Cancer
- Cachexia
- Electrolyte abnormalities
- Anemia
- Pneumonia
- Pulmonary aspiration
- Pulmonary emboli
- Neurologic paraneoplastic syndromes

Dyspnea Due to Cancer Treatment
- Surgery
- Radiation pneumonitis/fibrosis
- Chemotherapy-induced pulmonary disease
- Chemotherapy-induced cardiomyopathy
- Radiation-induced pericardial disease

Dyspnea Unrelated to Cancer
- Chronic obstructive pulmonary disease
- Asthma
- Congestive heart failure
- Interstitial lung disease
- Pneumothorax
- Anxiety
- Chest wall deformity
- Obesity
- Neuromuscular disorders
- Pulmonary vascular disease

Note. From "Dyspnea in Cancer Patients: Prevalence and Associated Factors," by D.J. Dudgeon, L. Kristjanson, J.A. Sloan, M. Lertzman, and K. Clement, 2001, *Journal of Pain and Symptom Management, 21*(2), p. 100. Copyright 2001 by Elsevier. Reprinted with permission.

---

either through external beam radiotherapy, brachytherapy, or airway stenting with or without laser ablation can palliate respiratory symptoms. Respiratory compromise from pleural effusions or ascites can be relieved temporarily with thoracentesis or paracentesis. In most instances, the fluid reaccumulates shortly after removal. If relief is obtained with pleural fluid drainage, pleurodesis with a sclerosing agent such as talc can obliterate the pleural space and prevent further accumulation of pleural fluid. Pleurodesis is created by instilling talc or other substance via a chest tube or by insufflation during thoracoscopy into the pleural space to fuse the visceral and parietal pleura ("Mediastinal and Pleural Disorders," 2006).

Talc causes inflammation that results in fibrosis and adherence of the serosal surfaces, which eliminates the pleural space. However, subsequent dyspnea described as a sense of lung restriction sometimes results from the pleurodesis procedure.

Dyspnea Indirectly Caused by Cancer

Two common complications of cancer as a chronic illness that may contribute to dyspnea are pneumonia and anemia. Chronic illness, as well as certain cancer therapies, can predispose an individual to secondary conditions, which may result in increased respiratory effort or discomfort. Pneumonia, an acute inflammation of the lung, can be treated with adequate antibiotic therapy and can lead to a degree of dyspnea relief. Anemia, a decrease from normal baseline of oxygen-carrying hemoglobin, may precipitate a feeling of breathing effort. If appropriate to the patient's condition, anemia can be relieved with red cell transfusion or erythropoietin therapy. Correcting anemia may or may not lessen dyspnea, and erythropoiesis-stimulating therapy is associated with risk of cardiovascular complications (U.S. Food and Drug Administration, 2007). Malnutrition, electrolyte and mineral imbalance, and overall deconditioning also seen in chronic illness can contribute to dyspnea. Again, depending upon the patient's status, attempts to correct these circumstances may improve dyspnea control.

Dyspnea Caused by Cancer Treatment

Either acute or chronic pneumonitis may be a consequence of radiation or some chemotherapy agents. An oral corticosteroid, usually prednisone starting at 40–60 mg daily for one to two weeks followed by a slow taper, such as reducing by 10 mg every one to two weeks, is the mainstay of therapy (Ghafoori, Marks, Vujaskovic, & Kelsey, 2008). Occasionally supplemental oxygen and bronchodilators are required to treat pneumonitis (Dudgeon, 2002).

Cardiomyopathy with risk of congestive heart failure (CHF) and shortness of breath can result from certain chemotherapy agents, such as doxorubicin. The risk of developing significant cardiomyopathy with doxorubicin is greatest when the total dose exceeds 550 mg/m^2 (Fischer et al., 2003, p. 110). Prevention of this cardiac toxicity is the key to success; once it develops, conventional therapy for CHF is indicated.

Palliative Treatment of Dyspnea

Symptomatic management of cancer-related dyspnea usually is based on a combination of pharmacologic therapy, oxygen therapy, and general supportive measures (Bruera & Ripamonti, 1998). Evidence derived solely in a cancer population for each of these modalities is scant. With some exception, evidence supporting use of specific interventions for cancer-related dyspnea is not strong because it comes from uncontrolled research conducted in small samples. Additional evidence comes from consensus opinion of experts. A synthesis of interventions for cancer-related dyspnea (DiSalvo, Joyce, Culkin, Tyson, & Mackay, 2007) is available from the Oncology Nursing Society as part of its Putting Evidence Into Practice (PEP) initiative. The evidence in the PEP synthesis is ranked and digested into categories such as *Recommended for Practice, Likely to Be Effective, Effectiveness Unlikely,* and *Not Recommended for Practice,* among others. Typically, most of the interventions for cancer-related dyspnea, with the exception of immediate-release opioids, lack sufficient evidence to be recommended and thus fall into the category of *Effectiveness Not Established.*

Pharmacologic Interventions

Opioids

Opioid mechanism of action to relieve dyspnea is presumably a respiratory depressive effect. Opioids may alleviate dyspnea by blunting perceptual responses, so that for a given stimulus, the intensity of a respiratory sensation is reduced (ATS, 1999). A Cochrane meta-analysis review (Jennings, Davies, Higgins, & Broadley, 2001) provided strong evidence in favor of using immediate-release oral or parenteral opioids such as morphine to palliate breathlessness in patients with any advanced disease. Three additional studies contributed support for opioid use to relieve dyspnea in patients with cancer (Allard, Lamontagne, Bernard, & Tremblay, 1999; Bruera, Macmillan, Pither, & MacDonald, 1990; Mazzocato, Buclin, & Rapin, 1999).

The opioid most frequently trialed in these studies was morphine, although others, such as codeine, dihydrocodeine, and diamorphine, also were used. Current common opioids such as oxycodone and fentanyl were not included in any of the oral or parenteral studies. No consistent morphine dose can be recommended because of the wide variety of doses trialed in the dyspnea studies. However, Allard et al. (1999) determined that 25%–50% of the four-hour opioid dose was equivalent in relieving dyspnea and recommended using the smaller dose to avoid adverse effects. No difference in opioid effect was seen when opioid-tolerant and opioid-naïve patients were compared in the previously described studies, primarily because of the limited number of participants. However, Jennings, Davies, Higgins, Gibbs, and Broadley (2002) reported that opioid adverse effects such as nausea, vomiting, constipation, dizziness, and drowsiness were more problematic in the opioid-naïve patients.

Two studies (one that involved people with cancer already on morphine [N = 15] and one predominantly with patients with COPD not previously treated with opioids [N = 38]) trialed the use of once-daily extended-release morphine and received conflicting results. The study in the cancer population failed to show a significant reduction in dyspnea (Boyd & Kelly, 1997), whereas a statistically significant reduction (p < 0.01) occurred in dyspnea ratings in the COPD group (Abernethy et al., 2003). Both studies had five to six participants withdraw because of unacceptable study drug side effects, namely sedation or dizziness.

The use of opioids to relieve dyspnea capitalizes upon the respiratory depressive action of the opioids. Although altered respiratory drive is the desired action to relieve dyspnea, severe decreases in respiratory rate (< 8 per minute) with unanticipated sedation or hypoxia may be an unexpected, untoward outcome. Cautious and slow titration of naloxone is available to treat severe respiratory depression associated with opioid use. Naloxone is an opiate antagonist, and standard doses cause abrupt opioid reversal precipitating severe pain and symptoms of opioid withdrawal (Payne, 1998). The 0.4 mg ampule of naloxone can be diluted in 10 ml of normal saline and injected intravenously slowly to titrate effect while monitoring the patient's level of consciousness and respiratory rate. Naloxone has a short duration of action, and the depressant effect of the opioid will recur at approximately 30–60 minutes, thus requiring close patient monitoring (Paice, 2007).

The addition of midazolam, a benzodiazepine, to morphine was tested in one randomized controlled study of 101 people with advanced cancer experiencing severe dyspnea during the last week of life (Navigante, Cerchietti, Castro, Lutteral, & Cabalar, 2006). Participants were randomized to receive either morphine or midazolam subcutaneously around the clock (ATC) with the alternate drug for breakthrough (BT) dyspnea. A third group received both morphine and midazolam ATC with morphine for BT dyspnea. Most participants (92%) who received both morphine and midazolam ATC reported dyspnea relief at 24 hours, compared with 69% (p < 0.01) of those who received morphine only ATC with midazolam for BT dyspnea and 46% (p = 0.03) of those who received midazolam only ATC with morphine for BT dyspnea. Additional evidence is needed to recommend this intervention for practice, but administration of both morphine and midazolam ATC with morphine for BT dyspnea appears promising as an intervention to relieve terminal dyspnea.

Benzodiazepines

Anxiolytic agents have the potential to relieve dyspnea by altering the emotional response (ATS, 1999), but evidence from clinical trials is scant. Expert opinion regarding the use of benzodiazepines is conflicting. Some recommend it to treat the anxiety associated with dyspnea (Campbell, 2004; National Comprehensive Cancer Network [NCCN], 2008); others claim the use of an anxiolytic is not supported for relief of cancer-related dyspnea (Dudgeon, 2002; Ripamonti, 1999). The evidence is based on small studies with negative results indicating no difference when a benzodiazepine was trialed to reduce dyspnea associated with exertion in people with COPD and does not support the regular use of benzodiazepines in the management of dyspnea (Bruera & Ripamonti, 1998). However, in some patients, a trial of benzodiazepine may be reasonable, particularly in those with morbid anxiety or history of respiratory panic attacks (ATS).

Nebulized Therapy

A nebulized route of different pharmacologic agents (morphine, fentanyl, furosemide, lidocaine) has been trialed to relieve dyspnea. Inhalation deposits a fine mist of aerosolized medication on the respiratory tract with potential for modification of dyspnea by local action. Specifically with respect to opioids, a local binding to pulmonary sensory receptors in the lung is thought to augment pulmonary effect and minimize systemic toxicity.

In general, scientific data are lacking to support the use of nebulized opioids in the treatment of dyspnea. A Cochrane database subgroup review of 9 out of 18 studies that compared the use of any opioid with a placebo as an intervention for dyspnea failed to show a positive effect of nebulized opioids (Jennings et al., 2001). An integrated synthesis of 20 studies including experimental trials, chart reviews, and case studies that examined the efficacy of nebulized opioids also concluded that further rigorous research stratifying patients into opioid-tolerant and opioid-naïve groups is needed before recommending that nebulized opioids be adopted into practice (Joyce, McSweeney, Carrieri-Kohlman, & Hawkins, 2004). Lower-level evidence tended to show benefit of nebulized opioids in samples that were mostly opioid tolerant with the theory being that presence of systemic opioids potentially influences the local pulmonary effect (Tanaka et al., 1999). In one small study of 17 subjects with cardiac or lung disease, all reported less dyspnea after nebulized therapy of either nebulized morphine or normal saline (Noseda, Carpiaux, Markstein, Meyvaert, & de Maertelaer, 1997). The lack of difference between the morphine and saline groups suggested a placebo or nonspecific effect of the treatment modality that bears further investigation.

Fentanyl (25 mcg in 2 ml of saline via nebulizer) was tested in an uncontrolled study of 35 patients with life-limiting illnesses complaining of dyspnea (Coyne, Viswanathan, & Smith, 2002). Eighty-one percent perceived improvement in their breathing, suggesting potential for efficacy if results could be duplicated in a controlled situation. Nebulized furosemide also was reported to decrease the sensation of dyspnea in a small study of 15 patients with advanced cancer (Kohara et al., 2003), suggesting potential but also needing confirmation with more rigorous research.

Oxygen

Researchers have postulated that supplemental oxygen may provide dyspnea relief through depressing the central hypoxic drive that is mediated through peripheral chemoreceptors in the carotid body (ATS, 1999). Reduced chemoreceptor activation and associated reduced ventilation effort is thought to be oxygen's primary mechanism to relieve dyspnea either at rest or during exercise. However, other factors also are thought to contribute to reduced dyspnea and may explain the variability in response to supplemental oxygen. One small study of 14 patients with terminal cancer provided evidence that those patients who are *hypoxemic* at rest on room air reported decreased dyspnea with supplemental oxygen (Bruera, de Stoutz, Velasco-Leiva, Schoeller, & Hanson, 1993). Patients in the trial received either oxygen or air at 5 L/min by face mask and then crossed over to receive the alternate therapy. All outcome measures (patients' ratings of dyspnea, oxygen saturation, respiratory rate and effort) improved with oxygen.

Evidence supporting the use of supplemental oxygen in *nonhypoxic* patients is inconclusive. In one study of 33 patients with cancer, subjects were randomized to either oxygen or air at 5 L/min via nasal cannula during a six-minute walk (Bruera et al., 2003). No statistically significant difference was found in dyspnea, fatigue, or distance walked with either oxygen or air. Another study of 51 patients with cancer with 24%–33% hypoxic patients (majority were nonhypoxic) examined the effect of oxygen and air on the relief of dyspnea (Philip et al., 2006). This study also demonstrated no significant difference between the two. On average, patients improved symptomatically with both air and oxygen. In the hypoxic subgroup, the mean oxygen saturation levels increased significantly with oxygen, but the mean change in VAS dyspnea scores did not differ significantly when oxygen or air were administered. This supports the multidimensional construct of dyspnea in that correction of the physiologic oxygen deficit alone may not be sufficient to relieve the symptom sensation.

Subjectively, some patients report benefit from oxygen and use it intermittently, such as at night during sleep or during activities that involve exertion. The prescription of oxygen in the absence of documented hypoxemia is problematic from a reimbursement perspective. Irrespective of patient report of decreased dyspnea, current Medicare guidelines require documented oxygen saturation percent less than or equal to 88% taken at rest to justify reimbursement (Centers for Medicare and Medicaid Services, 1993). However, because oxygen makes individual patients feel better (reporting less dyspnea), it behooves practitioners to assess the subjective benefit of this intervention irrespective of the physiologic findings, such as oxygen percent saturation, and seek alternative reimbursement. Supplemental oxygen without a specific hypoxic requirement usually is provided under the umbrella of a hospice homecare program.

One small study trialed the use of Heliox 28 (72% helium and 28% oxygen) compared to oxygen-enriched air (either 28% or 21.1% oxygen combined with nitrogen) to palliate dyspnea and improve exercise capacity in 12 patients with lung cancer (Ahmedzai, Laude, Robertson, Troy, & Vora, 2004). Helium has a low density with the potential of reducing the work of breathing and improving alveolar ventilation when replacing nitrogen in the air. The side effects of breathing helium-enriched air are a characteristic increase in the pitch of the voice and reduction of the core body temperature because helium is a better conductor of heat than nitrogen. Heliox 28 improved distances walked compared to both oxygen groups and significantly reduced dyspnea scores compared to the 21.1% oxygen group. A slight fall in the study participants' body temperature was noted that was statistically significant but not clinically significant. This finding suggests potential for the use of Heliox in practice but needs to be confirmed in a larger randomized controlled trial.

Ambient Airflow

Anecdotally, patients who are short of breath ask to sit near a fan or open window. It is thought that cold air directed across the cheek and through the nose can alter ventilation and reduce the perception of breathlessness, perhaps by affecting sensory receptors in the distribution of the trigeminal (fifth) cranial nerve that respond to both thermal and mechanical stimuli (Dudgeon, 2002). This is a low-cost and low-risk intervention that can be easily tried and thus recommended to see if it makes the patient feel better.

Supportive Care Measures

Evidence from a Cochrane systematic review (Lacasse, Goldstein, Lasserson, & Martin, 2006) supported the use of pulmonary rehabilitation in the care of patients with COPD. Pulmonary rehabilitation is defined as exercise training for least four weeks with or without education and/or psychological support. The analysis included 31 randomized controlled trials and found statistically significant improved exercise capacity and quality of life, including the domains of dyspnea, fatigue, and the patient's control over disease in people with COPD who completed pulmonary rehabilitation.

Evidence from one multicenter randomized controlled study and two smaller studies (one controlled and one uncontrolled) supported a similar rehabilitative intervention for people with cancer-related dyspnea. The intervention is described as a nurse-led program that trialed the use of a structured weekly approach that included assessment, education, and instruction in breathing control and coping techniques (Bredin et al., 1999; Corner, Plant, A'Hern, & Bailey, 1996; Hately, Laurence, Scott, Baker, & Thomas, 2003). Details of the nurse-led clinic are outlined in Figure 11-6. Patients with advanced cancer, the majority with a lung cancer diagnosis, were randomized to the intervention program or to usual standard care. At the eighth week, patients in the specialist program reported improved breathlessness, emotional and physical well-being, and performance status. A limitation of the multicenter study was significant attrition reportedly because some patients' clinical deterioration and other reasons; however, the overall conclusion was that patients benefited from the specialized program. Because the intervention contained many components, the exact contribution of each component remains unknown. A researchable question is whether all components of the breathing rehabilitation program are needed to achieve the same outcome or if one aspect of the intervention is more significant or essential.

Some alternative measures have shown success in the treatment of dyspnea. Williams (2006) reported that acupuncture and acupressure have been trialed successfully in three studies and suggested that this complementary therapy can be used to improve dyspnea in patients with COPD. However, Williams' analysis also cited two other studies that did not display a positive effect on dyspnea for patients with advanced cancer and other nonmalignant causes. In one small uncontrolled study of 20 patients with cancer-related dyspnea that was refractory to standard therapy, acupuncture was trialed with statistically significant reduction in dyspnea VAS and

---

FIGURE 11-6   **Specialized Nursing Intervention for Breathlessness**

- Detailed assessment of breathlessness and factors that ameliorate or exacerbate it
- Advice and support on ways of managing breathlessness
- Exploration of the meaning of breathlessness, disease, and feelings about the future
- Training in breathing control techniques, progressive muscle relaxation, and distraction exercises
- Goal setting to complement breathing and relaxation techniques, to help in the management of functional and social activities, and to support the development and adoption of coping strategies
- Early identification of problems needing pharmacologic or medical intervention

Note. From "Multicenter Randomized Controlled Trial of Nursing Intervention for Breathlessness in Patients With Lung Cancer," by M. Bredin, J. Corner, M. Krishnasamy, H. Plant, C. Bailey, and R. A'Hern, 1999, *BMJ, 318*(7188), p. 902. Copyright 1999 by BMJ Publishing Group. Adapted with permission.

improvement in relaxation and anxiety (Filshie, Penn, Ashley, & Davis, 1996). The acupuncture results may have been influenced by the fact that a nurse remained with the patient for 90 minutes. Clearly this intervention may be beneficial, but current evidence is lacking until more research about the effect of acupuncture and acupressure can confirm findings.

Expected Outcomes

Because dyspnea is a subjective symptom, similar to pain, patient report is the gold standard with respect to intensity and assessment of relief from any intervention. The exertional or paroxysmal nature of dyspnea also needs to be accounted for when evaluating outcomes. For example, many research assessments of dyspnea ask about its presence on average or in the past 24 hours or during the past week in addition to dyspnea "right now" to capture the symptom's variability. One clinical recommendation is that dyspnea ought to be measured with a quantitative measure such as VAS, NRS, or another reliable tool in a longitudinal manner so that the symptom may be monitored and addressed. One research recommendation is to publish reports of the use of specific tools to measure cancer-related dyspnea and associated psychometric data to build evidence about reliability and validity of the instrument in the cancer population.

Correction of abnormal physiologic parameters such as tachypnea, use of accessory muscles, cyanosis, or oxygen percent saturation will help care providers to assess resolution of clinical status with an understanding that the symptom of dyspnea may or may not resolve with return to normal parameters. The expectation of an intervention for dyspnea is that initial attempts to correct reversible causes will be made and attempts to palliate irreversible causes will be pursued to the goal that patients will report relief or comfort. However, given the refractory nature of dyspnea, NCCN (2008) recommends sedation, as needed, as a potential final intervention in terminal dyspnea.

Patient Teaching Points

Education about disease and symptoms is thought to provide patients with information and skills to understand and control symptoms, including dyspnea. The benefits of education have not been studied in cancer-related dyspnea. Education about dyspnea management in cardiopulmonary diseases is thought to be beneficial to enhance self-care strategies and coping with both acute and chronic dyspnea (ATS, 1999; Kohlman-Carrieri & Janson-Bjerklie, 1990). One meta-analysis of the effects of psychoeducational care in adults with COPD showed that pulmonary rehabilitation had a statistically significant effect on dyspnea (Hochstetter, Lewis, & Soares-Smith, 2005). A small sample of studies in that meta-analysis showed that education alone had a beneficial effect on healthcare utilization, and relaxation training alone had a statistically beneficial effect on dyspnea. Although this positive evidence of the benefit of psychoeducational care comes from the COPD patient population and should be retested in those with cancer-related dyspnea, it is reasonable to think the benefits also will transfer to patients with cancer.

Guidance for patient and caregiver teaching with respect to cancer-related dyspnea comes from general evidence and resources for oncology nursing care (Bruera & Ripamonti, 1998; Kohlman-Carrieri & Janson-Bjerklie, 1990). The main components of dyspnea education are knowledge of signs and symptoms to report to healthcare providers, understanding of medication regimens, and self-care strategies that range from recognizing maneuvers that precipitate dyspnea to maximizing body positions and breathing techniques to decrease breathlessness.

The symptom of dyspnea can change rapidly or insidiously. With an understanding that some causes of acute dyspnea are treatable or reversible even in the context of chronic dyspnea, patients should be informed and educated to report changes in baseline dyspnea, particularly increasing shortness of breath, fever, pain, and change in sputum production. Patients should be taught to avoid respiratory irritants such as primary or secondary tobacco smoke and exposure to individuals with respiratory infections. Nurses can advise about the prevention benefit of immunizations (if not contraindicated) such as pneumococcal vaccine and annual influenza vaccine.

Teaching patients and caregivers about medication regimens for dyspnea should include expected actions and side effects of medications and administration techniques. If nebulized medications are included in symptom management, this requires instruction and practice of using nebulizers to gain confidence in proper use. Proper and safe use of oxygen equipment is important information for patients to learn.

Use of specific breathing techniques may be helpful and require teaching; however, many people who experience dyspnea discover body positions and a variety of breathing techniques that improve their dyspnea from trial and error. Nonetheless, reinforcement of proper technique and encouragement to use breathing techniques in times of anxiety or distress are important teaching goals. Breathlessness management techniques commonly are taught in a rehabilitation program for people with chronic pulmonary disease and could be included in individualized teaching. These include (a) positioning, (b) pursed-lip breathing, (c) diaphragmatic breathing, (d) activity modification or energy conservation, and (e) relaxation training such as progressive muscle relaxation.

The "leaning forward" position enhances dyspnea relief. "This postural relief is thought to be due to an increase in the length-tension relationship of the diaphragm" (Kohlman-Carrieri & Janson-Bjerklie, 1990, p. 207). The resting length of the diaphragm is increased, thereby improving its ability to generate force (for exhalation). Common forward-leaning positions are pictured in Figures 11-7, 11-8, and 11-9.

Pursed-lip breathing is a technique that encourages a full-exhaled breath. Exhaling through pursed lips (the lip position to blow out a candle or to whistle) is thought to modify dyspnea

| FIGURE 11-7 | Forward-Lean Sitting Position |

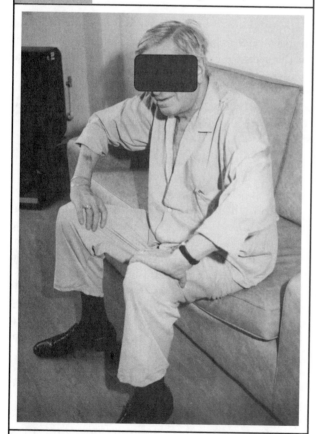

Note. From "An Investigation Into the Immediate Impact of Breathlessness Management on the Breathless Patient: Randomised Controlled Trial," by J. Hochstetter, J. Lewis, and L. Soares-Smith, 2005, *Physiotherapy, 91*(3), p. 180. Copyright 2005 by Elsevier. Reprinted with permission.

"by raising the pressure in the airway, stimulating positive end-expiratory pressure, and providing internal stability to the airways to prevent early closure" and causing "associated decrease in respiratory rate, and corresponding increase in tidal volume, leading to an increase in oxygen saturation" (Kohlman-Carrieri & Janson-Bjerklie, 1990, p. 208). Inhalation should occur at rest and exhalation during exertion. If a person cannot exhale through pursed lips, an alternative is to exhale through a fist held up to the mouth. Patients need to be taught to avoid exhaling too forcefully or hyperventilating, as this can be counterproductive (Gallo-Silver & Pollack, 2000).

Abdominal or diaphragmatic breathing actively uses the diaphragm rather than accessory muscles during inspiration. Diaphragmatic breathing also can promote a feeling of relaxation or stress reduction (Gallo-Silver & Pollack, 2000, p. 269). The potential benefits of diaphragmatic breathing are increased tidal volume, reduced functional residual capacity, and decreased oxygen cost of breathing (Kohlman-Carrieri & Janson-Bjerklie, 1990). A teaching tip for diaphragmatic breathing is "to emphasize that the more the abdomen moves when breathing, the more the lungs are being effectively

FIGURE 11-8   Forward-Lean Standing Position

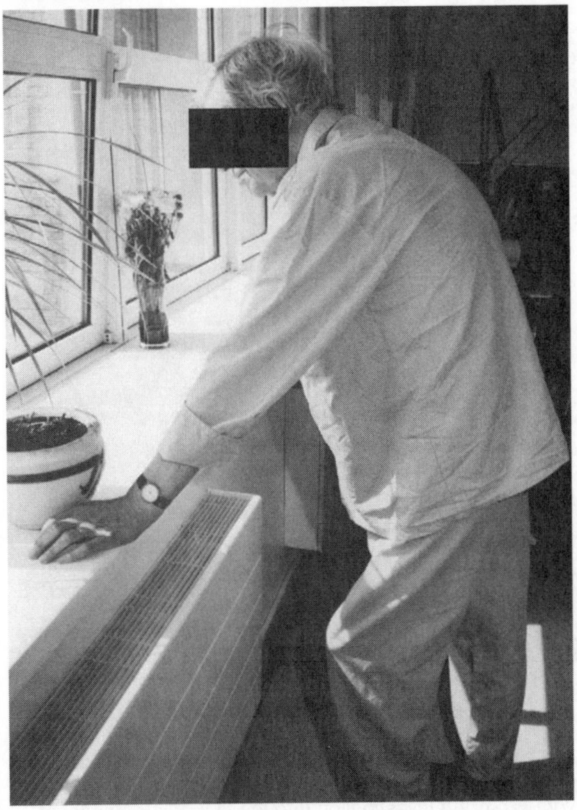

Note. From "An Investigation Into the Immediate Impact of Breathlessness Management on the Breathless Patient: Randomised Controlled Trial," by J. Hochstetter, J. Lewis, and L. Soares-Smith, 2005, *Physiotherapy, 91*(3), p. 181. Copyright 2005 by Elsevier. Reprinted with permission.

filled and emptied" (Gallo-Silver & Pollack, p. 269). A common diaphragmatic breathing exercise is as follows (Wikipedia, 2008): (a) Put one hand on your chest and one on your stomach. (2) Inhale slowly. (3) As you inhale, feel your stomach expand with your hand. (4) Slowly exhale. (5) Rest and repeat.

The benefit of pacing activities and slowing down to conserve energy is thought to regulate exertional dyspnea. For example, prioritizing essential actions and evenly pacing movements without sudden start-up or hurrying motion helps to control exertional dyspnea. Most people with dyspnea learn these regulatory mechanisms on their own, but discussion can support individuals to cope with lifestyle changes. Education about assistive devices or compensatory techniques to complete activities of daily living can teach patients how to perform activities more efficiently and function more independently. If feasible, consider referral to occupational therapy. This discipline specializes in educating patients in the performance of efficient and productive activities of daily living.

Although relaxation training is another recommended educational point that may be helpful in cancer-related dyspnea, as it has been shown to have utility in cardiopulmonary-related

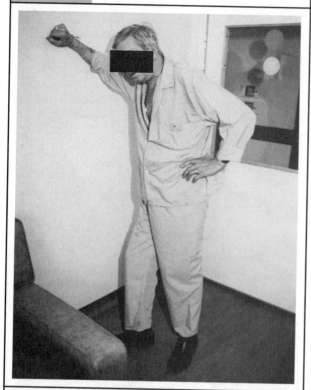

FIGURE 11-9	Side Leaning and Fixing Shoulder Girdle Against Wall

Note. From "An Investigation Into the Immediate Impact of Breathlessness Management on the Breathless Patient: Randomised Controlled Trial," by J. Hochstetter, J. Lewis, and L. Soares-Smith, 2005, *Physiotherapy, 91*(3), p. 181. Copyright 2005 by Elsevier. Reprinted with permission.

dyspnea (Hochstetter et al., 2005), one systematic review found no convincing evidence that relaxation and exercise are effective elements of a rehabilitation program in treatment of anxiety in people with COPD (Rose et al., 2002). However, Rose et al. noted secondary outcomes, including the positive impact of relaxation intervention on dyspnea, disability, and quality of life.

Many different approaches exist for relaxation training, including progressive muscle relaxation, visual imagery, biofeedback, and meditation. Relaxation is thought to be a behavioral self-care strategy that enhances sense of control during periods of increased breathlessness (Kohlman-Carrieri & Janson-Bjerklie, 1990). Relaxation can cause a patient to focus on sensations other than breathlessness and provides a response incompatible with anxiety and muscle tension based on the theory that individuals can only focus attention on one thing at a time (Kohlman-Carrieri & Janson-Bjerklie). Healthcare providers can work closely with patients and families to tailor a relaxation strategy to their situation. Instructional methods vary from live demonstrations to technologically delivered sessions. Encouragement and practice helps individuals to acquire the relaxation skill.

The goals of patient and caregiver education are to inform them about the symptom of dyspnea and empower self-care strategies to promote symptom reduction. This strategy is reinforced in multiple areas of oncology care. Nurses are important in the care of patients with dyspnea because symptom management education is an integral component of nurses' dialogue with patients and caregivers.

Need for Future Research

The symptom of dyspnea is a fertile area for research but, as noted in many research studies, is a difficult symptom area to study in a controlled manner because of the fragile clinical status of patients that often accompanies the symptom. Also, recruitment of patients to cancer-related dyspnea clinical trials is difficult because of patients' potentially unstable clinical status; thus, studies typically have small sample sizes. These recruitment and research design issues challenge researchers to collaborate or conduct multicenter trials to increase sample sizes and strengthen findings.

All areas of cancer-related dyspnea (description, assessment, measurement, and intervention) need further research. Qualitative description of the experience of general dyspnea exists, but description of cancer-related dyspnea is scarce. Description of the affective dimension of dyspnea is particularly lacking. The affective dimension of dyspnea is a component of the sensation that evokes distress and motivates behavior (ATS, 1999). Quantitative assessment of factors other than physiologic parameters that contribute to the symptom experience is lacking. Additionally, further testing of the reliability and validity of dyspnea measurement tools in cancer populations is needed, and the impact of cancer-related dyspnea on function and quality of life needs elaboration.

Intervention research is needed most. Replication of many studies that demonstrated a positive effect of dyspnea interventions in the COPD population should be conducted in the cancer population. The efficacy of newer opioids, such as oxycodone and fentanyl, in relieving dyspnea still needs to be trialed, and appropriate dose recommendations for other opioids still are needed.

Cognitive behavioral interventions for dyspnea need further testing so that specific recommendations for practice can be made. Cognitive behavioral therapy is an area where nursing-sensitive patient outcomes abound and recommended interventions could be integrated. Once research confirms the evidence, nurses could educate patients in complementary or alternative dyspnea management techniques. This area for nursing research is very fertile because results could readily be translated into daily bedside or outpatient practice.

Conclusion of Case Study

Because B.L. was taught to report breathing-related changes to his healthcare team and because previous dyspnea rating scores were documented, the nurse assessing him was alerted to the increase in his dyspnea. A chest x-ray was obtained, which revealed a new left pleural effusion. Because this is a potentially reversible cause of dyspnea, an ultrasound-guided thoracentesis was arranged to drain the pleural fluid. More than one liter of pleural fluid was removed, which significantly improved B.L.'s breathing. Unfortunately, the fluid rapidly reaccumulated over one week, and his dyspnea returned. While arrangements were being made for a pleurodesis procedure, B.L. was given a prescription for a short-acting immediate-release opioid to relieve the shortness of breath. Because he is taking 30 mg of sustained-release morphine, a 2.5 mg dose of immediate-release morphine (this is 25% of his four-hour dose) was ordered to relieve his dyspnea on an as-needed basis.

At his next visit to the cancer center, B.L.'s assessment parameters showed a hypoxic oxygen percent saturation of 87% obtained on room air at rest. In addition to this physiologic parameter, B.L. rated his breathlessness as a 7 out of 10 on the assessment NRS. His oxygen percent saturation improved to 94% with the use of supplemental oxygen at 2 L/min by nasal cannula. In addition to correcting the hypoxia, 15 minutes after the oxygen was applied B.L. noticed and reported a lower dyspnea score of 4. His ambulatory nurse arranged for home delivery of portable oxygen to be used both at rest and with exertion.

Because B.L. has a history of COPD, in addition to his newly diagnosed lung cancer, his treatment team thinks a referral to a pulmonary rehabilitation program might be of benefit to control his dyspnea. When asked if he was interested in such a program, B.L. says the idea sounds appealing and helpful, but he is concerned about his ability to participate because of fatigue and his debilitated state. Instead, he asks for education about breathing techniques that he could practice on his own. Not wanting to overwhelm him with information, his nurse chooses initially to teach him the forward-leaning position and the pursed-lip breathing technique. He also is given an audio-video program that demonstrates relaxation training. The nurse advises him to practice relaxation as a self-care strategy for times of dyspnea exacerbation.

These measures were successful in keeping B.L.'s dyspnea under control for several weeks. His disease did not respond to the systemic chemotherapy, and he was referred to a hospice homecare program. He maintained good symptom control until the last week of his life, when dyspnea again became a prominent symptom. A trial of nebulized morphine did not improve his breathing, as he was too weak to participate in the breathing treatment. Successive increases in the dose of immediate-release morphine were employed to palliate his dyspnea.

Conclusion

Because of the potential multiple causes of dyspnea and because dyspnea has both physiologic and reactive dimensions, it remains a complex symptom that requires thorough assessment and attention. A guiding principle is to treat reversible causes of dyspnea with specific therapies and to use nonspecific or palliative therapy to manage irreversible causes. Dyspnea often is a symptom that begs for intervention because of the distress it evokes in both the person experiencing it and the caregiver witnessing it. Although evidence is scant, use of the evidence-based interventions described in this chapter is essential, while research continues to discover the best methods to care for people with dyspnea.

References

Abernethy, A.P., Currow, D.C., Frith, P., Fazekas, B.S., McHugh, A., & Bui, C. (2003). Randomised, double blind, placebo controlled crossover trial of sustained release morphine for the management of refractory dyspnoea. *BMJ, 327*(7414), 523–528.

Ahmedzai, S.H., Laude, E., Robertson, A., Troy, G., & Vora, V. (2004). A double-blind, randomised, controlled phase II trial of Heliox28 gas mixture in lung cancer patients with dyspnoea on exertion. *British Journal of Cancer, 90*(2), 366–371.

Allard, P., Lamontagne, C., Bernard, P., & Tremblay, C. (1999). How effective are supplementary doses of opioids for dyspnea in terminally ill cancer patients? A randomized continuous sequential clinical trial. *Journal of Pain and Symptom Management, 17*(4), 256–265.

American Thoracic Society. (1999). Dyspnea. Mechanisms, assessment, and management: A consensus statement. *American Journal of Respiratory Critical Care Medicine, 159*(1), 321–340.

Bestall, J.C., Paul, E.A., Garrod, R., Garnham, R., Jones, P.W., & Wedzicha, J.A. (1999). Usefulness of the Medical Research Council (MRC) dyspnoea scale as a measure of disability in patients with chronic obstructive pulmonary disease. *Thorax, 54*(7), 581–586.

Borg, G.A. (1982). Psychophysical bases of perceived exertion. *Medicine and Science in Sports and Exercise, 14*(5), 377–381.

Boyd, K.J., & Kelly, M. (1997). Oral morphine as symptomatic treatment of dyspnoea in patients with advanced cancer. *Palliative Medicine, 11*(4), 277–281.

Bredin, M., Corner, J., Krishnasamy, M., Plant, H., Bailey, C., & A'Hern, R. (1999). Multicentre randomised controlled trial of nursing intervention for breathlessness in patients with lung cancer. *BMJ, 318*(7188), 901–904.

Bruera, E., de Stoutz, N., Velasco-Leiva, A., Schoeller, T., & Hanson, J. (1993). Effects of oxygen on dyspnoea in hypoxaemic terminal-cancer patients. *Lancet, 342*(8862), 13–14.

Bruera, E., Macmillan, K., Pither, J., & MacDonald, R.N. (1990). Effects of morphine on the dyspnea of terminal cancer patients. *Journal of Pain and Symptom Management, 5*(6), 341–344.

Bruera, E., & Ripamonti, C. (1998). Dyspnea in patients with advanced cancer. In A.M. Berger, R. Portenoy, & D. Weissman (Eds.), *Principles and practice of supportive oncology* (pp. 295–308). Philadelphia: Lippincott-Raven.

Bruera, E., Sweeney, C., Willey, J., Palmer, J.L., Strasser, F., Morice, R.C., et al. (2003). A randomized controlled trial of supplemental oxygen versus air in cancer patients with dyspnea. *Palliative Medicine, 17*(8), 659–663.

Brunelli, A., Xiume, F., Refai, M., Salati, M., Marasco, R., Sciarra, V., et al. (2007). Evaluation of expiratory volume, diffusion capacity, and exercise tolerance following major lung resection: A prospective follow-up analysis. *Chest, 131*(1), 141–147.

Campbell, M.L. (2004). Terminal dyspnea and respiratory distress. *Critical Care Clinics, 20*(3), 403–417.

Carrieri-Kohlman, V., Gormley, J.M., Douglas, M.K., Paul, S.M., & Stulbarg, M.S. (1996). Differentiation between dyspnea and its affective components. *Western Journal of Nursing Research, 18*(6), 626–642.

Carrieri-Kohlman, V.L., & Janson-Bjerklie, S. (1986). Dyspnea. In V.K. Carrieri, A.M. Lindsey, & C.M. West (Eds.), *Pathophysiological phenomena in nursing: Human responses to illness* (pp. 191–217). Philadelphia: Saunders.

Centers for Medicare and Medicaid Services. (1993, October 27). *Medicare coverage database national coverage determination (NCD) for home use of oxygen* [Publication Number 100-3, section 240.2, version 1]. Retrieved February 19, 2008, from http://www.cms.hhs.gov/mcd/viewncd.asp?ncd_id=240.2&ncd_version=1&basket=ncd%3A240%2E2%3A1%3AHome+Use+of+Oxygen

Corner, J., Plant, H., A'Hern, R., & Bailey, C. (1996). Non-pharmacological intervention for breathlessness in lung cancer. *Palliative Medicine, 10*(4), 299–305.

Coyne, P.J., Viswanathan, R., & Smith, T.J. (2002). Nebulized fentanyl citrate improves patients' perception of breathing, respiratory rate, and oxygen saturation in dyspnea. *Journal of Pain and Symptom Management, 23*(2), 157–160.

DiSalvo, W.M., Joyce, M., Culkin, A.E., Tyson, L.B., & Mackay, K. (2007). *Dyspnea.* Retrieved September 18, 2007, from http://www.ons.org/outcomes/volume2/dyspnea.shtml

Dudgeon, D.J. (2002). Managing dyspnea and cough. *Hematology/Oncology Clinics of North America, 16*(3), 557–577.

Dudgeon, D.J., Kristjanson, L., Sloan, J.A., Lertzman, M., & Clement, K. (2001). Dyspnea in cancer patients: Prevalence and associated factors. *Journal of Pain and Symptom Management, 21*(2), 95–102.

Dudgeon, D.J., & Lertzman, M. (1998). Dyspnea in the advanced cancer patient. *Journal of Pain and Symptom Management, 16*(4), 212–219.

Eakin, E.G., Resnikoff, P.M., Prewitt, L.M., Ries, A.L., & Kaplan, R.M. (1998). Validation of a new dyspnea measure: The UCSD Shortness of Breath Questionnaire. University of California, San Diego. *Chest, 113*(3), 619–624.

Farncombe, M. (1997). Dyspnea: Assessment and treatment. *Supportive Care in Cancer, 5*(2), 94–99.

Filshie, J., Penn, K., Ashley, S., & Davis, C. (1996). Acupuncture for the relief of cancer related breathlessness. *Palliative Medicine, 10*(2), 145–150.

Fischer, D., Knobf, M.T., Durivage, H., & Beaulieu, N. (Eds.). (2003). *The cancer chemotherapy handbook* (6th ed.). Philadelphia: Mosby.

Gallo-Silver, L., & Pollack, B. (2000). Behavioral interventions for lung cancer-related breathlessness. *Cancer Practice, 8*(6), 268–273.

Ghafoori, P., Marks, L., Vujaskovic, Z., & Kelsey, C. (2008). Radiation induced lung injury. *Oncology, 22*(1), 37–47.

Gift, A.G., & Narsavage, G. (1998). Validity of the numeric rating scale as a measure of dyspnea. *American Journal of Critical Care, 7*(3), 200–204.

Guyatt, G.H., Berman, L.B., Townsend, M., Pugsley, S.O., & Chambers, L.W. (1987). A measure of quality of life for clinical trials in chronic lung disease. *Thorax, 42*(10), 773–778.

Harver, A., & Mahler, D.A. (1990). The symptom of dyspnea. In D.A. Mahler (Ed.), *Dyspnea* (pp. 1–54). Mount Kisco, NY: Futura Publishing Co.

Hately, J., Laurence, V., Scott, A., Baker, R., & Thomas, P. (2003). Breathlessness clinics within specialist palliative care settings can improve the quality of life and functional capacity of patients with lung cancer. *Palliative Medicine, 17*(5), 410–417.

Hochstetter, J., Lewis, J., & Soares-Smith, L. (2005). An investigation into the immediate impact of breathlessness management on the breathless patient: Randomised controlled trial. *Physiotherapy, 91*(3), 178–185.

Houlihan, N.G., Inzeo, D., Joyce, M., & Tyson, L.B. (2004). Symptom management of lung cancer. In N.G. Houlihan (Ed.), *Site-specific cancer series: Lung cancer* (pp. 103–118). Pittsburgh, PA: Oncology Nursing Society.

Jennings, A.L., Davies, A.N., Higgins, J.P.T., & Broadley, K. (2001). Opioids for the palliation of breathlessness in terminal illness. *Cochrane Database of Systematic Reviews* 2001, Issue 3. Art. No.: CD002066. DOI: 10.1002/14651858.CD002066.

Jennings, A.L., Davies, A.N., Higgins, J.P., Gibbs, J.S., & Broadley, K.E. (2002). A systematic review of the use of opioids in the management of dyspnoea. *Thorax, 57*(11), 939–944.

Joyce, M., & Beck, S. (2005, March). *Measuring oncology nursing sensitive patient outcomes: Evidence-based summary.* Retrieved September 6, 2007, from http://www.ons.org/outcomes/measures/pdf/DyspneaTools.pdf

Joyce, M., McSweeney, M., Carrieri-Kohlman, V.L., & Hawkins, J. (2004). The use of nebulized opioids in the management of dyspnea: Evidence synthesis. *Oncology Nursing Forum, 31*(3), 551–561.

Kohara, H., Ueoka, H., Aoe, K., Maeda, T., Takeyama, H., Saito, R., et al. (2003). Effect of nebulized furosemide in terminally ill cancer patients with dyspnea. *Journal of Pain and Symptom Management, 26*(4), 962–967.

Kohlman-Carrieri, V., & Janson-Bjerklie, S. (1990). Coping and self-care strategies. In D.A. Mahler (Ed.), *Dyspnea* (pp. 201–230). Mount Kisco, NY: Futura Publishing Co.

Lacasse, Y., Goldstein, R., Lasserson, T.J., & Martin, S. (2006). Pulmonary rehabilitation for chronic obstructive pulmonary disease. *Cochrane Database of Systematic Reviews* 2006, Issue 4. Art. No.: CD003793. DOI: 10.1002/14651858.CD003793.pub2.

Lareau, S.C., Carrieri-Kohlman, V., Janson-Bjerklie, S., & Roos, P.J. (1994). Development and testing of the Pulmonary Functional Status and Dyspnea Questionnaire (PFSDQ). *Heart and Lung, 23*(3), 242–250.

Mack, J.M., & Altman G.B. (2004). Oxygenation. In G. Altman (Ed.), *Delmar's fundamental and advanced nursing skills.* Retrieved January 21, 2008, from http://www.statref.com

Mahler, D.A. (1990). Acute dyspnea. In D.A. Mahler (Ed.), *Dyspnea* (pp. 127–144). Mount Kisco, NY: Futura Publishing Co.

Mahler, D.A., Rosiello, R.A., Harver, A., Lentine, T., McGovern, J.F., & Daubenspeck, J.A. (1987). Comparison of clinical dyspnea ratings and psychophysical measurements of respiratory sensation in obstructive airway disease. *American Review of Respiratory Disease, 135*(6), 1229–1233.

Mahler, D.A., Weinberg, D.H., Wells, C.K., & Feinstein, A.R. (1984). The measurement of dyspnea: Contents, interobserver agreement, and physiologic correlates of two new clinical indexes. *Chest, 85*(6), 751–758.

Mahler, D.A., & Wells, C.K. (1988). Evaluation of clinical methods for rating dyspnea. *Chest, 93*(3), 580–586.

Mazzocato, C., Buclin, T., & Rapin, C.H. (1999). The effects of morphine on dyspnea and ventilatory function in elderly patients with advanced cancer: A randomized double-blind controlled trial. *Annals of Oncology, 10*(12), 1511–1514.

McCarley, C. (1999). A model of chronic dyspnea. *Image: The Journal of Nursing Scholarship, 31*(3), 231–236.

McGavin, C.R., Artvinli, M., Naoe, H., & McHardy, G.J. (1978). Dyspnoea, disability, and distance walked: Comparison of estimates of exercise performance in respiratory disease. *BMJ, 2*(6132), 241–243.

Mediastinal and pleural disorders. (2006). In *Merck manual of diagnosis and therapy* (18th ed.). Retrieved January 22, 2008, from http://www.statref.com

Medical Research Council's Committee on the Aetiology of Chronic Bronchitis. (1960). Standardized questionaries on respiratory symptoms. *BMJ, 2*(5213), 1665.

Meek, P.M. (2004). Measurement of dyspnea in chronic obstructive pulmonary disease: What is the tool telling you? *Chronic Respiratory Disease, 1*(1), 29–37.

National Comprehensive Cancer Network. (2008). *NCCN Clinical Practice Guidelines in Oncology™: Palliative care* [v.1.2009]. Retrieved December 1, 2008, from http://www.nccn.org/professionals/physician_gls/PDF/palliative.pdf

Navigante, A.H., Cerchietti, L.C., Castro, M.A., Lutteral, M.A., & Cabalar, M.E. (2006). Midazolam as adjunct therapy to morphine in the alleviation of severe dyspnea perception in patients with advanced cancer. *Journal of Pain and Symptom Management, 31*(1), 38–47.

Noseda, A., Carpiaux, J.P., Markstein, C., Meyvaert, A., & de Maertelaer, V. (1997). Disabling dyspnoea in patients with advanced disease: Lack of effect of nebulized morphine. *European Respiratory Journal, 10*(5), 1079–1083.

Paice, J.A. (2007). Opioid pharmacotherapy. In A.M. Berger, J.L. Shuster Jr., & J.H. VonRoenn (Eds.), *Principles and practice of palliative care and supportive oncology* (3rd ed.). Philadelphia: Lippincott Williams & Wilkins. Retrieved February 9, 2008, from http://ovidsp.tx.ovid.com

Payne, R. (1998). Pharmacologic management of pain. In A.M. Berger, R. Portenoy, & D. Weissman (Eds.), *Principles and practice of supportive oncology* (pp. 61–75). Philadelphia: Lippincott-Raven.

Philip, J., Gold, M., Milner, A., Di Iulio, J., Miller, B., & Spruyt, O. (2006). A randomized, double-blind, crossover trial of the effect of oxygen on dyspnea in patients with advanced cancer. *Journal of Pain and Symptom Management, 32*(6), 541–550.

Reuben, D.B., & Mor, V. (1986). Dyspnea in terminally ill cancer patients. *Chest, 89*(2), 234–236.

Ries, A.L., & Mahler, D.A. (1990). Chronic dyspnea. In D.A. Mahler (Ed.), *Dyspnea* (pp. 165–199). Mount Kisco, NY: Futura Publishing Co.

Ripamonti, C. (1999). Management of dyspnea in advanced cancer patient. *Supportive Care in Cancer, 7*(4), 233–243.

Ripamonti, C., Fulfaro, F., & Bruera, E. (1998). Dyspnoea in patients with advanced cancer: Incidence, causes and treatments. *Cancer Treatment Reviews, 24*(1), 69–80.

Ripamonti, C., & Fusco, F. (2002). Respiratory problems in advanced cancer. *Supportive Care in Cancer, 10*(3), 204–216.

Rose, C., Wallace, L., Dickson, R., Ayres, J., Lehman, R., Searle, Y., et al. (2002). The most effective psychologically-based treatments to reduce anxiety and panic in patients with chronic obstructive pulmonary disease (COPD): A systematic review. *Patient Education and Counseling, 47*(4), 311–318.

Shepherd, S., & Geraci, S. (1999). The differential diagnosis of dyspnea: A pathophysiologic approach. *Clinician Reviews, 9*(4), 52–72.

Tanaka, K., Akechi, T., Okuyama, T., Nishiwaki, Y., & Uchitomi, Y. (2000). Development and validation of the Cancer Dyspnoea Scale: A multidimensional, brief, self-rating scale. *British Journal of Cancer, 82*(4), 800–805.

Tanaka, K., Shima, Y., Kakinuma, R., Kubota, K., Ohe, Y., Hojo, F., et al. (1999). Effect of nebulized morphine in cancer patients with dyspnea: A pilot study. *Japanese Journal of Clinical Oncology, 29*(12), 600–603.

Thomas, J.R., & von Gunten, C.F. (2003). Management of dyspnea. *Journal of Supportive Oncology, 1*(1), 23–32.

U.S. Food and Drug Administration. (2007, March 9). *Information on erythropoiesis stimulating agents (ESA)*. Retrieved October 2, 2007, from http://www.fda.gov/cder/drug/infopage/RHE/default.htm

Vainio, A., & Auvinen, A. (1996). Prevalence of symptoms among patients with advanced cancer: An international collaborative study. Symptom Prevalence Group. *Journal of Pain and Symptom Management, 12*(1), 3–10.

Wikipedia. (2008). *Diaphragmatic breathing*. Retrieved November 23, 2008, from http://en.wikipedia.org/wiki/Diaphragmatic_breathing

Williams, C.M. (2006). Dyspnea. *Cancer Journal, 12*(5), 365–373.

Electrolyte Imbalances, Tumor Lysis Syndrome, and Syndrome of Inappropriate Antidiuretic Hormone

Sylvia C. Fairclough, RN, BSN, OCN®,
and Carlton G. Brown, PhD, RN, AOCN®

Case Study

T.C. is a 58-year-old man recently diagnosed with acute myeloid leukemia (AML) who has been admitted to the hospital to begin induction chemotherapy. Prior to his diagnosis being made, he exhibited a history of nausea, anorexia, fatigue, night sweats, and weight loss. He states that he has not been able to tolerate eating or drinking very much lately and has only been voiding once, maybe twice, a day. The results of his prechemotherapy laboratory test values are white blood cells: $107,000/mm^3$ with 82% blasts; hemoglobin: 7.9 g/dl; platelets: $145,000/mm^3$; electrolytes reveal sodium: 135 mEq/L; potassium: 5.2 mEq/L; chloride: 111 mEq/L. Additional studies reveal a blood urea nitrogen (BUN) of 48 mg/dl; creatinine of 2 mg/dl; lactate dehydrogenase (LDH) of 1,099 IU/L; and a uric acid level of 13.9 mg/dl.

T.C. appears to be at risk for potentially life-threatening electrolyte imbalances. This chapter will help oncology nurses to assess, identify treatments for, educate the patient on, and evaluate the outcomes of T.C.'s particular imbalance. This case study will be discussed again at the end of this chapter so that the reader can identify T.C.'s particular imbalance, determine and apply the specific treatment modalities indicated, and educate the patient on the related expected outcomes. Understanding electrolyte imbalances plays an important role in oncology nurses' approach of ensuring quality, holistic care for their patients and will enhance patients' quality of life and potential overall outcome through their cancer journey.

Electrolyte Imbalances
Overview

Electrolytes, to include sodium, chloride, potassium, magnesium, phosphorus, and calcium, are chemicals that regulate important physiologic functions within the body. They are

primarily responsible for the movement of nutrients into cells and the movement of wastes out of cells. Electrolytes, when dissolved in water, break up into positively and negatively charged ions. Nerve and muscle function and metabolic and fluid balances are dependent upon the proper exchange of these ions into and out of the cells. Electrolytes have a narrow range of normal functionality and serve a variety of critical functions within the body. Electrolytes are located primarily within one of two cellular compartments:
- Extracellular: sodium, chloride, and bicarbonate
- Intracellular: potassium, magnesium, and phosphate.

A membrane-bound sodium/potassium adenosine triphosphatase (ATPase) pump maintains the differentials between these cellular compartments. The fluid balances and distributions of electrolytes are dynamic and will change in response to losses or gains in any one department, creating a calibrated response within the body (Berk & Rana, 2006).

Electrolytes usually are measured per liter of blood, and the normal ranges and functions are listed in Table 12-1. Imbalances in these electrolytes, especially in patients with cancer, can be very serious if not prevented or treated promptly. For example, patients with breast cancer and metastasis to the bone could experience hypercalcemia leading to cardiac, neuromuscular, and gastrointestinal (GI) symptoms, which could be life threatening if left untreated.

Electrolyte imbalances occur for numerous reasons, including (a) treatment side effects, (b) disturbance in fluid balances, (c) malignancies with high tumor burdens, (d) alterations in kidney or liver functions, (e) hormone secretion from tumors, and (f) side effects of various drugs. These imbalances cause numerous symptoms with systemic effects creating a significant impact on the quality of life of patients with cancer. Therefore, oncology nurses need to understand the function of electrolytes, identify patients who are at risk for imbalances, recognize symptoms promptly, and provide appropriate and timely treatments. Although numerous electrolyte and metabolic imbalances can occur in patients with cancer, this chapter will focus primarily on symptom presentation and management of high and low levels of cal-

TABLE 12-1	Normal Values and Functions of Electrolytes					
Electrolyte	Sodium (Na⁺)	Chloride (Cl⁻)	Potassium (K⁺)	Magnesium (Mg⁺⁺)	Calcium (Ca⁺⁺)	
Normal adult range*	135–145 mEq/L	97–107 mEq/L	3.5–5.3 mEq/L	1.5–2.5 mEq/L	4.5–5.5 mEq/L	8.5–10.5 mg/dl
					Ionized 2.2–2.5	Ionized 4.6–5.3
Roles in body functions	Fluid balance; muscle contraction and nerve function	Fluid balance	Regulation of heart contraction; fluid balance	Muscle and nerve function; heart rhythm; bone strength; regulation of blood pressure; support for immune system; aid in control of blood sugar levels	Bone formation; nerve and brain function; muscle contraction; hormone secretion; kidney regulation	

*Ranges may vary slightly from different laboratories.

Note. Based on information from Berendt & D'Agostino, 2005; MedlinePlus, 2007.

cium, sodium, potassium, and magnesium, along with the conditions of syndrome of inappropriate antidiuretic hormone (SIADH) and tumor lysis syndrome (TLS).

Calcium Imbalances

Pathophysiology

Calcium is the fifth most abundant inorganic element in the body and is essential to the formation of bones, the maintenance of bones and teeth, muscle contractility, nerve impulse transmission, and normal clotting mechanisms. It also plays an important role in cardiac automaticity, enzyme reactions, white blood cell chemotaxis, and cell membrane permeability. Normal calcium levels are 4.5–5.5 mEq/L (8.5–10.5 mg/dl). When levels decrease, hypocalcemia develops, and when levels increase, hypercalcemia occurs.

Ninety-nine percent of all calcium is distributed and stored in the skeletal tissue, or bones, in the form of insoluble crystals, providing strength and durability. Bone tissue is constantly changing through a process known as *bone remodeling*. Bone remodeling involves *bone formation*, which is controlled by cells called osteoblasts, and *bone resorption*, or breakdown, which involves cells called osteoclasts. A number of hormones also are involved in the balance of bone remodeling. During normal bone remodeling, very little exchange of calcium actually occurs between bone and plasma (Gobel, 2005).

The remaining 1% of calcium is located in the serum. One-half of the serum calcium is ionized (physiologic active form or *free*), 40% is bound to protein, primarily albumin, and the remaining 10% is bound to anions such as phosphate, carbonate, citrate, lactate, and sulfate (Suneja, Muster, & Pegoraro, 2008). Ionized calcium is necessary for excitation of nerves and the function of cardiac muscle, voluntary skeletal muscles, and involuntary muscles of the gut (Gobel, 2005). Under normal conditions, the ionized calcium is in equilibrium with the protein-bound calcium. However, if changes in the protein level (serum albumin) occur, as is often found in the very ill, malnourished, or elderly, a direct effect on serum calcium levels will result. Therefore, serum calcium levels need to be corrected based on albumin levels to get an accurate view of the true calcium present in the serum (Myers, 2007). A formula for correction is included in Table 12-2.

Mechanisms for regulating calcium are through bone formation and resorption, GI absorption, and urinary excretion or absorption. These mechanisms are controlled by a complex balance of the following three hormones: the parathyroid hormone (PTH), calcitriol (1,25-dihydroxyvitamin D), and calcitonin. Extracellular calcium levels are balanced by actions of these hormones in the kidney (which filters and reabsorbs ionized calcium), in the gut (which absorbs dietary calcium and excretes it in feces), and in the bone (which acts as the storage depot for the body's supply of calcium). The balance of these hormones is controlled through a negative feedback loop in which individual hormones respond as needed to increases or decreases in the serum calcium concentration by altering the renal, GI, or bone absorption or release of calcium (Hemphill, 2006).

Hypercalcemia

Overview: Hypercalcemia is a metabolic disorder defined by a serum calcium level greater than 10.5 mg/dl. Ninety percent of hypercalcemia cases result from either primary hyperparathyroidism or malignancy. Other causes of hypercalcemia include immobility, granulomatous disorders, renal disease, infectious diseases, medication side effects, various endocrine disorders, and dietary disorders (Myers, 2007; Warrell, 2001). Hypercalcemia is a potentially

TABLE 12-2	Diagnostic Tests for Detection of Calcium Imbalances
Diagnostic Test	**Indications/Findings**
Serum calcium, ionized if possible	May need to do corrected (ionized) calcium Corrected (ionized) calcium = [total serum calcium level (mg/dl) + (4.0 − serum albumin level [g/dl])] × 0.8
Albumin	If albumin level is low and no ionized calcium levels were obtained, do corrected calcium calculation.
Serum magnesium (Mg^+)	May be low to normal
Serum phosphorus (PO_4)	May be low; has inverse relationship with calcium
Blood urea nitrogen/creatinine	To assess kidney function
Parathyroid hormone	Elevated if related to primary hyperparathyroidism; decreased or normal if malignant cause
Alkaline phosphatase	Will be elevated with bone metastasis and breast cancer
Urine calcium (Ca^{++}) and PO_4	Increased; may be present in urine before serum calcium levels are elevated
Chest x-ray	To rule out tumor, sarcoidosis, and any bony changes associated with hyperparathyroidism
Plain x-ray/bone scan	To determine bone metastasis or multiple myeloma
Electrocardiogram	To look for changes such as increased PR segment, shortened QT interval, and widening T wave

Note. Based on information from Hemphill, 2006; Myers, 2007; Smith, 2000a.

life-threatening disorder with a variable onset and often may go unnoticed until it is severe. Lack of treatment can lead to renal failure, coma, or cardiac arrest (Myers).

For hypercalcemia to develop, the normal calcium homeostasis between stored, ionized, and protein-bound calcium must be overwhelmed by an excess in PTH, calcitriol, some other serum factor that mimics these hormones, or an increased calcium load. The increased calcium load is the result of either a decreased ability of the kidneys to clear calcium from the blood, increased calcium absorption from the gut, or increased bone resorption (Gobel, 2005; Hemphill, 2006). Excessive calcium in the serum, or hypercalcemia, depresses neuromuscular function, causes increased contractility and irritability of the heart, interferes with antidiuretic hormone (ADH) action, and promotes blood clotting. It also can result in calcium deposits outside the skeletal system, especially in the kidneys.

The two primary causes of hypercalcemia can be divided into PTH-mediated or primary hypercalcemia, and non-PTH-mediated or malignant hypercalcemia disorders.

Primary hypercalcemia: Primary (PTH-mediated) hyperparathyroidism, the most common cause of hypercalcemia, often is asymptomatic and is seen mostly in the outpatient setting. Primary hypercalcemia is generally slow to develop and less severe than hypercalcemia associated with malignancy, or non-PTH-mediated hypercalcemia. Because the parathyroid glands are the primary regulators of calcium homeostasis, calcium elevations from hyperparathyroidism are directly related to the inappropriate or excess secretion of PTH by the parathyroid glands.

Malignant hypercalcemia: Malignant hypercalcemia is the most commonly occurring metabolic complication of cancer and is reported in 10%–20% of patients with cancer based on tumor type (Gobel, 2005; Myers, 2007). Eighty percent of malignancy-related hypercalcemia presents in patients with breast cancer, solid tumors, and lung cancer; the remaining 20% of cases are related to multiple myeloma, leukemia, lymphomas, or other related causes (Myers). Hypercalcemia often is seen in patients with advanced-stage disease and is a late complication of malignancy in 10%–40% of patients with cancer (Gobel).

Hypercalcemia associated with malignancy primarily develops because of increased bone resorption generated by osteoclastic activity. As a result, calcium is released into the extracellular fluid in amounts greater than the kidneys are able to adequately clear. The inadequate renal calcium clearance leads to potential polyuria, dehydration, decreased renal blood flow and glomerular filtration, and ultimately calcium precipitation into the renal tubules (National Cancer Institute [NCI], 2005). Hypercalcemia of malignancy can occur through several different mechanisms depending on the action and location of the cancer cells. However, two primary mechanisms exist: humoral hypercalcemia (HHM) and local osteolytic hypercalcemia (LOH).

HHM, which is responsible for 80% of cases of malignant hypercalcemia, is caused by the presence of humoral factors (hormones and/or cytokines), which are released or regulated ectopically by malignant cells. These humoral agents are not controlled by the same mechanisms as those present in normal cells. Hypercalcemia develops as a result of humoral agents inhibiting bone formation, stimulating bone resorption and osteoclastic activity, and increasing renal tubular reabsorption of calcium (Myers, 2007).

The most common malignancy-related humoral agent is PTH-related peptide (PTHrP). PTHrP-mediated hypercalcemia has been found in patients with solid tumors and is most common in squamous cell cancers and in 30%–50% of patients with breast cancer who have hypercalcemia (Warrell, 2001). Patients with HHM usually have little or no bone metastases. PTHrP-mediated hypercalcemia has not been found in hematologic cancers such as myeloma or lymphoma (Warrell). Other humoral factors associated with HHM are cytokines (interleukin-1), transforming growth factors, tumor necrosis factors (TNFs), osteoclast activation factors, colony-stimulating factors, and 1,25-dihydroxyvitamin D. Hypercalcemia related to hematologic malignancies such as myeloma tends to be related to the release of cytokines such as TNF alpha and beta and interleukins 1 and 6 (NCI, 2005; Warrell).

LOH, which accounts for approximately 20%–30% of patients with malignant hypercalcemia, is a result of direct bone destruction caused by the osteolytic activity of tumor cells either by direct tumor invasion or metastasis. An imbalance occurs in bone remodeling, osteoclastic activity increases, more destruction from metastatic disease occurs, and an excess of calcium is released into the serum. LOH often is associated with the formation of lytic lesions on the bone and occurs most frequently in breast cancers and multiple myeloma with bony metastases (Gobel, 2005).

Prolonged immobilization, dehydration, excessive use of certain vitamin supplements, renal failure, and prolonged use of thiazide diuretics also may contribute to or worsen hypercalcemia (Keenan & Wickham, 2005; Myers, 2007).

Clinical assessment: Conducting a thorough diagnostic workup is important to determine hypercalcemia using history, physical examination, and laboratory tests to differentiate the cause, type, and severity of hypercalcemia. Table 12-2 discusses the laboratory and diagnostic tests that should be obtained and reviewed to diagnose imbalances in calcium.

The nurse should obtain information about the patient's chief complaints, presenting symptoms, onset and duration of symptoms, diagnosis, and type of known cancer or metastases. Current chemotherapy or hormonal treatments and a list of all medications, including vitamins and supplements, should be obtained. A thorough pain assessment should be performed. Any mental status changes should be identified. A cardiac examination should be performed, including heart rate and rhythm, orthostatic blood pressures, and any electrocardiogram changes. Abdominal sounds should be assessed, and any signs of constipation, nausea, or vomiting should be noted. Signs of dehydration should be identified if present. Renal changes should be identified, such as polyuria, nocturia, or a history of kidney stones or flank pain. A neuromuscular examination should include reflexes, muscle tone and strength, and observation of a positive Chvostek or Trousseau sign (Keenan & Wickham, 2005; Myers, 2007).

Clinical manifestations: The signs and symptoms associated with hypercalcemia are nonspecific and vary according to degree, rate of onset, and underlying causes. They often may be misinterpreted as manifestations of terminal cancer or side effects from chemotherapy, radiation, or medications (Keenan & Wickham, 2005; Myers, 2007). Patients may be asymptomatic or may exhibit mild, moderate, or severe degrees of symptoms. Signs and symptoms are related directly to the underlying cause and the destruction of cellular activity on the involved body systems. General signs and symptoms associated with hypercalcemia can include lethargy, changes in mental status, vomiting, polyuria, constipation, abdominal or flank pain, muscle weakness and fatigue, hypertension, and cardiac arrhythmias. See Table 12-3 for signs and symptoms according to body system and degree of hypercalcemia.

Evidence-based interventions: Treatment for hypercalcemia is based on the severity, presenting symptoms, renal and cardiac function, and underlying cause or prognosis of disease. Controlling the malignancy is the most effective and only long-term treatment option for hypercalcemia related to malignancy. For example, initiating chemotherapy in a patient with multiple myeloma may produce a remission of the cancer cells, thereby decreasing the hypercalcemia because of the decrease in tumor cytokine release. If left untreated, cancer-induced

TABLE 12-3	Signs and Symptoms of Hypercalcemia by Degree and Systemic Effect		
Systemic Effect	Mild (< 12 mg/dl)	Moderate (12–15 mg/dl)	Severe (> 15 mg/dl)
Gastrointestinal	Anorexia, nausea, vomiting, vague abdominal pain	Constipation, increased pain, abdominal distention, bloating	Obstipation, ileus
Neurologic	Restlessness, indifference, difficulty concentrating, lethargy	Confusion, apathy, drowsiness, somnolence	Coma, seizures, death
Muscular	Fatigue, generalized muscle weakness, hyporeflexia	Bone pain, increased muscle weakness	Pathologic fractures, ataxia, severe muscle weakness
Cardiovascular	Possible hypertension, orthostatic hypotension	Electrocardiogram changes, cardiac dysrhythmias, hypertension	Cardiac arrest, death
Renal	Polyuria, nocturia, polydipsia, pruritus	Renal tubular acidosis, dehydration, renal calculi	Renal insufficiency, oliguric renal failure, azotemia

Note. Based on information from Myers, 2007; Shuey & Brant, 2004.

hypercalcemia is progressive, and death is usually inevitable from oliguric renal failure, coma, or cardiac arrest. In many cases, control of the malignancy may not be possible. A thorough evaluation of the patient's disease state should be performed with the patient, family, and medical team prior to initiation of treatment. Treatment options, in the case of advanced disease, should be directed at palliation and enhancing quality of life (Myers, 2007).

In addition to treating the underlying malignancy, medical management of hypercalcemia has three main goals: (a) to correct any dehydration, (b) to increase renal excretion of calcium, and (c) to inhibit calcium resorption from bone, usually with antiresorptive agents (Keenan & Wickham, 2005). The treatment for hypercalcemia is described in the following text based on the degree of hypercalcemia.

In patients with mild hypercalcemia (10.5–12 mg/dl) who are generally asymptomatic, rehydration is the primary treatment with continued monitoring and treatment of the underlying disease. Increasing oral fluid intake to 2–4 L/day may be sufficient to rehydrate and correct calcium levels (Smith, 2000a). Close monitoring of electrolytes should be continued and corrected along with monitoring of intake and output (I&O) and cardiac and renal function. Immobilization can be a contributing factor to hypercalcemia because it increases resorption of calcium from the bones. Therefore, weight-bearing exercise (walking, standing, etc.) should be encouraged (Myers, 2007). Pain management may need to be provided, as well as treatment for nausea and vomiting to promote fluid intake and increase mobility.

Patients with moderate hypercalcemia (12–14 mg/dl) who are symptomatic or are unable to tolerate oral fluids will need vigorous IV hydration with 0.9% normal saline to promote sodium diuresis and induce calcium excretion. The amount and rate of fluid administration depend on the degree of hypercalcemia, degree of dehydration, and renal and cardiac status. Fluid volume may range from 5–8 L over the first 24 hours and then decrease to 3 L daily until stabilized (Myers, 2007). It is important to closely monitor electrolytes, especially sodium, magnesium, and potassium, and replace as needed to prevent cardiac dysrhythmias.

Loop diuretics, such as furosemide, may be used to accelerate the elimination of calcium once rehydration has been achieved. Loop diuretics aid in blocking the reabsorption of calcium and help in the prevention of fluid overload from vigorous hydration, especially in patients for whom cardiac toxicity from hydration is a concern. Loop diuretics should be used cautiously because they may cause increased extracellular fluid losses promoting calcium reabsorption and the depletion of potassium and magnesium. Therefore, these electrolytes should be monitored frequently (Myers, 2007). Thiazide diuretics, such as hydrochlorothiazide, should be avoided completely because they inhibit renal excretion of calcium.

Antiresorptive therapy is the next step in the treatment of hypercalcemia to help restore calcium balance. Antiresorptive therapy includes the use of bisphosphonate drugs, such as pamidronate or zoledronic acid. These bisphosphonates, which are given intravenously, selectively concentrate in bone where they inhibit tumor cell binding in the bone and decrease bone resorption of calcium by altering osteoclastic activity through binding to the bone and preventing calcium from being released. They also may help to strengthen and stabilize bone. Antiresorptive therapy should start promptly after rehydration, particularly for patients whose corrected calcium is greater than 13 mg/dl (Keenan & Wickham, 2005). Table 12-4 describes the treatment indications and recommended doses for antiresorptive treatment options as well as the use of calcitonin, phosphates, and corticosteroids in the treatment of hypercalcemia.

The most common side effects of bisphosphonates include fever, flu-like syndrome, and venous irritation. Other side effects may include bone pain, nausea or vomiting, renal toxicity (zoledronic acid), and hypocalcemia. Most patients benefit substantially from the early introduction of bisphosphonates; this approach leads to more rapid clinical improvement, lower overall toxicity, and a decreased overall cost of treatment (Warrell, 2001).

For severe hypercalcemia (greater than 14–16 mg/dl), the hydration rate should be increased, if tolerated, in the first 24 hours and the use of loop diuretics as indicated previously should be initiated once rehydration has been obtained. In addition, antiresorptive agents should be started as soon as possible as indicated in Table 12-4. If the calcium level is greater than 16 mg/dl, which is considered life threatening, the use of calcitonin IV may be necessary. Calcitonin aids in reducing the calcium levels quickly, usually within four to six hours, by decreasing renal tubular reabsorption of calcium and by blocking osteoclast resorption. However, its effect is short term, and it rapidly loses effectiveness. Therefore, calcitonin should be given initially along with pamidronate, which is more long term. Dialysis, although rarely used in the treatment of hypercalcemia, may be a viable option for people who are experiencing renal insufficiency and severe hypercalcemia and have a relatively good prognosis with their malignancy (Keenan & Wickham, 2005; Myers, 2007).

TABLE 12-4	Antiresorptive Agents and Other Medications Used to Treat Hypercalcemia			
Medication	**Dose**	**Mode of Action**	**Adverse Reactions**	**Comments**
Bisphospho- nates				
• Zoledronic acid (3rd generation)	4 mg IV over 15 minutes; increase to 8 mg IV for relapsed or refractory cases	Inhibits action of osteo- clasts	**Renal toxicity;** skeletal pain, fever, flu-like syndrome Do not give with calcitonin. Hypophosphatemia; hypocalcemia Use caution with diuretics.	First-line treatment; superior efficacy and short infusion time Rapid results May repeat in 7 days, then every 4 weeks for ongoing management **Monitor serum creatinine with each dose.**
• Pamidronate (2nd generation)	60–90 mg IV over 2–24 hours	Inhibits action of osteo- clasts	Fever, flu-like syndrome, phlebitis	First-line therapy; highly effective and still used widely May be used with calcitonin Onset of action in 24 hours May repeat weekly until normal calcium then every 4 weeks for chronic management
Gallium nitrate	100–200 mg/ m^2 IV over 24 hours for up to 5 days	Antineoplastic; inhibits bone resorption without toxicity to bone cells; stabilizes bone crystals	Nephrotoxicity; anemia, nausea/ vomiting	Must be hospitalized; highly effective but slow onset; hydration must be maintained during use; duration of response is about 6 days. Not generally used because of expense, toxicities, and inconvenience.
Plicamycin (mithramycin)	15–25 mcg/kg IV over 4–6 hours for 3 days	Neoplastic agent; in- hibits RNA synthesis in osteoclasts	Nausea/vomiting; cumulative neph- rotoxicity; hepa- totoxicity; throm- bocytopenia	Onset in 1–2 days Duration of 2 weeks; third-line treatment; not recommended; rarely used

(Continued on next page)

TABLE 12-4	Antiresorptive Agents and Other Medications Used to Treat Hypercalcemia *(Continued)*			
Medication	**Dose**	**Mode of Action**	**Adverse Reactions**	**Comments**
Calcitonin	4 U/kg SC every 12 hours; 8 U/kg every 6 hours PRN if no response	Inhibits action of osteoclasts; decreased renal absorption of Ca^{++}	Allergic reaction; nausea/vomiting; flushing of face and hands; polyuria	Most rapid onset and short duration. Check serum Ca^{++} every 5–6 hours. Continue with hydration use of furosemide PRN; test dose intradermal recommended. May be given with pamidronate if serum Ca^{++} > 13 mg/dl.
Oral phosphates	0.5–3 g/day PO	Prevents gastrointestinal absorption; inhibits bone resorption	Diarrhea; contraindicated with renal failure	Used to correct hypophosphatemia and in chronic hypercalcemia
Corticosteroids • Hydrocortisone	100–300 mg IV/PO over 3–5 days	Inhibits lymphoid tissue growth	Hyperglycemia; sodium and water retention	Used with steroid-sensitive tumors (hematologic, breast); may enhance and prolong effect of calcitonin; never used alone or as primary treatment; no long-term use because of adverse effects
• Prednisone	40–100 mg/day	Inhibits regulation of steroid receptors; promotes urinary excretion of Ca^{++}	Same as above	Same as above

Note. Based on information from Hemphill, 2006; Myers, 2007; Smith, 2000a.

Expected outcomes: Hypercalcemia of malignancy is the most common complication of malignancy and is reversible in 80% of episodes if it is recognized promptly and aggressive treatment is initiated. However, the mortality rate is 50% in those not treated promptly (Myers, 2007). Most patients presenting with hypercalcemia of malignancy will require ongoing management and will be receiving treatment for their underlying malignancy. Hypercalcemia often occurs as a late complication of advanced cancer. Treatment of hypercalcemia in this instance is palliative, and the focus remains on enhancing quality of life (Keenan & Wickham, 2005).

Patient teaching points: Figure 12-1 describes teaching points that could be used to instruct patients on the management of hypercalcemia.

Hypocalcemia

Overview: Hypocalcemia is defined by a calcium level less than 8.5 mg/dl or an ionized calcium level less than 4.5 mg/dl (Berendt & D'Agostino, 2005). As previously described, the regulation of calcium levels is maintained through a complex balance of feedback loops between PTH, vitamin D, and calcitonin that act primarily on the bone and renal and GI systems. Magnesium, phosphorus, and albumin levels also affect calcium levels. Oncology nurs-

FIGURE 12-1	Teaching Points for Hypercalcemia

- Frequently assess fluid and electrolyte balance.
- Instruct patients to report early signs and symptoms such as nausea, vomiting, lethargy, restlessness, constipation, or changes in mental status.
- Maintain hydration at home; manage nausea if present.
- Maintain mobility and encourage weight-bearing exercise; provide appropriate pain management.
- Promote safety to reduce the risk of falls related to altered mental status, which may present at onset or be related to decreased bone strength.
- Determine whether patients require ongoing outpatient hypercalcemia treatment.
- Educate patients and caregivers about the increased risk of "flare"-type reactions of hypercalcemia with initial use of hormonal therapy (i.e., tamoxifen) in patients with breast cancer. This response is usually indicative of tumor response to the hormone.

es need to be aware of both the general mechanisms and the cancer-related mechanisms that can lead to hypocalcemia.

Numerous cancer-related causes of hypocalcemia exist, including chemotherapy agents such as high-dose cisplatin, fluorouracil/leucovorin combination therapies, and cetuximab. Bone metastases, the use of bisphosphonates, and adjuvant tamoxifen therapy for breast cancer also may lead to hypocalcemia. TLS, which will be discussed in detail later in this chapter, is associated with hypocalcemia, along with other electrolyte imbalances. Radiation treatments, especially to the thyroid gland or head and neck, may contribute to hypocalcemia. General causes of hypocalcemia may include hypoalbuminemia; hypoparathyroidism; hyperphosphatemia; deficiencies in vitamin D, magnesium, or dietary calcium; and chronic renal failure. In addition, chelating agents, hungry bone syndrome, blood citrates, and acute pancreatitis can cause hypocalcemia. Medication-induced causes of hypocalcemia may include aminoglycoside treatments; amphotericin B; loop diuretics; high doses of fluorides, glucose, insulin, and anticonvulsants such as phenobarbital and phenytoin; proton pump inhibitors; estrogen replacement therapies; and foscarnet used to treat cytomegalovirus or herpes infections (Beach, 2007; Suneja et al., 2008).

Clinical assessment: Table 12-5 describes the diagnostic test needed to evaluate the presence, degree, and potential underlying cause of hypocalcemia.

Oncology nurses should pay special attention to the following when obtaining a history on a person with suspected hypocalcemia: Identify any history of pancreatitis or liver or renal failure. Assess for recent thyroid, parathyroid, bowel, or head and neck surgery, trauma, or infection; treatment with radiation to the neck; or any recent blood or plasma infusions, chemotherapy, or bisphosphonate therapy. Inquire about current medications, including antibiotics, diuretics, estrogen therapies, anticonvulsants, and any type of supplements. Assess overall nutritional intake, especially calcium, vitamin D, magnesium, and phosphorus-containing foods or drinks. Inquire about alcohol intake. Assess for lack of sun exposure. Refer to Table 12-6 to identify important indicators in the physical assessment for the diagnosis and determination of causes for hypocalcemia.

Clinical manifestations: Signs and symptoms of hypocalcemia vary according to the underlying cause, onset, and acuity. Signs and symptoms of hypocalcemia are primarily related to the neurologic, muscular, and cardiac functions of calcium. The most common early sign of hypocalcemia is neuromuscular "irritability" exhibited by twitching muscles and spasms, leg or arm muscle cramps, and numbness or tingling in the perioral area or in the fingers and toes (Berendt & D'Agostino, 2005; Suneja et al., 2008).

Mild or chronic hypocalcemia can be asymptomatic; however, patients with chronic hypocalcemia may exhibit signs of chronic pruritus, cataracts, coarse hair, brittle nails, psoriasis, and dry skin (Beach, 2007). *Severe* hypocalcemia may lead to acute seizures, hallucinations, tetany, hypotension, cardiac arrhythmias, laryngospasm and bronchospasm, and ultimately heart failure and death (Berendt & D'Agostino, 2005). Therefore, rapid identification and correction of hypocalcemia are critical.

TABLE 12-5	Hypocalcemia Diagnostic Tests
Diagnostics	**Indications and Findings**
Serum electrolytes	Serum/ionized Ca^{++}: May need to correct for albumin Phosphorus: May be normal instead of elevated if related to vitamin D deficiency; calcium binds to phosphorus. Magnesium: Also may be decreased.
Blood urea nitrogen/creatinine	Assess for renal dysfunction.
Serum albumin	If decreased, will need to correct calcium level; hypoalbuminemia is the most common reason for general hypocalcemia.
Liver function tests (LFTs)	Assess for liver dysfunction or elevations of LFTs in rickets.
Parathyroid hormone (PTH)	Assess for parathyroid dysfunctions.
Vitamin D	If deficiency is suspected, check both 25(OH)D and 1,25(OH)2D levels to determine reason.
Urine calcium	May be decreased
Phosphorus	May be decreased with PTH deficiencies
Plain x-ray/bone scan	May be necessary to determine bone metastases
Electrocardiogram	May produce lengthened ST segment or prolonged QT intervals if severe hypocalcemia is present

Note. Based on information from Beach, 2007; Smith, 2000a; Suneja et al., 2008.

TABLE 12-6	Physical Assessment Indicators for Hypocalcemia
System	**Assessment Indicators**
Neuromuscular	Assess for muscle irritability, numbness, tingling, muscle spasms or cramps; assess for positive Chvostek or Trousseau sign with severe hypocalcemia.
Cardiovascular	Evaluate blood pressure and heart rate and rhythm, looking for evidence of hypotension, arrhythmias, or congestive heart failure.
Pulmonary	Auscultate breath sounds for evidence of stridor, wheezing caused by bronchospasms, rales, voice changes because of laryngospasms, or any dysphagia.
Gastrointestinal	Assess for hyperactive bowel sounds, intestinal colic, or recent diarrhea.
Neurologic	Assess for depression, irritability, personality changes, confusion, hallucinations, dementia, or extrapyramidal symptoms.
Skin	Assess for coarse hair, brittle nails, dry skin, pruritus, or psoriasis.

Evidence-based interventions: Treatment for hypocalcemia depends on the exact cause, the presence of symptoms, and the severity of the hypocalcemia. Severe, or acutely symptomatic, hypocalcemia generally is treated in a hospital setting with IV calcium administrations and close systemic monitoring. Mild, or asymptomatic, hypocalcemia can be treated with oral supplements and close monitoring of pertinent laboratory values.

Calcium supplements should be initiated at doses of a minimum of 1,000 mg/day up to 3,000 mg/day in divided doses two to four times a day (Beach, 2007; Suneja et al., 2008). Calcium in any form needs vitamin D to be absorbed by the GI tract, and many calcium supplements include vitamin D in their preparations. A general guideline for vitamin D supplementation is 400–800 mg/day to ensure that the calcium taken is absorbed. The least expensive form of calcium is calcium carbonate, but oral calcium gluconate, calcium citrate, or calcium lactate also may be used. Special attention should be paid to the actual amount of elemental calcium in each preparation. For example, calcium carbonate tablets 650 mg in size actually contain 250 mg of elemental calcium (Skugor & Milas, 2004). If calcium supplements alone do not improve the hypocalcemia, thiazide diuretics such as hydrochlorothiazide may be used cautiously because of their effect of increasing renal absorption of calcium. Serum calcium levels should be monitored closely to identify any resultant hypercalcemia.

The determination of supplement use will be partially dependant on the reason for the hypocalcemia. Additional vitamin D supplements may be necessary if the reason for hypocalcemia is related to vitamin D deficiencies. Determining the related cause for vitamin D deficiencies (i.e., secondary to chronic renal failure versus hypoparathyroidism) becomes especially important in determining the appropriate form of vitamin D to administer. Increasing exposure to sunlight, ensuring proper nutrition, and decreasing alcohol intake also may be important interventions in the treatment of vitamin D deficiencies.

Magnesium deficiencies, if present, must be corrected before the resulting hypocalcemia can be corrected. Hypocalcemia related to magnesium deficiencies is resistant to the administration of calcium and vitamin D. The recommended treatment for hypomagnesemia will be extensively discussed later in this chapter; however, oral or IV magnesium administration may be needed before an improvement is seen in calcium levels. Magnesium supplementation also may be used as a preventive measure to prevent magnesium wasting and resultant hypocalcemia. For example, magnesium sulfate often is given intravenously, mixed in hydration fluids, before and/or after cisplatin infusions to help prevent magnesium wasting and resultant hypocalcemia and hypomagnesemia.

If hyperphosphatemia is present, the reason (e.g., TLS, rhabdomyolysis) will need to be identified and corrected for the hypocalcemia to be resolved. Phosphate-binding antacids, such as calcium carbonate or aluminum hydroxide, may be given to decrease the GI absorption of phosphate. Caution should be used, especially with antacids containing aluminum, because of the risk of aluminum toxicity and in cases of renal failure (Smith, 2000a). Dietary restrictions of foods containing phosphate may be instituted. In acute cases of hyperphosphatemia, hydration with IV saline and acetazolamide as a diuretic may be used with special attention taken to prevent any further hypocalcemia (Skugor & Milas, 2004). If renal failure is present with hyperphosphatemia and hypocalcemia, dialysis may be required.

Severe cases of hypocalcemia (ionized calcium level less than 3 mg/dl) with symptoms of acute hypocalcemia require immediate evaluation and treatment. IV calcium gluconate 10% (93 mg of elemental calcium/10 ml) may be administered as a bolus infusion over 5–10 minutes for calcium replacement (Smith, 2000a; Suneja et al., 2008). The action is immediate but short lived, and a continuous calcium infusion often is recommended at 0.5–2 mg elemental calcium/kg/hr until the patient is stabilized. Frequent measuring of ionized calcium will be necessary. Calcium chloride is another alternative and has a higher percentage of ionized calcium (272 mg elemental calcium/10 ml), but it is recommended for only central venous access because of venous irritation and risk of tissue injury with extravasation. Seizure precautions should be instituted (Berendt & D'Agostino, 2005). In patients with cardiac arrhythmias or in patients on digoxin therapy, continuous electrocardiogram (ECG) monitoring is recommended and necessary during calcium infusions because calcium potentiates digitalis toxicities (Suneja et al.).

Expected outcomes: The prognosis for correcting acute hypocalcemia is excellent once the cause has been determined and it is treated promptly. The patient should be monitored closely for recurring hypocalcemia. Long-term (chronic) hypocalcemia can lead to irreversible eye damage, such as cataracts. Some patients, such as those with resistance to PTH or with chronic renal failure, may require long-term use of vitamin D, phosphorus, or calcium supplements. Occasionally, hemodialysis may be required.

Patient teaching points: Figure 12-2 describes teaching points that should be used to instruct patients on the management of hypocalcemia.

FIGURE 12-2	**Teaching Points for Hypocalcemia**

- Signs and symptoms of hypocalcemia include depression, irritability, muscle cramps in legs or arms, and numbness or tingling in fingers and toes.
- Identify patients who are at high risk for hypocalcemia; use preventive measures (i.e., IV magnesium sulfate prior to treatment) and frequent laboratory monitoring as necessary, especially in patients receiving cisplatin, cetuximab, zoledronic acid, pamidronate, and those with bone metastasis from breast cancer or those who are at risk for tumor lysis syndrome.
- Provide patients with a list of foods high in calcium and vitamin D. Dairy products contain the most calcium; however, leafy greens, fish such as sardines and salmon, soy products, red beans, and some calcium-fortified foods such as cereals and orange juice also are good sources. Teach patients the importance of reading labels and taking in proper nutrition.
- Advise patients to take calcium supplements one hour before meals and at bedtime to improve absorption (Smith, 2000a).
- Teach management techniques for constipation, as it is often common with calcium supplements.
- Inform patients that diarrhea may be experienced with magnesium supplements.
- Discuss increased risk for fractures, brittle bones, etc., because of the risk of bone thinning resulting from chronic low calcium levels.

Sodium Imbalances

Pathophysiology

Sodium is the major cation (positive ion) in the extracellular fluid. It has a principal role in the maintenance of serum osmolarity and fluid balance (Smith & Baird-Powell, 2000). It is indirectly regulated by alterations in total body water content by sensory receptors (osmoreceptors) that promote either the uptake of water or the excretion of urine (Berendt & D'Agostino, 2005). This uptake or excretion is accomplished by coordination with the central thirst mechanism, ADH, and renal sodium and water excretion.

In healthy individuals, the kidneys' regulation of urine concentration and production and regulation of the thirst response tightly control sodium levels. Under normal conditions, the balance between water intake and the combined water loss from renal excretion and respiratory, skin, and GI sources produces water homeostasis. The kidneys adjust urine concentration to match salt intake and loss to maintain salt homeostasis. In sodium imbalances, these adjustments, or homeostatic mechanisms, become disrupted (Stephanides, 2007).

Hypernatremia

Overview: Hypernatremia is defined as a high serum sodium level greater than 145 mEq/L. The most common cause is from lack of free water intake in adequate amounts to meet net losses. This leads to hypovolemia and an increased plasma osmolarity. This "hyperosmolarity" draws fluids from the intracellular to the extracellular compartments, leading to dehydration of the intracellular fluids and cell volume contraction. This dehydration is responsible for most of the symptoms of hypernatremia (Stephanides, 2007).

People with hypernatremia have either too much salt, too little water, or a combination of the two related to their total volume status. Proper treatment is dependant upon the particular associated volume status. Therefore, the type of hypernatremia must be determined. The three types are hypovolemic, euvolemic, or hypervolemic. Table 12-7 describes the various causes of hypernatremia based on volume status.

According to Stephanides (2007), hypernatremia occurs in approximately 1% of hospitalized patients and can increase up to 2% in debilitated patients, older adults, or breastfed infants. In addition, when severe hypernatremia occurs, it is associated with a high mortality rate—greater than 50% in some studies. Cancer rarely is a direct cause of hypernatremia. It most commonly is seen secondary to cancer or treatment-related symptoms, such as dehydration caused by lack of water intake, or in patients with severe diarrhea, vomiting, and high fever (Berendt & D'Agostino, 2005; Smith & Baird-Powell, 2000). In patients with cancer, hypernatremia is primarily hypovolemic in nature as a result of GI losses or increased sensible water loss (Berk & Rana, 2006).

Other causes of hypernatremia include diabetes insipidus resulting from either central nervous system (CNS) or nephrogenic causes, impaired renal function, burns, profuse sweating, CNS disorders or malignancies, excessive diuresis, and respiratory infections (Stephanides, 2007). The following medications also may cause hypernatremia: administration of hypertonic saline, sodium bicarbonate, or high-sodium parenteral nutrition, and long-term use of amphotericin-B, corticosteroids, antihypertensives, hydralazine, reserpine, lactulose, and lithium (Berendt & D'Agostino, 2005; Smith & Baird-Powell, 2000; Stephanides).

TABLE 12-7	Volemic States of Hypernatremia
Volemic State	**Findings**
Hypovolemic (water deficit > sodium deficit)	Extrarenal—diarrhea, vomiting, burns, sweating, fever Renal—osmotic diuresis, renal disease, diuretics, hyperglycosuria Hypodipsic—lack of or inability to respond to thirst Primary—destruction of thirst center in hypothalamus (tumors, central nervous system disorders, trauma) Secondary—inability to respond to thirst signals (older adults, infants, physically or mentally debilitated)
Hypervolemic (sodium gain > water gain)	Sodium bicarbonate or hypertonic solution administration Accidental salt ingestion Hyperaldosteronism
Euvolemic (increased pure water loss)	Extrarenal—increased insensible loss (hyperventilation, dermal or respiratory causes) Renal—Diabetes insipidus Central—lack of central stimulus (antidiuretic hormone [ADH]) to concentrate urine Nephrogenic—lack of renal response to stimulus of ADH secretion

Note. Based on information from Berk & Rana, 2006; Stephanides, 2007.

Clinical assessment: As with all electrolyte imbalances, a thorough history and physical examination and diagnostic and clinical assessment will be critical in the identification of imbalances. Those assessments that are particularly necessary in the determination of hypernatremia will be described in this section. Additional tests also might be needed if diabetes insipidus or adrenal insufficiency is suspected. Table 12-8 displays important diagnostic tests related to hypernatremia.

TABLE 12-8	Diagnostic Tests for Hypernatremia
Test	**Rationale and Findings**
Serum electrolytes (K^+, Cl^-, CO_2, Na^+)	To determine hydration status and acid-base balance Na^+ = 150–170 mEq/L indicates dehydration Na^+ > 170 mEq/L may indicate diabetes insipidus (DI) Na^+ > 190 mEq/L may indicate long-term salt ingestion
Blood urea nitrogen and creatinine	To determine kidney function; will be increased in renal insufficiency and dehydration
Urine: Na^+ Specific gravity Osmolarity (OsM)	To help to determine volemic state and whether associated with renal or nonrenal losses, DI, or insensible free water losses Urine Na^+ > 20 mEq/L and urine OsM normal = edema Urine Na^+ > 20 mEq/L and urine OsM low or normal = renal loss Urine Na^+ < 10 mEq/L and urine OsM high = nonrenal loss Urine Na^+ variable and urine OsM low = euvolemic, DI Urine Na^+ < 10 mEq/L and urine OsM high = euvolemic, insensible water loss
Serum glucose	To rule out hyperglycemia, diabetic ketoacidosis
Computed tomography scan or magnetic resonance imaging (severe hypernatremia)	To rule out intracranial hemorrhaging, dural sinus thrombosis, or to identify a central nervous system cause for hypernatremia

Note. Based on information from Smith & Baird-Powell, 2000; Stephanides, 2007.

History and physical assessment: Obtaining a thorough history is important because it often can lead to determining the cause of the hypernatremia. The history should include questions to determine any recent fluid losses (vomiting, diarrhea, fever, burns, profuse sweating), the patients' thirst response (excessive, no thirst mechanisms), fluid intake and urine output (polydipsia, polyuria, oliguria), their behavioral/physical ability to take in fluids, any recent intake of high-sodium products, and uses of tap water enemas. A review of current medications and treatments is important to determine any causes contributing to sodium overload, fluid restriction, or renal impairment, as well as any primary or secondary side effects that are related to specific medications (such as sodium bicarbonate) (Berendt & D'Agostino, 2005; Smith & Baird-Powell, 2000; Stephanides, 2007).

As hypernatremia develops, cell dehydration and cell volume contraction occur as water leaves the intracellular department. This cell dehydration leads to many of the signs and symptoms of hypernatremia. Vital signs should be obtained, and assessment should look at overall fluid status. A thorough neurologic examination should be performed to aid in determining any underlying cause and the severity of the hypernatremia, as neurologic changes are common in hypernatremia because of the cell dehydration (Berk & Rana, 2006; Smith & Baird-Powell, 2000).

Clinical manifestations: Physical findings associated with hypernatremia can be nonspecific and are based on the cause and severity of the sodium imbalance. Common symptoms of hypernatremia include lethargy, restlessness, irritability, muscle twitching, hyperactive reflexes, ataxia, tremors, seizures, and coma. Patients with hypotonic fluid losses will present with findings of dehydration: tachycardia, hypotension, decreased skin turgor, dry mucous membranes, and thick "doughy"-like skin.

Evidence-based interventions: Managing hypernatremia consists of a two-pronged approach: (1) restoring the serum sodium to normal and (2) diagnosing and treating the underlying cause. Correction of hypernatremia generally begins with the calculation of total free water deficits to include predicted insensible water losses and other ongoing losses. Rapid correction of hypernatremia should be avoided because of the risk of CNS swelling and subsequent neurologic effects, including cerebral edema and subdural hemorrhaging (Stephanides, 2007). The general recommendation is to correct half the total free water deficit in the first 24–36 hours; however, correction should occur at a rate no faster than a 0.5–1 mEq/L/hr decrease in serum sodium up to a maximum decrease of 12 mEq/L of serum sodium in 24 hours (Stephanides, 2007). It may take two to three days to correct the total free water deficit and restore sodium balance. In patients with chronic hypernatremia, correction may take longer in order to prevent any subsequent neurologic sequelae.

Medications, such as sodium bicarbonate, that contain sodium should be minimized or eliminated, and free water intake should be encouraged, if possible. Serum electrolyte values should be checked frequently (every one to two hours initially) to monitor sodium levels. Potassium also may need to be added to the IV solutions to prevent potassium depletion. Strict I&O records should be maintained (Berk & Rana, 2006; Smith & Baird-Powell, 2000).

The treatment for hypernatremia depends on the type of fluid volume state that is present with the sodium imbalance. Treatment guidelines based on the three volume states of hypovolemic, hypervolemic, and euvolemic hypernatremia are described in Figure 12-3.

FIGURE 12-3	Treatment Guidelines for Hypernatremia

Hypovolemic (water loss > sodium loss)	**Hypervolemic (Excess sodium)**	**Euvolemic (pure water loss)**
1. Treat dehydration: Volume expansion with 0.9% NS until hemodynamically stable (normal blood pressure and heart rate and urine output > 25 ml/hr), THEN 2. Correct free water deficits orally or by IV with hypotonic NS (0.45% in adults, 0.2% in children) or with D5W.	1. Remove excess sodium: Use loop diuretics (furosemide) combined with 2. IV D5W to replace free water losses. 3. Avoid sodium in foods, medications, and fluids. 4. If in acute renal failure, may need hemodialysis.	Correct free water deficits and excrete excess sodium by 1. Drinking increased amount of water (preferred method) or 2. IV fluids of D5W. **Central DI** — Replace ADH: Reduces free water loss and concentrates urine. Medications: 1. Vasopressin (short-term use) 2. Desmopressin (long-term use) **Nephrogenic DI** — Decrease urine volume: 1. Salt restrictions 2. Thiazide diuretics 3. Prostaglandin inhibitors

ADH—antidiuretic hormone; D5W—dextrose 5% in water; DI—diabetes insipidus; NS—normal saline

Note. Based on information from Berendt & D'Agostino, 2005; Berk & Rana, 2006; Smith & Baird-Powell, 2000; Stephanides, 2007.

Expected outcomes: Most patients survive an episode of hypernatremia. However, residual neurologic deficits have been reported in up to 30% of patients with acute hypernatremia. In addition, patients with a serum sodium level greater than 180 mEq/L or who have hypernatremia corrected too quickly often have residual CNS damage (Stephanides, 2007). Therefore, the goals of therapy are to detect hypernatremia quickly before sodium levels become greater than 160–170 mEq/L and to slowly correct elevated sodium levels to help prevent any residual neurologic sequelae.

Patient teaching points: Figure 12-4 describes teaching points that may be used to instruct patients on the management of hypernatremia.

FIGURE 12-4	**Teaching Points for Hypernatremia**

- Ensure adequate energy and nutritional intake.
- Assess daily weight and intake and output.
- Teach patients the signs of dehydration.
- Assess patients who are hypernatremic with dehydration on their ability to understand the importance of adequate and frequent water intake.
- Have patients verbalize understanding of foods to avoid (i.e., those high in sodium if patient is on sodium restrictions).
- Ensure that patients' social, behavioral, and physical abilities provide adequate access to regular water intake if the patient is an older adult, an infant, or debilitated or institutionalized.
- Instruct patients with nephrogenic diabetes insipidus on ways to avoid salt and to drink large amounts of water.
- Provide additional and ongoing medical support as needed if condition is chronic or if patient suffers from residual neurologic effects.

Note. Based on information from Berendt & D'Agostino, 2005; Stephanides, 2007.

Hyponatremia

Overview: In hyponatremia, the level of sodium in the plasma, or serum, is too low. Hyponatremia is defined by a serum sodium level less than 130 mEq/L and is the most common electrolyte imbalance among patients with cancer (Berendt & D'Agostino, 2005). It can occur as a result of diuretic therapies, abrupt withdrawal of steroids, development of SIADH, or as a resultant side effect of some chemotherapy drugs, including cyclophosphamide and vincristine (Berendt & D'Agostino).

Pathophysiology: When sodium levels drop in the fluids outside the cells, water will seep into the cells in an attempt to balance the concentration of salt outside the cells. The cells swell as a result of the excess water. The brain, however, cannot accommodate this swelling because of the confinement of the skull. This produces most of the symptoms of hyponatremia (MedlinePlus, 2005). This action also portrays the potential severity of this imbalance. Hyponatremia occurs in one of four volemic states (see Figure 12-5).

Clinical assessment: Hyponatremia is confirmed by history, physical examination, and baseline diagnostic laboratory studies. However, after a thorough assessment, additional testing may be deemed necessary to rule out additional causes. Initial laboratory studies are identified in Figure 12-6.

A complete medical history should be obtained that includes any history of cancer and identification of cancer treatments, including surgeries, radiation therapy, chemotherapy, and supportive drugs along with doses, dates of last infusions, and a list of current daily med-

FIGURE 12-5	Volemic States of Hyponatremia

- Hypovolemic: Water and sodium are both lost from the body, but sodium loss is greater. Related to vomiting, diarrhea, burns, adrenal insufficiency, gastrointestinal suctioning, malabsorption of sodium, use of diuretics, especially thiazides, or osmotic diuresis.
- Hypervolemic: Both sodium and water content in the body increase, but the water gain is greater. Related to liver disease, acute or chronic renal failure, congestive heart failure, or administration of dextrose 5% in water, causing rapidly metabolized dextrose.
- Euvolemic: Total body water increases, but sodium content remains constant because of either excessive water intake, impaired excretion of free water, or excessive inappropriate vasopressin (antidiuretic hormone) secretion. Related to syndrome of inappropriate antidiuretic hormone, hypothyroidism, central nervous system disorders, cortisol insufficiency, water intoxication, or chemotherapy drug infusions such as cisplatin, vinblastine, vincristine, and cyclophosphamide.
- Pseudohyponatremia: Reflects a measurement phenomenon rather than abnormal amounts of water and salt in the body; occurs with hyperlipidemia, hyperglycemia, and hyperproteinemia.

Note. Based on information from Berendt & D'Agostino, 2005; Smith & Baird-Powell, 2000.

FIGURE 12-6	Diagnostic Laboratory Tests for Hyponatremia

- Serum electrolytes (Na^+, K^+, Cl^-, CO_2): Look at imbalances and acid/base status
- Serum osmolality (OsM) (normal = 280–295 mOsm/kg): Will be decreased
- Urine sodium and OsM
  - Urine Na^+ < 10 mEq/L and urine OsM high or normal = edema
  - Urine Na^+ > 10 mEq/L and urine OsM normal = renal dehydration
  - Urine Na^+ < 10 mEq/L and urine OsM high = nonrenal dehydration
  - Urine Na^+ > 20 mEq/L and urine OsM high = syndrome of inappropriate antidiuretic hormone, euvolemic
- Urine specific gravity < 1.010
- Serum glucose: Hyperglycemia; may produce pseudohyponatremia
- Blood urea nitrogen/creatinine: Will be elevated with renal insufficiency and dehydration

Note. Based on information from Smith & Baird-Powell, 2000; University of Iowa, 2007.

ications, both prescribed and over the counter (Berendt & D'Agostino, 2005; Smith & Baird-Powell, 2000). A complete list of presenting symptoms should be obtained along with any changes in routines and abilities to perform activities of daily living. The underlying cause and onset of hyponatremia are the most important treatment indicators.

A thorough physical examination should be completed with special attention paid to the following: alterations in behavior and mental status, hydration status, vital signs, and assessment of skin, cardiac, GI, and neurologic systems. Determining patients' hydration status will help to determine the underlying cause as well as the necessary treatment for hyponatremia. For instance, *hypovolemic* patients with hyponatremia will present with dry mucous membranes, diminished skin turgor, tachycardia, and orthostatic hypotension because of increased loss of body fluids, whereas *hypervolemic* patients could present with pulmonary rales, jugular venous distention, peripheral edema, or ascites because of excess retention of sodium and free water (Craig, 2007).

Clinical manifestations: Signs and symptoms of hyponatremia range from mild or vague to severe and can vary according to degree and onset. Sodium balance is critical to the maintenance of blood pressure and the function of nerves and muscles and, as noted previously, the brain is sensitive to changes in the sodium level. Therefore, symptoms related to these functions occur first, such as lethargy, confusion, and headache. As hyponatremia becomes more severe, muscle twitching, loss of reflexes, and seizures may occur, which can lead to coma and death if not treated promptly. Signs and symptoms are grouped according to severity in Figure 12-7.

FIGURE 12-7	Symptom Presentation of Hyponatremia	
Mild **(125–135 mEq/L)** • May be asymptomatic • Anorexia, headache, nausea and vomiting, myalgias, fatigue, thirst, diarrhea	**Moderate** **(115–124 mEq/L)** • Nausea, weakness, anorexia, fatigue, combativeness, muscle cramps, irritability, confusion, personality changes	**Severe** **(< 115 mEq/L)** • Severe lethargy and weakness, psychosis, decreased deep tendon reflexes, seizures, coma (can occur rapidly over 1–2 days and is a medical emergency)

Note. Based on information from Berendt & D'Agostino, 2005; Smith & Baird-Powell, 2000.

Evidence-based interventions: The interventions used to treat hyponatremia are dependent on the degree, duration, and onset of the imbalance. The focus of treatment is on the underlying cause of hyponatremia, such as in cases of malignancy and SIADH, hypothyroidism, adrenal insufficiency, excessive fluid loss, or hyperglycemia.

Initial interventions are based on stabilizing the patient's sodium and water imbalance without adverse effects on the neurologic system. Sodium replacement must be done very carefully and slowly. If sodium levels rise too rapidly, brain damage could occur as a result of brain cell dehydration. Corrections in serum sodium levels should increase no faster than 0.5 mEq/L/hr or 12 mEq/L over 24 hours (Craig, 2007; Smith & Baird-Powell, 2000). Restrictions of water intake may be necessary along with the use of hypertonic IV solutions and medications that induce diuresis if severe or acute hyponatremia is present. Table 12-9 describes treatment recommendations based on severity and type of hyponatremia.

With all cases of hyponatremia, the nurse should monitor I&O and daily weights and offer comfort measures secondary to restricted water intake (e.g., routine mouth care, lip care, ice chips as directed), as well as offer supportive care for patients who may have an altered mental status or risk of seizures (Myers, 2007; Smith & Baird-Powell, 2000).

Expected outcomes: The goal of treatment is to correct the sodium and fluid imbalance and treat any underlying conditions contributing to the imbalance. Patients will require frequent laboratory studies until the electrolyte balance is stable. Acute-onset hyponatremia, occurring in 48 hours or less, is less common but more dangerous secondary to the brain not being able to compensate for the sudden increase of intracellular fluids or CNS swelling (Craig, 2007).

Patient teaching points: Figure 12-8 includes patient teaching points related to hyponatremia.

Potassium Imbalances

Pathophysiology

Potassium is the most abundant intracellular cation and is essential to cellular function, neuromuscular activity, and cardiac conduction. Very little potassium (2%–3%) is found in the extracellular fluids, where sodium is the major cation. Potassium plays an integral role in cell membrane potential through the maintenance of sodium and potassium con-

TABLE 12-9	Treatment Recommendations for Hyponatremia
Degree of Hyponatremia	**Treatment Indications**
Mild/asymptomatic (hypervolemia)	Maintain outpatient status, if possible. Restrict water intake (500–1,000 ml/day). Provide minimum level of sodium from 1–3 g/day. If related to congestive heart failure, loop diuretics and an angiotensin-converting enzyme inhibitor may be used.
Mild to moderate (hypovolemic)	Correct or treat underlying cause (diarrhea, administration of chemotherapy). Restore fluid loss, usually with isotonic saline (0.9%) at recommended rate of 0.5–1 mEq Na$^+$/L/hr until serum Na$^+$ = 120 mEq/L, then reduce to 0.5 mEq/L/hr.
Moderate	Restrict fluids (500–1,000 ml/day). Discontinue medications, except chemotherapy, that may contribute to hyponatremia (e.g., diuretics). Give demeclocycline (600–1,200 mg/day) if not responsive to fluid restrictions. Acts by stimulating diuresis. Used mostly with chronic syndrome of inappropriate antidiuretic hormone (SIADH). • Do NOT restrict fluids while on demeclocycline. • Monitor renal and hepatic function. May consider other drugs used to treat chronic SIADH, such as lithium, urea, and fludrocortisones.
Severe/acute	Continue water restrictions. Place patient in intensive care setting. Administer IV hypertonic saline (3% normal saline) at rate to increase Na$^+$ level by 4–6 mEq/L. (Goal is to stop seizures, severe confusion, coma, etc.) Give IV diuretics to increase water loss. Perform frequent urine and serum Na$^+$ levels, electrolytes, and neurologic assessments. Give supplemental oxygen. Implement seizure precautions.

Note. Based on information from Berendt & D'Agostino, 2005; Craig, 2007; Keenan, 2005; Smith & Baird-Powell, 2000.

centration balances via the sodium-potassium ATPase pump. The sodium-potassium pump, which is controlled by activation of insulin and beta-2 receptors, controls the minute-to-minute intracellular to extracellular exchanges of potassium (Garth, 2007). This cellular balance is critical for nerve impulse transmission, muscle contraction, and especially cardiac function.

Imbalances in potassium are potentially life threatening and require immediate investigation and treatment. Long-term potassium balance is achieved through a balance of GI intake and renal potassium excretion (Garth, 2007). Potassium is absorbed solely from the GI tract. Because the body is unable to store potassium, a daily minimum intake of 40–60 mEq/day of potassium must be acquired from nutrition. Foods rich in potassium include fruits, vegetables, nuts, whole grains, dairy products, and meats. Potassium excretion occurs primarily via the kidneys with a small amount being excreted by the gut and skin (Smith, 2000b). The regulation of renal excretion occurs at the collecting ducts of the kidneys where excretion is increased or decreased by aldosterone receptors, changes in sodium or potassium levels, acid-base balances, rates of urine flow, and degrees of renal function (Lederer, Ouseph, & Yazel, 2007).

FIGURE 12-8	Teaching Points for Hyponatremia

- Patients should be able to identify and report any changes on the following.
  - The signs and symptoms of hyponatremia, from mild to severe
  - Any changes in weight, loss or gain of more than 5% of body weight
  - Any critical or sudden changes in their condition, including severe vomiting or diarrhea, presence of any mental status changes, sudden changes in their urinary output or fluid intake
- Nurses should be aware of specific cancers and chemotherapy treatments that may predispose patients to hyponatremia.
- Patients may be on continued fluid restrictions or sodium dietary requirements. They should be able to read various food and drink labels and identify the amount of sodium in each.

Note. Based on information from Berk & Rana, 2006; Myers, 2007.

Cellular balance of potassium is maintained constantly by the movement of potassium across cell membranes regulated by several different factors. Potassium in the serum portrays the amount of potassium that has shifted from the intracellular to extracellular compartments but does not necessarily reflect the total body potassium stores. Therefore, an imbalance in cellular potassium levels can exist without a true loss or increase in total potassium stores. The healthcare team needs to identify any states of "pseudo" hyper- or hypokalemia prior to initiating treatment for imbalances (Lederer et al., 2007).

Hypokalemia

Overview: Hypokalemia is defined as a serum potassium level less than 3 mEq/L (Berendt & D'Agostino, 2005). Although severe hypokalemia (less than 2.5 mEq/L) is relatively uncommon, as many as 20% of hospitalized patients are mildly hypokalemic; of these patients, only about 4%–5% have clinically significant hypokalemia. Up to 14% of outpatients are mildly hypokalemic, and approximately 80% of patients who are receiving diuretics become hypokalemic (Garth, 2007).

Hypokalemia usually is related to multiple factors. Symptoms may be nonspecific and are predominantly related to cardiac or muscular dysfunctions. Weakness and fatigue are the most common initial complaints. Patients who have hypertension, are on diuretics, and/or have congestive heart failure are at a higher risk for hypokalemia (Berendt & D'Agostino, 2005). Hypokalemia occurs most often from an increased excretion of potassium but also occurs from poor intake or shifts of potassium from the extracellular to the intracellular spaces. If unidentified or untreated, severe hypokalemia can lead to paralysis, cardiac arrhythmias, and death.

Specific causes of hypokalemia are described in Figure 12-9 in relation to the mechanism of action that leads to hypokalemia.

Clinical assessment: Obtaining a thorough history and physical is important as it often identifies the most likely reason for the hypokalemia. The nurse should get a history of any cancer and all cancer treatments, a list of current medications both prescribed and over the counter (diuretics, laxatives, enemas), and a past medical history, including history of diabetes, kidney disease, GI disorders, congenital disorders, or hypertension. Any presenting symptoms should be identified, such as vomiting, diarrhea, polyuria, constipation, abdominal distention, muscle weakness, leg cramps, palpitations, or fatigue.

Table 12-10 describes the diagnostic tests that may be required in the determination of hypokalemia and may help identify the underlying causes leading to the potassium imbalance.

FIGURE 12-9   **Causes and Mechanism of Action Leading to Hypokalemia**

Poor Intake
- Eating disorders such as bulimia or anorexia
- Alcoholism
- Inability to chew or swallow
- Poor nutritional intake
- Use of K^+ poor total parenteral nutrition or K^+ free IV fluids

Increased Excretion
- Renal losses
  - Renal tubular acidosis
  - Osmotic diuresis
  - Hyperaldosteronism
  - Hypomagnesemia
  - Hypovolemia
  - Congenital disorders
  - Adrenal disorders or adenomas
  - Leukemia—nonlymphocytic type
- Drug-related losses
  - Diuretics (most common cause)
  - Insulin or glucose administration
  - Antibiotics—gentamicin, amphotericin B, carbenicillin
  - Bicarbonate ingestion, infusions
  - Steroids
  - Aminoglycosides
  - Theophylline
  - Chemotherapy—cisplatin because of decreased Mg^+, carmustine (BCNU), streptozotocin
- Gastrointestinal (GI) losses
  - Severe vomiting
  - Diarrhea
  - Laxative abuse
  - Long-term use of suctioning or intestinal drainage
  - Positive for *Clostridium difficile* or GI candidiasis

Cellular Shifts
- Release of insulin—can cause a shift of K^+ back into the cells, especially in diabetic ketoacidosis
- Acidosis—K^+ moves out of cell in exchange for H^+ (hydrogen), creating total body depletion of K^+ as the kidneys continue to excrete K^+
- Metabolic or respiratory alkalosis—K^+ loss caused by an increase in absorption of bicarbonate

Note. Based on information from Berendt & D'Agostino, 2005; Lederer et al., 2007; Smith, 2000b.

The physical examination should include a mental status assessment for drowsiness, general malaise, fatigue, mental depression, and confusion, and cardiopulmonary examination noting heart rate and rhythm. Initially, vital signs may be normal except for occasional tachycardia or tachypnea secondary to muscle weakness. The pulse may become weak and irregular, and hypotension (indicating diuretic or laxative use, bulimia, or tubular disorders) or hypertension (indicating primary aldosteronism, renal stenosis, or congenital or genetic hypertensive syndromes) can be present. If severe hypokalemia is present, the patient may have ventricular fibrillation, which could lead to respiratory paralysis and cardiac arrest. Physical examination also should include an abdominal examination to assess for decreased bowel sounds and abdominal distention as well as determination of bowel elimination patterns of diarrhea or laxative use. Musculoskeletal examination is performed to test muscle strength, as patients may have weakness or muscle cramps. Flaccid paralysis can occur if severe hypokalemia is present. Additionally, a neurologic examination is performed to assess for decreased or absent deep tendon reflexes (Berendt & D'Agostino, 2005; Lederer et al., 2007; Smith, 2000b).

TABLE 12-10	Diagnostic Tests and Indications for Hypokalemia
Test	**Rationale and Findings**
Serum electrolytes (Na^+, K^+, Cl^-, Mg^{++}, CO_2)	K^+: Decreased Na^+: Low level indicates thiazide diuretic use or gastrointestinal (GI) volume depletion. High level could indicate nephrogenic diabetes insipidus, primary hyperaldosteronism. Mg^{++}: If low, correct for magnesium first, then reassess K^+.
Arterial blood gas	pH: Looks at acid-base balance Acidosis: Suggests renal tubular acidosis, drug use such as amphotericin or gentamicin Alkalosis: Suggests vomiting, diuretics, mineralocorticoid excesses or congenital disorders
Urine potassium	< 20 mEq/L suggests poor intake, intracellular shifts, or GI loss > 40 mEq/L suggests renal loss of K^+
Urine sodium and osmolality (OsM)	OsM: Urine concentration affects the true value and presence of urine potassium wasting. Na^+: Helps refine results of urine potassium (high K^+ and low Na^+ indicates hyperaldosteronism)
24-hour urine potassium and creatinine	Helps to determine precise amount of potassium excretion over time; the kidneys are able to conserve up to 10–15 mEq/day of K^+.
Blood urea nitrogen/ creatinine	To assess kidney function
Electrocardiogram	To identify any dysrhythmias: Flat T wave, ST depression, U wave elevation may be seen with hypokalemia.
Glucose	Glucose tolerance can be impaired by long-term or severe K^+ loss; insulin production causes K^+ to shift intracellularly.
Digoxin levels (if applicable)	Decreased K^+ increases risk of digitalis toxicity.

Note. Based on information from Berendt & D'Agostino, 2005; Lederer et al., 2007; Smith, 2000b.

Evidence-based interventions: The goals of treatment are to determine the underlying cause of hypokalemia and restore the potassium balance to alleviate current and future toxicities. Treatment must be tailored to patients by identifying risks through a history and physical and by managing contributing factors of potassium imbalance to prevent further episodes.

The initial step in treatment should be to identify and stop ongoing losses of potassium. This may be accomplished by (a) controlling diarrhea or vomiting, (b) discontinuing diuretics or using potassium-sparing diuretics such as spironolactone or amiloride if diuretic treatment is required, (c) discontinuing laxatives, (d) restoring possible magnesium losses, and (e) controlling hyperglycemia if present (Lederer et al., 2007).

The second step of treatment should focus on restoring potassium losses. This may be accomplished with simple dietary replacement. However, oral potassium supplements often are required in cases of mild to moderate (3–3.5 mEq/L) potassium losses. For symptomatic or severe (less than 2.5 mEq/L) potassium losses, concurrent IV replacement also is necessary. Severe potassium losses will require cardiac monitoring, most often in a critical care setting. Adequate renal function must be present to ensure that excess potassium is secreted during potassium supplementation. If renal function is decreased, dialysis may be necessary. Concurrent use with angiotensin-converting enzyme (ACE) inhibitors and potassium-sparing diuretics can cause severe hyperkalemia, so potassium levels must be monitored closely. It is important to continue checking urine concentration and volume losses of potassium as well until the patient is stabilized.

Oral potassium supplements are readily absorbed via the GI tract. The main side effects are related to GI irritation, such as a bitter aftertaste, indigestion, or nausea and vomiting; they should be given with a full glass of water with or just after meals to help alleviate GI symptoms (Smith, 2000b). Oral supplements can be given safely with IV replacement.

Oral potassium chloride enhances reabsorption of potassium and chloride in exchange for sodium and bicarbonate for a more rapid correction. It is preferred for patients with metabolic alkalosis or for those on thiazide diuretics because they tend to lose chloride as well (Smith, 2000b). Doses range from 20–40 mEq twice a day to four times a day. Slow-release potassium chloride also may be given. In addition, potassium bicarbonate or potassium citrate tablets can be used in patients with metabolic acidosis, as they help to alkalinize imbalances.

ACE inhibitors, angiotensin II receptor blockers (ARBs), or selective aldosterone blockers also may be useful in some patients, particularly those with congestive heart failure, to decrease aldosterone secretion, thereby causing a decrease in renal potassium losses. They often are given concurrently with a low-sodium diet and potassium-sparing diuretics (Lederer et al., 2007).

IV potassium replacement is indicated when patients are unable to take oral supplements, when severe hypokalemia is present, or when cardiac arrhythmias exist. IV potassium is very irritating to veins and should be diluted in normal saline and administered slowly (10–20 mEq/hr in adults). Concentrations ≥ 40 mEq/L may be given in emergent cases, with cardiac monitoring, but should be administered via a central line. Never give potassium as an IV push, as it can cause heart irregularities and failure (Garth, 2007; Smith, 2000b).

Expected outcomes: Potassium imbalances create a great risk for patients secondary to the important cardiac effects that imbalances can cause. Patients with hypokalemia may need only a simple correction of potassium related to poor intake, dehydration, or medication side effects. However, many potassium imbalances are related to complex medical conditions such as leukemia, acid-base imbalances, unstable diabetes, renal function abnormalities, adrenal carcinomas or metastasis, or congenital disorders. These complex conditions require a collaborative, multidisciplinary medical team. This is an especially important time for the nurse to be an attentive patient advocate and educator.

Patient teaching points: The patient teaching points in Figure 12-10 describe important education points related to hypokalemia.

Hyperkalemia

Overview: Hyperkalemia, defined as an increase in serum potassium levels, occurs as a result of increased potassium intake, decreased potassium excretion, or cellular shifts of potassium into the extracellular spaces. Even small changes in extracellular potassium levels can have profound effects on the cardiac and neuromuscular systems. Patients with hyperkalemia initially may be asymptomatic or report vague symptoms of nausea, fatigue, muscle weakness, or tingling. However, if hyperkalemia progresses, electrical conduction is affected and can result in decreased and weakened pulses with ECG changes leading to cardiac arrest. In rare cases, muscular paralysis also can occur as a result of suppressed electrical activity in the muscles.

Hyperkalemia is defined as a serum potassium level greater than 5.5 mEq/L. Mild hyperkalemia ranges from 5.5–6 mEq/L; moderate hyperkalemia ranges from 6.1–7 mEq/L; and severe hyperkalemia is defined as any serum level greater than 7 mEq/L (Garth, 2007). Mild hyperkalemia, which generally is asymptomatic and often well tolerated, is diagnosed in up to 8% of hospitalized patients in the United States (Garth). However, even mild hyperkalemia needs to be managed to prevent continued increases to severe levels. If not recognized promptly or treated properly, severe hyperkalemia can result in cardiac arrest with a mortality rate of up to 67% (Garth; Stoppler, 2008).

FIGURE 12-10	**Teaching Points for Hypokalemia**

- Educate patients on diets with low sodium and/or high potassium and the importance of good nutrition.
- Educate patients on suspected side effects and proper administration of oral potassium supplements, angiotensin-converting enzyme inhibitors, or potassium-sparing diuretics.
- Treatment should be tailored to individual patients and based on their disease process.
- Educate patients regarding need for proper nutrition, decreased alcohol intake, or laxative use as appropriate.

Hyperkalemia is a result of one or more of the following conditions that cause increases in extracellular potassium: (a) increased potassium intake, including high-potassium foods such as bananas, oranges, tomatoes, and high-protein diets, (b) salt substitutes, which often contain high levels of potassium, (c) use of potassium supplements, either oral or IV (for the treatment of hypokalemia), and total parenteral nutrition fluids, and (d) use of herbal supplements that contain high levels of potassium (Hollander-Rodriguez & Calvert, 2006).

The most common reason for hyperkalemia is related to decreased potassium excretion and most often is related to impaired renal excretion secondary to acute or chronic renal failure. Decreased potassium excretion also can result from impaired renal excretion from acute or chronic renal insufficiency; glomerulonephritis or any other disease that affects the kidneys, such as lupus; or medications that may decrease potassium excretion, including ACE inhibitors, ARBs, potassium-sparing diuretics, nonsteroidal anti-inflammatory drugs (NSAIDs), cyclosporine, or pentamidine.

Additional causes of hyperkalemia include (a) conditions that move potassium into extracellular spaces, such as trauma, burns, potassium supplements, or hemolysis (e.g., venipuncture, blood transfusions, tumor lysis), (b) cellular shifts of potassium from intra- to extracellular spaces, such as in acidosis and effects from medications (digitalis toxicity, beta-blockers), or (c) pseudohyperkalemia resulting from incorrect handling of blood specimens, poor venipuncture technique, or errors in laboratory processing, and leukocytosis or thrombocytosis (Garth, 2007; Handy & Shen, 2005).

Clinical assessment: Identifying and monitoring patients who are at risk for hyperkalemia is important because hyperkalemia often can be asymptomatic or have vague clinical symptoms until it becomes severe. Obtaining a thorough history that includes all current medications, supplements, any cancer or cancer treatments, changes in activities of daily living, and past medical history is important in determining the risks for and a diagnosis of hyperkalemia. Presenting symptoms may provide clues toward risks of hyperkalemia, but often increased potassium levels are found incidentally with other laboratory findings.

Diagnostic tests for identifying the cause and presence of hyperkalemia are listed in Table 12-11. Additional diagnostic tests may be needed if diabetes is suspected (glucose), the patient is on digitalis (digoxin levels), or mineralocorticoid deficiencies are suspected (cortisol, aldosterone levels). It also is particularly important to avoid treating pseudohyperkalemia to prevent any potentially harmful interventions. If pseudohyperkalemia is suspected, plasma potassium levels should be drawn and serum potassium levels redrawn, avoiding excessive trauma during venipuncture to minimize hemolysis. The specimen must be in the correct

TABLE 12-11	Diagnostic Tests for Hyperkalemia
Diagnostic Tests	**Findings/Indicators**
Serum electrolytes (Na^+, K^+, Cl^-, Mg^{++}, CO_2, Ca^{++})	Identify K^+ levels and associated electrolyte imbalances. Hypocalcemia could exacerbate cardiac symptoms. Mg^{++} increases lead to K^+ increases. Na^+ decreased/K^+ increased = adrenocortical insufficiency.
Blood urea nitrogen and creatinine (Cr)	To assess renal function; if increased, hyperkalemia results.
Urine K^+, Cr, and osmolality	To assess kidney function and to determine if K^+ is being excreted renally; urine uric acid if tumor lysis syndrome suspected
Electrocardiogram	To determine presence of cardiac arrhythmias; prolonged PR intervals, wide QRS, tall T and flat P wave
Arterial blood gas	To assess for acidosis
Phosphorus, calcium, and uric acid levels, complete blood count	Particularly important in patients with cancer if tumor lysis, leukocytosis, or thrombocytosis is suspected.

Note. Based on information from Garth, 2007; Handy & Shen, 2005; Smith, 2000b.

tube and processed within 30 minutes of the blood draw, and the venipuncture site should not be near an infusion line. If pseudohyperkalemia is present, plasma potassium levels will be normal while serum potassium levels are elevated, and the patient will not exhibit clinical symptoms or changes on ECG (Handy & Shen, 2005).

Physical signs of hyperkalemia include the following (Berendt & D'Agostino, 2005; Garth, 2007; Smith, 2000b).
- Cardiac—irregular heartbeat, weakening pulse with progressive bradycardia, ventricular fibrillation, ECG changes as described in diagnostics
- Neuromuscular—generalized fatigue, muscle weakness, diminishing deep tendon reflexes, tingling, and paresthesias; in rare cases, muscle paralysis and hypoventilation
- GI—increased bowel sounds, abdominal cramps, diarrhea, nausea, or vomiting
- Renal—signs of decreasing kidney function (i.e., edema, skin changes, oliguria)
- Recent traumas such as burns, and injuries that might lead to rhabdomyolysis

Clinical manifestations: Physical symptoms of hyperkalemia often are vague until moderate or severe levels are reached. The most common symptoms, if present, are muscle weakness, tingling or twitching, paresthesias involving the face, tongue, feet, or hands, generalized fatigue, palpitations, and increased bowel sounds with diarrhea, nausea, or vomiting. As hyperkalemia progresses, oliguria, ascending flaccid paralysis, syncope, arrhythmias, bradycardia, and ECG changes will develop (Berendt & D'Agostino, 2005; Garth, 2007; Smith, 2000b). A slow-rising potassium level may be tolerated more easily without presenting symptoms, whereas an abrupt rise in potassium levels is more likely to cause symptoms. Information obtained in the history and presenting clinical symptoms may help to identify the underlying medical condition contributing to the hyperkalemia (i.e., patient with congestive heart failure who is on potassium-sparing diuretics or a patient who has had recent chemotherapy treatment for leukemia).

Evidence-based interventions: The initial goal of treatment is to protect the body from the effects of hyperkalemia, and then correct the potassium imbalance and treat the underlying cause. If mild, asymptomatic hyperkalemia is present, the patient may only require measures that lower the total body potassium, such as oral sodium polystyrene sulfonate or a low-potassium diet.

Moderate to severe hyperkalemia, identified by changes on ECG, a rapid rise in serum potassium and/or potassium levels greater than 6 mEq/L, decreased renal function, and the presence of significant acidosis, requires urgent treatment (Hollander-Rodriguez & Calvert, 2006). Urine potassium, creatinine, and osmolarity should be obtained prior to initiation of treatment to significantly alter serum potassium levels (Hollander-Rodriguez & Calvert).

When moderate to severe or symptomatic hyperkalemia exists, the following measures may be used for treatment.

- Stabilize myocardium: IV calcium chloride or gluconate acts quickly to reduce the risk of ventricular fibrillation and can be life saving; use as first-line treatment for severe hyperkalemia with ECG abnormalities (e.g., widening of QRS interval, loss of P wave, cardiac arrhythmias).
- Shift potassium intracellularly by using insulin and glucose, beta-2 antagonist (albuterol), and sodium bicarbonate for acidosis; these are temporary measures that promote shifts intracellularly but do not clear potassium from the body.
- Lower total body potassium via renal excretion (loop diuretics), GI excretion (sodium polystyrene sulfonate) that removes potassium from the gut in exchange for sodium, or hemodialysis in life-threatening situations or for those patients in renal failure (Berendt & D'Agostino, 2005; Garth, 2007; Smith, 2000b).

Expected outcomes: If not treated promptly, hyperkalemia can result in cardiac arrest or death. Even small changes in potassium levels can cause severe effects on the cardiac and neuromuscular systems. The most important elements in obtaining a positive patient outcome are prevention and identification of patients who are at risk for hyperkalemia and performing thorough patient assessments. Long-term treatments should be focused on the causes of the imbalance, such as treatment of renal failure, dietary changes, or medication management.

Patient teaching points: Additional patient teaching points relevant to hyperkalemia are presented in Figure 12-11.

FIGURE 12-11	**Teaching Points for Hyperkalemia**

- Explain foods for use on a low-potassium diet.
- Patients with a history of hyperkalemia or chronic renal failure should not use salt substitutes as part of a low-salt diet.
- Patients may need follow-up monitoring of potassium levels, as well as Ca^{++} and Mg^{++} if on sodium polystyrene sulfonate (Kayexalate®, Sanofi-Aventis), as it decreases these levels.
- May need long-term use of loop diuretics if renal failure is present. Educate patients on side effects of diuretic use.

Magnesium Imbalances

Pathophysiology

Magnesium is the second most abundant intracellular cation, after potassium, with 45%–49% of the body's magnesium being intracellular. The remaining 50% of magnesium is stored in the bone, leaving 1%–5% in the extracellular fluid. Of this extracellular magnesium, 25%–30% is bound to protein with the remaining portion being ionized, or free, in the serum. Normal serum levels should be 1.5–2.5 mEq/L (Konstantakos & Grisoni, 2006; Smith, 2000c).

Magnesium is important in a large number of cellular and enzyme reactions, including DNA and protein synthesis, ATP activation and production, nerve impulse transmission, hormone receptor binding, and the regulation of parathyroid production (Novello & Blumstein, 2007b; Smith, 2000c). Magnesium helps to regulate calcium absorption, aids in the structural integrity of bones and teeth, and regulates heart muscle contraction. It is necessary for proper heart cell function and plays an important role in the polarization function of the sodium-potassium ATPase pump and regulation of intracellular potassium. It also is important to the transmission of nerve impulses and neuromuscular activity, having a smooth muscle relaxation effect especially in the arterioles and bronchial and uterine muscles. It decreases blood coagulation and acts as a calcium channel blocker, aids in protein synthesis, and is involved in the activation of vitamin B complexes (Smith, 2000c).

The daily dietary requirement of magnesium is 200–300 mg. Magnesium can be found naturally in green leafy vegetables, chlorophyll, various fruits, cocoa derivatives, nuts, wheat, seafood, and meat. Less than 40% of dietary magnesium is absorbed, primarily by the ileum of the small intestine. The remaining unabsorbed magnesium is excreted through the feces (60%) and kidneys (40%). However, the regulation of *serum* magnesium, via excretion or absorption, is controlled mainly by the renal system (Novello & Blumstein, 2007b; Smith, 2000c). Overall magnesium balance is maintained by the kidneys, small intestine, and bone.

Hypomagnesemia

Overview: Magnesium deficiencies generally are caused by either malabsorption in the GI or renal systems, decreased nutritional intake, increases in renal elimination, or shifts in electrolyte balances. Magnesium imbalances rarely occur alone and usually are accompanied by imbalances in calcium, potassium, and phosphorus. For example, if serum potassium or phosphorus is decreased, magnesium will decrease; when magnesium is decreased, interference results in the peripheral action of PTH in the bone, causing a decreased release of calcium (Smith, 2000c).

Hypomagnesemia is common among hospitalized patients, especially in the intensive care setting, where up to 60% incidence has been found (Konstantakos & Grisoni, 2006; Novello & Blumstein, 2007b). It also is common among alcoholics and diabetics. Hypomagnesemia is defined as a serum magnesium level less than 1.5 mEq/L. It generally is related to losses of magnesium through GI (e.g., malnutrition, malabsorption) or renal (e.g., impaired renal absorption, renal magnesium wasting) losses.

In patients with cancer, hypomagnesemia most often is related to renal losses induced by administration of various chemotherapy drugs, most commonly cisplatin, which has had dose-dependent kidney damage reported in 100% of patients receiving it (Novello & Blumstein, 2007b). In addition, 5-fluorouracil/leucovorin combinations, cetuximab, panitumumab, and decitabine (approved for myelodysplastic syndrome) also can cause a decrease in magnesium levels. Other drug-related causes include diuretics (especially loop diuretics, because of their location of action in the kidney being the same as where magnesium is absorbed in the loop of Henle), antibiotics such as aminoglycosides, amphotericin B, and pentamidine, cyclosporin, digitalis, or fluoride poisoning.

Clinical assessment: In the assessment for hypomagnesemia, the nurse should obtain a thorough history that includes nutritional assessment, history of alcohol intake, diabetes, cardiac conditions, endocrine disorders, and GI and kidney disorders. A current list of all medications should be obtained, paying special attention to antibiotics, chemotherapy drugs (especially cisplatin), heart medications such as digitalis, and use of diuretics, especially loop diuretics, as well as any exposure to or ingestion of fluoride. Diagnostic laboratory values for hypomagnesemia are described in Table 12-12.

The physical examination for hypomagnesemia should include an evaluation of mental status looking for confusion, mood changes, vertigo, or nystagmus. Vital signs and a cardiac examination should be obtained, looking for dysrhythmias and hypertension. A neuromuscular workup should include assessment for deep tendon reflexes, tetany, or presence of a positive Chvostek or Trousseau sign (Novello & Blumstein, 2007b; Smith, 2000c).

TABLE 12-12	Diagnostic Tests for Hypomagnesemia
Diagnostic Test	**Findings/Indicators**
Serum magnesium, calcium, potassium, and phosphorus	A total body Mg^{++} deficit can be present with a normal serum Mg^{++}. An ionized serum magnesium level is recommended. Any low serum Mg^{++} level indicates a clear Mg^{++} deficiency. K^+, Na^+, and phosphorus may be decreased. Ca^{++} may be increased or decreased.
Blood urea nitrogen and creatinine	To assess kidney function
Urine magnesium	May indicate deficiencies from renal losses
Protein levels	To aid in interpreting "true" magnesium level, because extracellular magnesium is bound to protein
Glucose/parathyroid hormone/aldosterone levels	To determine link to diabetes or endocrine disorders Increases in aldosterone cause renal loss of Mg^{++}.
Electrocardiogram	To assess for cardiac arrhythmias, ventricular tachycardia; may be nonspecific to include ST segment depression, altered T waves, or loss of voltage

Note. Based on information from Berendt & D'Agostino, 2005; Konstantakos & Grisoni, 2006; Smith, 2000c.

Clinical manifestations: Signs and symptoms of hypomagnesemia may take several weeks to develop and often are similar to signs and symptoms of hypocalcemia (Smith, 2000c). Clinical effects are exhibited primarily as signs and symptoms of CNS hypersensitivity, neuromuscular irritability, and cardiac arrhythmias. Early symptoms may include painful muscle cramps, nausea, vomiting, lethargy, and mental confusion and can develop into seizures when magnesium levels are less than 1 mEq/L (Novello & Blumstein, 2007b; Smith, 2000c).

Evidence-based interventions: Treatment should be directed toward identifying and treating any underlying cause for hypomagnesemia (e.g., chronic diarrhea, recent chemotherapy treatments with cisplatin, cetuximab) and correcting the resultant magnesium levels.

Mild hypomagnesemia (i.e., serum magnesium levels greater than 1.2 mEq/L) can be treated with oral magnesium replacement (i.e., magnesium oxides, magnesium gluconates) as long as the patient is asymptomatic. Prescribed doses vary between 500–1,000 mg/day for adults (Konstantakos & Grisoni, 2006; Novello & Blumstein, 2007b). Oral absorption is variable, with 15%–50% of a dose being absorbed. Patients with normal renal function generally will excrete any excess magnesium without any problems; therefore, renal function should be assessed prior to replacement therapy to ensure safety of renal clearance. In cases of renal impairment, doses should be decreased and the patient should be monitored closely. The main side effect of oral replacement therapy is diarrhea; divided doses may decrease incidence of diarrhea, and adequate hydration should be maintained.

Moderate to severe hypomagnesemia (serum magnesium levels less than 1.2 mEq/L or symptomatic) should be treated with IV magnesium replacement such as magnesium sulfate. An initial bolus diluted to 5%–20% may be given over 30 minutes to an hour followed by a continuous infusion until immediate symptoms resolve (Smith, 2000c). Emergent administration of magnesium sulfate may be given in cases of cardiac arrhythmias, severe electrolyte imbalances, cases of preeclampsia in obstetric patients, and acute cases of asthma (Novello & Blumstein, 2007b). Rapid IV administration can be life threatening, causing sudden hypotension, hypermagnesemia, and hypocalcemia. IV infusions may cause sudden hypotension, dizziness and fainting, respiratory depression, or depletion of potassium (Konstantakos & Grisoni, 2006; Novello & Blumstein, 2007b).

It may take several days to correct intracellular magnesium. Continuous IV magnesium infusions may be recommended until symptoms resolve. Rates of infusion should be adjusted to maintain serum magnesium levels below 2.5 mEq/L (Smith, 2000c). Slow-release magnesium also may be helpful in elevating intracellular magnesium levels.

Magnesium sulfate infusions may be given to replace hypomagnesemia from renal wasting, especially with chemotherapy regimens. It often is standard procedure with pre- and post-hydration fluids in administration with platinum-based drugs, particularly cisplatin, and oncology nurses should be aware of this treatment indication.

Expected outcomes: Once the cause of hypomagnesemia has been identified, symptoms generally are reversible and patients have a very good prognosis. Symptoms of hypomagnesemia often are nonspecific and rarely occur in isolation from other electrolyte disturbances. Primary nutritional deficiencies, alcoholism, links to malnutrition or malabsorption, renal deficiencies, sequelae from drug-induced interactions, and endocrine disorders should all be considered as precursors to potential electrolyte imbalances related to hypomagnesemia.

Patient teaching points: Patient teaching points important for nurses to be aware of for hypomagnesemia are included in Figure 12-12.

FIGURE 12-12	**Teaching Points for Hypomagnesemia**

- High intakes of calcium, vitamin D, and protein may increase the requirement for magnesium.
- Several chemotherapy regimens may predispose patients to magnesium losses. Patients should be aware of early signs and symptoms of hypomagnesemia to report to the healthcare team.
- Proper nutrition, including consuming foods high in magnesium, decreasing or ceasing alcohol consumption, and controlling diabetic conditions, are all important in the control of magnesium levels.
- Diarrhea is the primary side effect of oral magnesium supplementation and should be reported to the healthcare team if developed.

Hypermagnesemia

Overview: Hypermagnesemia is defined as a serum magnesium level greater than 2.5 mEq/L. Hypermagnesemia is an uncommon electrolyte imbalance because the kidneys generally are very effective at eliminating excess magnesium by regulating the tubular reabsorption of magnesium to almost negligible amounts (Agraharkar, Workeneh, & Fahlen, 2006). As described previously, magnesium is absorbed via the GI tract and excreted primarily in the urine and stool. Therefore, elevated magnesium levels are found most often in patients with renal disease, kidney failure, or those who have ingested high amounts of magnesium.

The most common cause of hypermagnesemia is end-stage renal disease. However, it also occurs related to (a) increased ingestion or absorption via ingestion of magnesium-containing substances such as antacids, laxatives (milk of magnesia), or enemas, especially in those with chronic renal failure; IV magnesium infusion overdoses or administration rate errors; or decreased GI elimination and increased GI absorption related to decreased GI motility (because of use of narcotics or anticholinergics, bowel obstruction, chronic constipation), (b) renal causes such as acute renal failure without dialysis or lithium therapy, which decreases urinary excretion of magnesium, (c) endocrine causes, including adrenal insufficiencies or diabetic ketoacidosis, or (d) other causes such as electrolyte imbalances of potassium, calcium, uric acid, or phosphorus, or TLS related to rapid cell destruction and the subsequent release of intracellular components, including magnesium into the bloodstream (Agraharkar et al., 2006; Novello & Blumstein, 2007a; Smith, 2000c).

Clinical assessment: When magnesium levels increase significantly, the neuromuscular, cardiac, and central nervous systems are affected. Neuromuscular transmission is blocked, the conduction system of the heart and the sympathetic ganglia are depressed, the secretion of PTH decreases, and there is interference with blood clotting related to interference with platelet adhesiveness, thrombin time, and clotting time (Agraharkar et al., 2006).

The patient history should focus on identifying the reason for increased magnesium levels. It should include taking a history of any cancer and chemotherapy treatments; obtaining a list of current medications, especially narcotics, anticholinergics, or magnesium supplements; identifying changes in bowel habits or chronic bowel disease, including any use of antacids or laxatives; and looking at kidney function and current hydration status. Any recent hospitalizations should be identified, especially those in which the patient may have been treated for hypomagnesemia or other electrolyte imbalances, those in the intensive care unit, or those that included prescription of magnesium supplementation. The diagnostic tests described in Table 12-13 will aid in the diagnosis and determination of the related cause for hypermagnesemia.

The physical examination should include an assessment of mental status to look for drowsiness or any mental status changes; cardiac examination that includes vital signs to identify hypotension or any changes in heart rates or arrhythmias; and a neuromuscular examination to evaluate muscle strength and deep tendon reflexes (Smith, 2000c).

Clinical manifestations: Although symptomatic hypermagnesemia is rare, presenting early symptoms (magnesium levels of 2–4 mEq/L) are nausea, vomiting, sweating, confusion, muscle weakness, and a reduction in deep tendon reflexes. At higher magnesium levels (greater than 8 mEq/L), flaccid paralysis can develop along with hypotension proceeding to respiratory paralysis, arrhythmias, heart block, and eventually asystole, coma, or death (Novello & Blumstein, 2007a).

Evidence-based interventions: Prevention of hypermagnesemia should be the initial intervention in patients who are at higher risk, such as those receiving magnesium treatments, patients with cancer, and those who have reduced renal function. Mild hypermagnesemia often can be treated by discontinuing any magnesium supplements, reducing dietary intake of magnesium-rich foods, and avoiding laxatives or antacids that contain magnesium. Further treatment for hypermagnesemia depends on the presence of symptoms, renal impairment, and the level of serum magnesium.

TABLE 12-13	Diagnostic Tests for Hypermagnesemia
Diagnostic Tests	**Findings/Indicators**
Serum electrolyte panel to include Mg^{++}, K^+, Ca^{++}, PO_4	Will often find hyperkalemia and hypercalcemia If associated with tumor lysis syndrome, will find hyperkalemia, hyperuricemia, hyperphosphatemia, and resulting hypocalcemia.
Platelet count and thrombin time	Increased Mg^{++} levels can be associated with delayed thrombin formation and platelet clumping.
Blood urea nitrogen and creatinine, creatinine clearance (CrCl)	To assess kidney function Serum Mg^{++} rises when CrCl levels are less than 30 ml/min.
Arterial blood gas	May reveal respiratory acidosis with hypermagnesemia
Thyroid function tests	Hypothyroidism can be rare cause of hypermagnesemia.
Electrocardiogram	To assess for cardiac arrhythmias, bradycardia; generally nonspecific but may show prolongation of PR intervals

Note. Based on information from Agraharkar et al., 2006; Novello & Blumstein, 2007a.

The use of hydration fluids for volume expansion and diuretics are recommended as treatment for moderate hypermagnesemia but should only be given to patients with normal renal function. Isotonic IV fluids (normal saline or lactated Ringer's solution) work by diluting the extracellular magnesium, and diuretics (furosemide) act to promote the additional loss of magnesium through the kidneys. IV fluid rates will vary depending on the patient's status, and diuretics (furosemide 20–80 mg daily) should be given in divided doses. Close monitoring of cardiovascular and pulmonary function is necessary. IV fluids and diuretics should be stopped when the desired response is obtained or if pulmonary edema develops.

For patients with severe or life-threatening, symptomatic hypermagnesemia, calcium gluconate may be administered. It acts as a direct antagonist for the neuromuscular and cardiovascular effects of magnesium and should be reserved for patients with cardiac effects or respiratory distress from hypermagnesemia. The recommended dose is 10–20 ml (100–200 mg of elemental calcium) of 10% calcium gluconate IV over 10 minutes; it also may be infused for maintenance doses of 20 ml of 10% calcium gluconate in 1 liter of normal saline at 150–200 ml/hr in patients with normal renal function (Novello & Blumstein, 2007a; Smith, 2000c). Calcium gluconate is contraindicated in digitalized patients and those with respiratory failure, acidosis, or severe hyperphosphatemia (Novello & Blumstein, 2007a).

Glucose and insulin also can be given to help shift magnesium back into the cells and out of the extracellular spaces. It should always be administered with insulin to prevent hypoglycemia. Blood sugar levels should be monitored frequently. Suggested dosing is 10 U IV with 50 ml dextrose 50% in water bolus or 500 ml dextrose 10% in water over one hour. This is contraindicated in hypoglycemic patients, and caution should be used in those with thyroid, renal, endocrine, or hepatic disorders (Agraharkar et al., 2006).

A renal consult is necessary for patients with renal impairment. Dialysis may be used when serum levels exceed 8 mEq/L, life-threatening symptoms are present, or in patients with poor renal function.

Expected outcomes: Sudden elevations of magnesium are more likely to produce symptoms of hypermagnesemia than slow rises. The degree and severity of symptoms will have a direct effect on the outcome of treatment. However, prompt treatment of the underlying reason for elevations, symptom management, and correction of serum levels produce a positive outcome in most patients. Patients with end-stage renal disease may continue to need dialysis and require close management and monitoring.

Patient teaching points: Figure 12-13 describes teaching points that may be helpful for patients with hypermagnesemia.

FIGURE 12-13	Teaching Points for Hypermagnesemia

- Identify foods high in magnesium, which may need to be avoided, such as green leafy vegetables, chlorophyll-containing foods, various fruits, cocoa derivatives, nuts, wheat, seafood, and meat.
- Instruct patients to notify the healthcare team of severe constipation, nausea, vomiting, poor appetite, and any progressing muscle weakness.
- Follow-up electrolyte laboratory values will be necessary, with frequency based on patients' overall status and other contributing medical problems.

Syndrome of Inappropriate Antidiuretic Hormone

Overview

SIADH can present as a life-threatening oncologic emergency. It is rare in patients with cancer, developing in 1%–2% of all people with neoplasms. However, approximately two-thirds of all patients diagnosed with SIADH will have a neoplasm (Myers, 2007). The most common malignant disease associated with SIADH is lung cancer, and 80% of these cases are from small cell lung cancer (Keenan, 2005). Additional cancers associated with SIADH include cancers of the head and neck, esophagus, prostate, pancreas, bladder, or duodenum; lymphoma; thymoma; acute myeloid leukemia; and CNS tumors (Myers; Rafailov & Sinert, 2007).

SIADH is an endocrine-related syndrome causing an abnormal production or secretion of ADH (i.e., arginine vasopressin). Normally, the posterior pituitary gland releases ADH in response to increased osmolality or decreased plasma volume and sends signals to the collecting ducts of the kidneys to reabsorb water, concentrating the urine and normalizing serum osmolality (Ezzone, 2000). In SIADH, the production or secretion of ADH occurs even though osmolality is normal or low, resulting in an inappropriate reabsorption of free water by the kidneys (Ezzone; Keenan, 2005). This leads to decreased urine output, increased intravascular volume, excessive urine sodium excretion, and hyponatremia, which are the hallmark signs of SIADH (Ezzone; Keenan; Rafailov & Sinert, 2007). In SIADH, hyponatremia is a direct result of excess water, not a deficiency in sodium. The findings associated with SIADH occur in a *euvolemic* state, without edema or any history of diuretic therapy, and in the setting of otherwise normal cardiac, renal, thyroid, adrenal, and hepatic function (Rafailov & Sinert). The mechanisms of action and systemic effects of SIADH are described in Table 12-14.

Pathophysiology

Three pathophysiologic mechanisms generally are responsible for the inappropriate secretion of ADH. The first is primary inappropriate secretion of ADH (vasopressin) from the hypophyseal system within the hypothalamus, such as with CNS disorders, head trauma, brain tumor, CNS hemorrhage, shock, stroke, or any other condition causing an increase in intrathoracic pressure or a decrease in venous return. The second mechanism is ADH or ADH-like substances being secreted by cells outside of the hypophyseal system, referred to as ectopic secretion. This is the primary reason for cancer-related SIADH. The third pathophysiologic mechanism is enhanced action of ADH on the renal tubules by various drugs such as morphine, nicotine, thiazide diuretics, tricyclic antidepressants, barbiturates, chlorpropamide, selective serotonin reuptake inhibitors, NSAIDs, and carbamazepine. Various chemotherapy agents that can produce the same effect are cisplatin, cyclophosphamide, vinblastine, vincris-

TABLE 12-14	Systemic Effects of Syndrome of Inappropriate Antidiuretic Hormone
Mechanism of Action	**Resulting Effect**
Increased water reabsorption by renal tubules	Decreased serum osmolality; hyponatremia
Decreased excretion of water by renal tubules	Increased urine osmolality
Increased total water in intra- and extracellular fluids	Decreased serum osmolality
Decreased sodium plasma concentration secondary to excess water	Hyponatremia
Increased urine concentration	Increased urine osmolality
Increased sodium secretion by kidneys	Increased urine sodium

Note. Based on information from Flounders, 2003.

tine, ifosfamide, and melphalan (Keenan, 2005; Myers, 2007). Nausea, a common side effect of chemotherapy, also may stimulate ADH release leading to SIADH.

Clinical Assessment

A thorough clinical history and physical examination should be performed to determine whether the patient is experiencing SIADH versus another form of hyponatremia or electrolyte imbalance. Obtaining a history related to diagnosis and type of cancer or recent cancer treatments is important. Any ongoing side effects, current medications, presenting symptoms, and changes in activities or mental status should be noted, as well as a history of fluid I&O within the past 24 hours. A pulmonary assessment is important to identify any infection or pulmonary disease processes, as well as a neurologic examination to identify any changes in level of consciousness or loss of deep tendon reflexes (Ezzone, 2000; Gobel, 2005). SIADH is diagnosed based on the combination of the following: (a) hyponatremia with normal or increased intravascular volume, (b) decreased plasma osmolality, and (c) increased urine osmolality. The diagnostic tests described in Table 12-15 should be obtained to determine the diagnosis of SIADH.

Clinical Manifestations

Clinical signs and symptoms of SIADH are directly related to the rate of onset and severity of hyponatremia as well as the degree of water intoxication. In mild or chronic cases, patients may be asymptomatic. With an acute onset (within one to three days) or with a severe drop in serum sodium level (less than 110–115 mEq/L), SIADH symptoms will be related to the subsequent neurologic effects and will present an acute emergency.

The signs and symptoms are similar to those for hyponatremia (see Figure 12-7) and will vary in degree from mild to severe based on the degree of hyponatremia and water intoxication. However, SIADH usually will present with a normal blood pressure and pulse, normal skin turgor with moist mucous membranes, and none to very little peripheral edema. Patients with SIADH may present with thirst, anorexia, nausea, and vomiting, as well as oliguria (less

TABLE 12-15	Diagnostic Tests for Syndrome of Inappropriate Antidiuretic Hormone
Diagnostic Tests	**Findings/Indicators**
Serum electrolytes and osmolality (OsM)	Serum Na$^+$ and OsM (< 280 mOsm/kg): Decreased Serum K$^+$ and bicarbonate levels: Normal Serum phosphorus: May be decreased
Urine Na$^+$, OsM, and specific gravity	Urine Na$^+$ > 20 mEq/L Urine OsM > 100 mOsm/kg Urine specific gravity: Increased > 1.015
Blood urea nitrogen (BUN), creatinine, and uric acid	BUN, creatinine, and uric acid may all be decreased.
Renal, thyroid, and adrenal function	Will be normal with syndrome of inappropriate antidiuretic hormone
Chest x-ray	To identify any tumors or pulmonary disease
Computed tomography scan of head	To evaluate for anatomic lesions or evidence of cerebral edema

Note. Based on information from Amini & Schmidt, 2004; Gobel, 2005; Keenan, 2005; Myers, 2007.

than 400 ml/24 hours of urine), incontinence, and weight gain. They may have hypoactive reflexes, muscle weakness, myoclonus, tremors, and an unsteady gait. Left untreated, these symptoms could lead to seizures, coma, and eventually death (Ezzone, 2000; Myers, 2007).

Evidence-Based Interventions

Treatment for SIADH differs slightly from that of other types of hyponatremia because it is based on a euvolemic state; therefore, volume expansion should be avoided. The treatment of choice is to determine the underlying cause, as in the case of a tumor, drug, or disease causing the disorder, and eliminate or treat it (Amini & Schmidt, 2004; Myers, 2007). The patient's sodium level and neurologic status must be stabilized. Treatment decisions for SIADH should be based on correcting the hyponatremia as defined in Table 12-9 with the following guidelines being followed.

Patients with mild hyponatremia generally are asymptomatic. Fluid restrictions of 500–1,000 ml/day will promote a negative water balance, and the nurse should attempt to correct plasma sodium levels in three to five days (Myers, 2007). It is imperative to initiate or continue treatment for the underlying cause (e.g., malignancy) and to monitor and discontinue medication, if possible, that may be contributing to SIADH, such as thiazide diuretics or NSAIDs.

Mild to moderate hyponatremia may be chronic in nature. The treatment should include continued fluid restrictions and treatment of the underlying cause. The nurse should consider use of demeclocycline at doses of 600–1,200 mg/day if the patient is not responsive to continued fluid restrictions. Demeclocycline acts by inhibiting the action of ADH on the renal tubules so that water can be excreted. A response usually occurs in three to four days. Once the patient is receiving demeclocycline, fluid restrictions are not required. This medication should not be taken with food. Side effects generally are mild but may include nausea, photosensitivity, nephrotoxicity, and azotemia (Flounders, 2003; Myers, 2007).

Severe hyponatremia usually develops rapidly. Treatment will include instituting or continuing fluid restrictions and treatment of the underlying cause. Severe cases are treated with hypertonic saline. The same precautions for the treatment of severe hyponatremia (see Table 12-9) should be followed. Patients being treated with chemotherapy may present an especially difficult challenge. Chemotherapy agents such as cisplatin and cyclophosphamide may cause SIADH or contribute to SIADH because of their action or their need for increased hydration. Hydration with normal saline may need to be given sparingly, with the additional use of furosemide and electrolyte replacement. If the SIADH is severe, the neurologic complications will need to be stabilized before initiating any chemotherapy treatments (Ezzone, 2000; Gobel, 2005).

Expected Outcomes

SIADH, although not necessarily preventable, can be successfully treated. In cases associated with CNS and spine disorders, it can be self-limiting and remit spontaneously within two to three weeks (Amini & Schmidt, 2004). The goal of treatment is for the patient to be asymptomatic with a return to normal levels of serum osmolality, sodium and urine osmolality, and urine specific gravity. Neurologic impairment usually is reversible with appropriate treatment. SIADH often resolves with treatment of the underlying disease (e.g., tumor regression). However, it may return during stable disease while the patient is undergoing chemotherapy or with tumor progression and may require ongoing intermittent management (Keenan, 2005; Myers, 2007).

Patient Teaching Points

Patient teaching points should include those points already discussed in the management of hyponatremia as well as those in Figure 12-14.

FIGURE 12-14	Teaching Points for Syndrome of Inappropriate Antidiuretic Hormone (SIADH)

- Be aware of any medications, chemotherapy agents, or treatments that may predispose patients to SIADH.
- Conduct a thorough pain assessment because SIADH may be precipitated or worsened by pain and stress.
- Ensure that appropriate pain medications are used, or that substitutions are used for pain medications that may precipitate the release of antidiuretic hormone.
- When assessing the volume status of patients, nurses should be aware that signs and symptoms of hypervolemia or hypovolemia exclude the diagnosis of SIADH (Flounders, 2003).
- Continued assessment of physical symptoms and diagnostic findings is necessary to detect early signs of recurrent hyponatremia to prevent neurologic complications.

Tumor Lysis Syndrome

Overview

TLS is a potentially life-threatening electrolyte and metabolic complication and is considered an oncologic emergency. It occurs as a result of the metabolic consequences related to rapid tumor cell death, or tumor lysis. In TLS, as tumor cells die, they release their intracellular components into the bloodstream so rapidly and at such high concentrations that the body is not able to eliminate them fast enough. This accumulation of intracellular contents produces the hallmark electrolyte and metabolic disturbance combinations of TLS: hyperkalemia, hyperuricemia, hyperphosphatemia, and resulting hypocalcemia. If not prevented, detected, or treated early, TLS can lead to neurologic and GI complications, cardiac arrhythmias, acute renal failure, and eventual death (Gobel, 2005; Myers, 2007).

TLS is most commonly found in bulky, rapidly growing tumors with high growth fractions or those with highly sensitive responses to cancer treatment. TLS occurs most frequently in patients with high-grade lymphomas, such as Burkitt lymphoma, and those with high white blood cell counts, as in acute lymphoblastic leukemia (ALL). It also can present in AML, chronic myeloid leukemia in blast crisis, some solid tumors such as small cell lung cancer, metastatic breast cancer, metastatic medulloblastoma, soft tissue sarcomas, and other related hematologic malignancies, such as advanced myeloma or myelodysplastic disease (Del Toro, Morris, & Cairo, 2005; Myers, 2007). Patients with an elevated LDH level associated with high tumor volume, preexisting renal dysfunction, splenomegaly, or lymphadenopathy also may be vulnerable to TLS (Cope, 2004; Lydon, 2005; Myers).

Although most commonly associated with chemotherapy, TLS can occur with any form of treatment that causes rapid cell death and necrosis of tumor mass, such as radiation, immunotherapy or hormonal therapy, surgery, and hyperthermia (Lydon, 2005). Although rare, TLS can occur spontaneously prior to initiation of cancer treatment, especially in patients with leukemia and lymphoma because of the high proliferative tumor rate or the large, bulky tumors associated with these cancers (Vachani, 2006). In previous studies of the frequency of TLS occurrence in high-grade lymphomas in adults and ALL in children, laboratory-evidenced TLS occurred in 42% of adults and 70% of children, but clinically significant TLS occurred in only 6% of adults and 3% of children (Krishnan & Hammad, 2006).

TLS can occur within 24 hours to seven days after chemotherapy is initiated but is most often seen 48–72 hours after initiation and usually resolves within seven days if treated. In the early stages, TLS is a preventable and treatable condition. Therefore, the primary focus of TLS is early identification of those at risk, prevention, and early treatment. By analyzing the three categories of risk factors associated with TLS (see Figure 12-15), oncology nurses can identify patients who are at higher risk.

Mato et al. (2006) created the Penn Predictive Score (PPS) in conjunction with findings from their research, which assisted in the identification of those patients who are at highest risk for TLS. The PPS identifies higher levels of LDH and uric acid and male gender as indicators for higher risk of TLS. Nurses and other healthcare providers can use the PPS as a tool to successfully identify patients who are at high risk for TLS.

FIGURE 12-15	Associated Risks for Tumor Lysis Syndrome	
Tumor Risks	**Treatment Risks**	**Patient Risks**
• Lymphoma	• Chemotherapy (e.g., cisplatin,	• Increased uric acid, phosphate,
• Leukemia	etoposide, cytarabine [Ara-C],	K+, lactate dehydrogenase prior
• High growth fraction	paclitaxel, fludarabine, hy-	to and/or after initiation of treat-
• Large and/or bulky mass	droxyurea, intrathecal metho-	ment
• B-cell/activated T-cell pheno-	trexate)	• Elevated white blood cell count
types	• Immunotherapy (e.g., inter-	• Preexisting renal impairment
• Metastatic disease	ferons, interleukins, tumor	• Splenomegaly
• Tumor sensitivity to chemo-	necrosis factors, monoclonal	• Extensive lymphadenopathy
therapy	antibodies [rituximab])	• Dehydration
	• Hormonal therapy (tamoxifen)	• Ascites
	• Corticosteroids	• Pleural effusion
	• Radiation	• Superior vena cava syndrome
	• Surgery	
Note. Based on information from Del Toro et al., 2005; Lydon, 2005.		

Pathophysiology

When tumor cells are killed, potassium, phosphorus, and nucleic acids are released into the bloodstream. The liver then converts the nucleic acids to uric acid, and the kidneys excrete the resulting uric acid. The kidneys also act as filters for necessary electrolytes, reabsorbing the amount needed and excreting the excess into the urine.

In the development of TLS, the associated high rate of tumor lysis produces rapid release of these intracellular contents into the bloodstream. As a result of the sudden serum potassium, phosphorus, and uric acid elevations, the kidneys become overwhelmed and are unable to sufficiently excrete these byproducts of cell death. The resulting electrolyte imbalances of hyperkalemia, hyperphosphatemia, and hyperuricemia occur. Because of the inverse relationship between calcium and phosphorus, as phosphorus levels increase, calcium levels decrease.

Some tumor cells, such as in lymphoblastic leukemia, may have more than four times the amount of phosphorus than normal cells and also may be richer in purine nucleic acids, which convert to uric acid when released. Therefore, these additional tumor characteristics may further increase the elevations of phosphorus and uric acid with rapid tumor lysis.

Hyperuricemia, the most common complication of TLS, causes uric acid crystals to form in the collecting ducts of the kidneys and ureters, thereby causing obstruction, increased pressure, and decreased glomerular filtration, which all lead to renal failure (Vachani, 2006). Hyperphosphatemia results in the binding of phosphorus and calcium to create calcium-phosphate salts, which contributes to the blockage of the kidneys and resultant kidney failure.

Hyperkalemia, often the first life-threatening sign of electrolyte imbalance in TLS, leads to cardiac arrhythmias, respiratory failure, and neuromuscular dysfunction if not detected and treated and also contributes to renal failure (Krishnan & Hammad, 2006). Hypocalcemia, a consequence of acute hyperphosphatemia, can cause cardiac arrhythmias and heart dysfunctions as well as contribute to the neuromuscular and renal side effects of TLS (Krishnan & Hammad).

Clinical Assessment

Prevention and early detection of risks and symptoms are key factors in preventing the life-threatening consequences of TLS. Prior to initial treatment for cancer, baseline serum electrolytes, especially potassium, phosphorus, calcium, and uric acid levels, should be obtained. Renal function studies (BUN, creatinine, urine pH) and liver function tests (LDH, aspartate aminotransferase, alanine aminotransferase) should be obtained for baseline studies as well as to identify any preexisting abnormalities. Monitoring of laboratory values may be necessary several times a day for the first 48–72 hours in patients who are at high risk for TLS. Baseline and daily weights, vital signs, and I&O measurements should be obtained during the initial treatment phase to aid in monitoring renal and cardiac conditions.

The history should include nutritional and hydration status, past and current medications, a history of any chronic health problems or past organ dysfunctions, such as kidney or liver problems, and any recent cancer treatments. A baseline echocardiogram may be recommended before initiation of cancer treatment and in those at high risk for or with hyperkalemia (Gobel, 2005; Krishnan & Hammad, 2006).

Clinical Manifestations

Initial symptoms of TLS include nausea, vomiting, shortness of breath, irregular heartbeat, clouding of urine, lethargy, and joint discomfort or muscle aches. Continued progression of TLS leads to increased GI symptoms; neurologic impairments, which may lead to hallucinations, muscle tetany, and seizures; cardiac complications of high blood pressure, tachycardia then bradycardia, and possible ventricular arrhythmias; and progressive renal impairments, including azotemia and anuria (Gobel, 2005; Lydon, 2005; Myers, 2007). If TLS is not recognized and treated promptly, progression may lead to acute kidney failure, stimulation of disseminated intravascular coagulation, cardiac arrest, and death (Gobel; Myers). Early and late symptom presentations are described in Table 12-16 for each imbalance present with TLS.

Evidence-Based Interventions

The most important key to managing TLS is to identify patients who are at highest risk and initiate preventive or prophylactic measures prior to any treatments for cancer. Close monitoring of laboratory values and associated symptoms of imbalances is crucial to identify abnormalities before they become life threatening (Myers, 2007; Vachani, 2006). Patients considered to be at high risk for TLS should be placed in a specialized oncology or intensive care setting and may benefit from having central venous access before initiation of treatment for cancer (Krishnan & Hammad, 2006; Vachani).

TABLE 12-16	Symptom Presentation of Tumor Lysis Syndrome			
Imbalance Presentation	**Gastrointestinal**	**Neuromuscular**	**Cardiac**	**Renal**
Hyperkalemia	Nausea, diarrhea, vomiting	**Early** Twitching, cramping, muscle weakness, paresthesias **Late** Ascending flaccid paralysis, positive Chvostek sign, positive Trousseau sign	**Early** Hypertension, tachycardia, electrocardiogram (ECG) changes **Late** ECG changes, bradycardia, heart block, asystole	–
Hyperphosphatemia	–	–	Hypertension	Azotemia, oliguria, anuria, renal failure
Hyperuricemia	Nausea, vomiting, diarrhea, anorexia	**Early** Fatigue, lethargy, pruritus **Late** Acute articular distress (similar to gout)	–	**Early** Mild azotemia, flank pain, oliguria, increased urine osmolarity **Late** Edema, crystalluria, hematuria, profound azotemia, anuria, renal failure
Hypocalcemia	–	**Early** Restlessness, irritability, impaired memory, muscle cramps, twitching, muscle weakness, paresthesias **Late** Positive Chvostek sign, positive Trousseau sign, seizures, tetany	Hypotension, heart block, cardiac arrest	–

Note. Based on information from Lydon, 2005; Myers, 2007.

The preventive measures and treatments for TLS are multifaceted and include laboratory monitoring, adequate hydration, forced diuresis, alkalinization of urine (controversial), control of hyperuricemia, and treatment of electrolyte alterations.

Laboratory monitoring should include obtaining potassium, phosphorus, calcium, uric acid, BUN, creatinine, and LDH levels at baseline, and levels should be drawn every 6–8 hours daily during the first 48–72 hours after induction of treatment in high-risk patients. If TLS develops, laboratory values should be checked at least twice daily and then decreased according to risk and response to treatment. A baseline ECG also might be indicated, especially in patients with identified hyperkalemia, along with frequent cardiac assessment to monitor changes that may be caused by hyperkalemia and hypocalcemia (Krishnan & Hammad, 2006; Lydon, 2005).

Hydration should be aggressive and begin 24–48 hours prior to chemotherapy and continue for at least 72 hours after treatment. Approximately $3 L/m^2/day$ of isotonic or hypotonic fluid to maintain urine output of at least $100 ml/m^2/day$ is the accepted rate (Gobel, 2005; Vachani, 2006). Aggressive hydration will enhance renal blood flow, glomerular filtration, and urine volume, thus decreasing the concentration of soluble acids in the urine. Nurses should monitor patients for symptoms of fluid overload by assessing frequent vital signs to look for changes in blood pressure and heart rate, identifying any signs of edema, maintaining strict I&O, monitoring for respiratory or cardiac changes, and weighing the patients daily.

Urinary alkalinization is a controversial intervention that historically was one of the primary focuses of prevention of TLS. Some controversy exists as to whether alkalinization should be continued once treatment has been started because alkalinization also can lead to the precipitation of calcium and phosphate in the renal tubules, contributing to hypocalcemia and hyperphosphatemia (Krishnan & Hammad, 2006; Myers, 2007; Vachani, 2006), and can lead to the precipitation of xanthine crystals in the renal tubules. However, some practitioners still use alkalinization, which is obtained with the addition of sodium bicarbonate to IV fluids at a rate of 50–100 mEq/L to maintain urine pH levels greater than or equal to 7. Urine alkalinization helps to prevent uric acid from forming into insoluble crystals in the tubules of the kidney. Therefore, urine alkalinization often is recommended to be stopped once uric acid levels stabilize, the urine pH is greater than 7.5, or serum bicarbonate levels reach 30 mEq/L (Krishnan & Hammad; Myers).

Forced diuresis with loop diuretics, such as furosemide, may be helpful to prevent fluid overload, maintain urinary output, and promote the excretion of potassium, phosphate, and uric acid in the urine. However, diuretics should be used only with patients who are well hydrated.

Control of hyperuricemia also is used in prevention and treatment of TLS. When high uric acid levels (greater than or equal to 8 mg/dl) develop, uric acid converts into insoluble crystals formed of sodium urate. These crystals can block the tubules throughout the kidney, preventing proper filtration and causing acute kidney damage, ultimately leading to kidney failure. Treatment for hyperuricemia includes aggressive hydration, urinary alkalinization, and the use of diuretics. In addition, allopurinol and rasburicase often are used in the prevention and treatment of TLS. These drugs block the formation of uric acid.

Allopurinol is a xanthine oxidase inhibitor and works by interfering with purine metabolism and inhibiting xanthine oxidase enzyme, which is essential for converting nucleic acid into uric acid (Kaplow, 2002). This also decreases the deposits of uric acid in the kidneys, but it cannot decrease uric acids that have already formed prior to its initiation. It can be given orally (Zyloprim®, Prometheus Laboratories) in adults at 600–900 mg/day (up to a maximum dose of $500 mg/m^2/day$) for prophylaxis and treatment of TLS (Krishnan & Hammad, 2006). It is critical for oncology nurses to be aware of those patients who are at high risk for TLS so that prophylactic treatment can be initiated as appropriate. Treatment should be initiated one to two days before treatment for cancer and should continue for two to three days following treatment (Doane & Gobel, 2004; Krishnan & Hammad, 2006). For patients unable to tolerate oral dosages, allopurinol may be given IV (Aloprim™, Bioniche Pharma) as a single dose or in equally divided doses at 6-, 8-, or 12-hour intervals at total dosages of 200–400 $mg/m^2/day$ (up to maximum dose of 600 mg/day) with the same initiation times as oral allopurinol (Spratto & Woods, 2004). Doses may need to be reduced in patients with impaired renal function or patients taking mercaptopurine, 6-thioguanine, or azathioprine because of interference with the metabolism of these drugs (Krishnan & Hammad).

Oncology nurses should educate themselves and their patients on precautions associated with taking allopurinol, such as dietary restrictions related to foods high in purine, the potential risk of allergic reactions, including Stevens-Johnson syndrome, and drug incompatibilities. Possible side effects include nausea and vomiting, rash, fever, and renal failure and insufficiency. If a rash develops, the drug should be stopped (Gobel, 2005; Spratto & Woods, 2004).

Rasburicase (Elitek™, Sanofi-Aventis) is a relatively new and more costly drug being used when uric acid levels cannot be lowered efficiently or quickly enough with standard approaches. It is a recombinant urate oxidase enzyme that converts circulating uric acid into a water-soluble metabolite, therefore quickly decreasing both plasma and urinary uric acid levels (Krishnan & Hammad, 2006; Ueng, 2005). The U.S. Food and Drug Administration has approved rasburicase for use in the management of hyperuricemia in *pediatric* patients who are receiving chemotherapy for leukemia, lymphoma, or solid tumors and are anticipated to develop tumor lysis and elevated uric acid levels (Sanofi-Aventis, 2007). *Adult* use of this drug is being investigated in the United States and has already shown effectiveness in other places such as Europe, Canada, and Australia (Krishnan & Hammad). Rasburicase is given at 0.15–0.20 mg/kg IV as a single daily dose for five days starting 4–24 hours prior to chemotherapy. It should be given as an infusion over 30 minutes and should not be administered as a bolus (Sanofi-Aventis).

When patients are receiving rasburicase, nurses should be aware that only one course of treatment is recommended, and results often are seen in decreasing uric acid levels as soon as four hours after administration. Patients receiving rasburicase do not need urine alkalinization prior to use. A risk of anaphylactic reaction is present with each dose, so appropriate medications should be at the bedside and the patient monitored closely. Although generally well tolerated, additional side effects may include headache, nausea and vomiting, fever, abdominal pain with diarrhea or constipation, mucositis, and rash. The use of rasburicase in patients with a glucose-6-phosphate dehydrogenase (G6PD) deficiency is contraindicated because of the risk of severe hemolysis. Patients considered to be at high risk for G6PD deficiency (i.e., patients of African or Mediterranean ancestry) may need to be screened for this deficiency prior to the use of rasburicase (Gobel, 2005; Sanofi-Aventis, 2007; Ueng, 2005). Measures should be taken to place blood specimens for testing of uric acid levels immediately on ice after the initiation of rasburicase in order to prevent the breakdown of uric acid in the specimen, which results in inaccurate laboratory results (Sanofi-Aventis; Vachani, 2006).

Control of Electrolyte Disturbances Associated With Tumor Lysis Syndrome

Hyperkalemia can be a very serious electrolyte disturbance causing irregular cardiac rhythms and neuromuscular dysfunctions, especially when it develops in conjunction with oliguria or anuria. Therefore, careful monitoring and prompt treatment of elevated potassium levels should be initiated as soon as possible. Refer to the section on treatment of hyperkalemia for management recommendations. Alkalinization of urine, as previously discussed, also will help to neutralize the effects of hyperkalemia. Hyperphosphatemia can be managed with oral phosphate binders, such as phosphate-binding antacids, or aluminum antacid gels, such as aluminum hydroxide, which will form an insoluble complex that is then excreted by the bowel. Hypertonic infusions of glucose and insulin, as used in the treatment of hyperkalemia, also may help to lower severely elevated phosphate levels (Gobel, 2005; Krishnan

& Hammad, 2006). Medications containing phosphate should be discontinued, and phosphate-rich foods may be restricted. Close monitoring of electrolytes, especially calcium levels with hyperphosphatemia, is critical because of the reciprocal relationship of calcium and phosphorus.

Hypocalcemia often will resolve itself as hyperphosphatemia is corrected. Concurrent diuretic therapy for TLS helps to promote the excretion of phosphorus, thereby aiding in the normalization of calcium levels. Krishnan and Hammad (2006) recommended that hypocalcemia not be corrected unless evidence of neuromuscular irritability exists. If it is necessary to treat specific hypocalcemia, refer to the section on hypocalcemia for treatment recommendations.

In cases of acute renal failure or severe or persistent electrolyte abnormalities, hemodialysis should be initiated promptly. Dialysis most often is temporary and will help to avoid irreversible renal failure. Critical parameters that may indicate the need for dialysis include levels of potassium greater than 6 mEq/L, phosphate greater than 10 mg/dl, or uric acid greater than 10 mg/dl (Myers, 2007). Persistent hyperkalemia and hyperphosphatemia, fluid overload, uremia, and symptomatic hypocalcemia also can be critical indications for dialysis (Krishnan & Hammad, 2006).

Expected Outcomes

TLS, if treated promptly, can be managed and the sequelae reversed. However, prevention of TLS is the main goal, and oncology nurses play a critical role in the detection and prevention of TLS. Thorough assessments, close laboratory monitoring, knowledge of signs and symptoms related to the hallmark electrolyte disturbances of TLS, and identification of high-risk patients are all critical in preventing TLS. Working with other members of the healthcare team to screen patients and initiate prophylactic treatments can aid in the prevention of this oncologic emergency.

Patient Teaching Points

Refer to Figure 12-16 for teaching points related to TLS.

FIGURE 12-16	Teaching Points for Tumor Lysis Syndrome

- Diet history: Patients may need to be on a renal diet low in potassium and phosphorus. Potassium-rich foods include oranges, bananas, orange juice, tomatoes, and chocolate; foods with phosphorus include milk, meat, cheese, eggs, bread, fish, nuts, poultry, legumes, cereal, chocolate, and carbonated drinks (Doane & Gobel, 2004).
- Medication history: Avoid medications high in potassium (e.g., potassium-sparing diuretics), phosphate (e.g., clindamycin), or those that have a propensity to increase uric acid levels (e.g., thiazide diuretics, aspirin).
- Nurses should be aware of nephrotoxic agents, such as amphotericin B, aminoglycoside antibiotics, or nonsteroidal anti-inflammatory drugs, which may need to be avoided in high-risk patients.
- Explain the need for aggressive hydration before and after chemotherapy treatments.
- Closely monitor intake and output; teach symptoms of fluid overload such as shortness of breath, peripheral edema, distended neck veins, and "rattling" in lungs.
- Use of allopurinol as directed: Patients should be instructed on the importance of following the medication regimen. Foods high in purine, such as organ meats, sardines in oil, salmon, scallops, anchovies, fish roes, mincemeat, and meat extracts, may need to be avoided while taking allopurinol.

Note. Based on information from Spratto & Woods, 2004.

Conclusion of Case Study

T.C. is most at risk for TLS. He is about to receive chemotherapy for a highly proliferative malignancy of AML. He is already dehydrated, has poor urine output, and an elevated BUN and creatinine, potentially indicating poor renal function, as well as having elevated LDH and uric acid levels. The first response would be to give T.C. aggressive hydration with isotonic or hypotonic IV fluids to restore hydration status, encourage renal blood flow, and decrease acidic concentration of the urine. Strict I&O should be maintained along with frequent vital sign monitoring to detect any early signs of TLS. Oral or IV allopurinol should be initiated one to two days prior to chemotherapy administration and continue for up to two to three days following chemotherapy. Electrolytes should be checked frequently along with BUN, creatinine, LDH, and uric acid levels. Nurses should be particularly aware of the signs and symptoms of developing hyperkalemia, hypophosphatemia, hyperuricemia, and hypocalcemia, the hallmark signs of TLS. Initiation of preventive measures, thorough patient assessment, and knowledge related to the risks and identifying symptoms of TLS are all critical in providing quality patient care for the prevention and successful treatment of TLS.

Conclusion

Oncology nurses need to understand the dynamic balance in the body that exists with electrolytes, their importance in cellular function, and their metabolic implications of function throughout the entire body. In patients with cancer, who may also be suffering from numerous side effects of the disease and the treatment modalities, oncology nurses must be aware of preventive measures and high-risk situations that patients may encounter throughout their disease management that could put them at risk for electrolyte imbalances, TLS, or SIADH. It is critical for oncology nurses to be aware of the indicators, preventive measures, assessment tools, and treatment modalities discussed in this chapter. Patient education should be provided at the time of diagnosis and frequently reviewed and revised as necessary as patients progress through their treatment. Nurses are vital in identifying the risks, signs, and symptoms that may indicate an electrolyte imbalance or emergency, providing treatment and support, and instructing patients with cancer about electrolyte imbalances.

References

Agraharkar, M., Workeneh, B., & Fahlen, M. (2006, May). *Hypermagnesemia.* Retrieved April 15, 2008, from http://www.emedicine.com/med/TOPIC3383.htm

Amini, A., & Schmidt, M. (2004). Syndrome of inappropriate secretion of antidiuretic hormone and hyponatremia after spinal surgery. *Neurosurgical Focus Journal, 16*(4), E10. Retrieved August 3, 2007, from http://www.medscape.com/viewarticle/474907_3

Beach, C. (2007). *Hypocalcemia.* Retrieved February 25, 2008, from http://www.emedicine.com/emerg/Topic271.htm

Berendt, M.C., & D'Agostino, S. (2005). Alterations in nutrition: Electrolyte imbalances. In J.K. Itano & K.N. Taoka (Eds.), *Core curriculum for oncology nursing* (4th ed., pp. 300–306). St. Louis, MO: Elsevier Saunders.

Berk, L., & Rana, S. (2006, March). Hypovolemia and dehydration in the oncology patient. *Journal of Supportive Oncology, 4*(9), 447–454.

Cope, D. (2004). Tumor lysis syndrome. *Clinical Journal of Oncology Nursing, 8*(4), 415–416.

Craig, S. (2007, January). *Hyponatremia.* Retrieved August 2, 2007, from http://www.emedicine.com/emerg/topic275.htm

Del Toro, G., Morris, E., & Cairo, M.S. (2005). Tumor lysis syndrome: Pathophysiology, definition, and alternative treatment approaches. *Clinical Advances in Hematology and Oncology, 3*(1), 54–61.

Doane, L., & Gobel, B. (2004, May). *Tumor lysis syndrome: Pathophysiology, signs, and symptoms.* Paper presented at the Oncology Nursing Society 29th Annual Congress, Anaheim, CA. Abstract retrieved June 19, 2007, from http://www.ons.org/publications/journals/pdfs/spotlight43.pdf

Ezzone, S. (2000). Syndrome of inappropriate antidiuretic hormone. In D. Camp-Sorrell & R. Hawkins (Eds.), *Clinical manual for the oncology advanced practice nurse* (pp. 571–575). Pittsburgh, PA: Oncology Nursing Society.

Flounders, J.A. (2003). *Syndrome of inappropriate antidiuretic hormone* [Online exclusive]. *Oncology Nursing Forum, 30*(3), E63–E70. Retrieved July 2, 2007, from http://www.ons.org/publications/journals/ONF/Volume30/Issue3/3003381.asp

Garth, D. (2007, February). *Hyperkalemia.* Retrieved April 16, 2008, from http://www.emedicine.com/EMERG/topic261.htm

Gobel, B. (2005). Metabolic emergencies: Tumor lysis syndrome, hypercalcemia, and syndrome of inappropriate secretion of antidiuretic hormone. In J.K. Itano & K.N. Taoka (Eds.), *Core curriculum for oncology nursing* (4th ed., pp. 395–412). St. Louis, MO: Elsevier Saunders.

Handy, B., & Shen, Y. (2005). Evaluation of potassium values in a cancer patient population. *Laboratory Medicine, 36*(2), 95–97.

Hemphill, R. (2006, May). *Hypercalcemia.* Retrieved July 9, 2007, from http://www.emedicine.com/emerg/topic260.htm

Hollander-Rodriguez, J., & Calvert, J. (2006, January). Hyperkalemia. *American Family Physician, 73*(2), 283–289.

Kaplow, R. (2002). Clinical Q&A: Intravenous allopurinol. *Clinical Journal of Oncology Nursing, 6*(2), 110.

Keenan, A. (2005). Syndrome of inappropriate antidiuretic hormone. In C.H. Yarbro, M.H. Frogge, & M. Goodman (Eds.), *Cancer nursing: Principles and practice* (6th ed., pp. 940–945). Sudbury, MA: Jones and Bartlett.

Keenan, A.K.M., & Wickham, R. (2005). Hypercalcemia. In C.H. Yarbro, M.H. Frogge, & M. Goodman (Eds.), *Cancer nursing: Principles and practice* (6th ed., pp. 791–807). Sudbury, MA: Jones and Bartlett.

Konstantakos, A., & Grisoni, E. (2006, May). *Hypomagnesemia.* Retrieved March 12, 2008, from http://www.emedicine.com/ped/topic1122.htm

Krishnan, K., & Hammad, A. (2006, December). *Tumor lysis syndrome.* Retrieved September 14, 2007, from http://www.emedicine.com/MED/topic2327.htm

Lederer, E., Ouseph, R., & Yazel, L. (2007, March). *Hypokalemia.* Retrieved April 16, 2008, from http://www.emedicine.com/MED/topic1124.htm

Lydon, J. (2005). Tumor lysis syndrome. In C.H. Yarbro, M.H. Frogge, & M. Goodman (Eds.), *Cancer nursing: Principles and practice* (6th ed., pp. 947–958). Sudbury, MA: Jones and Bartlett.

Mato, A.R., Miltiades, A.N., Guo, M., Heitjan, D.F., Carroll, M.P., Loren, A.W., et al. (2006). Reproducibility of the Penn predictive score of tumor lysis syndrome (PPS-TLS) in acute myelogenous leukemia (AML) [Abstract]. *Proceedings of the American Society of Clinical Oncology Annual Meeting, 24*(Suppl. 18), Abstract No. 6577.

MedlinePlus. (2005). *Medical encyclopedia: Hyponatremia.* Retrieved July 23, 2007, from http://www.nlm.nih.gov/medlineplus/ency/article/000394.htm

MedlinePlus. (2007, February). *Medical encyclopedia: Chem-20.* Retrieved July 24, 2007, from http://www.nlm.nih.gov/medlineplus/ency/article/003468.htm

Myers, J. (2007). Complications of cancer and cancer treatment: Hypercalcemia. In M. Langhorne, J. Fulton, & S. Otto (Eds.), *Oncology nursing* (5th ed., pp. 402–453). St Louis, MO: Elsevier Mosby.

National Cancer Institute. (2005). *Hypercalcemia (PDQ®).* Retrieved August 13, 2007, from http://www.cancer.gov/cancertopics/pdq/supportivecare/hypercalcemia/healthprofessional/allpages

Novello, N., & Blumstein, H. (2007a, October). *Hypermagnesemia.* Retrieved April 15, 2008, from http://www.emedicine.com/EMERG/topic262.htm

Novello, N., & Blumstein, H. (2007b, October). *Hypomagnesemia.* Retrieved March 12, 2008, from http://www.emedicine.com/emerg/topic274.htm

Rafailov, A., & Sinert, R. (2007, May). *Syndrome of inappropriate antidiuretic hormone secretion.* Retrieved August 2, 2007, from http://www.emedicine.com/emerg/topic784.htm

Sanofi-Aventis. (2007). Elitek [Package insert]. Bridgewater, NJ: Author.

Shuey, K.M., & Brant, J.M. (2004). Hypercalcemia of malignancy: Part II. *Clinical Journal of Oncology Nursing, 8*(3), 321–323.

Skugor, M., & Milas, M. (2004). *Hypocalcemia: The Cleveland Clinic Disease Management Project.* Retrieved July 9, 2007, from http://www.clevelandclinicmeded.com/medicalpubs/diseasemanagement/endocrinology/hypocal/hypocal.htm

Smith, W. (2000a). Hypocalcemia/hypercalcemia. In D. Camp-Sorrell & R. Hawkins (Eds.), *Clinical manual for the oncology advanced practice nurse* (pp. 849–858). Pittsburgh, PA: Oncology Nursing Society.

Smith, W. (2000b). Hypokalemia/hyperkalemia. In D. Camp-Sorrell & R. Hawkins (Eds.), *Clinical manual for the oncology advanced practice nurse* (pp. 859–867). Pittsburgh, PA: Oncology Nursing Society.

Smith, W. (2000c). Hypomagnesemia/hypermagnesemia. In D. Camp-Sorrell & R. Hawkins (Eds.), *Clinical manual for the oncology advanced practice nurse* (pp. 869–873). Pittsburgh, PA: Oncology Nursing Society.

Smith, W., & Baird-Powell, S. (2000). Hyponatremia/hypernatremia. In D. Camp-Sorrell & R. Hawkins (Eds.), *Clinical manual for the oncology advanced practice nurse* (pp. 875–881). Pittsburgh, PA: Oncology Nursing Society.

Spratto, G., & Woods, A. (2004). Allopurinol. In *PDR®: Nurse's drug handbook* (2004 ed., pp. 30–33). New York: Thomson Delmar Learning.

Stephanides, S. (2007, August). *Hypernatremia.* Retrieved August 9, 2007, from http://www.emedicine.com/emerg/TOPIC263.htm

Stoppler, M. (2008, March). *Hyperkalemia.* Retrieved April 16, 2008, from http://www.medicinenet.com/hyperkalemia/article.htm

Suneja, M., Muster, H.A., & Pegoraro, A.A. (2008, January). *Hypocalcemia.* Retrieved February 26, 2008, from http://www.emedicine.com/med/topic1118.htm

Ueng, S. (2005). Rasburicase (Elitek): A novel agent for tumor lysis syndrome. *Baylor University Medical Center Proceedings Journal, 18*(3), 275–279.

University of Iowa. (2007). *Fluid and electrolyte: Diagnosis and management; disorders of sodium concentration.* Retrieved August 3, 2007, from http://www.int-med.uiowa.edu/patients/bonemarrow/healthpro/fluidelectrolyte/sodium.htm

Vachani, C. (2006, April). *Tumor lysis syndrome.* Retrieved November 1, 2007, from http://www.oncolink.org/resources/article.cfm?c=16&s=46&ss=205&id=886

Warrell, R. (2001). Metabolic emergencies. In V.T. DeVita Jr., S. Hellman, & S.A. Rosenberg (Eds.), *Cancer: Principles and practice of oncology* (6th ed., pp. 2633–2645). Philadelphia: Lippincott Williams & Wilkins.

CHAPTER 13

Cancer-Related Fatigue

Sandra A. Mitchell, PhD, CRNP, AOCN®

Case Study

J.B. is a single 46-year-old African American woman admitted for vertebroplasty and to receive her first cycle of chemotherapy (vincristine, doxorubicin [Adriamycin®, Bedford Laboratories], dexamethasone [VAD]) for newly diagnosed stage IIIA IgG kappa multiple myeloma complicated by compression fractures of thoracic vertebrae T4–T8. She has severe bone pain, which is currently well managed with controlled-release narcotic agents. After four cycles of VAD chemotherapy given at monthly intervals, if her disease response is satisfactory, the plan is for her to receive high-dose melphalan chemotherapy followed by autologous peripheral blood stem cell transplantation.

With the new diagnosis of multiple myeloma, she admits to feeling anxious, fearful, and somewhat discouraged, and she is tearful as she discusses her concerns. She is worried about how she will maintain her job and health insurance, given the anticipated need for intensive treatment over several months. She is sleeping poorly because of the stress of the diagnosis and hospitalization, pain, and sleep disruptions resulting from treatment with dexamethasone. She tells the oncology nurse that her most bothersome issues are difficulty sleeping and severe fatigue. She rates the severity of her fatigue as an 8 on a 0–10 scale, where higher values indicate more severe fatigue. In gathering a history, the nurse learns that the fatigue had predated her diagnosis for approximately three to four months, and excessive fatigue was one of the reasons she had originally presented to her primary care provider for evaluation. On examination, she is mildly cachectic, with point tenderness of the spine in the thoracic region. Laboratory data reveal a hemoglobin level of 9.4 g/dl and a serum creatinine level of 1.7 g/dl.

Overview

Cancer-related fatigue (CRF) is recognized as one of the most common symptoms in patients receiving treatment for cancer, often persisting beyond the conclusion of active treatment and at the end of life (Mystakidou, Parpa, Katsouda, Galanos, & Vlahos, 2006; Prue, Rankin, Allen, Gracey, & Cramp, 2006). Longitudinal and comparative studies indicate that fatigue also may be a significant problem for cancer survivors, with many survivors reporting fatigue scores higher than that of an age-matched general population (Braun, Greenberg, & Pirl, 2008). Depending upon how fatigue is defined and measured, prevalence estimates of fatigue vary from 25%–99% (Lawrence, Kupelnick, Miller, Devine, & Lau, 2004; Servaes, Verhagen, & Bleijenberg, 2002b). A survey of more than 500 patients and nearly 100 clinicians found that across all cancer types, fatigue was ranked as the most important symptom or concern (Butt, Rosenbloom, et al., 2008). Fatigue may occur both as an isolated symptom and as one element in a cluster of symptoms, such as depression, pain, sleep disturbance, and menopausal symptoms (Beck, Dudley, & Barsevick, 2005; Bender, Ergyn, Rosenzweig, Cohen, & Sereika, 2005; Chow, Fan, Hadi, & Filipczak, 2007; Francoeur, 2005; Glaus et al., 2006; Walsh & Rybicki, 2006).

Fatigue is distressing to patients and has adverse effects on functional status, mood, and well-being. Studies suggest that CRF is a multifaceted condition characterized by diminished energy and an increased need to rest, disproportionate to any recent change in activity level, and accompanied by a range of other characteristics, including generalized weakness, diminished mental concentration, insomnia or hypersomnia, and emotional reactivity (Cella, Peterman, Passik, Jacobsen, & Breitbart, 1998). Consequences of CRF include decrements in physical, social, and vocational functioning (Curt, 2000; Curt & Johnston, 2003; de Jong, Candel, Schouten, Abu-Saad, & Courtens, 2006; Mallinson, Cella, Cashy, & Holzner, 2006), mood (Dimeo et al., 2004), and sleep disturbances (Andrykowski, Curran, & Lightner, 1998; Lindqvist, Widmark, & Rasmussen, 2004; Magnusson, Moller, Ekman, & Wallgren, 1999), as well as emotional and spiritual distress for both the patients and their family members (Magnusson et al.; Mystakidou et al., 2006; Servaes, Verhagen, & Bleijenberg, 2002a; Wang et al., 2002).

Despite its prevalence, consequences, and importance to patients and those who care for them, published reports suggest that fatigue is underrecognized and undertreated, perhaps in part because patients may hesitate to discuss fatigue treatment options with their healthcare team (Vogelzang et al., 1997) or may be unaware of interventions that have shown to be effective in the management of fatigue (Passik et al., 2002). Improved communication between patients and the healthcare team about CRF (Butt, Wagner, et al., 2008) and efforts to reduce the barriers clinicians encounter in translating evidence-based fatigue interventions into clinical practice (Borneman et al., 2007) are critical to improving clinical outcomes for patients with CRF.

Although a universally accepted definition of CRF does not exist, the National Comprehensive Cancer Network (NCCN) defines CRF as a distressing, persistent, and subjective sense of tiredness or exhaustion that is not proportional to recent activity and interferes with usual functioning (NCCN, 2008). Based on the defined criteria for the diagnosis of CRF (see Figure 13-1), CRF is of a markedly different quality and severity from ordinary fatigue, adversely affects function, and is unrelieved by rest or sleep (Cella, Lai, Chang, Peterman, & Slavin, 2002). To make the diagnosis of CRF, fatigue must be persistent and accompanied by associated symptoms such as increasing need for rest, limb heaviness, diminished concentration, inertia, emotional lability, and postexertional malaise. One must also be fairly certain that the underlying cause is cancer or its treatment.

The etiology and clinical expression of CRF are multidimensional. An inherently subjective condition, fatigue may be experienced and reported differently by each individual. Qualitative studies of fatigue underscore the fact that the cancer fatigue experience is unlike any other fatigue patients have previously experienced, and patients emphasize that its unpredictability and refractoriness to previously effective self-management strategies make it a particularly distressing symptom (Glaus, Crow, & Hammond, 1996; Wu & McSweeney, 2007). Personality and coping style also may influence the experience of CRF (Andrykowski, Schmidt, Salsman, Beacham, & Jacobsen, 2005). Some patients complain of a loss of efficiency, mental fogginess, inertia, and that sleep is not restorative, whereas others describe an excessive need to rest, the inability to recover promptly from exertion, or muscle heaviness and weakness. Further research is needed to determine whether these represent variable features of

FIGURE 13-1	**International Classification of Diseases, 10th Edition (ICD-10) Proposed Criteria for Cancer-Related Fatigue**

A. Six (or more) of the following symptoms have been present every day or nearly every day during the same 2-week period in the past month, and at least one of the symptoms is (1) significant fatigue.
   1. Significant fatigue, diminished energy, or increased need to rest, disproportionate to any recent change in activity level;
   2. Complaints of generalized weakness or limb heaviness;
   3. Diminished concentration or attention;
   4. Decreased motivation or interest to engage in usual activities;
   5. Insomnia or hypersomnia;
   6. Experience of sleep as unrefreshing or nonrestorative;
   7. Perceived need to struggle to overcome inactivity;
   8. Marked emotional reactivity (e.g., sadness, frustration, irritability) to feeling fatigued;
   9. Difficulty completing daily tasks attributed to feeling fatigued;
   10. Perceived problems with short-term memory;
   11. Post-exertional malaise lasting several hours;
B. The symptoms cause clinically significant distress or impairment in social, occupational, or other important areas of functioning.
C. There is evidence from the history, physical examination, or laboratory findings that the symptoms are a consequence of cancer or cancer therapy.
D. The symptoms are not primarily a consequence of co-morbid psychiatric disorders such as major depression, somatization disorder, somatoform disorder, or delirium.

Note. From "Progress Toward Guidelines for the Management of Fatigue," by D. Cella, A. Peterman, S. Passik, P. Jacobsen, and W. Breitbart, 1998, *Oncology, 12*(11A), p. 374. Copyright 1998 by CMPMedica LLC. Reprinted with permission.

fatigue, suggest the presence of fatigue subtypes, or are the cause or sequelae of fatigue (Sadler et al., 2002; Tchekmedyian, Kallich, McDermott, Fayers, & Erder, 2003). Efforts continue to be directed toward clarifying the defining features of fatigue (Jacobsen, Donovan, & Weitzner, 2003) and determining how CRF can be distinguished from syndromes, such as depression, cognitive dysfunction, or asthenia, that have overlapping symptoms (Capuron et al., 2002; Hinshaw, Carnahan, & Johnson, 2002; Lai et al., 2005; Reuter & Harter, 2004; Valentine & Meyers, 2001; Van Belle et al., 2005) or may share neurophysiologic mechanisms (Bower, Ganz, & Aziz, 2005; Lee et al., 2004).

A large body of research describes the relationships between the occurrence and severity of CRF and treatment type, stage of tumor, time since treatment completion, and clinical and demographic factors. However, because of the variability in the association between CRF and disease- and treatment-related variables, few conclusions can be drawn (Prue et al., 2006). Understanding is further limited by the fact that although fatigue symptoms are known to fluctuate across the course of cancer treatment, much of the research has been conducted using cross-sectional study designs. Despite these limitations, the literature suggests that 40%–90% of patients undergoing chemotherapy or radiation therapy experience fatigue (Lawrence et al., 2004; Prue et al.; Ryan et al., 2007).

Longitudinal studies suggest that in patients receiving cyclic chemotherapy, fatigue is most severe during the first three days after chemotherapy is administered and gradually improves until approximately the next treatment cycle. During a course of fractionated radiation therapy, fatigue is often cumulative, and its peak of severity may occur after radiation is concluded. Severe fatigue is almost universal with the use of biologic response modifiers, including interferon alfa and the interleukins (ILs), and following autologous or allogeneic hematopoietic stem cell transplantation. Little is known, however, concerning the prevalence of fatigue in patients receiving molecularly targeted agents such as tyrosine kinase inhibitors and agents that promote apoptosis. Moreover, the trajectory of fatigue experienced by individuals undergoing surgery for cancer has not been well characterized. Little consistent association between treatment-related variables, such as dose intensity, radiation fractionation schedule, and time since treatment completion, has been observed (Prue et al., 2006).

The correlates of fatigue also appear to vary across the disease trajectory. For example, during active cancer treatment, fatigue has been shown to correlate with the presence of other distressing symptoms, such as pain, sleep disturbances, dyspnea, and anorexia (Davis, Khoshknabi, & Yue, 2006; Yennurajalingam, Palmer, Zhang, Poulter, & Bruera, 2008). In cancer survivors, an association between depression or psychological distress and fatigue has been demonstrated; however, in patients who are in the terminal phases of their disease, fatigue was not associated with depression. Associations between the occurrence and severity of CRF and demographic variables such as sex, age, marital status, and employment status have not been consistently identified. Studies suggest that fatigue may be related to anemia, mood disorder, concurrent symptoms such as pain, sleep disturbances, electrolyte disturbances, cardiopulmonary, hepatic or renal dysfunction, hypothyroidism, hypogonadism, adrenal insufficiency, infection, malnutrition, deconditioning, and the sedative side effects of drugs that act on the central nervous system, such as opioid analgesics, benzodiazepines, or anticonvulsants (Iop, Manfredi, & Bonura, 2004; Morrow, Shelke, Roscoe, Hickok, & Mustian, 2005; Nail, 2002, 2004; Servaes et al., 2002b; Stasi, Abriani, Beccaglia, Terzoli, & Amadori, 2003; Strasser et al., 2006; Tavio, Milan, & Tirelli, 2002; Wagner & Cella, 2004). A number of metabolic and endocrine disorders can exacerbate CRF, including hypothyroidism, hypogonadism, adrenal insufficiency, hypercalcemia, hypomagnesemia, and dehydration (Strasser et al.). Cancer anorexia-cachexia and resultant protein-calorie malnutrition leads to increased proteolysis in skeletal muscles, producing muscle wasting, weakness/asthenia, and reduced endurance (Kalman & Villani, 1997).

Accumulated evidence also suggests that gene polymorphisms, altered circadian rhythmicity, immune dysregulation, and proinflammatory cytokine activity may directly or indirectly contribute to CRF (Ancoli-Israel et al., 2006; Berger, Farr, Kuhn, Fischer, & Agrawal, 2007; Bower, Ganz, Dickerson, et al., 2005; Collado-Hidalgo, Bower, Ganz, Cole, & Irwin, 2006; Fernandes, Stone, Andrews, Morgan, & Sharma, 2006; Massacesi et al., 2006; Schubert, Hong, Natarajan, Mills, & Dimsdale, 2007; Wood, Nail, Gilster, Winters, & Elsea, 2006). Factors associated with CRF are listed in Figure 13-2.

FIGURE 13-2   Etiologic Factors for Cancer-Related Fatigue

- Underlying disease
- Cancer treatment
- Anemia
- Hypothyroidism
- Adrenal insufficiency
- Hypogonadism
- Infection
- Malnutrition
- Depletion of vitamins B_1, B_6, and B_{12}
- Electrolyte disturbances (calcium, magnesium, phosphorus)
- Cardiopulmonary, hepatic, or renal dysfunction
- Deconditioning
- Generalized inflammation
- Side effects of medications that act on central nervous system (e.g., narcotics, anxiolytics, antiemetics)
- Concurrent symptoms (e.g., pain, dyspnea)
- Impaired sleep quality
- Psychological distress (depression, anxiety)

Note. Based on information from Radbruch et al., 2008.

Pathophysiology

The precise pathophysiology of CRF is poorly understood. In some instances, fatigue is temporally related to treatment and resolves after its completion. However, fatigue also may persist for months or even years after treatment concludes. In any one individual, the etiology of CRF is likely to be multifactorial, and across the disease trajectory, the relative contribution of each etiology will fluctuate.

Although study findings are not consistent, perhaps in part because of the challenges in studying the mechanisms of fatigue in humans (Andrews, Morrow, Hickok, Roscoe, & Stone, 2004), evidence suggests that elevated circulating levels of inflammatory cytokines are one of the major contributing factors to fatigue. Elevated concentrations of inflammatory cytokines such as IL-1 receptor antagonist, IL-6, and neopterin in association with fatigue have been described in patients receiving chemotherapy and radiation therapy and in long-term survivors (Schubert et al., 2007). The precise mechanisms by which proinflammatory cytokines initiate or promote CRF are a topic of continued study, but evidence suggests that a proinflammatory state may lead to fatigue by alteration of muscle metabolism, dysregulation of the hypothalamic-pituitary-adrenal (HPA) axis, and via direct effects on the mechanisms of arousal within the central nervous system (Gutstein, 2001; Miller, Ancoli-Israel, Bower, Capuron, & Irwin, 2008). The concept of *sickness behavior* may be particularly relevant to understanding the link between proinflammatory cytokine elevations, arousal and affect, and CRF (Dantzer, O'Connor, Freund, Johnson, & Kelley, 2008; Johnson, 2002; Miller, 2003). The indicators of sickness behavior include a loss of energy and motivation, changes in sleep and appetite, and a decrease in exploratory and mating behaviors. During recovery from acute inflammation, such as occurs with infection, sickness behavior is part of an adaptive motivational state that focuses the organism's priorities on recovery. However, in patients whose immune system is chronically activated, sickness behavior may be among the pathophysiologic mechanisms for CRF. In support of the importance of sickness behavior in CRF is the fact that proinflammatory cytokines also play a role in cachexia, anemia, sleep disturbances, depression, fever, and infection, all of which can worsen fatigue (Jacobsen et al., 2003; Kurzrock, 2001).

Proinflammatory cytokines also result in altered serotonin metabolism within the brain, and serotonin is involved in many biologic processes, including muscle contraction. Alterations in synaptic levels of serotonin or in serotonin receptor function within the brain have been associated with a reduction in the capacity for voluntary activation of muscle and the sensation of a reduced capacity to perform physical work (Jager, Sleijfer, & van der Rijt, 2008). It may be, then, that serotonin dysregulation is a contributing factor to CRF and perhaps is responsible for the sensation of muscular weakness or the sense that greater effort is required to accomplish a task, which many patients with CRF describe (Ryan et al., 2007).

Disturbed sleep also may be an intermediary factor that explains the relationship between CRF and one or more of the mechanisms discussed previously, including disruptions in the HPA axis and circadian rhythms, serotonin metabolism, and proinflammatory cytokine expression. Studies suggest that cancer and its therapy dysregulate the HPA axis and adversely affect the secretion of corticotropin-releasing hormone (Ryan et al., 2007). Changes in this essential neuroendocrine hormonal milieu can impair several aspects of sleep, including depth of sleep, slow-wave sleep, rapid eye movement sleep, and waking (Parker et al., 2008). These adverse changes in sleep architecture act together with psychological stressors to produce significant sleep disturbances in patients with cancer (Akechi et al., 2007).

Altered energy metabolism within skeletal muscle also has been postulated as a cause of CRF. Substances in the muscle, including calcium, potassium, hydrogen adenosine diphosphate, and adenosine triphosphate (ATP), all affect skeletal muscle energy metabolism, thereby influencing the ability of the muscle to perform mechanical work. Cancer, its treatment with chemotherapy and radiation therapy, and any resulting anemia or cachexia may contribute directly or indirectly to altered skeletal muscle energy metabolism and to reductions in the capacity for muscle contraction via the accumulation of metabolites, deprivation of nutrients, the disruption of mitochondrial synthesis of ATP, or diminished oxygen delivery to muscle cells.

Several different conceptual models of the pathophysiology of CRF have been proposed. Although many of these models use similar constructs, the models can be differentiated based on the extent to which they emphasize fatigue as caused by disturbances in energy balance, stress responses, or neuroendocrine regulation. Energy balance/energy analysis models depict energy as the major variable in fatigue and propose that alterations in the balance among intake, metabolism, and expenditure of energy are factors in producing fatigue. Examples of this thematic group of models include Piper's integrated fatigue model (Piper, Lindsey, & Dodd, 1987), Irvine's energy analysis model (Irvine, Vincent, Graydon, Bubela, & Thompson, 1994), and Winningham's psychobiologic-entropy model (Winningham, 2001). Models that postulate fatigue as a response to stress posit that tiredness, fatigue, and exhaustion form an adaptational continuum of response to stress. Each state along this continuum from tiredness to exhaustion can be distinguished by different behavioral and symptom patterns. Examples of models in this thematic class include fatigue models proposed by Aistars (1987), Rhoten (1982), Glaus (1998), and Olson (2007). Lastly, neuroendocrine regulatory fatigue models hypothesize that the multiple dimensions of fatigue are explained by dysregulation in the functioning of the regulatory systems controlling the neurologic, endocrine, and immune systems, including the HPA axis, circadian rhythms, and neuroimmune system transmitter secretion and function (Miller et al., 2008). Examples of fatigue models based on neuroendocrine dysregulation include those proposed by Lee et al. (2004); Payne (2004); Morrow, Andrews, Hickok, Roscoe, and Matteson (2002); and Schubert et al. (2007). These conceptual models may be helpful in generating testable hypotheses for continued research into the problem of CRF and in guiding the development and evaluation of interventions to limit and manage fatigue and to reduce its deleterious impact on health-related quality of life.

Assessment

Identifying patients who are experiencing CRF is the first step in improving fatigue evaluation and management. Studies suggest that CRF is underdiagnosed, that assessment of fatigue in patients with cancer is suboptimal, and that healthcare professionals may not fully appreciate the degree of distress and functional loss that fatigue produces (Hockenberry-Eaton & Hinds, 2000; Knowles, Borthwick, McNamara, Miller, & Leggot, 2000; Vogelzang et al., 1997). Identified barriers to communication between patients and their clinicians about fatigue include the clinicians' failure to offer interventions (47%), patients' lack of awareness of effective treatments for fatigue (43%), patients' desire to treat fatigue without medications (40%), and patients' tendency to be stoic about fatigue to avoid being labeled as a "complainer" (28%) (Curt, 2000; Passik et al., 2002).

Assessment of CRF includes two aspects: (a) routine, periodic screening of all patients to identify the presence of CRF and gauge its severity, and (b) detailed evaluation of the characteristics, consequences, and potential contributing factors in patients with moderate or severe CRF. A wide range of approaches to the assessment of CRF exist in the literature, including single items that gauge fatigue severity; single items or subscales relevant to fatigue and drawn from measures of quality of life, psychosocial adjustment, mood, or self-reported health status; and instruments that were designed specifically to evaluate CRF from a multidimensional perspective.

Although no consensus currently exists concerning the optimal method or frequency to screen for CRF in the clinical or research setting (Davis, Lai, Hahn, & Cella, 2008), evidence of the widespread occurrence of CRF supports a conclusion that routine screening for CRF should occur at regular intervals throughout treatment, follow-up, and long-term follow-up. Accumulating evidence demonstrates that single-item measures to screen for fatigue are rapid and sensitive and can be applied efficiently in the clinic to identify patients who would benefit from more systematic evaluation (Danjoux, Gardner, & Fitch, 2007; Hwang, Chang, & Kasimis, 2003; Kirsh, Passik, Holtsclaw, Donaghy, & Theobald, 2001; Temel, Pirl, Recklitis, Cashavelly, & Lynch, 2006). In screening for fatigue in the clinic, consideration also must be given to the response frame (e.g., past 24 hours, past 7 days, past month) that has the most clinical relevance for a specific patient population and would be least affected by biases of recall or by transient changes in CRF severity. Streamlined approaches to screening may be offered by new technologies that use electronic or Web-based applications and emphasize real-time assessments of fatigue (Hacker & Ferrans, 2007) or computer-adapted testing (Cella, Gershon, Lai, & Choi, 2007). Figure 13-3 proposes a screening measure for CRF that nurses can apply in their clinical setting to identify patients who warrant further evaluation and clinical intervention.

Although a single-item measure may provide rapid assessment of general fatigue or serve as a screening tool, evidence suggests that single-item measures do not fully capture all the dimensions of fatigue (Banthia et al., 2006). More than 20 self-report measures (including

---

FIGURE 13-3	**Screening Questions for Cancer-Related Fatigue**

1. On how many days in the past week have you felt somewhat to quite fatigued?
   ☐ None   ☐ 1–2 days   ☐ 3–5 days   ☐ More than 5 days

2. In the past week, on a scale of 0 to 10, what is the "worst" fatigue you have experienced?

None										Worst
0	1	2	3	4	5	6	7	8	9	10

Within the past week, to what extent has fatigued interfered with:

	Not at all	A little bit	Somewhat	Quite a bit	Very much
3. Performing the activities you need or want to do	0	1	2	3	4
4. Relationships with other people	0	1	2	3	4
5. Mood	0	1	2	3	4

6. Have you been experiencing any of the following symptoms during the past 7 days? Select all that apply:
   ☐ I have no symptoms.
   ☐ Pain
   ☐ Nausea
   ☐ Poor appetite
   ☐ Difficulty sleeping
   ☐ Shortness of breath
   ☐ Difficulty moving around
   ☐ Problem with bowels
   ☐ Other_____

7. Would you like to discuss your fatigue with a member of your healthcare team?
   ☐ No   ☐ Yes

single-item measures, multi-item unidimensional scales, and multidimensional inventories) have been developed to measure fatigue in patients with cancer (Mota & Pimenta, 2006; Wagner & Cella, 2001). These measures are summarized in Table 13-1.

Unidimensional fatigue measures typically focus on severity of fatigue, although multi-item unidimensional scales also may ask about the severity of other symptoms, such as exhaustion, tiredness, or weakness. Examples of unidimensional measures of fatigue include quality-of-life measures, such as the Functional Assessment of Cancer Therapy–General (FACT-G) and the European Organisation for Research and Treatment of Cancer Quality of Life Questionnaire (EORTC QLQ C-30), and measures of symptoms, health, mood state, or psychosocial adjustment, such as the Medical Outcomes Study Short Form-36 (SF-36), Profile of Mood States, Rotterdam Symptom Checklist, Brief Symptom Inventory, and Symptom Distress Scale, which includes single items that address fatigue or subscales that reflect fatigue, vigor, or vitality. In evaluating a potential measurement approach to fatigue assessment, it is important to keep in mind that other subjective descriptors such as weakness and tiredness or the absence of vigor are not necessarily equated with the measurement of fatigue.

Good consensus exists in the literature that fatigue generally consists of a sensory dimension (fatigue severity, persistence), a physiologic dimension (e.g., leg weakness, diminished mental concentration), and a performance dimension (reduction in performance of needed or valued activities). Multidimensional fatigue measures provide information about this full range of characteristics other than simply intensity. Consideration of the measurement properties and strengths and limitations of these instruments, including reliability, validity, specificity, sensitivity to change, recall period, respondent burden, translation in multiple languages, and the availability of normed values to aid interpretation, should be used to guide decisions about the utility of a measure for specific clinical or research purposes (Lai et al., 2005; Meek et al., 2000; Nail, 2002; Schwartz, 2002; Varricchio, 2000; Wu & McSweeney, 2001). Ecologic momentary assessment of fatigue (a technique that offers real-time measurement of a phenomenon as it occurs in a naturalistic setting) may overcome some of the methodologic limitations of fatigue assessment, including recall bias and the influence of current context on self-report of fatigue (Hacker & Ferrans, 2007).

The NCCN guidelines recommend that CRF be assessed using a two-tiered approach (Mock et al., 2007). First, every patient should be screened for the presence or absence of fatigue, and if present, fatigue should be assessed quantitatively on a 0–10 scale (0 = no fatigue and 10 = worst fatigue imaginable). Patients with a severity of more than 4 should be further evaluated by history and physical examination, including an evaluation of whether disease progression or recurrence could be among the causes of fatigue. Components of fatigue assessment include its presence, intensity, persistence or pervasiveness, course over time, exacerbating and relieving factors, and the impact on functioning and level of distress. Clinicians can obtain valuable information about the consequences of CRF by exploring the effects of CRF on self-esteem, mood, and the ability to perform activities of daily living, fulfill important roles as parent, spouse, and worker, and relate to family and friends. Also important to the evaluation is an assessment of what interventions the patients are using to manage their fatigue and the effectiveness of these interventions.

The presence of any treatable contributing factors, such as concurrent distressing symptoms, emotional distress, sleep disturbances, anemia, nutritional compromise, and inactivity/physical deconditioning, should be identified (Mock, 2004; Shafqat et al., 2005). Current medications (including over-the-counter medications and herbal supplements) should be reviewed to identify any agents or medication interactions that may contribute to worsening fatigue. In evaluating patients with CRF, screening for etiologic or potentiating factors is important, including hypothyroidism, hypogonadism, adrenal insufficiency, cardiomyopathy,

TABLE 13-1	Instruments to Measure Cancer-Related Fatigue				
Measure	**Dimensions of Fatigue Evaluated**	**Number of Items**	**Scaling**	**Source for More Information**	**Comments**
Brief Fatigue Inventory	Severity and impact of fatigue	9	11-point Likert scale	Mendoza et al., 1999	Available in multiple languages
Fatigue Numerical Scale	Severity of fatigue	2	100 mm linear analog scale	Okuyama et al., 2000	–
Cancer-Related Fatigue Distress Scale	Consequences of fatigue relative to physical, social, and psychospiritual distress	20	11-point Likert scale	Holley, 2000	–
Chalder Fatigue Scale	Fatigue severity, associated distress, self-efficacy for coping, and the extent to which fatigue was overwhelming, uncontrollable, unpredictable, and abnormal	7	100 mm linear analog scale	Armes et al., 2007	–
Functional Assessment of Cancer Therapy–Fatigue	Physical, affective, and cognitive dimensions of fatigue and consequences for daily functioning	13	5-point Likert scale	Yellen et al., 1997	Available in multiple languages Norms for comparison with health and cancer samples available
Cancer Fatigue Scale	Physical, affective, and cognitive dimensions of fatigue	15	5-point Likert scale	Okuyama et al., 2000	Available in multiple languages
Fatigue Symptom Inventory	Severity, frequency, daily pattern of fatigue, and its interference with quality of life	13	11-point Likert scale	Hann et al., 1998	–
Fatigue Severity Scale	Single-item fatigue severity score and impact of fatigue on daily functioning	10	7-point Likert scale for impact items; single-item 100 mm linear analog scale for severity	Krupp et al., 1989	–

(Continued on next page)

TABLE 13-1	Instruments to Measure Cancer-Related Fatigue *(Continued)*				
Measure	**Dimensions of Fatigue Evaluated**	**Number of Items**	**Scaling**	**Source for More Information**	**Comments**
Fatigue Scale–Adolescent	Multiple dimensions of fatigue, including affective, behavioral, somatic, and cognitive aspects of fatigue and consequences for daily functioning	14	5-point Likert scale	Hinds et al., 2007	–
Multidimensional Fatigue Symptom Inventory	Multiple dimensions of fatigue: global experience, somatic symptoms, cognitive symptoms, affective symptoms, and behavioral symptoms	83	5-point Likert scale	Stein et al., 1998	–
Multidimensional Fatigue Inventory	Multiple dimensions of fatigue: global experience, somatic symptoms, cognitive symptoms, affective symptoms, and behavioral symptoms	20	5-point Likert scale	Smets et al., 1995	Available in multiple languages
Multidimensional Assessment of Fatigue	Fatigue severity, timing, distress, and interference	16	100 mm linear analog scale; 2 additional items are multiple choice	Belza, 1995	–
Piper Fatigue Scale–Revised	Multiple dimensions of fatigue, including severity/behavioral, sensory, affective meaning, cognitive/mood	22	11-point Likert scale	Piper et al., 1998	–
Rhoten Fatigue Scale	Fatigue	1	Linear analog scale scaled from 0–10	Schneider, 1998	–
Schwartz Cancer Fatigue Scale	Physical and perceptual fatigue	6	5-point Likert scale	Schwartz, 1998	–
Lee Fatigue Scale	Fatigue, energy	18	Linear analog scale scaled from 0–10	Lee et al., 1991	–

Note. Based on information from Ahlberg et al., 2003; Beck et al., 2004; Jacobsen, 2004; Meek et al., 2000; Piper, 2004; Schwartz, 2002; Winstead-Fry, 1998.

pulmonary dysfunction, anemia, sleep disturbance, fluid and electrolyte imbalances, emotional distress, and uncontrolled concurrent symptoms. The medication profile also should be reviewed to identify specific classes of medications with a sedative side effect profile. Medications with a sedative side effect profile include opioid analgesics, sedative-hypnotic agents such secobarbital, benzodiazepines such as lorazepam, and anxiolytics such as buspirone. A number of antidepressants, antiemetics, antihistamines, and anticonvulsant agents such as gabapentin, phenobarbital, and carbamazepine also have the potential to produce sedation, daytime sleepiness, and fatigue. Certain cardiac medications (e.g., beta-blockers) may contribute to fatigue by causing bradycardia. Medications such as corticosteroids may cause fatigue by disrupting sleep. The coadministration of multiple agents with sedative, cardiac, or sleep-disrupting side effects may significantly compound fatigue symptoms. Figure 13-4 lists the dimensions of the fatigue experience to explore when evaluating patients with CRF.

FIGURE 13-4	Dimensions to Include in an Assessment of Fatigue

Fatigue is a common problem for patients with cancer. It is a feeling of weariness, tiredness, or exhaustion that can include a loss of physical and/or emotional energy. Many factors can contribute to the fatigue that a person with cancer experiences.

- On a scale of 0–10, where 0 is no fatigue and 10 is the worst fatigue imaginable, how severe has your fatigue been in the past 7 days?
- Would you say that your fatigue is mild, moderate, or severe?
- When did the fatigue start?
- Duration of fatigue: _____ days per week or _____ hours per day
- To what extent have you, because of fatigue, had to limit social activity, had difficulty getting things done, or felt like fatigue was making it difficult to maintain a positive outlook?
- To what extent does fatigue interfere with relationships or fulfilling responsibilities at work or in the home?
- What makes your fatigue better?
- What makes your fatigue worse?
- What do you do to help with fatigue or manage fatigue?
- Does rest relieve your fatigue?
- Do you have any trouble sleeping?
- Do you have other symptoms, such as pain, difficulty breathing, nausea, or vomiting?
- Do you experience anxiety? If yes, how often?
- Do you feel discouraged, blue, or sad? If yes, how often?
- Have you discussed your fatigue with anyone on your healthcare team?
- Have you ever been given any recommendations for managing your fatigue?

Evidence-Based Interventions

Because fatigue typically has several different causes in any one patient, the treatment plan needs to be individualized. It is helpful to work with the patients and family caregivers to improve assessment of fatigue and identify management strategies. Open communication among patients, family members, and the caregiving team will facilitate discussion about the experience of fatigue and its effects on daily life. General supportive care recommendations for patients with fatigue include encouraging a balanced diet with adequate intake of fluid, calories, protein, carbohydrates, fat, vitamins, and minerals, and balancing rest with physical activity and attention-restoring activities, such as exposure to natural environments, and pleasant distractions such as music (NCCN, 2008). The results of trials of interventions to reduce or manage fatigue are summarized in Figure 13-5, and selected findings are discussed in the following sections.

FIGURE 13-5	Evidence-Based Interventions for Managing Cancer-Related Fatigue

Interventions With Strong and Consistent Evidence Supporting Effectiveness
- Exercise
- Screen for potential etiologic factors and manage as appropriate
- Energy conservation and activity management
- Measures to optimize sleep quality
- Education/information provision
- Relaxation
- Massage and healing touch

Interventions With Some Evidence to Support Effectiveness
- Structured rehabilitation
- Cognitive behavioral therapy for fatigue
- Cognitive behavioral treatment for other concurrent symptoms, including depression
- Complementary therapies such as hypnosis, progressive muscle relaxation
- Distraction—virtual reality immersion
- Nutritional supplementation with omega-3 fatty acids or levocarnitine

Interventions With Evidence Supporting Effectiveness But With Risk for Harm
- Correction of anemia with erythropoiesis-stimulating agents

Interventions for Which Effectiveness Has Not Been Established
- Individual and group psychotherapy
- Expressive writing
- Paroxetine
- Methylphenidate
- Donepezil
- Bupropion sustained-release
- Modafinil
- Venlafaxine
- Anticytokine agents (infliximab, etanercept)
- Yoga
- Combination therapy: Aromatherapy, footsoak, and reflexology
- Dietary supplementation with soy protein, lipid replacement, antioxidant combinations
- Mindfulness-based stress reduction
- Acupuncture

Interventions Supported by Expert Opinion
- Work with patients and family caregivers to improve assessment of fatigue and identify management strategies
- Promote open communication among patients, family members, and caregiving team to facilitate discussions about the experience of fatigue and its effects on daily life
- Consider attention-restoring activities, such as exposure to natural environments, and pleasant distractions such as music
- Encourage a balanced diet with adequate intake of fluid, calories, protein, carbohydrates, fat, vitamins, and minerals
- Low-dose corticosteroids

Note. Based on information from Mitchell et al., 2009.

Pharmacologic Measures

More than 15 pharmacologic agents or nutritional supplements either alone or in combinations have been evaluated for their effectiveness in reducing fatigue during and following cancer treatment, including paroxetine, bupropion, amisulpride, methylphenidate, sertraline, multiple vitamins, high-dose vitamin C supplementation, and omega-3 fatty acid supplementation. These agents have been studied in randomized controlled trials as well as single-arm, open-label studies with small samples, and a recent Cochrane review has summarized the results of trials of a number of different pharmacologic agents for the management of CRF (Minton, Stone, Richardson, Sharpe, & Hotopf, 2008). Four trials have examined the effectiveness of the antidepressant paroxetine in treating fatigue during and following cancer treatment, with mixed findings. In two large multicenter, randomized, double-blind placebo-controlled trials, paroxetine 20 mg PO daily did not have an effect on fatigue (Morrow et al., 2003; Roscoe et al., 2005), although improvements in depression and overall mood were noted in the paroxetine treatment group. However, two small trials have shown a trend toward a possible benefit of paroxetine in treating fatigue in women with hot flashes (n = 13) (Weitzner, Moncello, Jacobsen, & Minton, 2002) and patients receiving interferon alfa (n = 18) (Capuron et al., 2002). One randomized controlled trial and five open-label, single-arm trials with small samples have examined the use of psychostimulant methylphenidate in reducing fatigue. Although the five open-label, single-arm trials reported improvements in fatigue in most of their participants as a result of the methylphenidate intervention, a randomized controlled trial of a patient-controlled dosing schedule for methylphenidate did not demonstrate improvement in the outcome of fatigue (Bruera et al., 2006). Furthermore, in one study (Sarhill et al., 2001), more than half of the patients experienced side effects such as insomnia, agitation, anorexia, nausea and vomiting, or dry mouth. The antidepressants bupropion, sertraline, and venlafaxine also have been studied with mixed results. Bupropion sustained-release at a dose of 100–150 mg/day has been found to be efficacious in the management of fatigue in two uncontrolled trials in small samples of patients with mixed tumor types (N < 25 in each trial) (Cullum, Wojciechowski, Pelletier, & Simpson, 2004; Moss, Simpson, Pelletier, & Forsyth, 2006). In the patients who derived benefit, the improvement occurred within two to four weeks. Controlled studies are necessary to establish the efficacy of this intervention in larger and more homogeneous samples of patients with cancer and to determine whether this effect of bupropion is separate from its action as an antidepressant. However, in a randomized controlled trial in nondepressed patients, the antidepressant sertraline did not result in improvement. Antidepressant treatment with venlafaxine, however, did produce improvement in fatigue, but only in those patients who experienced significant improvement in the severity and degree of interference from hot flashes (Carpenter et al., 2007).

Donepezil is a centrally acting reversible acetylcholinesterase inhibitor currently used to treat Alzheimer disease. In two open-label trials in patients with cancer, donepezil 5–10 mg/day was found to be effective in limiting CRF (Bruera et al., 2003; Shaw et al., 2006). However, in a double-blind, randomized trial, fatigue outcomes were not significantly different between the donepezil-treated and placebo-controlled groups (Bruera et al., 2007). Randomized controlled trials in a larger sample are needed to more thoroughly evaluate the efficacy of donepezil and to characterize its toxicity profile. In a case report regarding the use of modafinil (at a dose of 100 mg once a day or BID), improvements in daytime wakefulness and normalization of the sleep-wake cycle were reported in two older adult patients with advanced cancer (Caraceni & Simonetti, 2004). No side effects were reported. Expert opinion (Cox & Pappagallo, 2001) has supported the potential usefulness of the psychostimulant modafinil (at a dose of 100–400 mg in a daily or divided dose) in treating CRF. It also is supported by two reports of a small case series in patients with advanced cancers (Radbruch, Elsner, Krumm, Peuckmann, & Trottenberg, 2007; Reineke-Bracke, Radbruch, & Elsner, 2006) and an open-label trial in a small sample of patients receiving treatment with interferon (Martin, Krahn, Balan, & Rosati, 2007). A large phase III trial of this agent to manage fatigue in patients receiving chemotherapy is ongoing.

Several nutritional supplements have been explored, either as single agents or as part of a combination therapy. The safety and potential efficacy of levocarnitine supplementation in treating fatigue in patients with cancer who have low serum carnitine levels have been suggested by four small open-label trials (Cruciani et al., 2004, 2006; Gramignano et al., 2006; Graziano et al., 2002). Levocarnitine is a naturally occurring substance that facilitates fatty acid entry into cellular mitochondria, thereby optimizing the delivery of the main substrate for energy production in skeletal and cardiac muscle. Although interpretation of the results of these studies is limited by the small sample size and the absence of a double-blind randomized controlled design, preliminary results of a phase III trial suggest that levocarnitine may be effective in treating CRF (Mantovani et al., 2008).

Erythropoiesis-Stimulating Agents

Seven meta-analyses, systematic reviews, or evidence-based guidelines concluded that although erythropoiesis-stimulating agents may improve fatigue in patients with cancer who have hemoglobin levels less than 10 g/dl, the effects appear to be small (Bohlius et al., 2006; Kimel, Leidy, Mannix, & Dixon, 2008; Melosky, 2008; Mikhael, Melosky, Cripps, Rayson, & Kouroukis, 2007; Rizzo et al., 2008; Rodgers, 2006; Wilson et al., 2007). Moreover, most recent evidence suggests that erythropoiesis-stimulating agents are associated with risks for thromboembolic disease and may negatively affect disease control and overall survival. Although the most recent guidelines suggest that patients receiving recombinant human erythropoietin to correct anemia less than 10 g/dl may experience increased vigor and diminished fatigue, only limited evidence has shown that erythropoietin improves fatigue when anemia is less severe. Data suggest that a target hemoglobin level of 11–12 g/dl will produce the greatest gains in fatigue and other quality-of-life outcomes (Stasi et al., 2005). Although clinical circumstances may necessitate earlier treatment (e.g., patients with substantially reduced exercise capacity or ability to carry out activities of daily living), evidence is lacking to recommend initiating erythropoiesis-stimulating agents at hemoglobin levels greater than 10 g/dl. Guidelines from the American Society of Clinical Oncology (ASCO) recommend that hemoglobin only be raised to (or near) a concentration of 12 g/dl, at which time the dosage should be titrated to maintain that level (Rizzo et al.). Dose reductions also are recommended when the hemoglobin exceeds 11 g/dl or when the hemoglobin increases more than 1 g/dl in a two-week period. Iron stores should be monitored also, and iron intake should be supplemented in patients receiving erythropoiesis-stimulating agents. The ASCO guidelines urge prescribers to use these agents cautiously in patients with an elevated risk for thromboembolic complications, and they caution against the use of these agents to treat anemia associated with malignancy or the anemia of cancer in patients with solid or nonmyeloid malignancies who are not receiving concurrent chemotherapy because recent trials reported increased thromboembolic risks and decreased survival under these circumstances (Rizzo et al.).

Although both epoetin and darbepoetin generally are well tolerated, use of these agents specifically for the management of fatigue requires consideration of safety issues, including an increased risk of thrombotic events, hypertension, pure red cell aplasia, and theoretical concerns that epoetin may support or extend tumor growth in certain tumor types (Glaspy, 2005; Littlewood & Collins, 2005; Stasi et al., 2005; Steensma & Loprinzi, 2005). Overall, better quality evidence is needed to unequivocally support the use of recombinant human erythropoietin solely as an intervention to improve patient-reported outcomes such as fatigue in patients with cancer who have anemia (Bottomley, Thomas, Van Steen, Flechtner, & Djulbegovic, 2002; Littlewood, Cella, & Nortier, 2002).

Exercise

Meta-analyses of randomized trials support the benefits of exercise in the management of fatigue during and following cancer treatment in patients with breast cancer or solid tumors or in those undergoing hematopoietic stem cell transplantation, although effects generally are small and positive results for the outcome of fatigue have not been observed consistently across studies. The exercise modalities that have been applied differ in content (walking, cycling, swimming, resistive exercise, or combined exercise), frequency (ranging from two times per week to two times daily), intensity (with most programs at 50%–90% of the estimated VO_2 maximum heart rate), degree of supervision (fully supervised group versus self-directed exercise), and duration (from two weeks up to one year). The type, intensity, and duration of physical exercise that will be most beneficial in reducing fatigue at different stages of disease and treatment are not known (Humpel & Iverson, 2005), and more research is needed to systematically assess the safety of exercise (both aerobic exercise and strength training) in cancer subpopulations.

Psychoeducational Interventions

Several adequately powered randomized controlled trials and a meta-analysis (Jacobsen, Donovan, Vadaparampil, & Small, 2007) support a conclusion that educational interventions and psychological support have an important role in supporting positive coping in patients with CRF during and following treatment, and that such interventions decrease fatigue severity and its interference with daily functioning. Across studies, a number of common elements were incorporated into the psychoeducational interventions. These included anticipatory guidance about patterns of fatigue; tailored recommendations for self-management of fatigue, including increased activity or exercise and measures to address sleep dysregulation; coaching to enhance motivation and empower self-care and active coping; and praise and encouragement to promote self-efficacy and augment feelings of control. Other elements of effective psychoeducational interventions for fatigue included supportive counseling (to support in coping with fear of disease recurrence and to augment social support in patients with low social support), the use of a fatigue diary to record the affective consequences of fatigue, and cognitive restructuring to help normalize CRF and to identify and manage negative thought patterns (e.g., this fatigue is so terrible, I can't cope, I am helpless, there is nothing I can do) that diminish mood and interfere with goal setting and incremental goal attainment. Programs that are lengthy or involve frequent treatment sessions may exacerbate fatigue levels in some patient populations, such as those receiving radiation therapy or those with advanced cancers (Brown et al., 2006).

Many of the effective psychoeducational interventions included components of energy conservation and activity management (ECAM). ECAM is a self-management intervention that teaches patients to apply the principles of energy conservation and activity management and provides coaching to integrate these activities into their daily lifestyle. Figure 13-6 summarizes the principles of ECAM.

Studies have indicated that cognitive behavioral interventions designed to improve sleep quality also have a beneficial effect on fatigue. These interventions to improve sleep quality can be delivered individually or in a group setting and include relaxation training, along with sleep consolidation strategies (avoiding long or late afternoon naps, limiting time in bed to actual sleep time), stimulus control therapy (going to bed only when sleepy, using bed/bedroom for sleep and sexual activities only, having a consistent time to lie down and get up, avoiding caffeine and stimulating activity in the evening), and strategies to reduce cognitive-emotional arousal (keeping at least an hour to relax before going to bed and establishing a presleep routine to be used every night).

| FIGURE 13-6 | Energy Conservation and Activity Management for Cancer-Related Fatigue |

Energy conservation means looking at your daily routines to find ways to reduce the amount of effort needed to perform certain tasks, eliminating other tasks, and alternating rest periods with activities throughout the day to prevent bursts of activity and to discourage physical inactivity. Although not every technique will work for you, these are suggestions that you can consider.

Rearrange Your Environment
- Keep frequently used items in easily accessible places.
- Adjust work spaces, such as raising a tabletop, to eliminate awkward positions; bad posture drains energy.
- Sit rather than stand whenever possible—while preparing meals, washing dishes, ironing, etc.
- Use adaptive equipment to make tasks easier; try a jar opener, a reacher, or a shower chair to allow you to sit while bathing,
- Soak your dishes before washing, then let them air dry, or use paper plates and napkins.
- Use prepared foods when possible.
- Get a rolling cart to transport things around the house rather than carrying them.
- See if your grocery store will deliver your groceries.
- Use store-provided wheelchairs or scooters when shopping.

Plan Ahead
- Gather all the supplies you need for a task or project before starting so that everything is in one place.
- Call ahead to stores to make sure the items you need are available.
- Cook in larger quantities, and refrigerate or freeze extra portions for later.
- Work rest breaks into activities as often as possible. Take a break before you get tired.
- Schedule enough time for activities—rushing takes more energy.
- Try keeping a daily activity journal for a few weeks to identify times of day or certain tasks that result in more fatigue.

Prioritize
- Eliminate or reduce tasks that are not important to you.
- Delegate tasks to friends or family members who offer help.
- Consider hiring professionals, such as a cleaning or lawn care service, to cut down your workload.

Alternate Activity With Rest
- Avoid bursts of activity or prolonged activity that induces severe fatigue.
- With permission of your healthcare team, begin a program of physical activity such as walking or cycling. Begin with 5 or 10 minutes twice daily, and increase the time by 1 minute a day.
- Do not be tempted to overdo it in exercising, but rather strive for consistency.

Complementary Therapies

Preliminary evidence supports the efficacy of a wide array of complementary and alternative therapies for CRF, including yoga, relaxation, mindfulness-based stress reduction strategies, acupuncture, expressive writing, progressive muscle relaxation, massage, and music therapy. Several combined modality interventions also have shown promise, including aromatherapy, lavender foot soak, and reflexology, and yoga or Tai Chi combined with walking; however, disentangling the effects of the separate components involved in these combined modality therapies is a limitation. Many of these techniques share an emphasis on progressive muscle relaxation, mindfulness, meditation, and controlled movement. These interventions have also been delivered in groups, and thus shared group experience and mutual support may be an additional mechanism for the improvements noted in fatigue. Recent results obtained with progressive muscle relaxation, mindfulness-based stress reduction, and yoga are particularly encouraging because these self-management techniques are relatively inexpensive to deliver and once learned can continue to produce beneficial outcomes without side effects. Mindfulness-based stress reduction typically includes gentle yoga (stretches, poses, breathing, and meditation), mindfulness (the practice of becoming more aware of the present moment rather than dwelling in the past or projecting into the future), and a heightened awareness of one's breathing and the sensations of the body, coupled with relaxation and meditation. Three single-arm trials (Bauer-Wu et al., 2008; Carlson & Garland, 2005; Carlson, Speca, Patel, & Goodey, 2003) and a randomized controlled trial (Speca, Carlson, Goodey, & Angen, 2000) have demonstrated the preliminary effectiveness of mindfulness-based stress reduction interventions in reducing fatigue in patients with mixed tumor types and undergoing active treatment. Follow-up studies have suggested that the clinical improvements achieved with mindfulness-based stress reduction can be sustained (Carlson, Speca, Faris, & Patel, 2007).

Most of these studies are limited by their open-label, uncontrolled design and small samples, making it difficult to draw firm conclusions about efficacy. Of note, the studies evaluating acupuncture, expressive writing, and the combined aromatherapy, foot soak, and reflexology intervention included patients with advanced cancer and at the end of life. If found to be effective in larger randomized controlled trials, these approaches may offer treatment options for patients with advanced cancer and those at the end of life for whom other fatigue interventions, such as exercise, may not be feasible. Despite these limitations, and with acknowledgment that inclusion of controls such as double-blinding presents methodologic challenges (Elam, Carpenter, Shu, Boyapati, & Friedmann-Gilchrist, 2006), results suggest these complementary therapies have potential in the treatment of fatigue in patients with cancer.

Expected Outcomes

Expected outcomes of effective fatigue management include a reduction in fatigue severity and corollary improvements in the psychological distress and functional interference associated with fatigue. In some clinical situations (for example, patients undergoing hematopoietic stem cell transplantation or beginning a course of radiation therapy), the achievable clinical goal is to attenuate the worsening of fatigue severity, distress, and interference across the course of treatment. Programmatic outcomes of an effective fatigue management program include that all patients with cancer are screened for fatigue during each encounter with the healthcare team while on active treatment and during long-term follow-up, and that in patients with moderate to severe fatigue, the presence of the factors contributing to CRF (concurrent symptoms, emotional distress, sleep disturbances, anemia, nutritional alterations, inactivity or deconditioning, and comorbidities such as hypothyroidism and cardiomyopathy) and the management plan to address these issues are documented at regular intervals.

NCCN has published evidence-based guidelines to support the achievement of these expected outcomes (Mock et al., 2007), and the Oncology Nursing Society has developed Putting Evidence Into Practice resources for fatigue (Mitchell, Beck, Hood, Moore, & Tanner, 2006).

Patient and Family Teaching Points

Education concerning fatigue and its anticipated characteristics, pattern of onset, duration, and consequences for mood and role function should be provided to all patients as they begin any fatigue-inducing treatment and reinforced at regular intervals across the treatment course. Patients receiving biotherapy or intensive chemoradiotherapy or undergoing hematopoietic stem cell transplantation should be aware that they may develop moderate to severe fatigue. All patients and their families should be educated that interventions such as energy conservation, exercise, relaxation and stress management, psychosocial support, and measures to optimize sleep quality and reduce concurrent symptoms have been shown to be effective in limiting the severity of fatigue during treatment. Based on an understanding of the effectiveness of these interventions, patients should be encouraged to develop their own individualized plan for fatigue self-management. The importance of remaining active and participating in a consistent program of gentle exercise, individualized to the patient's age, condition, and physical fitness level, should be communicated. Referral to physical therapy or physical medicine and rehabilitation should be considered, especially for patients with significant comorbidities and deconditioning. Nurses should provide anticipatory guidance that fatigue develops or worsens as a direct result of treatment, and that this does not necessarily indicate that a treatment is ineffective or that the disease is progressing. Monitoring fatigue levels daily and recording these in a log or diary can be helpful not only in identifying times of peak energy but also in exploring the factors that may contribute to intensified fatigue, such as sleep disturbance, concurrent symptoms, or boredom.

The transition to long-term follow-up is another important point at which to provide anticipatory guidance concerning the pace at which fatigue symptoms may be expected to improve and energy levels normalize. Cancer survivors and their families should be prepared for the fact that resolution of moderate to severe fatigue may require several months to even a year of recovery, and a subset of patients continue to experience levels of fatigue that interfere with function. The development of a survivorship care plan offers an opportunity to review strategies that may be effective for long-term fatigue management during survivorship (e.g., exercise, cognitive behavioral and psychosocial support interventions, screening for hypothyroidism, measures to improve sleep quality).

Individuals with fatigue who have advanced cancer or who may be at the end of life and those who care for them will benefit from education to understand the multiple causes and consequences of fatigue at this point in the disease trajectory. It may be helpful to normalize that fatigue may increase substantially or become more unpredictable as the disease progresses and that the effects of fatigue (e.g., sadness, isolation, fear) on well-being may become more prominent. Intervention strategies that may have worked in the past (e.g., distraction, exercise) may no longer be feasible, and patients and their families benefit from guidance about options such as massage, yoga, aromatherapy, relaxation, acupuncture, counseling, and aggressive management of concurrent symptoms that may help in managing fatigue and alleviating suffering at the end of life.

Need for Future Research

A wide range of pharmacologic and nonpharmacologic interventions for fatigue have been studied, although a recent systematic review concluded that many have only been tested in uncontrolled or pilot studies (Mitchell, Beck, Hood, Moore, & Tanner, 2007). Interventions for fatigue that are supported by one or more well-designed randomized trials include exercise, psychoeducational interventions, and measures to optimize sleep quality and to correct anemia less than 10 g/dl, as well as relaxation, massage, and healing touch. Preliminary evidence or inconclusive evidence has suggested that pharmacologic agents, including paroxetine, methylphenidate, donepezil, bupropion sustained-release, modafinil, and levocarnitine, have a role in the management of fatigue, but systematic drug development studies are needed to define the optimal dosing, gauge the toxicity profile, and determine the effectiveness of these agents in specific populations. Interventions supported by preliminary evidence of effectiveness include individual and group psychotherapy and complementary therapies such as yoga and acupuncture. Urgent need exists for rigorously designed and adequately powered randomized controlled trials of therapies that have shown initial promise. Research focused on developing and testing interventions specifically for patients with fatigue in the setting of advanced cancer and at the end of life is imperative.

With a substantial body of evidence now accumulating regarding rehabilitative and psychoeducational interventions that are effective for CRF, questions remain concerning how best to deliver these programs on a widespread basis, to which patient populations, and at which phase in the illness trajectory. The role of strategies such as motivational interviewing and nurse coaching in helping patients to make behavior and lifestyle changes also deserves exploration.

Conclusion of Case Study

As an initial step in the management of CRF in J.B., who has moderate to severe fatigue (based on her severity rating of 8 out of 10), a comprehensive assessment of her fatigue is conducted. This assessment includes tracking the persistence of the fatigue across the course of the day and the week, noting any fluctuations and exacerbating or relieving factors, and gauging the impact on functioning and level of distress. J.B. tearfully relates her fear that the continued persistent fatigue indicates that the VAD chemotherapy will not be effective in treating her disease. She rates her pain as 2 out of 10 at most times but is most bothered by pain when she tries to go to sleep and admits she has slept for a only few hours in the past several nights, in part because of her treatment with dexamethasone. In addition to sleep disturbance and pain, J.B. admits to feeling profound sadness and discouragement and to feeling somewhat helpless to improve her current situation. In screening her for contributing factors for CRF, the nurse notes that she has renal insufficiency and moderate anemia, as well as psychological distress, sleep disturbance, and suboptimally managed concurrent symptoms. An initial plan of management for fatigue includes measures to improve pain management, particularly at night. To improve sleep quality, the nurse explores strategies with the patient, including progressive muscle relaxation with imagery and sleep hygiene measures, such as daytime sleep restriction, a warm shower, and a quiet, restful routine prior to sleep. During these conversations, the nurse has an opportunity to provide guidance that fatigue is often a presenting symptom of multiple myeloma, and its continued presence arises from different causes (e.g., sleep problems, pain) than the original causative factors (often anemia). The nurse also provides coaching and encouragement for the positive steps (goal setting, self-management) the patient is taking to relieve fatigue. At the weekly team conference, the oncology nurse can discuss the use of an erythropoiesis-stimulating agent to improve anemia and sleep quality, along with the possibility of administering daily doses of dexamethasone in the morning to limit the effect on sleep.

As the patient prepares for discharge from the hospital, the nurse's anticipatory guidance emphasizes the importance of hydration and improved nutrition. The patient is encouraged to keep a diary of her fatigue severity and its correlates to facilitate continued dialogue with the healthcare team regarding fatigue management interventions. As she returns to the home setting for continued monthly VAD treatments and to prepare for autologous transplantation, referrals are initiated for physical therapy to design and supervise an exercise program. To enhance her limited social support in the community, the patient also can begin participating in the monthly myeloma support group. Her fatigue severity is monitored every two weeks at her clinic visits for blood counts and clinical evaluation. She has noted some improvement in her level of fatigue (peak fatigue severity of 7 out of 10 in the past two weeks, despite onset of mild neutropenia), and she verbalizes greater self-efficacy in coping with fatigue and with her diagnosis. Sleep quality remains a problem, and she must continue to work on strategies of daytime sleep restriction, improved nighttime pain control, and stress management.

Conclusion

CRF is a prevalent, often persistent symptom during and following cancer treatment, producing marked effects on functional status, symptom burden, psychosocial adjustment, and well-being. Effective management of CRF requires that the clinician assess patients' fatigue levels regularly, offer anticipatory guidance and ongoing education about fatigue and strategies for its management, and define a therapeutic plan with both pharmacologic and non-pharmacologic interventions. Based on the multiple etiologies and contributing factors, optimal management of CRF must employ the skills of an interdisciplinary team. Research has identified a number of promising approaches for the treatment of CRF, although many of these require further evaluation in randomized controlled trials. As evidence-based treatment strategies for CRF continue to evolve, clinicians are challenged to synthesize this evidence base and to implement the interventions with the greatest likelihood of producing benefit. To achieve a rational approach to CRF management, continued research is needed to clarify the physiologic and psychological causes of CRF in specific disease- and treatment-related subpopulations and at each phase along the illness continuum and to develop and test mechanism-targeted interventions for CRF.

References

Ahlberg, K., Ekman, T., Gaston-Johansson, F., & Mock, V. (2003). Assessment and management of cancer-related fatigue in adults. *Lancet, 362*(9384), 640–650.

Aistars, J. (1987). Fatigue in the cancer patient: A conceptual approach to a clinical problem. *Oncology Nursing Forum, 14*(6), 25–30.

Akechi, T., Okuyama, T., Akizuki, N., Shimizu, K., Inagaki, M., Fujimori, M., et al. (2007). Associated and predictive factors of sleep disturbance in advanced cancer patients. *Psycho-Oncology, 16*(10), 888–894.

Ancoli-Israel, S., Liu, L., Marler, M.R., Parker, B.A., Jones, V., Sadler, G.R., et al. (2006). Fatigue, sleep, and circadian rhythms prior to chemotherapy for breast cancer. *Supportive Care in Cancer, 14*(3), 201–209.

Andrews, P., Morrow, G.R., Hickok, J., Roscoe, J., & Stone, P. (2004). Mechanisms and models of fatigue associated with cancer and its treatment: Evidence from preclinical and clinical studies. In J. Armes, M. Krishnasamy, & I. Higginson (Eds.), *Fatigue in cancer* (pp. 51–87). New York: Oxford University Press.

Andrykowski, M.A., Curran, S.L., & Lightner, R. (1998). Off-treatment fatigue in breast cancer survivors: A controlled comparison. *Journal of Behavioral Medicine, 21*(1), 1–18.

Andrykowski, M.A., Schmidt, J.E., Salsman, J.M., Beacham, A.O., & Jacobsen, P.B. (2005). Use of a case definition approach to identify cancer-related fatigue in women undergoing adjuvant therapy for breast cancer. *Journal of Clinical Oncology, 23*(27), 6613–6622.

Armes, J., Chalder, T., Addington-Hall, J., Richardson, A., & Hotopf, M. (2007). A randomized controlled trial to evaluate the effectiveness of a brief, behaviorally oriented intervention for cancer-related fatigue. *Cancer, 110*(6), 1385–1395.

Banthia, R., Malcarne, V.L., Roesch, S.C., Ko, C.M., Greenbergs, H.L., Varni, J.W., et al. (2006). Correspondence between daily and weekly fatigue reports in breast cancer survivors. *Journal of Behavioral Medicine, 29*(3), 269–279.

Bauer-Wu, S., Sullivan, A.M., Rosenbaum, E., Ott, M.J., Powell, M., McLoughlin, M., et al. (2008). Facing the challenges of hematopoietic stem cell transplantation with mindfulness meditation: A pilot study. *Integrative Cancer Therapies, 7*(2), 62–69.

Beck, S.L., Dudley, W.N., & Barsevick, A. (2005). Pain, sleep disturbance, and fatigue in patients with cancer: Using a mediation model to test a symptom cluster. *Oncology Nursing Forum, 32*(3), 542.

Beck, S.L., Erickson, J., & Shun, S.C. (2004). *Measuring oncology nursing-sensitive patient outcomes: Evidence-based summary.* Retrieved June 15, 2008, from http://onsopcontent.ons.org/toolkits/evidence/Clinical/pdf/Fatigue2.pdf

Belza, B.L. (1995). Comparison of self-reported fatigue in rheumatoid arthritis and controls. *Journal of Rheumatology, 22*(4), 639–643.

Bender, C.M., Ergyn, F.S., Rosenzweig, M.Q., Cohen, S.M., & Sereika, S.M. (2005). Symptom clusters in breast cancer across 3 phases of the disease. *Cancer Nursing, 28*(3), 219–225.

Berger, A.M., Farr, L.A., Kuhn, B.R., Fischer, P., & Agrawal, S. (2007). Values of sleep/wake, activity/rest, circadian rhythms, and fatigue prior to adjuvant breast cancer chemotherapy. *Journal of Pain and Symptom Management, 33*(4), 398–409.

Bohlius, J., Wilson, J., Seidenfeld, J., Piper, M., Schwarzer, G., Sandercock, J., et al. (2006). Recombinant human erythropoietins and cancer patients: Updated meta-analysis of 57 studies including 9353 patients. *Journal of the National Cancer Institute, 98*(10), 708–714.

Borneman, T., Piper, B.F., Sun, V.C., Koczywas, M., Uman, G., & Ferrell, B. (2007). Implementing the fatigue guidelines at one NCCN member institution: Process and outcomes. *Journal of the National Comprehensive Cancer Network, 5*(10), 1092–1101.

Bottomley, A., Thomas, R., Van Steen, K., Flechtner, H., & Djulbegovic, B. (2002). Erythropoietin improves quality of life—a response. *Lancet Oncology, 3*(9), 527.

Bower, J.E., Ganz, P.A., & Aziz, N. (2005). Altered cortisol response to psychologic stress in breast cancer survivors with persistent fatigue. *Psychosomatic Medicine, 67*(2), 277–280.

Bower, J.E., Ganz, P.A., Dickerson, S.S., Petersen, L., Aziz, N., & Fahey, J.L. (2005). Diurnal cortisol rhythm and fatigue in breast cancer survivors. *Psychoneuroendocrinology, 30*(1), 92–100.

Braun, I.M., Greenberg, D.B., & Pirl, W.F. (2008). Evidenced-based report on the occurrence of fatigue in long-term cancer survivors. *Journal of the National Comprehensive Cancer Network, 6*(4), 347–354.

Brown, P., Clark, M.M., Atherton, P., Huschka, M., Sloan, J.A., Gamble, G., et al. (2006). Will improvement in quality of life (QOL) impact fatigue in patients receiving radiation therapy for advanced cancer? *American Journal of Clinical Oncology, 29*(1), 52–58.

Bruera, E., El Osta, B., Valero, V., Driver, L.C., Pei, B.L., Shen, L., et al. (2007). Donepezil for cancer fatigue: A double-blind, randomized, placebo-controlled trial. *Journal of Clinical Oncology, 25*(23), 3475–3481.

Bruera, E., Strasser, F., Shen, L., Palmer, J.L., Willey, J., Driver, L.C., et al. (2003). The effect of donepezil on sedation and other symptoms in patients receiving opioids for cancer pain: A pilot study. *Journal of Pain and Symptom Management, 26*(5), 1049–1054.

Bruera, E., Valero, V., Driver, L., Shen, L., Willey, J., Zhang, T., et al. (2006). Patient-controlled methylphenidate for cancer fatigue: A double-blind, randomized, placebo-controlled trial. *Journal of Clinical Oncology, 24*(13), 2073–2078.

Butt, Z., Rosenbloom, S.K., Abernethy, A.P., Beaumont, J.L., Paul, D., Hampton, D., et al. (2008). Fatigue is the most important symptom for advanced cancer patients who have had chemotherapy. *Journal of the National Comprehensive Cancer Network, 6*(5), 448–455.

Butt, Z., Wagner, L.I., Beaumont, J.L., Paice, J.A., Straus, J.L., Peterman, A.H., et al. (2008). Longitudinal screening and management of fatigue, pain, and emotional distress associated with cancer therapy. *Supportive Care in Cancer, 16*(2), 151–159.

Capuron, L., Gumnick, J.F., Musselman, D.L., Lawson, D.H., Reemsnyder, A., Nemeroff, C.B., et al. (2002). Neurobehavioral effects of interferon-alpha in cancer patients: Phenomenology and paroxetine responsiveness of symptom dimensions. *Neuropsychopharmacology, 26*(5), 643–652.

Caraceni, A., & Simonetti, F. (2004). Psychostimulants: New concepts for palliative care from the modafinil experience? *Journal of Pain and Symptom Management, 28*(2), 97–99.

Carlson, L.E., & Garland, S.N. (2005). Impact of mindfulness-based stress reduction (MBSR) on sleep, mood, stress and fatigue symptoms in cancer outpatients. *International Journal of Behavioral Medicine, 12*(4), 278–285.

Carlson, L.E., Speca, M., Faris, P., & Patel, K.D. (2007). One year pre-post intervention follow-up of psychological, immune, endocrine and blood pressure outcomes of mindfulness-based stress reduction (MBSR) in breast and prostate cancer outpatients. *Brain, Behavior, and Immunity, 21*(8), 1038–1049.

Carlson, L.E., Speca, M., Patel, K.D., & Goodey, E. (2003). Mindfulness-based stress reduction in relation to quality of life, mood, symptoms of stress, and immune parameters in breast and prostate cancer outpatients. *Psychosomatic Medicine, 65*(4), 571–581.

Carpenter, J.S., Storniolo, A.M., Johns, S., Monahan, P.O., Azzouz, F., Elam, J.L., et al. (2007). Randomized, double-blind, placebo-controlled crossover trials of venlafaxine for hot flashes after breast cancer. *Oncologist, 12*(1), 124–135.

Cella, D., Gershon, R., Lai, J.S., & Choi, S. (2007). The future of outcomes measurement: Item banking, tailored short-forms, and computerized adaptive assessment. *Quality of Life Research, 16*(Suppl. 1), 133–141.

Cella, D., Lai, J.S., Chang, C.H., Peterman, A., & Slavin, M. (2002). Fatigue in cancer patients compared with fatigue in the general United States population. *Cancer, 94*(2), 528–538.

Cella, D., Peterman, A., Passik, S., Jacobsen, P., & Breitbart, W. (1998). Progress toward guidelines for the management of fatigue. *Oncology, 12*(11A), 369–377.

Chow, E., Fan, G., Hadi, S., & Filipczak, L. (2007). Symptom clusters in cancer patients with bone metastases. *Supportive Care in Cancer, 15*(9), 1035–1043.

Collado-Hidalgo, A., Bower, J.E., Ganz, P.A., Cole, S.W., & Irwin, M.R. (2006). Inflammatory biomarkers for persistent fatigue in breast cancer survivors. *Clinical Cancer Research, 12*(9), 2759–2766.

Cox, J.M., & Pappagallo, M. (2001). Modafinil: A gift to portmanteau. *American Journal of Hospice and Palliative Care, 18*(6), 408–410.

Cruciani, R.A., Dvorkin, E., Homel, P., Culliney, B., Malamud, S., Shaiova, L., et al. (2004). L-carnitine supplementation for the treatment of fatigue and depressed mood in cancer patients with carnitine deficiency: A preliminary analysis. *Annals of the New York Academy of Sciences, 1033,* 168–176.

Cruciani, R.A., Dvorkin, E., Homel, P., Malamud, S., Culliney, B., Lapin, J., et al. (2006). Safety, tolerability and symptom outcomes associated with L-carnitine supplementation in patients with cancer, fatigue, and carnitine deficiency: A phase I/II study. *Journal of Pain and Symptom Management, 32*(6), 551–559.

Cullum, J.L., Wojciechowski, A.E., Pelletier, G., & Simpson, J.S. (2004). Bupropion sustained release treatment reduces fatigue in cancer patients. *Canadian Journal of Psychiatry. Revue Canadienne de Psychiatrie, 49*(2), 139–144.

Curt, G. (2000). Impact of fatigue on quality of life in oncology patients. *Seminars in Hematology, 37*(4, Suppl. 6), 14–17.

Curt, G., & Johnston, P.G. (2003). Cancer fatigue: The way forward. *Oncologist, 8*(Suppl. 1), 27–30.

Danjoux, C., Gardner, S., & Fitch, M. (2007). Prospective evaluation of fatigue during a course of curative radiotherapy for localized prostate cancer. *Supportive Care in Cancer, 15*(10), 1169–1176.

Dantzer, R., O'Connor, J.C., Freund, G.G., Johnson, R.W., & Kelley, K.W. (2008). From inflammation to sickness and depression: When the immune system subjugates the brain. *Nature Reviews Neuroscience, 9*(1), 46–56.

Davis, K.M., Lai, J.S., Hahn, E.A., & Cella, D. (2008). Conducting routine fatigue assessments for use in clinical oncology practice: Patient and provider perspectives. *Supportive Care in Cancer, 16*(4), 379–386.

Davis, M.P., Khoshknabi, D., & Yue, G.H. (2006). Management of fatigue in cancer patients. *Current Pain and Headache Report, 10*(4), 260–269.

de Jong, N., Candel, M.J., Schouten, H.C., Abu-Saad, H.H., & Courtens, A.M. (2006). Course of the fatigue dimension "activity level" and the interference of fatigue with daily living activities for patients with breast cancer receiving adjuvant chemotherapy. *Cancer Nursing, 29*(5), E1–E13.

Dimeo, F., Schmittel, A., Fietz, T., Schwartz, S., Kohler, P., Boning, D., et al. (2004). Physical performance, depression, immune status and fatigue in patients with hematological malignancies after treatment. *Annals of Oncology, 15*(8), 1237–1242.

Elam, J.L., Carpenter, J.S., Shu, X.O., Boyapati, S., & Friedmann-Gilchrist, J. (2006). Methodological issues in the investigation of ginseng as an intervention for fatigue. *Clinical Nurse Specialist, 20*(4), 183–189.

Fernandes, R., Stone, P., Andrews, P., Morgan, R., & Sharma, S. (2006). Comparison between fatigue, sleep disturbance, and circadian rhythm in cancer inpatients and healthy volunteers: Evaluation of diagnostic criteria for cancer-related fatigue. *Journal of Pain and Symptom Management, 32*(3), 245–254.

Francoeur, R.B. (2005). The relationship of cancer symptom clusters to depressive affect in the initial phase of palliative radiation. *Journal of Pain and Symptom Management, 29*(2), 130–155.

Glaspy, J.A. (2005). The development of erythropoietic agents in oncology. *Expert Opinion in Emerging Drugs, 10*(3), 553–567.

Glaus, A. (1998). Fatigue in patients with cancer. Analysis and assessment. *Recent Results in Cancer Research, 145,* I–XI, 1–172.

Glaus, A., Boehme, C., Thurlimann, B., Ruhstaller, T., Hsu Schmitz, S.F., Morant, R., et al. (2006). Fatigue and menopausal symptoms in women with breast cancer undergoing hormonal cancer treatment. *Annals of Oncology, 17*(5), 801–806.

Glaus, A., Crow, R., & Hammond, S. (1996). A qualitative study to explore the concept of fatigue/tiredness in cancer patients and in healthy individuals. *European Journal of Cancer Care, 5*(Suppl. 2), 8–23.

Gramignano, G., Lusso, M.R., Madeddu, C., Massa, E., Serpe, R., Deiana, L., et al. (2006). Efficacy of l-carnitine administration on fatigue, nutritional status, oxidative stress, and related quality of life in 12 advanced cancer patients undergoing anticancer therapy. *Nutrition, 22*(2), 136–145.

Graziano, F., Bisonni, R., Catalano, V., Silva, R., Rovidati, S., Mencarini, E., et al. (2002). Potential role of levocarnitine supplementation for the treatment of chemotherapy-induced fatigue in non-anaemic cancer patients. *British Journal of Cancer, 86*(12), 1854–1857.

Gutstein, H.B. (2001). The biologic basis of fatigue. *Cancer, 92*(Suppl. 6), 1678–1683.

Hacker, E.D., & Ferrans, C.E. (2007). Ecological momentary assessment of fatigue in patients receiving intensive cancer therapy. *Journal of Pain and Symptom Management, 33*(3), 267–275.

Hann, D.M., Jacobsen, P.B., Azzarello, L.M., Martin, S.C., Curran, S.L., Fields, K.K., et al. (1998). Measurement of fatigue in cancer patients: Development and validation of the Fatigue Symptom Inventory. *Quality of Life Research, 7*(4), 301–310.

Hinds, P.S., Hockenberry, M., Tong, X., Rai, S.N., Gattuso, J.S., McCarthy, K., et al. (2007). Validity and reliability of a new instrument to measure cancer-related fatigue in adolescents. *Journal of Pain and Symptom Management, 34*(6), 607–618.

Hinshaw, D.B., Carnahan, J.M., & Johnson, D.L. (2002). Depression, anxiety, and asthenia in advanced illness. *Journal of the American College of Surgeons, 195*(2), 271.

Hockenberry-Eaton, M., & Hinds, P.S. (2000). Fatigue in children and adolescents with cancer: Evolution of a program of study. *Seminars in Oncology Nursing, 16*(4), 261–272.

Holley, S.K. (2000). Evaluating patient distress from cancer-related fatigue: An instrument development study. *Oncology Nursing Forum, 27*(9), 1425–1431.

Humpel, N., & Iverson, D.C. (2005). Review and critique of the quality of exercise recommendations for cancer patients and survivors. *Supportive Care in Cancer, 13*(7), 493–502.

Hwang, S.S., Chang, V.T., & Kasimis, B.S. (2003). A comparison of three fatigue measures in veterans with cancer. *Cancer Investigation, 21*(3), 363–373.

Iop, A., Manfredi, A.M., & Bonura, S. (2004). Fatigue in cancer patients receiving chemotherapy: An analysis of published studies. *Annals of Oncology, 15*(5), 712–720.

Irvine, D., Vincent, L., Graydon, J.E., Bubela, N., & Thompson, L. (1994). The prevalence and correlates of fatigue in patients receiving treatment with chemotherapy and radiotherapy. A comparison with the fatigue experienced by healthy individuals. *Cancer Nursing, 17*(5), 367–378.

Jacobsen, P.B. (2004). Assessment of fatigue in cancer patients. *Journal of the National Cancer Institute Monographs, 2004*(32), 93–97.

Jacobsen, P.B., Donovan, K.A., Vadaparampil, S.T., & Small, B.J. (2007). Systematic review and meta-analysis of psychological and activity-based interventions for cancer-related fatigue. *Health Psychology, 26*(6), 660–667.

Jacobsen, P.B., Donovan, K.A., & Weitzner, M.A. (2003). Distinguishing fatigue and depression in patients with cancer. *Seminars in Clinical Neuropsychiatry, 8*(4), 229–240.

Jager, A., Sleijfer, S., & van der Rijt, C.C. (2008). The pathogenesis of cancer related fatigue: Could increased activity of pro-inflammatory cytokines be the common denominator? *European Journal of Cancer, 44*(2), 175–181.

Johnson, R.W. (2002). The concept of sickness behavior: A brief chronological account of four key discoveries. *Veterinary Immunology and Immunopathology, 87*(3–4), 443–450.

Kalman, D., & Villani, L.J. (1997). Nutritional aspects of cancer-related fatigue. *Journal of the American Dietetic Association, 97*(6), 650–654.

Kimel, M., Leidy, N.K., Mannix, S., & Dixon, J. (2008). Does epoetin alfa improve health-related quality of life in chronically ill patients with anemia? Summary of trials of cancer, HIV/AIDS, and chronic kidney disease. *Value in Health, 11*(1), 57–75.

Kirsh, K.L., Passik, S., Holtsclaw, E., Donaghy, K., & Theobald, D. (2001). I get tired for no reason: A single item screening for cancer-related fatigue. *Journal of Pain and Symptom Management, 22*(5), 931–937.

Knowles, G., Borthwick, D., McNamara, S., Miller, M., & Leggot, L. (2000). Survey of nurses' assessment of cancer-related fatigue. *European Journal of Cancer Care, 9*(2), 105–113.

Krupp, L.B., LaRocca, N.G., Muir-Nash, J., & Steinberg, A.D. (1989). The fatigue severity scale. Application to patients with multiple sclerosis and systemic lupus erythematosus. *Archives of Neurology, 46*(10), 1121–1123.

Kurzrock, R. (2001). The role of cytokines in cancer-related fatigue. *Cancer, 92*(Suppl. 6), 1684–1688.

Lai, J.-S., Cella, D., Dineen, K., Bode, R., Von Roenn, J., Gershon, R.C., et al. (2005). An item bank was created to improve the measurement of cancer-related fatigue. *Journal of Clinical Epidemiology, 58*(2), 190–197.

Lawrence, D.P., Kupelnick, B., Miller, K., Devine, D., & Lau, J. (2004). Evidence report on the occurrence, assessment, and treatment of fatigue in cancer patients. *Journal of the National Cancer Institute Monographs, 2004*(32), 40–50.

Lee, B.N., Dantzer, R., Langley, K.E., Bennett, G.J., Dougherty, P.M., Dunn, A.J., et al. (2004). A cytokine-based neuroimmunologic mechanism of cancer-related symptoms. *Neuroimmunomodulation, 11*(5), 279–292.

Lee, K.A., Hicks, G., & Nino-Murcia, G. (1991). Validity and reliability of a scale to assess fatigue. *Psychiatry Research, 36*(3), 291–298.

Lindqvist, O., Widmark, A., & Rasmussen, B.H. (2004). Meanings of the phenomenon of fatigue as narrated by 4 patients with cancer in palliative care. *Cancer Nursing, 27*(3), 237–243.

Littlewood, T., & Collins, G. (2005). Epoetin alfa: Basic biology and clinical utility in cancer patients. *Expert Review of Anticancer Therapy, 5*(6), 947–956.

Littlewood, T.J., Cella, D., & Nortier, J.W. (2002). Erythropoietin improves quality of life. *Lancet Oncology, 3*(8), 459–460.

Magnusson, K., Moller, A., Ekman, T., & Wallgren, A. (1999). A qualitative study to explore the experience of fatigue in cancer patients. *European Journal of Cancer Care, 8*(4), 224–232.

Mallinson, T., Cella, D., Cashy, J., & Holzner, B. (2006). Giving meaning to measure: Linking self-reported fatigue and function to performance of everyday activities. *Journal of Pain and Symptom Management, 31*(3), 229–241.

Mantovani, G., Maccio, A., Madeddu, C., Gramignano, G., Serpe, R., Massa, E., et al. (2008). Randomized phase III clinical trial of five different arms of treatment for patients with cancer cachexia: Interim results. *Nutrition, 24*(4), 305–313.

Martin, K., Krahn, L., Balan, V., & Rosati, M. (2007). Modafinil's use in combating interferon-induced fatigue. *Digestive Diseases and Sciences, 52*(4), 893–896.

Massacesi, C., Terrazzino, S., Marcucci, F., Rocchi, M.B., Lippe, P., Bisonni, R., et al. (2006). Uridine diphosphate glucuronosyl transferase 1A1 promoter polymorphism predicts the risk of gastrointestinal toxicity and fatigue induced by irinotecan-based chemotherapy. *Cancer, 106*(5), 1007–1016.

Meek, P.M., Nail, L.M., Barsevick, A., Schwartz, A.L., Stephen, S., Whitmer, K., et al. (2000). Psychometric testing of fatigue instruments for use with cancer patients. *Nursing Research, 49*(4), 181–190.

Melosky, B.L. (2008). Erythropoiesis-stimulating agents: Benefits and risks in supportive care of cancer. *Current Oncology, 15*(Suppl. 1), S10–S15.

Mendoza, T.R., Wang, X.S., Cleeland, C.S., Morrissey, M., Johnson, B.A., Wendt, J.K., et al. (1999). The rapid assessment of fatigue severity in cancer patients: Use of the Brief Fatigue Inventory. *Cancer, 85*(5), 1186–1196.

Mikhael, J., Melosky, B., Cripps, C., Rayson, D., & Kouroukis, C.T. (2007). Canadian supportive care recommendations for the management of anemia in patients with cancer. *Current Oncology, 14*(5), 209–217.

Miller, A.H. (2003). Cytokines and sickness behavior: Implications for cancer care and control. *Brain, Behavior, and Immunity, 17*(1, Suppl. 1), S132–S134.

Miller, A.H., Ancoli-Israel, S., Bower, J.E., Capuron, L., & Irwin, M.R. (2008). Neuroendocrine-immune mechanisms of behavioral comorbidities in patients with cancer. *Journal of Clinical Oncology, 26*(6), 971–982.

Minton, O., Stone, P., Richardson, A., Sharpe, M., & Hotopf, M. (2008). Drug therapy for the management of cancer related fatigue. *Cochrane Database of Systematic Reviews* 2008, Issue 1. Art. No.: CD006704. DOI: 10.1002/14651858.CD006704.pub2.

Mitchell, S., Beck, S., Hood, L., Moore, K., & Tanner, E. (2006). *Putting evidence into practice: Fatigue detailed PEP card.* Retrieved June 15, 2008, from http://www.ons.org/outcomes/volume1/fatigue/pdf/FATIGUE-Detailed PEPCard4-28-06.pdf

Mitchell, S.A., Beck, S.L., Hood, L.E., Moore, K., & Tanner, E.R. (2007). Putting evidence into practice: Evidence-based interventions for fatigue during and following cancer and its treatment. *Clinical Journal of Oncology Nursing, 11*(1), 99–113.

Mitchell, S.A., Beck, S.L., Hood, L.E., Moore, K., & Tanner, E.R. (2009). ONS PEP resource: Fatigue. In L.H. Eaton & J.M. Tipton (Eds.), *Putting evidence into practice: Improving oncology patient outcomes* (pp. 155–174). Pittsburgh, PA: Oncology Nursing Society.

Mock, V. (2004). Evidence-based treatment for cancer-related fatigue. *Journal of the National Cancer Institute Monographs, 2004*(32), 112–118.

Mock, V., Atkinson, A., Barsevick, A.M., Berger, A.M., Cimprich, B., Eisenberger, M.A., et al. (2007). Cancer-related fatigue. Clinical practice guidelines in oncology. *Journal of the National Comprehensive Cancer Network, 5*(10), 1054–1078.

Morrow, G.R., Andrews, P.L., Hickok, J.T., Roscoe, J.A., & Matteson, S. (2002). Fatigue associated with cancer and its treatment. *Supportive Care in Cancer, 10*(5), 389–398.

Morrow, G.R., Hickok, J.T., Roscoe, J.A., Raubertas, R.F., Andrews, P.L., Flynn, P.J., et al. (2003). Differential effects of paroxetine on fatigue and depression: A randomized, double-blind trial from the University of Rochester Cancer Center Community Clinical Oncology Program. *Journal of Clinical Oncology, 21*(24), 4635–4641.

Morrow, G.R., Shelke, A.R., Roscoe, J.A., Hickok, J.T., & Mustian, K. (2005). Management of cancer-related fatigue. *Cancer Investigation, 23*(3), 229–239.

Moss, E.L., Simpson, J.S., Pelletier, G., & Forsyth, P. (2006). An open-label study of the effects of bupropion SR on fatigue, depression and quality of life of mixed-site cancer patients and their partners. *Psycho-Oncology, 15*(3), 259–267.

Mota, D.D., & Pimenta, C.A. (2006). Self-report instruments for fatigue assessment: A systematic review. *Research and Theory for Nursing Practice, 20*(1), 49–78.

Mystakidou, K., Parpa, E., Katsouda, E., Galanos, A., & Vlahos, L. (2006). The role of physical and psychological symptoms in desire for death: A study of terminally ill cancer patients. *Psycho-Oncology, 15*(4), 355–360.

Nail, L.M. (2002). Fatigue in patients with cancer. *Oncology Nursing Forum, 29*(3), 537.

Nail, L.M. (2004). My get up and go got up and went: Fatigue in people with cancer. *Journal of the National Cancer Institute Monographs, 2004*(32), 72–75.

National Comprehensive Cancer Network. (2008). *NCCN Clinical Practice Guidelines in Oncology™: Cancer-related fatigue* [v.1.2008]. Retrieved November 18, 2008, from http://www.nccn.org/professionals/physician_gls/PDF/fatigue.pdf

Okuyama, T., Akechi, T., Kugaya, A., Okamura, H., Imoto, S., Nakano, T., et al. (2000). Factors correlated with fatigue in disease-free breast cancer patients: Application of the Cancer Fatigue Scale. *Supportive Care in Cancer, 8*(3), 215–222.

Olson, K. (2007). A new way of thinking about fatigue: A reconceptualization. *Oncology Nursing Forum, 34*(1), 93–99.

Parker, K.P., Bliwise, D.L., Ribeiro, M., Jain, S.R., Vena, C.I., Kohles-Baker, M.K., et al. (2008). Sleep/wake patterns of individuals with advanced cancer measured by ambulatory polysomnography. *Journal of Clinical Oncology, 26*(15), 2464–2472.

Passik, S.D., Kirsh, K.L., Donaghy, K., Holtsclaw, E., Theobald, D., Cella, D., et al. (2002). Patient-related barriers to fatigue communication: Initial validation of the fatigue management barriers questionnaire. *Journal of Pain and Symptom Management, 24*(5), 481–493.

Payne, J.K. (2004). A neuroendocrine-based regulatory fatigue model. *Biological Research for Nursing, 6*(2), 141–150.

Piper, B.F. (2004). Measuring fatigue. In M. Frank-Stromborg & S.J. Olsen (Eds.), *Instruments for clinical health-care research* (3rd ed., pp. 538–553). Sudbury, MA: Jones and Bartlett.

Piper, B.F., Dibble, S.L., Dodd, M.J., Weiss, M.C., Slaughter, R.E., & Paul, S.M. (1998). The revised Piper Fatigue Scale: Psychometric evaluation in women with breast cancer. *Oncology Nursing Forum, 25*(4), 677–684.

Piper, B.F., Lindsey, A.M., & Dodd, M.J. (1987). Fatigue mechanisms in cancer patients: Developing nursing theory. *Oncology Nursing Forum, 14*(6), 17–23.

Prue, G., Rankin, J., Allen, J., Gracey, J., & Cramp, F. (2006). Cancer-related fatigue: A critical appraisal. *European Journal of Cancer, 42*(7), 846–863.

Radbruch, L., Elsner, F., Krumm, N., Peuckmann, V., & Trottenberg, P. (2007). Drugs for the treatment of fatigue in palliative care (Protocol). *Cochrane Database of Systematic Reviews* 2007, Issue 4. Art. No.: CD006788. DOI: 10.1002/14651858.CD006788.

Radbruch, L., Strasser, F., Elsner, F., Goncalves, J.F., Loge, J., Kaasa, S., et al. (2008). Fatigue in palliative care patients—an EAPC approach. *Palliative Medicine, 22*(1), 13–32.

Reineke-Bracke, H., Radbruch, L., & Elsner, F. (2006). Treatment of fatigue: Modafinil, methylphenidate, and goals of care. *Journal of Palliative Medicine, 9*(5), 1210–1214.

Reuter, K., & Harter, M. (2004). The concepts of fatigue and depression in cancer. *European Journal of Cancer Care, 13*(2), 127–134.

Rhoten, D. (1982). Fatigue and the postsurgical patient. In C. Norris (Ed.), *Conceptual clarification in nursing* (pp. 277–300). Rockville, MD: Aspen.

Rizzo, J.D., Somerfield, M.R., Hagerty, K.L., Seidenfeld, J., Bohlius, J., Bennett, C.L., et al. (2008). Use of epoetin and darbepoetin in patients with cancer: 2007 American Society of Clinical Oncology/American Society of Hematology clinical practice guideline update. *Journal of Clinical Oncology, 26*(1), 132–149.

Rodgers, G.M. (2006). Guidelines for the use of erythropoietic growth factors in patients with chemotherapy-induced anemia. *Oncology, 20*(8, Suppl. 6), 12–15.

Roscoe, J.A., Morrow, G.R., Hickok, J.T., Mustian, K.M., Griggs, J.J., Matteson, S.E., et al. (2005). Effect of paroxetine hydrochloride (Paxil) on fatigue and depression in breast cancer patients receiving chemotherapy. *Breast Cancer Research and Treatment, 89*(3), 243–249.

Ryan, J.L., Carroll, J.K., Ryan, E.P., Mustian, K.M., Fiscella, K., & Morrow, G.R. (2007). Mechanisms of cancer-related fatigue. *Oncologist, 12*(Suppl. 1), 22–34.

Sadler, I.J., Jacobsen, P.B., Booth-Jones, M., Belanger, H., Weitzner, M.A., & Fields, K.K. (2002). Preliminary evaluation of a clinical syndrome approach to assessing cancer-related fatigue. *Journal of Pain and Symptom Management, 23*(5), 406–416.

Sarhill, N., Walsh, D., Nelson, K.A., Homsi, J., LeGrand, S., & Davis, M.P. (2001). Methylphenidate for fatigue in advanced cancer: A prospective open-label pilot study. *American Journal of Hospice and Palliative Care, 18*(3), 187–192.

Schneider, R.A. (1998). Reliability and validity of the Multidimensional Fatigue Inventory (MFI-20) and the Rhoten Fatigue Scale among rural cancer outpatients. *Cancer Nursing, 21*(5), 370–373.

Schubert, C., Hong, S., Natarajan, L., Mills, P.J., & Dimsdale, J.E. (2007). The association between fatigue and inflammatory marker levels in cancer patients: A quantitative review. *Brain, Behavior and Immunity, 21*(4), 413–427.

Schwartz, A.H. (2002). Validity of cancer-related fatigue instruments. *Pharmacotherapy, 22*(11), 1433–1441.

Schwartz, A.L. (1998). The Schwartz Cancer Fatigue Scale: Testing reliability and validity. *Oncology Nursing Forum, 25*(4), 711–717.

Servaes, P., Verhagen, S., & Bleijenberg, G. (2002a). Determinants of chronic fatigue in disease-free breast cancer patients: A cross-sectional study. *Annals of Oncology, 13*(4), 589–598.

Servaes, P., Verhagen, C., & Bleijenberg, G. (2002b). Fatigue in cancer patients during and after treatment: Prevalence, correlates and interventions. *European Journal of Cancer, 38*(1), 27–43.

Shafqat, A., Einhorn, L.H., Hanna, N., Sledge, G.W., Hanna, A., Juliar, B.E., et al. (2005). Screening studies for fatigue and laboratory correlates in cancer patients undergoing treatment. *Annals of Oncology, 16*(9), 1545–1550.

Shaw, E.G., Rosdhal, R., D'Agostino, R.B., Jr., Lovato, J., Naughton, M.J., Robbins, M.E., et al. (2006). Phase II study of donepezil in irradiated brain tumor patients: Effect on cognitive function, mood, and quality of life. *Journal of Clinical Oncology, 24*(9), 1415–1420.

Smets, E.M., Garssen, B., Bonke, B., & De Haes, J.C. (1995). The Multidimensional Fatigue Inventory (MFI) psychometric qualities of an instrument to assess fatigue. *Journal of Psychosomatic Research, 39*(3), 315–325.

Speca, M., Carlson, L.E., Goodey, E., & Angen, M. (2000). A randomized, wait-list controlled clinical trial: The effect of a mindfulness meditation-based stress reduction program on mood and symptoms of stress in cancer outpatients. *Psychosomatic Medicine, 62*(5), 613–622.

Stasi, R., Abriani, L., Beccaglia, P., Terzoli, E., & Amadori, S. (2003). Cancer-related fatigue: Evolving concepts in evaluation and treatment. *Cancer, 98*(9), 1786–1801.

Stasi, R., Amadori, S., Littlewood, T.J., Terzoli, E., Newland, A.C., & Provan, D. (2005). Management of cancer-related anemia with erythropoietic agents: Doubts, certainties, and concerns. *Oncologist, 10*(7), 539–554.

Steensma, D.P., & Loprinzi, C.L. (2005). Erythropoietin use in cancer patients: A matter of life and death? *Journal of Clinical Oncology, 23*(25), 5865–5868.

Stein, K.D., Martin, S.C., Hann, D.M., & Jacobsen, P.B. (1998). A multidimensional measure of fatigue for use with cancer patients. *Cancer Practice, 6*(3), 143–152.

Strasser, F., Palmer, J.L., Schover, L.R., Yusuf, S.W., Pisters, K., Vassilopoulou-Sellin, R., et al. (2006). The impact of hypogonadism and autonomic dysfunction on fatigue, emotional function, and sexual desire in male patients with advanced cancer: A pilot study. *Cancer, 107*(12), 2949–2957.

Tavio, M., Milan, I., & Tirelli, U. (2002). Cancer-related fatigue (review). *International Journal of Oncology, 21*(5), 1093–1099.

Tchekmedyian, N.S., Kallich, J., McDermott, A., Fayers, P., & Erder, M.H. (2003). The relationship between psychologic distress and cancer-related fatigue. *Cancer, 98*(1), 198–203.

Temel, J.S., Pirl, W.F., Recklitis, C.J., Cashavelly, B., & Lynch, T.J. (2006). Feasibility and validity of a one-item fatigue screen in a thoracic oncology clinic. *Journal of Thoracic Oncology, 1*(5), 454–459.

Valentine, A.D., & Meyers, C.A. (2001). Cognitive and mood disturbance as causes and symptoms of fatigue in cancer patients. *Cancer, 92*(Suppl. 6), 1694–1698.

Van Belle, S., Paridaens, R., Evers, G., Kerger, J., Bron, D., Foubert, J., et al. (2005). Comparison of proposed diagnostic criteria with FACT-F and VAS for cancer-related fatigue: Proposal for use as a screening tool. *Supportive Care in Cancer, 13*(4), 246–254.

Varricchio, C.G. (Ed.). (2000). *Measurement and assessment: What are the issues?* Sudbury, MA: Jones and Bartlett.

Vogelzang, N.J., Breitbart, W., Cella, D., Curt, G.A., Groopman, J.E., Horning, S.J., et al. (1997). Patient, caregiver, and oncologist perceptions of cancer-related fatigue: Results of a tripart assessment survey. *Seminars in Hematology, 34*(3, Suppl. 3), 4–12.

Wagner, L., & Cella, D. (2001). Cancer-related fatigue: Clinical screening, assessment, and management. In M. Marty & S. Pecorelli (Eds.), *ESO scientific updates: Fatigue, asthenia, exhaustion and cancer* (5th ed., pp. 201–214). Oxford, England: Elsevier Science.

Wagner, L., & Cella, D. (2004). Fatigue and cancer: Causes, prevalence and treatment approaches. *British Journal of Cancer, 91*(5), 822–828.

Walsh, D., & Rybicki, L. (2006). Symptom clustering in advanced cancer. *Supportive Care in Cancer, 14*(8), 831–836.

Wang, X.S., Giralt, S.A., Mendoza, T.R., Engstrom, M.C., Johnson, B.A., Peterson, N., et al. (2002). Clinical factors associated with cancer-related fatigue in patients being treated for leukemia and non-Hodgkin's lymphoma. *Journal of Clinical Oncology, 20*(5), 1319–1328.

Weitzner, M.A., Moncello, J., Jacobsen, P.B., & Minton, S. (2002). A pilot trial of paroxetine for treatment of hot flashes and associated symptoms in women with breast cancer. *Journal of Pain and Symptom Management, 23*(4), 337–345.

Wilson, J., Yao, G.L., Raftery, J., Bohlius, J., Brunskill, S., Sandercock, J., et al. (2007). A systematic review and economic evaluation of epoetin alfa, epoetin beta and darbepoetin alfa in anaemia associated with cancer, especially that attributable to cancer treatment. *Health Technology Assessment, 11*(13), 1–220.

Winningham, M.L. (2001). Strategies for managing cancer-related fatigue syndrome: A rehabilitation approach. *Cancer, 92*(Suppl. 4), 988–997.

Winstead-Fry, P. (1998). Psychometric assessment of four fatigue scales with a sample of rural cancer patients. *Journal of Nursing Measurement, 6*(2), 111–122.

Wood, L.J., Nail, L.M., Gilster, A., Winters, K.A., & Elsea, C.R. (2006). Cancer chemotherapy-related symptoms: Evidence to suggest a role for proinflammatory cytokines. *Oncology Nursing Forum, 33*(3), 535–542.

Wu, H.S., & McSweeney, M. (2001). Measurement of fatigue in people with cancer. *Oncology Nursing Forum, 28*(9), 1371–1384.

Wu, H.S., & McSweeney, M. (2007). Cancer-related fatigue: "It's so much more than just being tired". *European Journal of Oncology Nursing, 11*(2), 117–125.

Yellen, S.B., Cella, D.F., Webster, K., Blendowski, C., & Kaplan, E. (1997). Measuring fatigue and other anemia-related symptoms with the Functional Assessment of Cancer Therapy (FACT) measurement system. *Journal of Pain and Symptom Management, 13*(2), 63–74.

Yennurajalingam, S., Palmer, J.L., Zhang, T., Poulter, V., & Bruera, E. (2008). Association between fatigue and other cancer-related symptoms in patients with advanced cancer. *Supportive Care in Cancer, 16*(10), 1125–1130.

Hot Flashes

Christine Engstrom, PhD, CRNP, AOCN®

Case Study

C.L. is a 45-year-old African American man with a history of advanced prostate cancer. Six months ago he received a diagnosis of adenocarcinoma of the prostate, Gleason score of 4 + 4 = 8, tumor-node-metastasis staging of T3N0M1. Prostate-specific antigen (PSA) level was 229 ng/ml at the time of diagnosis. He immediately began treatment with total androgen blockade after the staging workup was completed. He began taking daily oral bicalutamide and subcutaneous goserelin acetate every three months. C.L. was in excellent health until six months ago when he complained of urinary hesitancy to his primary care nurse practitioner. PSA testing was ordered, and a prostate biopsy confirmed the diagnosis of prostate cancer. C.L. then was referred to medical oncology and urology for treatment. A computed tomography scan of the chest/abdomen/pelvis did not demonstrate evidence of metastatic disease; however, a bone scan revealed lesions in the right pelvis and at T11 and T12. The patient was given the option of surgical castration versus medical castration and opted for medical treatment. C.L. is a financial adviser in a large banking firm meeting with clients daily and leading business meetings with his staff weekly. He is present at the clinic today for his second injection of goserelin acetate and is complaining of profuse sweating during the day and at night that is sometimes accompanied by palpitations and feelings of anxiety.

Overview

Hot flashes in both men and women have been physiologically defined as the sensation of heat that is associated with objective signs of cutaneous vasodilation and a subsequent drop in core temperature (Stearns et al., 2002). It also has been defined in women subjectively as a recurrent, transient period of flushing, sweating, and a sensation of heat, often accompanied by palpitations and a feeling of anxiety and sometimes followed by chills (Carpenter, Johnson, Wagner, & Andrykowski, 2002).

Men with prostate cancer frequently are treated with androgen ablation that can be defined as either medical or surgical castration. Androgen ablation is associated with unpleasant side effects or symptoms, including hot flashes/flushes in up to 70%–80% of patients (Clark, Wray, & Ashton, 2001), with more than 50% developing hot flashes severe enough to warrant treatment (Charig & Rundle, 1989) and which can persist for up to eight years (Karling, Hammar, & Varenhorst, 1994).

Hot flashes are difficult to measure because of their transient and unpredictable nature and have been the object of very little investigation. Studies have been conducted using an ambulatory hot flash monitor device in women to record skin conductance levels on sternal skin in breast cancer survivors, which was found to be a feasible method for objectively assessing hot flashes (Carpenter, Andrykowski, Freedman, & Munn, 1999). A controlled clinical trial evaluated the feasibility and psychometric properties of the sternal skin conductance monitor measuring the frequency of hot flashes in 19 patients with breast cancer and 5 premenopausal matched healthy women. Findings indicated a 30% false-negative rate with the monitor and a 31%–33% false-positive rate with subjective measures of hot flashes (Carpenter et al., 1999). Based on the research of hot flashes in patients with breast cancer, Carpenter (2005) has defined an objective hot flash as "an increase in skin conductance of 2 micromhos or more within a 30-second period" (p. 9).

Risk Factors

Few published studies have examined risk factors for hot flashes in women, and only one study has been done on men and hot flashes. Figure 14-1 lists the nonmodifiable risk factors, such as age and race, and other risk factors that are associated with lifestyle, such as smoking, increased body mass index (BMI), and alcohol intake, that may influence hot flashes (Glaus et al., 2006; Gold et al., 2006; Hardy, Kuh, & Wadsworth, 2000; Staropoli, Flaws, Bush, & Moulton, 1998; Whiteman, Staropoli, Benedict, Borgeest, & Flaws, 2003; Whiteman, Staropoli, Langenberg, et al., 2003). Gold et al.'s longitudinal study reported that lower socioeconomic status and less than a high school education also were predictors of hot flashes. These risk factors have been supported by another study of 468 perimenopausal women. One study showed that after controlling for age, race, use of oral contraceptives and hormone replacement therapy (HRT), and depression, correlates of hot flashes in perimenopausal women were BMI ≥ 25 kg/m^2 (adjusted overall risk [OR] = 1.03 per unit of increase; 95% confidence interval [CI] = 1.01–1.04) and increasing age (adjusted OR = 1.17; 95% CI = 1.13–1.21) (Riley, Inui, Kleinman, & Connelly, 2004). Therefore, as the women aged and had a higher BMI, the risk of hot flashes increased. A case-controlled study of women ages 45–54 found that alcohol use actually decreased the severity and frequency of hot flashes, contrary to previous findings (Schilling et al., 2005).

Patients with breast cancer have a high prevalence of vasomotor symptoms related to estrogen deprivation (Carpenter, 2000; Zibecchi, Greendale, & Ganz, 2003). Hot flashes have been observed in patients with breast cancer who are on tamoxifen (Carpenter, 2000; Carpenter et al., 1998; Carpenter, Johnson, et al., 2002) or letrozole (Femara®, Novartis Pharmaceuticals Corp.) compared with placebo (Whelan et al., 2005) and less in patients taking anastrozole (Arimidex®, AstraZeneca Pharmaceuticals) compared with tamoxifen (Fallowfield et al., 2004). Chemotherapy type and dosage increase the induction of amenorrhea or ovarian failure with adjuvant chemotherapy by reducing the number and quality of

FIGURE 14-1	Risk Factors for Hot Flashes

- Age
- African American women
- Lack of exercise
- Smoking
- Low socioeconomic status
- Less than high school education
- Chemotherapy
- Current use of tamoxifen
- Current use of aromatase inhibitors
- Androgen ablation
- Breast cancer
- Prostate cancer

oocytes available in the ovaries (Partridge et al., 2007; Schover, 2008). Increasing doses of alkylating agents such as cyclophosphamide increase the risk of premenopausal amenorrhea compared to therapy with anthracycline-based regimens such as doxorubicin and cyclophosphamide (AC). However, when taxanes are added to the AC regimen, a slight increase occurs in the risk of amenorrhea (Petrek et al., 2006). Therefore, the regimen of cyclophosphamide, methotrexate, and 5-fluorouracil (5-FU) and the regimen of cyclophosphamide, epirubicin, and 5-FU are associated with a higher risk of ovarian failure that leads to a prevalence of hot flashes.

In older men, decreasing levels of testosterone have been associated with hot flashes (Matsumoto, 2002; Thompson, Shanafelt, & Loprinzi, 2003). Although the physiologic mechanism is not well understood, men with prostate cancer also may experience hot flashes (Weldon, Neuwirth, & Bennett, 2005).

Hot flashes have a wide variety of potential triggers, such as reports of either hot or cold drinks, minor changes in room temperature, emotional flushing, alcohol and drugs, and flushing associated with food additives and spicy foods. The disease process of cancers, such as carcinoid syndrome, pheochromocytoma, medullary carcinoma of the thyroid, pancreatic islet-cell tumor, and renal cell carcinoma, also may cause hot flashes (Mohyi, Tabassi, & Simon, 1997).

Few qualitative studies have explained the experience of hot flashes in patients with cancer. Researchers conducting interviews with patients with and survivors of breast cancer found similar themes of loss of control and vulnerability (Fenlon & Rogers, 2007) as well as behavioral responses, such as changing clothing and bed linen (Finck, Barton, Loprinzi, Quella, & Sloan, 1998). Only one qualitative study of hot flashes has been performed in men. This study described the severity of hot flashes from the perspective of 59 patients with prostate cancer (Quella, Loprinzi, & Dose, 1994). This gap in the literature related to the hot flash experience in men lends itself to exploration of the phenomenon in a qualitative study.

Overall health-related quality of life (HRQOL) and symptom distress can be measured using a wide variety of tools. No specific quality-of-life instruments are available to assess hot flashes; the frequency, intensity, and severity are recorded in self-report diaries. Men treated with hormonal therapy have demonstrated a decreased overall HRQOL (Herr, Kornblith, & Ofman, 1993). Most of the studies of this group of patients described the overall global decline in HRQOL (Kouriefs, Georgiou, & Ravi, 2002; van Andel & Kurth, 2003) but did not specifically address the impact of hot flashes on HRQOL. British researchers asked 129 men with locally advanced prostate cancer to evaluate their quality of life on multiple symptoms and found that the men were willing to give up increased life expectancy (0.5 months) to avoid hot flashes (Sculpher et al., 2004).

Pathophysiology

The exact physiologic mechanisms of hot flashes are unknown; however, both animal and human studies have shed some light on this complex phenomenon. The following discussion reviews mechanisms of hot flashes in the thermoregulatory system and the potential future role of genetics in this phenomenon. Most studies in hot flashes have been conducted in postmenopausal women, women with breast cancer, and breast cancer survivors (Carpenter, 2001; Carpenter et al., 1999; Carpenter, Gautam, Freedman, & Andrykowski, 2001; Carpenter, Gilchrist, Chen, Gautam, & Freedman, 2004). Researchers monitored nine breast cancer survivors for 24 hours in a temperature- and humidity-controlled room and found that changes in core body temperature (0.09°C increase) occurred 7–20 minutes before the hot flashes started (Carpenter et al., 2004).

The central control of thermoregulation is the preoptic/anterior area in the brain. This area of the brain can be likened to a thermostat; heat dissipation occurs when it is too hot, and heat conservation or heat generation occurs when it is too cold. Human control of the thermostat is a negative feedback loop as depicted in Figure 14-2. The negative signs refer to the correction or change in skin or internal temperature; increases in internal or skin temperature sensed in the anterior pituitary results in dissipation through cutaneous vasodilation and sweating, resulting in the resetting of the thermostat. Conversely, decreased internal or skin temperature results in cutaneous vasoconstriction and increased heat generation via shivering to correct for the decrease in temperature, again resetting the thermostat. This feedback control loop is a set of physiologic control mechanisms that are vital to the maintenance of thermal homeostasis (Charkoudian, 2003). Hot flashes occur when the thermoregulatory zone is disrupted in human beings.

Core body temperature is regulated between an upper threshold for sweating and a lower threshold for shivering. A neutral zone lies between the upper and lower thresholds, an area in which no sweating or shivering occurs (Savage & Brengelmann, 1996). This theory postulates that heat dissipation responses of the hot flash (sweating and peripheral dilation) would be triggered if core body temperature (T_c) were elevated to the extent the threshold would be crossed. Researchers have demonstrated that small elevations in T_c occurred prior to most hot flashes (Freedman, 1989; Freedman, Norton, Woodward, & Cornelissen, 1995). A subsequent study measured the thermoneutral zone in 12 symptomatic and 8 asymptomatic postmenopausal women using ambient heating and cooling (Freedman & Krell, 1999). T_c was measured using a rectal probe and an ingested radiotelemetry pill, which determined the sweating thresholds for each group and a group of people who were exercising. The measured thermoneutral zone for all groups was 0°C in the symp-

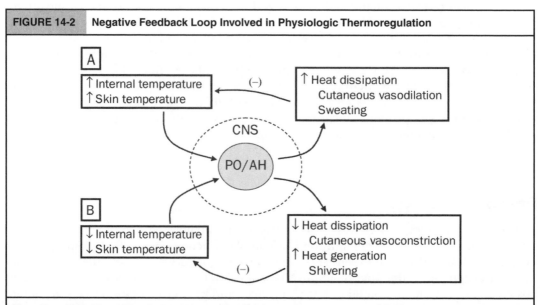

FIGURE 14-2   Negative Feedback Loop Involved in Physiologic Thermoregulation

A
↑ Internal temperature
↑ Skin temperature

(−)

↑ Heat dissipation
Cutaneous vasodilation
Sweating

CNS

PO/AH

B
↓ Internal temperature
↓ Skin temperature

(−)

↓ Heat dissipation
Cutaneous vasoconstriction
↑ Heat generation
Shivering

Note. From "Skin Blood Flow in Adult Human Thermoregulation: How It Works, When It Does Not, and Why," by N. Charkoudian, 2003, *Mayo Clinic Proceedings, 78*(5), p. 604. Copyright 2003 by Mayo Foundation for Medical Education and Research. Reprinted with permission.

tomatic women and 0.4°C in the asymptomatic women. The sweating thresholds were the same for the heating and exercise group and were accompanied by objective and subjective hot flashes in all cases. Sweat rates in the symptomatic women were twice those of the asymptomatic women, and no hot flashes occurred in the asymptomatic women. Therefore, the authors postulated that hot flashes are triggered by T_c elevations acting within a greatly reduced thermoneutral zone in symptomatic menopausal women (Freedman & Krell). The sensation of the hot flash may be caused by the temperature fluctuations that lead to sweating and shivering.

Assessment

Hot flashes can be measured both subjectively and objectively. Subjective measures of hot flash frequency, severity, intensity, and bother can be collected using self-reported data from the patient. The practitioner may simply ask patients if they do or do not have hot flashes or may ask patients to complete a hot flash diary. A number of self-reported instruments are available to measure vasomotor symptoms (hot flashes); however, very few have been validated and are sometimes poorly described.

The Loprinzi and Sloan daily diary (see Figure 14-3) method has been validated on breast cancer survivors. Patients record a summary of events once a day that notes the number and severity of hot flashes. The score is computed multiplying the frequency by the severity (Sloan et al., 2001). Another tool, the Hot Flash-Related Daily Inference Scale (HFRDIS), a 10-item scale designed to measure the extent to which hot flashes interfere with overall quality of life, has been validated in breast cancer survivors (Carpenter, 2001; Carpenter, Johnson, et al., 2002).

Sternal skin conductance has been validated as an objective measure of hot flash frequency in patients with breast and prostate cancer (Carpenter et al., 1999; Hanisch, Palmer, Donahue, & Coyne, 2007). Sternal skin conductance is a measure of the skin's ability to conduct electricity (Dawson, Schell, & Filion, 2000) and is not influenced by anxiety or emotion; therefore, it is a better measure of conductance than the palms of the hands or soles of the feet, which produce sweat during emotional times. A constant voltage current applied to the sternum between two electrodes to measure a brisk increase in skin conductance detects the hot flash occurrence (Carpenter et al., 1999; Freedman & Krell, 1999). The sternal skin conductance monitor is a small ambulatory unit worn by the patient for up to 24 hours to measure hot flash activity.

In summary, two hot flash assessment tools or measures are validated to assess subjective hot flash frequency, duration, and intensity: the daily diary method tested in breast cancer survivors and the HFRDIS for hot flash interference on measures of activities of daily living and quality of life. Sternal skin conductance is a valid instrument to assess objective measures of hot flash frequency in patients with breast and prostate cancer.

Evidence-Based Interventions

Various treatment options, including both pharmacologic and nonpharmacologic therapies, are available for patients with cancer who experience hot flashes. These treatments comprise lifestyle changes, hormonal and nonhormonal agents, and complementary and alternative therapies. Appropriate interventions should be selected by the best evidence available based upon research in patients with cancer, along with patient preference. The

FIGURE 14-3	Patient-Reported Hot Flash Diary

FIRST STUDY WEEK (BASELINE)

DAILY PATIENT QUESTIONNAIRE: DOUBLE-BLIND PHASE

No tablets this week

Date week started: ___ ___ / ___ ___ / ___ ___ ___ ___
         m m   d d   y y y y

	Day 1	Day 2	Day 3	Day 4	Day 5	Day 6	Day 7**
Number of today's hot flashes that were mild, moderate, severe, or very severe?	__ mild __ moderate __ severe __ very severe	__ mild __ moderate __ severe __ very severe	__ mild __ moderate __ severe __ very severe	__ mild __ moderate __ severe __ very severe	__ mild __ moderate __ severe __ very severe	__ mild __ moderate __ severe __ very severe	__ mild __ moderate __ severe __ very severe
Total number of hot flashes today*							

* One day should be considered to be a 24 hour period (i.e. 7:00 a.m. to 7:00 a.m. or midnight to midnight).

Date week stopped: ___ ___ / ___ ___ / ___ ___ ___ ___
        m m   d d   y y y y

Do you have any of the following symptoms?:

appetite loss	__ no	__ yes	abnormal sweating	__ no	__ yes
sleepiness	__ no	__ yes	constipation	__ no	__ yes
nausea	__ no	__ yes	trouble sleeping	__ no	__ yes
dizziness	__ no	__ yes	nervousness	__ no	__ yes
tiredness (fatigue)	__ no	__ yes	mood changes	__ no	__ yes
dry mouth	__ no	__ yes			
other	__ no	__ yes, please describe _____			

Comments: _____

Blood Pressure _____ / _____   Date blood pressure obtained: ___ ___ / ___ ___ / ___ ___ ___ ___
                                      m m   d d   y y y y

** Please complete the next 3 pages on Day 7

Note. From "Methodologic Lessons Learned From Hot Flash Studies," by J.A. Sloan, C.L. Loprinzi, P.J. Novotny, D.L. Barton, B.I. Lavasseur, and H. Windschitl, 2001, *Journal of Clinical Oncology, 19*(23), pp. 4280–4290 (Appendix A). Used with permission of Charles L. Loprinzi, MD, Mayo Clinic, Rochester, MN.

following interventions are evaluated using the classification schema developed by the Oncology Nursing Society (ONS) (Ciliska, Cullum, & Marks, 2001; Hadorn, Baker, Hodges, & Hicks, 1996; ONS, 2007; Ropka & Spencer-Cisek, 2001; Rutledge, DePalma, & Cunningham, 2004).

Pharmacologic Interventions

Hormonal Therapies

Historically, estrogen and progesterone supplementation has been the mainstay in reducing hot flashes in both women and men (Neff, 2004). Hormonal therapy is contraindicated in patients with hormone-dependent tumors such as breast cancer (Holmberg & Anderson, 2004). The HABITS (Hormonal Replacement Therapy After Breast Cancer—Is It Safe?) study consisted of two randomized clinical trials conducted in Scandinavia addressing whether HRT was safe for women with a previous diagnosis of breast cancer. The studies were stopped early because a significant increase in breast cancer recurrence rate occurred in those randomized to estrogen (Holmberg & Anderson), showing that hormonal therapy may not be safe to use in breast cancer survivors.

Tibolone is a steroid with progestogenic activity (Landgren, Helmond, & Engelen, 2005) that has demonstrated a reduction in hot flashes compared to placebo in healthy postmenopausal women (Landgren et al., 2005) and in a randomized, double-blind, placebo-controlled trial in postmenopausal women receiving tamoxifen after surgery for breast cancer (p = 0.031) (Kroiss et al., 2005). However, as with other estrogens and progesterones, the safety profiles in patients with cancer are not clear.

Megestrol acetate may be effective in relieving hot flashes in women and men (Barton, La, et al., 2002; Barton, Loprinzi, et al., 2002; Loprinzi et al., 2006; Loprinzi, Michalak, et al., 1994). However, the safety evidence is conflicting for the use of this drug. Megestrol acetate may promote tumor growth in men with prostate cancer (Sartor & Eastham, 1999). The safety in breast cancer survivors has not yet been determined. In vitro models have demonstrated that progestational agents such as megestrol acetate increased or accelerated breast cancer development (Eden, 2003). Therefore, hormonal therapies generally are not recommended for patients with breast or prostate cancer. Definitive safety data from large, long-term, randomized, controlled clinical trials are needed to show the safety record of megestrol acetate.

Nonhormonal Therapies

Many prospective randomized clinical trials have demonstrated the effectiveness of the selective serotonin reuptake inhibitor/serotonin and norepinephrine reuptake inhibitor (SSRI/SNRI) family, such as venlafaxine, paroxetine, and sertraline, to reduce hot flashes by as much as 50%–60% (Stearns, 2006). Table 14-1 is a summary of evidence for therapies that are recommended for practice. The underlying hypothesis is that serotonin is strongly involved in the pathogenesis of hot flashes by the interaction of estrogens and progestins with the serotonergic system in the brain. Stimulation of the 5-HT_{2A} drug receptors in the hypothalamus change the T_c set rate, resulting in a hot flash. The premise is that blocking of 5-HT_{2A} receptors (inhibition of serotonin reuptake) may be effective in the treatment of hot flashes (Berendsen, 2000). Three recent meta-analyses on the treatment of hot flashes recommended venlafaxine, paroxetine, fluoxetine, and sertraline in the treatment of hot flashes in breast cancer survivors (Kimmick, Lovato, McQuellon, Robinson, & Muss, 2006; Loprinzi et al., 2002; Stearns et al., 2005) and venlafaxine (Loprinzi et al., 2000) and paroxetine in patients with prostate cancer (Nelson et al., 2006; Stearns, 2006; Stricker, 2007).

Gabapentin is a gamma-aminobutyric acid analog whose mechanism of action in hot flashes is unclear. However, it is hypothesized to be related to upregulation of gabapentin binding sites caused by estrogen withdrawal (Pandya et al., 2005). A few randomized clinical tri-

TABLE 14-1	Summary of Hot Flash Interventions That Are Recommended for Practice						
Lead Author	Journal	Year	Study Design	Sample Size	Cancer*	Medication	Dose Per Day
Loprinzi	*Mayo Clinic Proceedings*	2004	Pilot	24	P	Paroxetine	37.5 mg
Stearns	*Journal of Clinical Oncology*	2005	Randomized	151	B	Paroxetine	10 mg/20 mg
Kimmick	*Breast Journal*	2006	Randomized	47	B	Sertraline	50 mg
Loprinzi	*Lancet*	2000	Randomized	191	B	Venlafaxine	37.5 mg/75 mg
Loprinzi	*Journal of Clinical Oncology*	2002	Randomized	81	B	Fluoxetine	20 mg
Pandya	*Lancet*	2005	Randomized	347	B	Gabapentin	900 mg

* P = prostate cancer; B = breast cancer

als have evaluated the efficacy and safety in gabapentin only (Loprinzi, 2006; Pandya et al., 2005) or in combination with an antidepressant such as venlafaxine or paroxetine (Loprinzi et al., 2007). In one study, gabapentin 900 mg/day (versus 300 mg/day or placebo) was found to be significant ($p < 0.0001$) in reducing the frequency of hot flashes by 41% and the severity of hot flashes by 49% in patients with breast cancer (Pandya et al., 2005). Adverse effects of somnolence and dizziness are reported with gabapentin, which might limit its use in relieving hot flashes (Baber, Hickey, & Kwik, 2005).

A pilot study to evaluate the efficacy and safety of mirtazapine 30 mg/m^2 in 40 patients with breast cancer showed a significant reduction (55.6%; $p = 0.05$) in the frequency of hot flashes. Mirtazapine is a potent antagonist of 5-HT$_2$, 5-HT$_3$, and histamine receptors (Biglia et al., 2007). The alpha adrenergic agent clonidine acts peripherally to reduce vasodilation, therefore reducing hot flashes. Results from studies in breast cancer survivors on tamoxifen and patients with prostate cancer who also took clonidine have demonstrated effectiveness in reducing hot flashes (Loprinzi, Goldberg, et al., 1994; Pandya et al., 2000). A double-blind, randomized phase III study in 64 patients with breast cancer experiencing hot flashes compared venlafaxine to clonidine in reducing hot flashes. The study found venlafaxine to be superior to clonidine ($p = 0.025$) in decreasing the frequency of hot flashes compared to baseline (Loibl et al., 2007). Significant dose-related side effects of increased constipation, dry mouth, and drowsiness limit the use of clonidine for symptom control (Baber et al., 2005).

Centrally active agents, such as venlafaxine, paroxetine, and gabapentin, seem to be the most promising of the nonhormonal treatments for hot flashes in patients and survivors of breast cancer and are recommended for practice. A randomized trial of 11 patients with breast cancer taking gabapentin alone versus gabapentin and an antidepressant (venlafaxine or paroxetine) demonstrated no significant difference in the groups (Loprinzi et al., 2007). Nurses should be cautioned to screen patients for clinical depression, monitor patients who are already on antidepressants, observe for antidepressant polypharmacy, and determine undertreatment of depression.

Nonpharmacologic Interventions

Complementary and Alternative Medicine Approaches

Black cohosh is an herbaceous perennial plant thought to have multiple mechanisms of action, including potential phytoestrogenic properties that have caused some concern about its use by patients with hormone-sensitive cancer (Walji, Boon, Guns, Oneschuk, & Younus, 2007). It commonly is used to treat hot flashes and other symptoms associated with menopause. A recent meta-analysis of clinical (n = 5) and preclinical (n = 21) studies of black cohosh and cancer (breast and prostate) to treat hot flashes found that black cohosh seems not to exhibit phytoestrogenic activity and is possibly an inhibitor of tumor growth (Walji et al.). A large randomized placebo-controlled study of black cohosh using a crossover design (N = 132) showed that black cohosh did not reduce hot flashes any more than placebo (Pockaj et al., 2006)—the same results as previous trials (Jacobson et al., 2001). Therefore, black cohosh is not recommended for practice.

Soy phytoestrogens are weak estrogens found in many plants, vegetables, and fruits. No evidence has shown that soy is better than placebo in controlling hot flashes in patients with breast cancer in randomized controlled clinical trials (MacGregor, Canney, Patterson, McDonald, & Paul, 2005; Nikander et al., 2003; Nikander, Metsa-Heikkila, Ylikorkala, & Tiitinen, 2004; Quella et al., 2000; Van Patten et al., 2002). MacGregor et al. conducted a study of 72 patients with breast cancer taking soy compound versus placebo in a randomized, double-blind controlled trial. Results did not support the use of soy supplements for the treatment of hot flashes, nor was any change noted in the quality of life between the two groups (Walji et al., 2007). The main side effects of soy compounds are bloating, constipation, and nausea (Baber et al., 2005). No longitudinal studies have been conducted to determine the effects of soy in patients with breast or prostate cancer or the risk of recurrent breast cancer; therefore, it cannot be recommended for practice at this time.

Vitamin E has been found to be a safe, mildly effective intervention for hot flashes based on anecdotal information and pilot study information. Only one randomized, placebo-controlled study of vitamin E has been conducted. Researchers in this study, which was performed by the North Central Cancer Treatment Center, determined that 105 survivors of breast cancer with hot flashes did not prefer vitamin E over the placebo (Barton et al., 1998). Therefore, this treatment is not currently recommended.

Hypnosis is an intervention that has been hypothesized to help alleviate hot flashes. However, only one pilot study has been performed using hypnosis in breast cancer survivors (N = 16), which indicated a 59% decrease in total daily hot flashes (Elkins, Marcus, Stearns, & Rajab, 2007). In a study of magnet therapy in breast cancer survivors, results failed to reach significance (Carpenter, Wells, et al., 2002).

A recent randomized study of true acupuncture versus sham acupuncture (sham needles do not puncture the skin, and instead retract back into the handle) measured flash frequency in 72 women with breast cancer and found no significant difference between the true and sham acupuncture groups (Deng, Vickers, Yeung, & Cassileth, 2007). These results conflicted with a previous study of 31 patients with breast cancer who were randomized to relaxation or acupuncture, in which symptoms were significantly reduced (Nedstrand, Wijma, Wyon, & Hammar, 2005). One study of six patients with prostate cancer receiving acupuncture reported a substantial decrease in the number of hot flashes (average 70% after 10 weeks) (Hammar et al., 1999).

No head-to-head studies have compared nonhormonal therapy to hormonal therapy for the relief of hot flashes, and only a limited number of well-designed complementary and alternative studies exist. Therefore, at this time, none of these approaches can be recommended for practice.

Patient Teaching Points

Treatment modalities should be individualized to each patient, considering potential risks and benefits of treatment. Patients should be assured that hot flashes are not an inevitable symptom or side effect of being a patient with breast cancer or prostate cancer. Treatment should begin after a thorough assessment of the severity and frequency of hot flashes. Hot flashes may occur in a cluster of symptoms, such as sleep-wake disturbances, alterations in cognition, anxiety or depression, or decreased quality of life (Engstrom, 2005). Nurses should encourage patients to report symptom interference with social activities, activities of daily living, rest and sleep, and overall quality of life.

Patient education should focus on the potential benefits, risks, and scientific uncertainties of each treatment option (Stearns, 2007) while underscoring the potential for drug-drug interactions with SSRI/SNRI medications. For example, paroxetine and fluoxetine are inhibitors of the cytochrome P450 (CYP) 2D6 pathway, lowering the efficacy of tamoxifen (Loprinzi, Stearns, & Barton, 2005).

Using personal hot flash diaries or journals to record the number, frequency, severity, and timing of hot flashes will assist both patients and nurses in an ongoing assessment of interventions. Teach patients to anticipate or recognize personal triggers for hot flashes (e.g., ambient room temperature, hot or cold beverages, anxiety) and to record these in the diary. Some patients may benefit from avoiding spicy foods, alcohol, caffeine, or hot, humid weather. Dressing in layers may help to reduce the intensity of hot flashes.

Patient teaching should discuss the value of lifestyle modifications that may reduce hot flashes, such as decreasing BMI, smoking cessation, and limiting alcohol usage. Referral to support groups such as the American Cancer Society's *I Can Cope* or *Man to Man* programs may help some patients to cope with the side effects of treatment.

Need for Future Research

Currently, no standardized guidelines exist for the treatment of hot flashes in the oncology patient population. Advances in the development of treatment modalities will depend on increased knowledge about the physiologic mechanism of hot flashes, thus leading to possible targeted therapies with favorable safety profiles. More research is needed to better elucidate the role of environmental factors, such as room temperature, and genetic predisposing factors such as estradiol and catecholamine (single nucleotide polymorphisms of genes involved in estrogen function to vasomotor symptoms) and the responses that might allow for better individual tailoring of interventions (Crandall, Crawford, & Gold, 2006).

Future studies examining the multiple effects of mirtazapine or gabapentin on hot flash symptom clusters, including sleep-wake disturbances and quality of life, would add to the armamentarium for nurses. More studies also are needed to evaluate alternative therapies such as acupuncture. Studies have demonstrated that longer and more intense acupuncture intervention could produce a larger reduction of these symptoms.

Few treatment options are available for men and women with hot flashes apart from hormonal therapies, which may cause myriad side effects. Interventions or therapies need to be tailored to patients individually, taking into consideration the comorbidities and other medications that patients may be taking.

Conclusion of Case Study

The nurse must obtain a comprehensive database on C.L. to ascertain the etiology of his symptoms. A detailed history and review of systems will help in determining pertinent positive and negative symptoms related to his complaints and in considering possible interventions. He denies a history of diabetes, tuberculosis, thyroid disease, cardiac disease, or generalized anxiety disorder. C.L. is concerned with the sweating that has occurred for the past five to six months with each episode lasting from one to five minutes. He has noticed that if he drinks coffee, he breaks out in a sweat "that drips down my face and neck and is embarrassing when I am with customers." He has tried carrying a small battery-operated fan with him to cool off, but it has had minimal effect. He denies fever or chills, nausea or vomiting, weight loss, or signs and symptoms of an infection or other cancers. C.L. says he is quite anxious about the "heart pounding" during the hot flashes. He denies fatigue, chest pain, shortness of breath, dyspnea on exertion, dizziness, cough, peripheral edema, or change in medications.

The most likely diagnosis for C.L. is hot flashes related to the hormonal treatment for prostate cancer. Infection, cardiac disease, respiratory disease, diabetes, and thyroid disease most likely can be ruled out by the pertinent negatives in the review of symptoms, physical examination, and diagnostic testing.

The nurse explains to C.L. that his symptoms are most likely the result of side effects from his hormonal treatment for prostate cancer. He and his wife have had all of the treatment options explained to them, including possible side effects. He does not want to take medications for the hot flashes; however, he is interested in participating in a clinical trial for hot flashes and would like to further investigate treatment with alternative therapy using either magnets or acupuncture. He was given contact information for a National Cancer Institute study of acupuncture in the treatment of hot flashes in men receiving androgen ablation as well as for a pharmaceutical company–sponsored study of cyproterone acetate.

Conclusion

Hot flashes and hot flash clusters of symptoms are commonly reported side effects of hormonal treatment for men and women. Reliable evaluation tools are needed to accurately measure both subjective and objective hot flashes. Interventions should match the frequency, distress, and severity of the symptoms. The only recommended therapy with sufficient evidence in the treatment of hot flashes is with one of the SSRIs/SNRIs, venlafaxine, paroxetine, or gabapentin. Future research studies may provide evidence to treat patients with alternative therapies such as acupuncture or dietary supplements.

References

Baber, R., Hickey, M., & Kwik, M. (2005). Therapy for menopausal symptoms during and after treatment for breast cancer: Safety considerations. *Drug Safety, 28*(12), 1085–1100.

Barton, D., La, V.B., Loprinzi, C., Novotny, P., Wilwerding, M.B., & Sloan, J. (2002). Venlafaxine for the control of hot flashes: Results of a longitudinal continuation study. *Oncology Nursing Forum, 29*(1), 33–40.

Barton, D., Loprinzi, C., Quella, S., Sloan, J., Pruthi, S., & Novotny, P. (2002). Depomedroxyprogesterone acetate for hot flashes. *Journal of Pain and Symptom Management, 24*(6), 603–607.

Barton, D.L., Loprinzi, C.L., Quella, S.K., Sloan, J.A., Veeder, M.H., Egner, J.R., et al. (1998). Prospective evaluation of vitamin E for hot flashes in breast cancer survivors. *Journal of Clinical Oncology, 16*(2), 495–500.

Berendsen, H.H. (2000). The role of serotonin in hot flushes. *Maturitas, 36*(3), 155–164.

Biglia, N., Kubatzki, F., Sgandurra, P., Ponzone, R., Marenco, D., Peano, E., et al. (2007). Mirtazapine for the treatment of hot flushes in breast cancer survivors: A prospective pilot trial. *Breast Journal, 13*(5), 490–495.

Carpenter, J.S. (2000). Hot flashes and their management in breast cancer. *Seminars in Oncology Nursing, 16*(3), 214–225.

Carpenter, J.S. (2001). The Hot Flash Related Daily Interference Scale: A tool for assessing the impact of hot flashes on quality of life following breast cancer. *Journal of Pain and Symptom Management, 22*(6), 979–989.

Carpenter, J.S. (2005). Physiological monitor for assessing hot flashes. *Clinical Nurse Specialist, 19*(1), 8–10.

Carpenter, J.S., Andrykowski, M.A., Cordova, M., Cunningham, L., Studts, J., McGrath, P., et al. (1998). Hot flashes in postmenopausal women treated for breast carcinoma: Prevalence, severity, correlates, management, and relation to quality of life. *Cancer, 82*(9), 1682–1691.

Carpenter, J.S., Andrykowski, M.A., Freedman, R.R., & Munn, R. (1999). Feasibility and psychometrics of an ambulatory hot flash monitoring device. *Menopause, 6*(3), 209–215.

Carpenter, J.S., Gautam, S., Freedman, R.R., & Andrykowski, M. (2001). Circadian rhythm of objectively recorded hot flashes in postmenopausal breast cancer survivors. *Menopause, 8*(3), 181–188.

Carpenter, J.S., Gilchrist, J.M., Chen, K., Gautam, S., & Freedman, R.R. (2004). Hot flashes, core body temperature, and metabolic parameters in breast cancer survivors. *Menopause, 11*(4), 375–381.

Carpenter, J.S., Johnson, D.H., Wagner, L.J., & Andrykowski, M.A. (2002). Hot flashes and related outcomes in breast cancer survivors and matched comparison women. *Oncology Nursing Forum, 29*(3), E16–E25. Retrieved December 27, 2007, from http://ons.metapress.com/content/6616786818742847/fulltext.pdf

Carpenter, J.S., Wells, N., Lambert, B., Watson, P., Slayton, T., Chak, B., et al. (2002). A pilot study of magnetic therapy for hot flashes after breast cancer. *Cancer Nursing, 25*(2), 104–109.

Charig, C.R., & Rundle, J.S. (1989). Flushing. Long-term side effect of orchiectomy in treatment of prostatic carcinoma. *Urology, 33*(3), 175–178.

Charkoudian, N. (2003). Skin blood flow in adult human thermoregulation: How it works, when it does not, and why. *Mayo Clinic Proceedings, 78*(5), 603–612.

Ciliska, D., Cullum, N., & Marks, S. (2001). Evaluation of systematic reviews of treatment or prevention interventions. *Evidence-Based Nursing, 4*(4), 100–104.

Clark, J.A., Wray, N.P., & Ashton, C.M. (2001). Living with treatment decisions: Regrets and quality of life among men treated for metastatic prostate cancer. *Journal of Clinical Oncology, 19*(1), 72–80.

Crandall, C.J., Crawford, S.L., & Gold, E.B. (2006). Vasomotor symptom prevalence is associated with polymorphisms in sex steroid-metabolizing enzymes and receptors. *American Journal of Medicine, 119*(9, Suppl. 1), S52–S60.

Dawson, M.E., Schell, A.M., & Filion, D.L. (2000). The electrodermal system. In J.T. Cacioppo, L.G. Tassinary, & G.G. Berntson (Eds.), *Handbook of psychophysiology* (2nd ed., pp. 200–223). New York: Cambridge University Press.

Deng, G., Vickers, A., Yeung, S., & Cassileth, B. (2007). Randomized, controlled trial of acupuncture for the treatment of hot flashes in breast cancer patients. *Journal of Clinical Oncology, 25*(35), 5584–5590.

Eden, J. (2003). Progestins and breast cancer. *American Journal of Obstetrics and Gynecology, 188*(5), 1123–1131.

Elkins, G., Marcus, J., Stearns, V., & Rajab, M.H. (2007). Pilot evaluation of hypnosis for the treatment of hot flashes in breast cancer survivors. *Psycho-Oncology, 16*(5), 487–492.

Engstrom, C. (2005). Hot flash experience in men with prostate cancer: A concept analysis. *Oncology Nursing Forum, 32*(5), 1043–1048.

Fallowfield, L., Cella, D., Cuzick, J., Francis, S., Locker, G., & Howell, A. (2004). Quality of life of postmenopausal women in the Arimidex, Tamoxifen, Alone or in Combination (ATAC) Adjuvant Breast Cancer Trial. *Journal of Clinical Oncology, 22*(21), 4261–4271.

Fenlon, D.R., & Rogers, A.E. (2007). The experience of hot flushes after breast cancer. *Cancer Nursing, 30*(4), E19–E26.

Finck, G., Barton, D.L., Loprinzi, C.L., Quella, S.K., & Sloan, J.A. (1998). Definitions of hot flashes in breast cancer survivors. *Journal of Pain Symptom and Management, 16*(5), 327–333.

Freedman, R.R. (1989). Laboratory and ambulatory monitoring of menopausal hot flashes. *Psychophysiology, 26*(5), 573–579.

Freedman, R.R., & Krell, W. (1999). Reduced thermoregulatory null zone in postmenopausal women with hot flashes. *American Journal of Obstetrics and Gynecology, 181*(1), 66–70.

Freedman, R.R., Norton, D., Woodward, S., & Cornelissen, G. (1995). Core body temperature and circadian rhythm of hot flashes in menopausal women. *Journal of Clinical Endocrinology and Metabolism, 80*(8), 2354–2358.

Glaus, A., Boehme, C., Thurlimann, B., Ruhstaller, T., Hsu Schmitz, S.F., Morant, R., et al. (2006). Fatigue and menopausal symptoms in women with breast cancer undergoing hormonal cancer treatment. *Annals of Oncology, 17*(5), 801–806.

Gold, E.B., Colvin, A., Avis, N., Bromberger, J., Greendale, G.A., Powell, L., et al. (2006). Longitudinal analysis of the association between vasomotor symptoms and race/ethnicity across the menopausal transition: Study of women's health across the nation. *American Journal of Public Health, 96*(7), 1226–1235.

Hadorn, D.C., Baker, D., Hodges, J.S., & Hicks, N. (1996). Rating the quality of evidence for clinical practice guidelines. *Journal of Clinical Epidemiology, 49*(7), 749–754.

Hammar, M., Frisk, J., Grimas, O., Hook, M., Spetz, A.C., & Wyon, Y. (1999). Acupuncture treatment of vasomotor symptoms in men with prostatic carcinoma: A pilot study. *Journal of Urology, 161*(3), 853–856.

Hanisch, L.J., Palmer, S.C., Donahue, A., & Coyne, J.C. (2007). Validation of sternal skin conductance for detection of hot flashes in prostate cancer survivors. *Psychophysiology, 44*(2), 189–193.

Hardy, R., Kuh, D., & Wadsworth, M. (2000). Smoking, body mass index, socioeconomic status and the menopausal transition in a British national cohort. *International Journal of Epidemiology, 29*(5), 845–851.

Herr, H.W., Kornblith, A.B., & Ofman, U. (1993). A comparison of the quality of life of patients with metastatic prostate cancer who received or did not receive hormonal therapy. *Cancer, 71*(Suppl. 3), 1143–1150.

Holmberg, L., & Anderson, H. (2004). HABITS (hormonal replacement therapy after breast cancer-is it safe?), a randomised comparison: Trial stopped. *Lancet, 363*(9407), 453–455.

Jacobson, J.S., Troxel, A.B., Evans, J., Klaus, L., Vahdat, L., Kinne, D., et al. (2001). Randomized trial of black cohosh for the treatment of hot flashes among women with a history of breast cancer. *Journal of Clinical Oncology, 19*(10), 2739–2745.

Karling, P., Hammar, M., & Varenhorst, E. (1994). Prevalence and duration of hot flushes after surgical or medical castration in men with prostatic carcinoma. *Journal of Urology, 152*(4), 1170–1173.

Kimmick, G.G., Lovato, J., McQuellon, R., Robinson, E., & Muss, H.B. (2006). Randomized, double-blind, placebo-controlled, crossover study of sertraline (Zoloft) for the treatment of hot flashes in women with early stage breast cancer taking tamoxifen. *Breast Journal, 12*(2), 114–122.

Kouriefs, C., Georgiou, M., & Ravi, R. (2002). Hot flushes and prostate cancer: Pathogenesis and treatment. *BJU International, 89*(4), 379–383.

Kroiss, R., Fentiman, I.S., Helmond, F.A., Rymer, J., Foidart, J.M., Bundred, N., et al. (2005). The effect of tibolone in postmenopausal women receiving tamoxifen after surgery for breast cancer: A randomised, double-blind, placebo-controlled trial. *British Journal of Gynecology, 112*(2), 228–233.

Landgren, M.B., Helmond, F.A., & Engelen, S. (2005). Tibolone relieves climacteric symptoms in highly symptomatic women with at least seven hot flushes and sweats per day. *Maturitas, 50*(3), 222–230.

Loibl, S., Schwedler, K., von Minckwitz, G., Strohmeier, R., Mehta, K.M., & Kaufmann, M. (2007). Venlafaxine is superior to clonidine as treatment of hot flashes in breast cancer patients—a double-blind, randomized study. *Annals of Oncology, 18*(4), 689–693.

Loprinzi, C.L. (2006). 900 mg daily of gabapentin was effective for hot flashes in women with breast cancer. *ACP Journal Club, 144*(2), 41.

Loprinzi, C.L., Barton, D.L., Carpenter, L.A., Sloan, J.A., Novotny, P.J., Gettman, M.T., et al. (2004). Pilot evaluation of paroxetine for treating hot flashes. *Mayo Clinic Proceedings, 79*(10), 1274–1251.

Loprinzi, C.L., Goldberg, R.M., O'Fallon, J.R., Quella, S.K., Miser, A.W., Mynderse, L.A., et al. (1994). Transdermal clonidine for ameliorating post-orchiectomy hot flashes. *Journal of Urology, 151*(3), 634–636.

Loprinzi, C.L., Kugler, J.W., Barton, D.L., Dueck, A.C., Tschetter, L.K., Nelimark, R.A., et al. (2007). Phase III trial of gabapentin alone or in conjunction with an antidepressant in the management of hot flashes in women who have inadequate control with an antidepressant alone: NCCTG N03C5. *Journal of Clinical Oncology, 25*(3), 308–312.

Loprinzi, C.L., Kugler, J.W., Sloan, J.A., Mailliard, J.A., LaVasseur, B.I., Barton, D.L., et al. (2000). Venlafaxine in management of hot flashes in survivors of breast cancer: A randomised controlled trial. *Lancet, 356*(9247), 2059–2063.

Loprinzi, C.L., Levitt, R., Barton, D., Sloan, J.A., Dakhil, S.R., Nikcevich, D.A., et al. (2006). Phase III comparison of depomedroxyprogesterone acetate to venlafaxine for managing hot flashes: North Central Cancer Treatment Group Trial N99C7. *Journal of Clinical Oncology, 24*(9), 1409–1414.

Loprinzi, C.L., Michalak, J.C., Quella, S.K., O'Fallon, J.R., Hatfield, A.K., Nelimark, R.A., et al. (1994). Megestrol acetate for the prevention of hot flashes. *New England Journal of Medicine, 331*(6), 347–352.

Loprinzi, C.L., Sloan, J.A., Perez, E.A., Quella, S.K., Stella, P.J., Mailliard, J.A., et al. (2002). Phase III evaluation of fluoxetine for treatment of hot flashes. *Journal of Clinical Oncology, 20*(6), 1578–1583.

Loprinzi, C.L., Stearns, V., & Barton, D. (2005). Centrally active nonhormonal hot flash therapies. *American Journal of Medicine, 118*(Suppl. 12B), 118–123.

MacGregor, C.A., Canney, P.A., Patterson, G., McDonald, R., & Paul, J. (2005). A randomised double-blind controlled trial of oral soy supplements versus placebo for treatment of menopausal symptoms in patients with early breast cancer. *European Journal of Cancer, 41*(5), 708–714.

Matsumoto, A.M. (2002). Andropause: Clinical implications of the decline in serum testosterone levels with aging in men. *Journal of Gerontology: Medical Sciences, 57*(2), M76–M99.

Mohyi, D., Tabassi, K., & Simon, J. (1997). Differential diagnosis of hot flashes. *Maturitas, 27*(3), 203–214.

Nedstrand, E., Wijma, K., Wyon, Y., & Hammar, M. (2005). Vasomotor symptoms decrease in women with breast cancer randomized to treatment with applied relaxation or electro-acupuncture: A preliminary study. *Climacteric, 8*(3), 243–250.

Neff, M.J. (2004). NAMS releases position statement on the treatment of vasomotor symptoms associated with menopause. *American Family Physician, 70*(2), 393–394, 396, 399.

Nelson, H.D., Vesco, K.K., Haney, E., Fu, R., Nedrow, A., Miller, J., et al. (2006). Nonhormonal therapies for menopausal hot flashes: Systematic review and meta-analysis. *JAMA, 295*(17), 2057–2071.

Nikander, E., Kilkkinen, A., Metsa-Heikkila, M., Adlercreutz, H., Pietinen, P., Tiitinen, A., et al. (2003). A randomized placebo-controlled crossover trial with phytoestrogens in treatment of menopause in breast cancer patients. *Obstetrics and Gynecology, 101*(6), 1213–1220.

Nikander, E., Metsa-Heikkila, M., Ylikorkala, O., & Tiitinen, A. (2004). Effects of phytoestrogens on bone turnover in postmenopausal women with a history of breast cancer. *Journal of Clinical Endocrinology and Metabolism, 89*(3), 1207–1212.

Oncology Nursing Society. (2007). *ONS PEP Putting Evidence Into Practice: Classification schema.* Retrieved December 27, 2007, from http://www.ons.org/publications/journals/CJON

Pandya, K.J., Morrow, G.R., Roscoe, J.A., Zhao, H., Hickok, J.T., Pajon, E., et al. (2005). Gabapentin for hot flashes in 420 women with breast cancer: A randomised double-blind placebo-controlled trial. *Lancet, 366*(9488), 818–824.

Pandya, K.J., Raubertas, R.F., Flynn, P.J., Hynes, H.E., Rosenbluth, R.J., Kirshner, J.J., et al. (2000). Oral clonidine in postmenopausal patients with breast cancer experiencing tamoxifen-induced hot flashes: A University of Rochester Cancer Center Community Clinical Oncology Program study. *Annals of Internal Medicine, 132*(10), 788–793.

Partridge, A., Gelber, S., Gelber, R.D., Castiglione-Gertsch, M., Goldhirsch, A., & Winer, E. (2007). Age of menopause among women who remain premenopausal following treatment for early breast cancer: Long-term results from International Breast Cancer Study Group Trials V and VI. *European Journal of Cancer, 43*(11), 1646–1653.

Petrek, J.A., Naughton, M.J., Case, L.D., Paskett, E.D., Naftalis, E.Z., Singletary, S.E., et al. (2006). Incidence, time course, and determinants of menstrual bleeding after breast cancer treatment: A prospective study. *Journal of Clinical Oncology, 24*(7), 1045–1051.

Pockaj, B.A., Gallagher, J.G., Loprinzi, C.L., Stella, P.J., Barton, D.L., Sloan, J.A., et al. (2006). Phase III double-blind, randomized, placebo-controlled crossover trial of black cohosh in the management of hot flashes: NCCTG Trial N01CC1. *Journal of Clinical Oncology, 24*(18), 2836–2841.

Quella, S., Loprinzi, C.L., & Dose, A.M. (1994). A qualitative approach to defining "hot flashes" in men. *Urology Nursing, 14*(4), 155–158.

Quella, S.K., Loprinzi, C.L., Barton, D.L., Knost, J.A., Sloan, J.A., LaVasseur, B.I., et al. (2000). Evaluation of soy phytoestrogens for the treatment of hot flashes in breast cancer survivors: A North Central Cancer Treatment Group Trial. *Journal of Clinical Oncology, 18*(5), 1068–1074.

Riley, E., Inui, T.S., Kleinman, K., & Connelly, M.T. (2004). Differential association of modifiable health behaviors with hot flashes in perimenopausal and postmenopausal women. *Journal of General Internal Medicine, 19*(7), 740–746.

Ropka, M.E., & Spencer-Cisek, P. (2001). PRISM: Priority Symptom Management Project phase I: Assessment. *Oncology Nursing Forum, 28*(10), 1585–1594.

Rutledge, D.N., DePalma, J.A., & Cunningham, M. (2004). A process model for evidence-based literature syntheses. *Oncology Nursing Forum, 31*(3), 543–550.

Sartor, O., & Eastham, J.A. (1999). Progressive prostate cancer associated with use of megestrol acetate administered for control of hot flashes. *Southern Medical Journal, 92*(4), 415–416.

Savage, M.V., & Brengelmann, G.L. (1996). Control of skin blood flow in the neutral zone of human body temperature regulation. *Journal of Applied Physiology, 80*(4), 1249–1257.

Schilling, C., Gallicchio, L., Miller, S.R., Babus, J.K., Lewis, L.M., Zacur, H., et al. (2005). Current alcohol use is associated with a reduced risk of hot flashes in midlife women. *Alcohol and Alcoholism, 40*(6), 563–568.

Schover, L.R. (2008). Premature ovarian failure and its consequences: Vasomotor symptoms, sexuality, and fertility. *Journal of Clinical Oncology, 26*(5), 753–758.

Sculpher, M., Bryan, S., Fry, P., de Winter, P., Payne, H., & Emberton, M. (2004). Patients' preferences for the management of non-metastatic prostate cancer: Discrete choice experiment. *BMJ, 328*(7436), 382.

Sloan, J.A., Loprinzi, C.L., Novotny, P.J., Barton, D.L., Lavasseur, B.I., & Windschitl, H. (2001). Methodologic lessons learned from hot flash studies. *Journal of Clinical Oncology, 19*(23), 4280–4290.

Staropoli, C.A., Flaws, J.A., Bush, T.L., & Moulton, A.W. (1998). Predictors of menopausal hot flashes. *Journal of Women's Health, 7*(9), 1149–1155.

Stearns, V. (2006). Serotonergic agents as an alternative to hormonal therapy for the treatment of menopausal vasomotor symptoms. *Treatments in Endocrinology, 5*(2), 83–87.

Stearns, V. (2007). Clinical update: New treatments for hot flushes. *Lancet, 369*(9579), 2062–2064.

Stearns, V., Slack, R., Greep, N., Henry-Tilman, R., Osborne, M., Bunnell, C., et al. (2005). Paroxetine is an effective treatment for hot flashes: Results from a prospective randomized clinical trial. *Journal of Clinical Oncology, 23*(28), 6919–6930.

Stearns, V., Ullmer, L., Lopez, J.F., Smith, Y., Isaacs, C., & Hayes, D. (2002). Hot flushes. *Lancet, 360*(9348), 1851–1861.

Stricker, C.T. (2007). Endocrine effects of breast cancer treatment. *Seminars in Oncology Nursing, 23*(1), 55–70.

Thompson, C.A., Shanafelt, T.D., & Loprinzi, C.L. (2003). Andropause: Symptom management for prostate cancer patients treated with hormonal ablation. *Oncologist, 8*(5), 474–487.

van Andel, G., & Kurth, K.H. (2003). The impact of androgen deprivation therapy on health related quality of life in asymptomatic men with lymph node positive prostate cancer. *European Urology, 44*(2), 209–214.

Van Patten, C.L., Olivotto, I.A., Chambers, G.K., Gelmon, K.A., Hislop, T.G., Templeton, E., et al. (2002). Effect of soy phytoestrogens on hot flashes in postmenopausal women with breast cancer: A randomized, controlled clinical trial. *Journal of Clinical Oncology, 20*(6), 1449–1455.

Walji, R., Boon, H., Guns, E., Oneschuk, D., & Younus, J. (2007). Black cohosh (*Cimicifuga racemosa* [L.] Nutt.): Safety and efficacy for cancer patients. *Supportive Care in Cancer, 15*(8), 913–921.

Weldon, V.E., Neuwirth, H., & Bennett, P.M. (2005, August). *Marin urology.* Retrieved August 4, 2005, from http://www.marinurology.com/articles/cap/learning/hormonal.htm

Whelan, T.J., Goss, P.E., Ingle, J.N., Pater, J.L., Tu, D., Pritchard, K., et al. (2005). Assessment of quality of life in MA.17: A randomized, placebo-controlled trial of letrozole after 5 years of tamoxifen in postmenopausal women. *Journal of Clinical Oncology, 23*(28), 6931–6940.

Whiteman, M.K., Staropoli, C.A., Benedict, J.C., Borgeest, C., & Flaws, J.A. (2003). Risk factors for hot flashes in midlife women. *Journal of Women's Health, 12*(5), 459–472.

Whiteman, M.K., Staropoli, C.A., Langenberg, P.W., McCarter, R.J., Kjerulff, K.H., & Flaws, J.A. (2003). Smoking, body mass, and hot flashes in midlife women. *Obstetrics and Gynecology, 101*(2), 264–272.

Zibecchi, L., Greendale, G.A., & Ganz, P.A. (2003). Continuing education: Comprehensive menopausal assessment: An approach to managing vasomotor and urogenital symptoms in breast cancer survivors. *Oncology Nursing Forum, 30*(3), 393–407.

CHAPTER 15

Lymphedema

Joyce A. Marrs, MS, FNP-BC, AOCNP®

Case Study

L.J. is a 56-year-old woman who was diagnosed in 2001 with a stage I intraductal carcinoma of the right breast. She underwent a lumpectomy with a sentinel lymph node biopsy. The tumor was 0.8 cm in size, intermediate grade with the sentinel lymph node negative for metastasis. Prognostic indicators for estrogen receptors and progesterone receptors were negative. HER2/neu was also negative. Because the sentinel lymph node was negative for metastatic disease, she did not need further axillary dissection.

Following surgery, L.J. received adjuvant chemotherapy that included the use of an anthracycline and a taxane. When chemotherapy was completed, she received radiation therapy. She had been followed on a regular basis without any evidence of disease recurrence. She was in good health and reported no ongoing side effects or complications from prior treatment.

Overview

Lymphedema in the oncology setting can be a lifelong concern. Lymphedema occurs when the flow of fluid in the lymphatic system is obstructed. The obstruction causes a chronic, persistent swelling in the affected extremity or body part. The presence of lymphedema can result in pain, decreased mobility, altered body image, infection, and diminished quality of life. Signs of lymphedema include tightness of the affected limb, swelling, puffiness, pain, or stiffness. Patients and healthcare providers often overlook the first signs of lymphedema because the changes may be subtle (Holcomb, 2006). Oncology nurses can affect patient outcomes through having basic knowledge of the condition, monitoring for its presence, educating the patient about prevention, and assisting in treatment measures. Lymphedema is classified as either primary or secondary.

Primary Lymphedema

Primary lymphedema is caused by a lack of or an abnormality in the lymphatic tissue (Dell & Doll, 2006; Holcomb, 2006). Three types of primary lymphedema exist: congenital lymphedema, lymphedema praecox, and lymphedema tarda. One million to two million people in the United States are affected with primary lymphedema (Holcomb). In primary lymphedema, fluid accumulation generally is bilateral with lower extremities affected more often than upper extremities, and women are more likely than men to have the disorder (Holcomb; Story, 2005; Williams, Franks, & Moffatt, 2005). The age at onset determines the type of primary lymphedema. The cause and presentation of each primary lymphedema type differ.

- *Congenital lymphedema* is present at birth and represents 10%–25% of primary lymphedema cases. With congenital lymphedema, the subcutaneous lymphatic trunks are absent (Revis, 2005). Milroy disease, a familial sex-linked inherited disorder, is a classification of congenital lymphedema and accounts for 2% of all primary lymphedema cases (Revis).
- *Lymphedema praecox* can present from birth to age 35. Lymphedema praecox is the most common primary type and is accountable for 65%–80% of primary lymphedema cases. In lymphedema praecox, the number and diameter of lymphatic channels are reduced (Revis, 2005).
- *Lymphedema tarda* typically does not develop until after the age of 35. Also known as Meige disease, this is the rarest form of primary lymphedema (Dell & Doll, 2006; Holcomb, 2006). The lymphatic vessels are tortuous and often have incompetent or missing valves (Revis, 2005).

Secondary Lymphedema

Secondary lymphedema affects two to three million people in the United States (Holcomb, 2006). It develops when lymphatic structures are damaged, which results in fluid accumulation (International Society of Lymphology [ISL], 2003; Muscari, 2004). Anatomic changes in the lymph system rise from physical disruption, compression, or closure of the lymphatic channel. For example, a woman who has had lymph nodes removed as part of breast cancer treatment may develop secondary lymphedema when surgery physically disrupts the lymph system. This same woman may develop fibrosis following radiation. The fibrosis then compresses the lymphatic vessels. Finally, the woman may later develop metastatic cancer in the axilla that obstructs or closes the existing lymphatic channels. Figure 15-1 lists specific causes for secondary lymphedema. The most common cause worldwide for secondary lymphedema is filariasis, a parasitic infection of the lymph nodes (Holcomb).

In the oncology setting, the two most common causes for secondary lymphedema are radiation therapy and lymph node dissection (Muscari, 2004). Figure 15-2 depicts a patient with a history of bilateral upper-extremity lymphedema that was brought about by treatment with both radiation therapy and lymph node dissection. The anatomic changes in the lymphatic system from radiation therapy and lymph node dissection lead to an increased lifetime risk of developing secondary lymphedema (Armer & Stewart, 2005; Muscari). In addition to an increased lifetime risk for secondary lymphedema from radiation and lymph node dissection, some patients may be predisposed to development of secondary lymphedema because of additional situations that alter the lymphatic flow (Cohen, Payne, & Tunkel, 2001). Figure 15-3 identifies a list of risk factors that may affect the development or worsening of secondary lymphedema through impairment of the lymphatic load. Nurses can assist patients in identification of these risk factors and provide pre-

FIGURE 15-1	Causes of Secondary Lymphedema

- Alteration in the lymphatic system
- Trauma, such as burns
- Surgery that dissects or removes lymph nodes
- Radiation therapy
- Infection
- Tumor growth or metastasis to lymph nodes
- Scarring
- Chronic disease, such as cerebrovascular accident, rheumatoid arthritis, and spina bifida
- Filariasis, a parasitic infection

Note. Based on information from Holcomb, 2006; Story, 2005; Williams et al., 2005.

ventive measures, such as weight loss for obesity, regular exercise, and tight glucose control for those with diabetes. In addition to the list of risk factors provided, nurses should advise patients to avoid wearing tight-fitting clothing that causes constriction of the extremity and to avoid increasing their body temperature through the use of hot tubs, heating pads, or hot showers, which may contribute to the development of lymphedema (Muscari).

With secondary lymphedema, the problem may present in an acute or chronic phase. Four types of acute lymphedema exist (Holcomb, 2006). The following provides the description of presentation and most effective treatment for each type of acute lymphedema.

| FIGURE 15-2 | Bilateral Lymphedema |

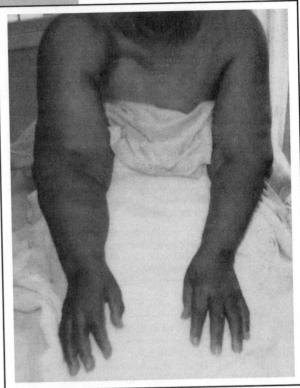

Note. The left arm is status post modified radical mastectomy and axillary lymph node dissection. The right arm is status post radical mastectomy and lymph node dissection.

Note. From "Lymphedema: Responding to Our Patients' Needs," by E. Muscari, 2004, *Oncology Nursing Forum*, *31*(5), p. 910. Copyright 2004 by Oncology Nursing Society. Reprinted with permission.

1. The first type is a mild acute lymphedema that occurs a few days following surgery. The lymphedema happens because lymphatic vessels have been either manipulated or cut during surgery. Symptoms for mild acute lymphedema are swelling, warmth, and erythema. The mild acute type is not usually associated with pain. This form is transient and responds to elevation and muscle contraction to improve blood flow to the extremity.

2. A second type occurs six to eight weeks after surgery or radiation therapy. Acute lymphedema occurs as a result of inflammation such as lymphangitis or phlebitis without thrombosis. The limb may be red, warm, and tender. Treatment involves elevation of extremity and anti-inflammatory agents.

3. The third type is an erysipeloid form that occurs following a minor trauma or insect bite. The area will be have redness, be hot to touch, and painful. Treatment necessitates antibiotics and elevation.

4. The fourth type can occur 18–24 months after surgery, yet also may appear many years later. Patients will note an insidious onset of pain that generally is associated with soft tissue stretching or postural changes from limb weight. Pain medication and anti-inflammatory medications may be used to provide relief of symptoms.

Acute lymphedema may become chronic. Chronic lymphedema happens when the lymphatic system is unable to handle the demands of lymphatic fluid flow. The amount of fluid removed is less than the amount produced, leading to an excessive accumulation.

FIGURE 15-3	Risk Factors for Lymphedema

- Obesity
- Lack of exercise
- Overuse of an affected extremity
- Hematomas
- Seromas
- Cellulitis
- Wounds
- Tight or constrictive clothes
- Airplane travel
- Long distance travel
- Infection in or trauma to an affected extremity
- Prolonged standing
- Diabetes

Note. Based on information from Dell & Doll, 2006; Story, 2005.

From "Lymphedema and Implications for Oncology Nursing Practice," by J. Marrs, 2007, *Clinical Journal of Oncology Nursing, 11*(1), p. 19. Copyright 2007 by Oncology Nursing Society. Reprinted with permission.

FIGURE 15-4	Prevalence of Lymphedema

Upper-Extremity Lymphedema
- Occurs in 15%–28% of breast cancer survivors
- Occurs in 5%–10% of patients who have undergone radical mastectomy
- Most common in patients having axillary lymph node dissection
- Can occur 1–20 years postsurgery

Lower-Extremity Lymphedema
- Commonly misdiagnosed as edema
- Seen in as many as 80% of patients with a history of lymph node dissection of the groin
- Occurs in patients who have compression of pelvic or inguinal lymph nodes

Note. Based on information from Story, 2005.

From "Lymphedema and Implications for Oncology Nursing Practice," by J. Marrs, 2007, *Clinical Journal of Oncology Nursing, 11*(1), p. 20. Copyright 2007 by Oncology Nursing Society. Reprinted with permission.

Chronic lymphedema can affect both upper and lower extremities, depending on the causative factor (Story, 2005). Figure 15-4 presents the prevalence of distribution patterns in upper- and lower-extremity lymphedema. Patients complain of heaviness, pain, aching, weakness, fullness, puffiness, and skin changes with chronic lymphedema (Marrs, 2007). Lymphedema has the potential to be a lifelong problem; therefore, quality of life can be greatly affected.

Quality of Life

The long-term consequences of lymphedema can affect cancer survivors physically and emotionally (Cohen et al., 2001). For example, the physical changes from lymphedema cannot be disguised cosmetically, and the disfigurement is a constant reminder of cancer and fear of recurrence. The effects of discomfort, pain, and pressure can compromise quality of life. Altered body image can affect sexuality, and impaired motor skills can affect activity, especially with work- or home-related tasks (Muscari, 2004; Ryan et al., 2003; Rymal, 2003). The long-term consequences of lymphedema are listed in Figure 15-5. Some of these include self-image changes, altered interpersonal relationships, improperly fitting clothes or shoes, and altered function of the extremity. Ryan et al. completed a retrospective survey that described women's experiences with lower limb edema. A total of 487 women depicted how lymphedema affected their daily life, and the final sample for analysis was 82 women who had confirmed lower limb lymphedema and agreed to be interviewed. The participants reported that the lymphedema caused financial burden (27%, n = 22), changed wardrobe habits (79%, n = 65), and altered activities of daily living (51%, n = 42) (Ryan et al.). Oncology nurses need to be aware of the impact that lymphedema has on quality of life and take appropriate actions to prevent or treat the disorder.

Pathophysiology

The lymphatic system is present extensively throughout the body. The purpose of the system is to remove waste and foreign materials that are the byproducts of the body clearing infection and disease (Marrs, 2007). The network of fine vessels begins just beneath the surface of the skin, and the fine vessels then merge to become larger vessels in the tissue. The system is responsible for removing 10% of the interstitial fluid that the circulatory system does not eliminate (Muscari, 2004; Ridner, 2002). The fluid exchange occurs at the blood capillary-interstitial-lymphatic vessel surface (see Figure 15-6). The small lymphatic vessels have one-way valves that transport the fluid into larger lymphatic vessels that connect to lymphatic trunks that run through territories or quadrants into lymph node basins and eventually terminate in the venous system (Muscari; Ridner; Rymal, 2003). Movement through the lymphatic system is dependent on three mechanisms: contraction of segments between valves when full, compression of vessels from external pressure such as muscle contractions, and intrinsic contractile filaments in the endothelial cells of lymph vessels (Muscari). Figure 15-7 depicts the normal lymph transport system. Fluid accumulation (lymphedema) occurs because the

FIGURE 15-5	Consequences of Lymphedema

- Pain
- Altered sensations and function
- Need for nontailored, large-sized clothing and shoes
- Repeated, persistent infections
- Fatigue
- Altered interpersonal relationships
- Functional disability
- Self-image alterations

Note. From "Lymphedema: Responding to Our Patients' Needs," by E. Muscari, 2004, *Oncology Nursing Forum, 31*(5), p. 907. Copyright 2004 by Oncology Nursing Society. Reprinted with permission.

FIGURE 15-6	Blood Capillary-Interstitial-Lymphatic Vessel Interface

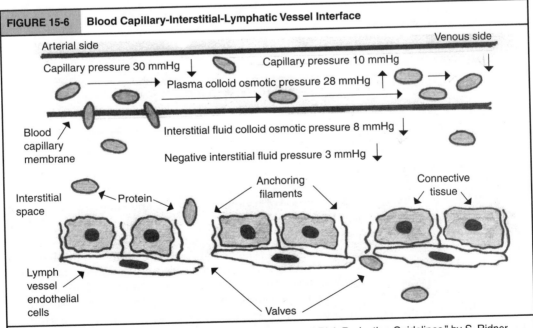

Note. From "Breast Cancer Lymphedema: Pathophysiology and Risk Reduction Guidelines," by S. Ridner, 2002, *Oncology Nursing Forum, 29*(9), p. 1287. Copyright 2002 by Oncology Nursing Society. Reprinted with permission.

FIGURE 15-7	Diagram of Peripheral and Central Lymph Transport

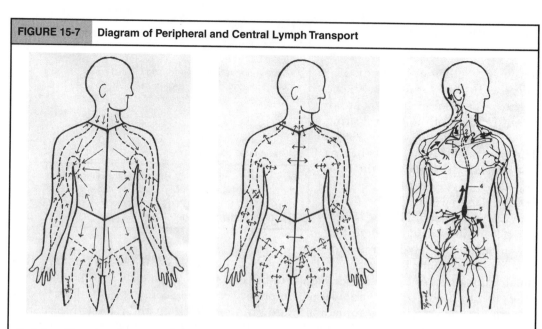

Peripheral lymph transport under normal conditions
Solid lines—Quadrant watersheds
Broken lines—Secondary watersheds

Peripheral lymph transport across watersheds
Allows for transport away from congestion and around obstructions

Central lymph transport
1—Internal jugular veins
2—Lymphovenous anastomoses
3—Subclavian veins
4—Thoracic duct
5—Cisterna chyli

Note. From "Lymphedema Therapy During Adjuvant Therapy for Cancer," by C. Rymal, 2003, *Clinical Journal of Oncology Nursing, 7*(4), p. 450. Copyright 2003 by Oncology Nursing Society. Reprinted with permission.

---

lymph transport system is unable to handle the capacity of fluid produced (ISL, 2003; Morrell et al., 2005; Muscari).

Fluid in the lymphatic system is composed of protein, water, fats, and cellular waste. Lymph vessels are thin, allowing larger proteins to filter through easily. An obstruction in lymphatic flow allows the large proteins to filter through the vessels and invade the surrounding interstitial tissue (ISL, 2003; Marrs, 2007; Morrell et al., 2005; Muscari, 2004). When this happens, the highly concentrated protein-filled fluid in the interstitial space causes inflammation and subsequent skin changes along with fibrosis. The amount of accumulation determines the severity or stage of lymphedema. Early detection and treatment may prevent progression to later stages, which will affect quality-of-life indicators. Nurses need to identify early symptoms of lymphedema.

Staging is based on physical examination and measurement of the extremity (ISL, 2003; Morrell et al., 2005; Muscari, 2004; Ridner, 2002). See Table 15-1 for the stages of lymphede-

TABLE 15-1	Stages of Lymphedema	
Grade	Description	Measurement
Stage 0	Patients have no obvious signs or symptoms. Impaired lymph drainage is subclinical. Lymphedema (LE) may be present for months to years before progressing to later stages.	Edema is not evident. Clinical detection of edema does not occur until the normal interstitial volume increases by 30% or more.
Stage I	Swelling is present. An affected area pits with pressure. Elevation relieves swelling. Skin texture is smooth. LE is spontaneously reversible.	< 3 cm difference between extremities
Stage II	Skin tissue is firmer. Skin may look tight and shiny. Pitting may or may not occur. Elevation does not completely alleviate the swelling. Hair loss or nail changes may be experienced in an affected extremity. LE is spontaneously irreversible. Assistance will be needed to reduce edema.	3–5 cm difference between extremities
Stage III	LE has progressed to the elephantiasis stage. An affected area is nonpitting with a permanent edema. Skin is firm and thick. Hyperkeratosis, fat deposits, and acanthosis are present. Skin folds develop. Patients may be at risk for cellulitis, infections, or ulcerations. An affected area may ooze fluid. LE is irreversible. Elevation will not alleviate symptoms.	≥ 5 cm difference between extremities

Note. Based on information from Dell & Doll, 2006; Holcomb, 2006; Quan & Petrek, 2004; Story, 2005. From "Lymphedema and Implications for Oncology Nursing Practice," by J. Marrs, 2007, *Clinical Journal of Oncology Nursing, 11*(1), p. 21. Copyright 2007 by Oncology Nursing Society. Reprinted with permission.

ma. Fortunately, early stages of lymphedema are reversible. As the disorder progresses into later stages, the condition will become irreversible (ISL; Morrell et al.; Muscari). Survivors with progressive, chronic, irreversible changes are susceptible to cellulitis, lymphangitis, elephantiasis, and a rare angiosarcoma (Stewart-Treves syndrome), all of which will affect patients' quality of life.

Assessment

Nursing assessment should include inspection of the affected limb for color, warmth, texture, and presence of any scars, injuries, wounds, or skin changes (Dell & Doll, 2006; Holcomb, 2006; Muscari, 2004). The nurse should verify whether swelling is relieved with elevation. The extremity should be measured on a regular basis, comparing the affected limb to the unaffected limb and documenting results in the patient's record (Dell & Doll; Holcomb; Story, 2005).

Several measurement techniques are available to assess the extent of lymphedema. *Water displacement* uses the amount of water displaced to determine the volume of the limb (Armer & Stewart, 2005; Brown, 2004). Although water displacement is sensitive and accurate, the process is cumbersome and may not be used with open skin wounds. *Circumferential measurement* is easy to use in the clinical setting. A tape measure is the only tool required. Measurements of the upper extremity should be taken 5 cm and 10 cm above and below the olecranon process (see Figure 15-8), for a total of four measurements per extremity. These four

FIGURE 15-8	Circumferential Measurement

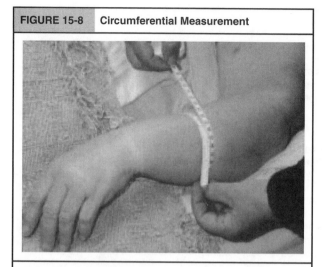

Note. From "Lymphedema: Responding to Our Patients' Needs," by E. Muscari, 2004, *Oncology Nursing Forum, 31*(5), p. 907. Copyright 2004 by Oncology Nursing Society. Reprinted with permission.

measurements are recorded and compared over time. The lower extremity should be measured at calf level (Story, 2005). A newer technique, *bioelectric impedance,* uses electrical current to measure the amount of fluid in a limb. This technique requires the use of expensive equipment (Armer & Stewart; Brown). Limb measurement provides the foundation for diagnosis of lymphedema.

The diagnosis of lymphedema may be based on the patient history and a physical examination; however, further testing might be conducted to eliminate other possible causes (Holcomb, 2006; ISL, 2003; Petropoulos, 2005). Workup should include evaluation for disease recurrence because of compression from tumor or lymphatic obstruction (Morrell et al., 2005; Muscari, 2004). Tests that can be performed include lymphoscintigraphy, computed tomography (CT) scan, magnetic resonance imaging (MRI), lymphangiography, and evaluation of lymph fluid for protein content.

- Lymphoscintigraphy is a nuclear medicine test that has 100% sensitivity and specificity for the detection of lymphedema.
- A CT scan or MRI can be used to check for disease recurrence.
- Lymphangiography may be used if surgery is being considered.

The lymph fluid may be evaluated for protein content. Determination of protein content differentiates the underlying cause of edema. A protein level of 1–5.5 g/dl indicates lymphedema, and a level of 0.1–0.9 g/dl indicates venous or cardiac edema (Holcomb, 2006). Other testing useful in lymphedema evaluation includes venous Doppler ultrasound to check for thrombus formation and laboratory tests to measure liver function, albumin level, kidney function, or urine analysis. Once the diagnosis is confirmed, treatment measures will be initiated.

Treatment

Treatment of lymphedema depends on the stage at presentation. Most management will involve nonpharmacologic measures. The Oncology Nursing Society Putting Evidence Into Practice research team published a comprehensive report on lymphedema interventions in 2008 that will assist nurses with reduction and treatment for lymphedema (Poage, Singer, Shellabarger, & Poundal, 2008). As with all interventions, prevention is a primary nursing concern.

Risk Reduction

The National Lymphedema Network (NLN) has developed guidelines designed to reduce the risk for development of lymphedema (Ridner, 2002). These guidelines are based more on expert opinion than on evidence-based studies. However, once lymphedema develops, the problem is chronic, and interventions that can reduce development should be considered, although research is needed to provide evidence. See Table 15-2 for a list of the physiologic bases for the NLN guidelines. The guidelines recommend meticulous skin care, exercise, lifestyle changes, avoidance of constriction in the limb, use of compression garments, and

TABLE 15-2	Physiologic Bases for Guidelines		
Guideline	**Infection/ Inflammation**	**Reduced Risk of Increased Lymphatic Load**	**Pressure Changes[a]**
Report swelling of limb.	X	—	—
No blood draw or injection	X	—	X
No blood pressure	—	X	X
Keep arm clean and dry; apply lotion after bathing.	X	—	—
Avoid vigorous repetitive movement against resistance.	—	X	X
No lifting of heavy objects	—	X	X
No tight jewelry or elastic bands	—	X	X
Avoid extreme temperature changes.	—	X	X
Avoid cuts or abrasions.	X	—	—
Do not cut cuticles.	X	—	—
Do not over exercise.	—	X	X
Rest arm if it begins to ache.	—	X	—
Wear a compression sleeve when flying.	—	—	X
Wear lightweight breast prostheses.	—	—	X
Use an electric razor when shaving axilla.	X	—	—
Report rash, itching, pain, redness, or warmth.	X	—	—
Maintain ideal body weight; avoid smoking and alcohol.	—	—	X
If you have lymphedema, wear a compression sleeve during waking hours.	—	—	X

[a] at blood capillary-interstitial-lymphatic vessel interface

Note. From "Breast Cancer Lymphedema: Pathophysiology and Risk Reduction Guidelines," by S. Ridner, 2002, *Oncology Nursing Forum, 29*(9), p. 1290. Copyright 2002 by Oncology Nursing Society. Reprinted with permission.

minimizing temperature exposure to reduce lymphedema risk (NLN, 2004, 2005a, 2005b). Nurses should explain that meticulous skin care will reduce the risk of infection; exercise will improve lymphatic flow through muscle contractions and deep breathing; compression garments that fit well will support the affected limb; exposure to cold will cause rebound edema; and the patient should not be in a sauna or hot tub for longer than 15 minutes because of vasodilation from the increase in skin temperature.

Pharmacologic Measures

Medications used in the treatment of lymphedema are limited to supportive measures. In general, medications are used to treat secondary problems of lymphedema, such as infection and thrombosis, and for pain relief (Smith & Zobec, 2001).

Diuretics have been used historically on a short-term basis for other causes of edema in the affected limb, not necessarily the lymphedema itself. However, the use of diuretics is not recommended on a long-term basis because the treatment does nothing to remove the underlying cause of protein accumulation in the interstitial tissue (ISL, 2003). Fluid and electrolyte imbalances may occur as a result of inappropriate diuretic use.

Benzopyrones, specifically coumarin, are available in Europe and are used to treat lymphedema (ISL, 2003; Morrell et al., 2005). However, the use of benzopyrones is not approved in the United States. The drug's mechanism of action is attributed to a breakdown of proteins that helps to decrease the fluid accumulation. However, studies have failed to demonstrate benefit, and coumarin (not to be confused with Coumadin® [Bristol-Myers Squibb Co.]) causes liver toxicities.

Selenium has been studied as a treatment for radiation-induced lymphedema and secondary lymphedema from breast cancer surgery. Radiation causes fibrosis of the tissue surrounding the lymph vessels, producing compression with subsequent fluid accumulation. The hypothesis is that selenium will consume oxygen radicals that will subsequently decrease the lymph system damage (Holcomb, 2006). The drug has only been evaluated in a small population of survivors. Although the small study showed a reduction in arm circumference in 83% (10 of 12) of patients, the evidence is not strong enough to recommend the use of selenium for lymphedema at this time (Morrell et al., 2005). Although selenium often is considered nontoxic, it may cause side effects. The side effects are nausea, vomiting, diarrhea, and elevated heart rate (Holcomb; Morrell et al.).

Antibiotic therapy is recommended for use when an infection, such as cellulitis, is present (ISL, 2003; Twycross & Wilcock, 2006). Indications that an infection is present include fever, redness, pain, tenderness, blisters, increased swelling, and possibly nausea and vomiting. The presence of erythema alone does not always indicate infection. Although more than one organism may cause cellulitis, most infections in patients with lymphedema result from Group A *Streptococci* (Twycross & Wilcock). Antimicrobial agents used for infectious episodes include amoxicillin, penicillin V, amoxicillin plus clavulanate, clindamycin, erythromycin, or ciprofloxacin.

Nonpharmacologic Measures

The main treatments for lymphedema are nonpharmacologic. In considering the appropriate modalities to use, providers need to recognize barriers that may interfere with treatment (Rymal, 2003). Barriers to treatment include patient fatigue, the time involved for therapy, the chronicity of the condition, and limitations from insurance carriers.

The various modalities used to treat lymphedema are termed *complete decongestive therapy* (CDT) (NLN, 2006) and are recommended for use with lymphedema. Components of CDT include (a) manual lymph drainage (MLD), (b) compression bandaging, (c) exercise, and (d) compression garments.

MLD involves the movement of lymph fluid from a nonfunctioning region to an adjacent region that is draining effectively (Muscari, 2004; NLN, 2006). Figure 15-9 shows MLD of the thorax, done prior to moving fluid from distal regions. Although MLD technique appears to be similar to massage, the method uses lighter pressure. Figure 15-10 demonstrates how the hands are placed to stretch the skin during MLD. MLD should not be used on patients with open wounds, skin infections, or thrombosis (Smith & Zobec, 2001). Initially, in the acute phase of treatment, MLD involves daily therapy lasting 60–90 minutes in length for up to 15 sessions (Muscari). The subsequent maintenance phase involves self-care activities for patients to complete on a regular basis. During the acute phase, application of compression bandages follows the completion of an MLD session.

Compression bandaging involves the application of multiple layers of short stretch bandages from distal to proximal regions (Muscari, 2004; NLN, 2006). Compression bandaging promotes the movement of fluid along a pressure gradient to reduce the potential for refilling of the nondraining lymphatic tissue. Figure 15-11 depicts a patient wearing compression bandaging. Multilayered compression bandages are intricately wrapped using bandages similar to ACE® (Becton Dickenson and Co.) bandages. Compression bandaging is worn up to 22 hours a day during the acute phase of

| FIGURE 15-9 | Manual Lymph Drainage Pathways |

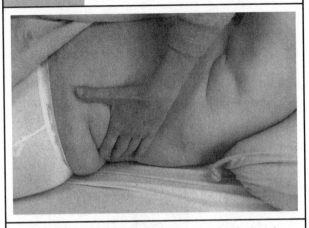

Note. From "Lymphedema: Responding to Our Patients' Needs," by E. Muscari, 2004, *Oncology Nursing Forum,* 31(5), p. 909. Copyright 2004 by Oncology Nursing Society. Reprinted with permission.

| FIGURE 15-10 | Stretching Skin Perpendicular to the Lymph Pathways Running From Elbow to Shoulder |

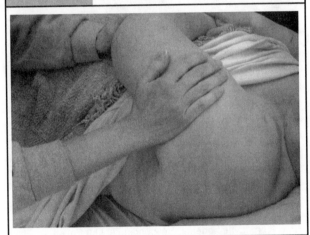

Note. From "Lymphedema: Responding to Our Patients' Needs," by E. Muscari, 2004, *Oncology Nursing Forum,* 31(5), p. 908. Copyright 2004 by Oncology Nursing Society. Reprinted with permission.

treatment. Figure 15-12 shows the effect of MLD and compression bandaging therapy in a patient with lower-extremity lymphedema. Once the acute phase of treatment has ended and maximum reduction in fluid has taken place, the patient will be fitted for a garment.

Compression garments are used for long-term control of lymphedema. Compression garments use the application of pressure at a level of 20–60 mm Hg to prevent recurrence

FIGURE 15-11	Compression Bandaging

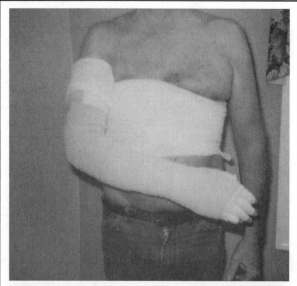

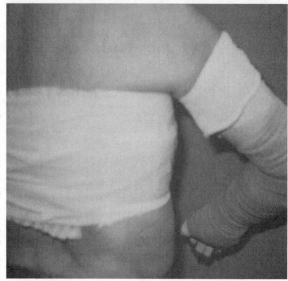

Note. From "Lymphedema: Responding to Our Patients' Needs," by E. Muscari, 2004, *Oncology Nursing Forum, 31*(5), p. 910. Copyright 2004 by Oncology Nursing Society. Reprinted with permission.

(ISL, 2003). Compression garments provide a gradient pressure that prevents backflow of lymph fluid into distal tissue (Cohen et al., 2001). Nurses should advise patients that they will be measured and fitted for the compression garment by a person properly trained in fitting the garment. The compression garment is worn during waking hours to maintain a reduction in chronic lymphedema. A properly fitting compression garment will be close-fit without a tourniquet-like effect, easy to apply, and comfortable to wear during activities of daily life. Garments should be washed regularly and replaced every six months. Proper care of garments will ensure better control of lymphedema.

Other components of lymphedema treatment include therapeutic exercises, mechanical pumps, elevation, and surgery (ISL, 2003; Morrell et al., 2005; Muscari, 2004; NLN, 2006). The use of mechanical pumps involves an air compression pump that applies pressure along an extremity (NLN, 2006). Different types of devices exist. Older models provided even pressure over an extremity that allowed for backflow of lymph fluid into the distal tissue (Petrek, Pressman, & Smith, 2000). Newer models have more options available. Sequential systems deliver higher pressure in the distal portion of the device with lower pressure in the medial region (Cohen et al., 2001). The average gradient pressure applied is 40 mm Hg. Pressures applied at 50–60 mm Hg and higher may cause injury to lymphatic vessels. Nurses should advise patients that using a mechanical pump involves a minimum of 60 minutes per session. Although the control of chronic lymphedema may be challenging, mechanical pumps are not as likely to be effective in maintaining control over lymphedema as MLD and compression garments (Smith & Zobec, 2001). In addition, mechanical pumps can cause swelling in the area adjacent to the pump sleeve. Therefore, the use of mechanical pumps for chronic lymphedema is controversial as a standardized treatment recommendation.

FIGURE 15-12   **Bilateral Lower-Extremity Lymphedema**

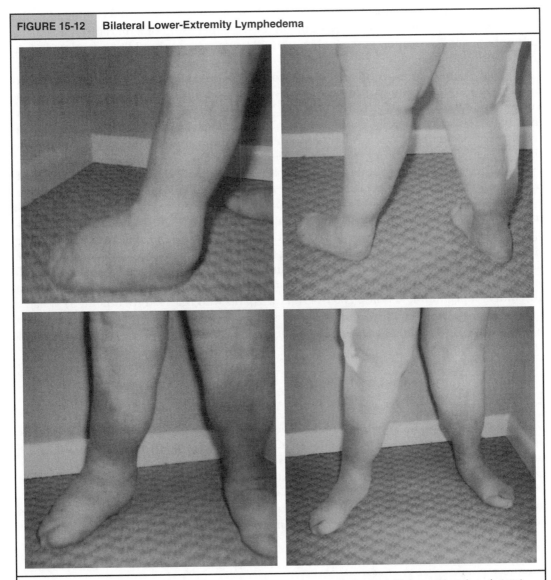

Note. The photos on the left were taken pretreatment. The patient underwent 12 manual lymph node treatments and compression bandaging and experienced a 50% reduction in the size of the lower extremities (as depicted in the photos on the right).

Note. From "Lymphedema: Responding to Our Patients' Needs," by E. Muscari, 2004, *Oncology Nursing Forum, 31*(5), p. 911. Copyright 2004 by Oncology Nursing Society. Reprinted with permission.

Remedial exercises are recommended (NLN, 2005a, 2006), and patients should conduct muscle contractions, which increase the interstitial pressure in the limb and thus encourage movement of lymph fluid in the area. Flexibility exercises provide for mild stretching of muscles and soft tissue, reducing the tightening and fibrosis that impairs lymphatic flow. Resistive exercises done in a gradual manner based on individual fitness level will promote increased muscle tone that will improve the flow of lymph fluid. Patients should be cautioned that exercise can increase local blood flow, which in turn can increase the fluid load in the lymphatic system. Exercise should be done under the supervision of a therapist specializing in lymphedema. To counteract the increased fluid load, exercise should be completed while the limb is bandaged (Morrell et al., 2005).

Surgical treatment for lymphedema is performed under advanced circumstances that do not respond to CDT. Surgery does not cure lymphedema. It provides a reduction in tissue and weight of the affected limb (ISL, 2003; NLN, 2006). Surgical procedures involve debulking the extremity through excision of skin and subcutaneous tissue, liposuction, or reconstruction of the lymph system. Patients who undergo surgical procedures will need to continue the use of compression garments following surgery.

Laser therapy is a newer tool used to control lymphedema. The U.S. Food and Drug Administration approved low-level laser therapy for use in patients with postmastectomy lymphedema (Carati, 2007). The therapy affects fibroblasts and macrophage cells and has been postulated to promote lymphangiogenesis and stimulate the immune system. Lymph drainage therefore is improved because new lymph pathways are produced; fibrosis and scarring is reduced; and blood flow is altered, resulting in a reduction in accumulation of fluid in the tissue. The laser therapy unit has been tested in a double-blind, placebo-controlled trial with a small sample size (N = 64, with 37 in the treatment arm and 27 in the control arm) (Carati, Anderson, Gannon, & Piller, 2003). Of participants who received treatment, 31% had a reduction in lymphedema three months after starting therapy. Although this therapy shows some promise for treatment of postmastectomy lymphedema, effectiveness has not been established for a broad range of use.

Expected Outcomes

The outcomes with lymphedema are based on whether the condition has developed. The primary goal is to prevent the development of lymphedema. Nurses should complete measurements of the extremities on a regular basis to identify the effectiveness of risk reduction interventions. When measurements of the extremity are taken regularly, the development of lymphedema will be detected early, and treatment can be initiated quickly and can effect long-term outcomes that reduce further progression. Prevention and early detection are the keys to lessen the effects of lymphedema and improve quality of life.

Patient Teaching Points

Education is essential to the prevention and treatment of lymphedema. Interventions include the following (Dell & Doll, 2006; Holcomb, 2006; Muscari, 2004; Story, 2005).
- Maintain lifelong preventive measures (see Table 15-2).
- Exercise regularly and maintain proper weight.
- Avoid injury to the affected extremity by averting cuts, abrasions, and insect bites.
- Avoid tight clothing, jewelry, or elastic bands on the affected extremity.
- Avoid blood pressure measurements, blood draws, and IV insertions in the affected extremity.
- Report signs of redness, warmth, pain, swelling, or change in fit of clothes in the affected extremity.
- Report feelings of heaviness or aching in the affected extremity.
- Avoid carrying a purse or briefcase on the affected side.

- Wear a compression garment when traveling by plane.
- Use an electric razor to shave an affected limb or axilla.
- Keep nails clean and short. Avoid cutting the skin when trimming nails, and avoid artificial nails.
- Avoid use of sharp objects, such as knives, needles, or scissors, on the affected side.
- If lymphedema is in lower extremities, avoid standing or sitting for long periods and do not cross legs.
- Use compression garments, stockings, and devices as directed by a healthcare provider trained in lymphedema management.
  The following patient and provider resources may be helpful.
- Breastcancer.org: www.breastcancer.org/tips/lymphedema/index.jsp
- Lymphology Association of North America: www.clt-lana.org
- MayoClinic.com: www.mayoclinic.com/health/lymphedema/DS00609
- NLN: www.lymphnet.org, 800-541-3259
- Oncology Nursing Society Lymphedema Management Special Interest Group: http://lymphedema.vc.ons.org

Need for Future Research

Although great strides have been achieved in the area of lymphedema, much work remains. Research is needed in a variety of aspects with regard to lymphedema (ISL, 2003; Morrell et al., 2005; Muscari, 2004). Lymphedema remains an underidentified problem. Epidemiology studies need to be conducted to identify the extent of the problem. Preventive measures, although based on sound physiologic thought, lack evidence-based studies to support their effectiveness. Thus, all interventions previously discovered need to have supporting data and research. One such recommendation is the avoidance of blood draws, blood pressure measurements, and IV insertions in the affected limb. Further studies need to be done to clarify the risk of these procedures in order to adequately educate survivors. Specific measurement techniques and imaging studies that are clinically useful and accurate and that require minimal time and expense are needed. Healthcare providers need to support all efforts that will have an impact on this chronic, debilitating disorder.

Conclusion of Case Study

L.J. called the office to report a week-long history of right arm edema. At the time, she was six years out from diagnosis and treatment. She described the arm as feeling tight and heavy. She denied any redness, tenderness, or warmth. She had not had any recent airline travel, blood pressure measurement, or needle sticks. Her hobbies include gardening. She denied any cuts, insect bites, or injuries. L.J. was instructed to elevate the extremity and wrap with an ACE bandage during the day. An appointment was made for evaluation with a healthcare provider.

At the evaluation, a review of her medical history, social history, and family history is completed. The subjective review of systems is negative except for the new onset of right-sided arm swelling. On physical examination, the breasts are supple bilaterally, a lumpectomy scar is present in the right breast, and no lumps or masses are palpable. No palpable adenopathy is present. The right arm is visibly edematous, and the skin feels smooth. No evidence of pitting is present. Measurements reveal a 2.5 cm difference in size between the right and left arms. Swelling decreased some with elevation. L.J. is suspected of having stage I lymphedema. Further workup is required.

L.J. undergoes a breast MRI to determine whether disease recurrence could be the cause for the new onset of lymphedema. The MRI is negative. A Doppler ultrasound does not show thrombosis. Because no evidence of underlying disease exists, she is referred to a certified lymphedema specialist for follow-up evaluation and treatment. L.J. is shown how to massage the limb to decrease the swelling and is provided education about to how to care for her extremity. She will continue to receive routine follow-up on a regular basis.

Conclusion

Lymphedema is an often debilitating condition in cancer survivors. Nurses can make a tremendous impact on survivors' quality of life through sound knowledge of the condition. Nurses need to provide education in prevention of lymphedema, conduct ongoing assessment for the presence of lymphedema, and refer patients promptly for current lymphedema management interventions.

References

Armer, J., & Stewart, B. (2005). A comparison of four diagnostic criteria for lymphedema in a post-breast cancer population. *Lymphatic Research and Biology, 3*(4), 208–217.

Brown, J. (2004). A clinically useful method for evaluating lymphedema. *Clinical Journal of Oncology Nursing, 8*(1), 35–38.

Carati, C. (2007, May). Laser therapy cleared for use in lymphedema. *Lymphedema Management Special Interest Group Newsletter, 18*(1). Retrieved July 28, 2007, from http://onsopcontent.ons.org/publications/signewsletters/lym/lym18.1.html#story4

Carati, C.J., Anderson, S.N., Gannon, B.J., & Piller, N.B. (2003). Treatment of postmastectomy lymphedema with low-level laser therapy: A double blind, placebo-controlled trial. *Cancer, 98*(6), 1114–1122.

Cohen, S.R., Payne, D.K., & Tunkel, R.S. (2001). Lymphedema: Strategies for management. *Cancer, 92*(Suppl. 4), 980–987.

Dell, D.D., & Doll, C. (2006). Caring for a patient with lymphedema. *Nursing, 36*(6), 49–51.

Holcomb, S.S. (2006). Identification and treatment of different types of lymphedema. *Advances in Skin and Wound Care, 19*(2), 103–108.

International Society of Lymphology. (2003). The diagnosis and treatment of peripheral lymphedema: Consensus document of the International Society of Lymphology. *Lymphology, 36*(2), 84–91.

Marrs, J. (2007). Lymphedema and implications for oncology nursing practice. *Clinical Journal of Oncology Nursing, 11*(1), 19–21.

Morrell, R., Halyard, M., Schild, S., Ali, M., Gunderson, L., & Pockaj, B. (2005). Breast cancer–related lymphedema. *Mayo Clinic Proceedings, 80*(11), 1480–1484.

Muscari, E. (2004). Lymphedema: Responding to our patients' needs. *Oncology Nursing Forum, 31*(5), 905–912.

National Lymphedema Network. (2004). *Position statement of the National Lymphedema Network. Topic: Air travel.* Retrieved July 28, 2007, from http://www.lymphnet.org/pdfDocs/nlnairtravel.pdf

National Lymphedema Network. (2005a). *Position statement of the National Lymphedema Network. Topic: Exercise.* Retrieved July 28, 2007, from http://www.lymphnet.org/pdfDocs/nlnexercise.pdf

National Lymphedema Network. (2005b). *Position statement of the National Lymphedema Network. Topic: Lymphedema risk reduction practices.* Retrieved July 28, 2007, from http://www.lymphnet.org/pdfDocs/nlnriskreduction.pdf

National Lymphedema Network. (2006). *Position statement of the National Lymphedema Network. Topic: Treatment.* Retrieved July 28, 2007, from http://www.lymphnet.org/pdfDocs/nlntreatment.pdf

Petrek, J., Pressman, P., & Smith, R. (2000). Lymphedema: Current issues in research and management. *CA: A Cancer Journal for Clinicians, 50*(5), 292–306.

Petropoulos, P. (2005). Lymphedema. In F.F. Ferri (Ed.), *Ferri's clinical advisor: Instant diagnosis and treatment* (pp. 490–491). St. Louis, MO: Elsevier Mosby.

Poage, E.G., Singer, M., Shellabarger, M.J., & Poundall, M.D. (2008). *Putting evidence into practice: Lymphedema.* Pittsburgh, PA: Oncology Nursing Society.

Quan, M., & Petrek, J. (2004). Lymphedema. In S. Singletary, G.L. Robb, & G.N. Hortobagyi (Eds.), *Advanced therapy of breast disease* (2nd ed., pp. 772–780). Hamilton, Canada: BC Decker.

Revis, D.R. (2005). *Lymphedema.* Retrieved February 1, 2008, from http://www.emedicine.com/MED/topic2722.htm

Ridner, S. (2002). Breast cancer lymphedema: Pathophysiology and risk reduction guidelines. *Oncology Nursing Forum, 29*(9), 1285–1291.

Ryan, M., Stainton, M.C., Jaconelli, C., Watts, S., MacKenzie, P., & Mansberg, T. (2003). The experience of lower limb lymphedema for women after treatment for gynecologic cancer. *Oncology Nursing Forum, 30*(3), 417–423.

Rymal, C. (2003). Lymphedema therapy during adjuvant therapy for cancer. *Clinical Journal of Oncology Nursing, 7*(4), 449–451.

Smith, J., & Zobec, A. (2001). Lymphedema. In B. Ferrell & N. Coyle (Eds.), *Textbook of palliative nursing* (pp. 192–203). New York: Oxford University Press.

Story, K.T. (2005). Alterations in circulation. In J.K. Itano & K.N. Taoka (Eds.), *Core curriculum for oncology nursing* (4th ed., pp. 364–379). St. Louis, MO: Elsevier Saunders.

Twycross, R., & Wilcock, A. (Eds.). (2006). Acute inflammatory episodes in a lymphedematous limb. *Hospice and Palliative Care Formulary USA* (pp. 285–288). Nottingham, United Kingdom: Palliativedrugs.com.

Williams, A.F., Franks, P.J., & Moffatt, C.J. (2005). Lymphoedema: Estimating the size of the problem. *Palliative Medicine, 19*(4), 300–313.

CHAPTER 16

Oral Mucositis

Carlton G. Brown, PhD, RN, AOCN®

Case Study

G.B. is a 64-year-old man diagnosed with adenocarcinoma of the colon. Next week he is scheduled to begin four to six cycles of leucovorin and bolus fluorouracil (5-FU), which will be administered over five days every four weeks. G.B. and his wife ask the nurse who is providing chemotherapy teaching what will likely be the most significant symptom for him during the treatment. The nurse knows that oral mucositis will be a severe problem for G.B.

Overview

Oral mucositis (OM), sometimes referred to as stomatitis, is one of the most incapacitating, painful, and menacing side effects of cancer therapies such as chemotherapy and radiation therapy. According to Eilers and Million (2007), "Mucositis refers to the inflammatory process involving the mucous membranes of the oral cavity and gastrointestinal tract" (p. 201). OM is a somewhat common and treatment-limiting side effect of cancer therapy (Scully, Sonis, & Diz, 2006). It is said to be a side effect that is dose limiting in that OM generally disappears a few days or weeks after the chemotherapy or radiation is discontinued.

The American Cancer Society (1999) estimated that of the 1.2 million patients who receive antineoplastic treatment for cancer, more than 400,000 patients will develop OM. OM can be characterized by ulceration in the oro-esophageal mucosa and results in an acutely painful toxicity of treatment (Scully et al., 2006). The varying degrees of mucositis range from mild changes in sensation to more major changes including acute oral pain, bleeding, infection, xerostomia (dry mouth), and ulcerative, bleeding lesions (Eilers & Million, 2007). Patients who encounter OM also complain of a "sore mouth" and are sometimes subjected to a variety of physical sequelae along with pain, including difficulty eating and drinking, difficulty talking, depression, sleep disturbances, weight loss, and hospitalization (Rose-Ped et al., 2002). Because it can be painful for patients with OM to eat and drink, nutritional shortfalls such as anorexia, dehydration, weight loss, and malnutrition frequently develop (Wilkes, 1998). Not all mucositis is confined to the oral cavity but presents throughout the entire gastrointestinal tract and commonly is referred to as alimentary mucositis (Keefe, Peterson, & Schubert, 2006).

Patients may find OM so painful and unbearable that they may prematurely terminate their cancer therapy. Sonis et al. (2004) estimated that more than half of patients with OM have temporary delays in treatment, and more than one-third of patients with OM discontinued treatment altogether. According to Elting et al. (2003), the potential for having a dose reduction in chemotherapy is almost doubled for patients with OM.

Although OM is certainly a detriment to a patient's quality of life, this debilitating side effect can be financially costly as well. An episode of OM may increase a patient's chances for hospitalization, and the length of stay may be extended because of fever and infection or the necessity for pain management and parenteral nutrition (Rubenstein et al., 2004). An estimated 62% of patients with OM are hospitalized and 70% require tube feedings to maintain acceptable hydration and nutrition (Sonis et al., 2004).

Peterman, Cella, Glandon, Dobrez, and Yount (2001), in their retrospective study of costs associated with an episode of OM, found that patients with head and neck cancer who had OM had statistically higher medical costs and that these were associated with OM severity. Elting et al. (2003) estimated that the incremental cost of hospitalization was $2,725 to manage patients with grades I and II OM and $5,565 to manage patients with grades III and IV OM.

Risk Factors and Associated Incidence

Variance exists in OM incidence and severity depending on patient-related and treatment- or therapy-related risk factors. Patient-related factors (see Figure 16-1) that may increase the incidence of OM include age, sex, and level of oral health. Vokurka et al. (2006) reported a higher incidence of chemotherapy-induced OM in females when compared with males. Raber-Durlacher et al. (2000) suggested that patients older than 50 years develop OM that is more severe and has a longer duration. They proposed that this more intense and prolonged OM might be related to a decline in renal function in patients older than 50.

Examples of treatment-related risk factors (see Table 16-1) include the particular chemotherapy agents and dosage of medication, the frequency of the treatment schedule, the use of radiation therapy, and resultant neutropenia (Avritscher, Cooksley, & Elting, 2004; Barasch & Peterson, 2003; Peterson & Cariello, 2004). The radiation- and chemotherapy-associated risk factors will now be discussed in further detail.

Radiation

The occurrence of OM fluctuates noticeably depending on the different types of treatments for cancer (Peterson & Cariello, 2004). In patients receiving radiation, especially those treated for head and neck cancer, the incidence of OM is almost 100% (National Cancer Institute [NCI], 2008). The incidence of radiation-induced OM is particularly high in (a) patients with primary tumors of the oral cavity, orophar-

FIGURE 16-1	Patient-Related Risk Factors for Oral Mucositis

- Age: Children/older adults
- Oral health/hygiene: Poor oral health/hygiene
- Salivary secretion function: Reduced salivary flow increases susceptibility to oral mucositis (OM).
- Genetic factors: Patients who express high levels of cytokines may be at higher risk.
- Body mass index (BMI): Low body mass (BMI < 20 for males and < 19 for females)
- Renal function: Decreased renal function
- Smoking
- Previous cancer treatment
- Nutritional status: Patients with low body weight
- Oral microflora: Incidence of OM is higher in patients with higher levels of microflora.
- Inflammation: Role of inflammation in development of OM is unclear but suspect.

Note. Based on information from Avritscher et al., 2004; Barasch & Peterson, 2003.

TABLE 16-1	Treatment-Related Risk Factors for Oral Mucositis
Factor	**Comment**
Chemotherapy agent	5-fluorouracil (5-FU), methotrexate, and etoposide produce high rate of mucositis.
Chemotherapy dose	High-dose chemotherapy regimens and continuous infusion (5-FU) are associated with higher incidence and severity of mucositis.
Type of transplant	Allogeneic stem cell transplant recipients experience higher rates of mucositis than autologous bone marrow transplant recipients.
Radiation site	Radiation administered directly to the head and neck, thorax, and abdomen produce higher rates of mucositis.
Combined modality	The use of chemotherapy in conjunction with radiation therapy is associated with increased risk and severity of mucositis.

Note. Based on information from Avritscher et al., 2004; Barasch & Peterson, 2003.

ynx, or nasopharynx, (b) those who have received concomitant chemotherapy, (c) those who received greater than 5,000 centigray (cGy) of radiation, and (d) those treated with more than one radiation treatment per day (Lalla, Sonis, & Peterson, 2008). Patients receiving radiation for head and neck cancers tend to develop erythema around the second week of treatment or when doses reach approximately 2,000 cGy (Shih, Miaskowski, Dodd, Stotts, & MacPhail, 2003). Thereafter, severity of OM generally worsens over the next weeks of radiation treatment and does not subside until the treatment is terminated. Unfortunately, radiation causes permanent tissue damage not only to the oral mucosa but also to the salivary glands, muscles, and bone, thus resulting in permanent chronic problems such as xerostomia. Patients who receive radiotherapy and chemotherapy concurrently for head and neck cancer have marked OM (Peterson & Cariello). Shih et al. reported that when radiation and chemotherapy are given together, severe OM increases from 60% up to 100%.

Chemotherapy

Receiving a particular chemotherapy regimen puts patients at higher risk for OM. Certain chemotherapeutic agents have a higher potential to cause OM than others, and not all chemotherapy agents cause OM (Beck, 2004). NCI (2008) estimated that 10% of patients receiving adjunctive and 40% of patients receiving primary chemotherapy experience OM. Figure 16-2 presents an overview of chemotherapeutic agents with a high likelihood of causing OM. The following chemotherapy agents have a tendency to be more likely to cause OM: busulfan, cyclophosphamide, liposomal doxorubicin, mechlorethamine, high-dose methotrexate, and capecitabine (Wilkes, 1998). A common drug used in the treatment of colon cancer, 5-FU, especially when given continuously over an extended period (as opposed to bolus), can cause higher incidence of grade 3–4 OM to greater than 15% (Sonis et al., 2004). Of course, higher doses of chemotherapy agents frequently administered for stem cell transplantation and induction therapy for leukemia are likely to cause more severe mucositis related to more extensive cellular damage to the mucosa (Beck). Chemotherapy-induced OM can be detected anywhere from 2–14 days following drug administration. Mucositis induced by chemother-

FIGURE 16-2	Chemotherapeutic Agents With Affinity to Cause Oral Mucositis

- Actinomycin D
- Bleomycin
- Busulfan*
- Capecitabine*
- Cyclophosphamide*
- Cytosine arabinoside
- Daunomycin
- Daunorubicin
- Docetaxel
- Doxil*
- Doxorubicin
- Etoposide
- 5-fluorouracil*
- Floxuridine
- High-dose methotrexate
- Hydroxyurea
- Mechlorethamine*
- Melphalan
- Mitomycin
- Mitoxantrone
- Paclitaxel
- Procarbazine
- 6-mercaptopurine
- 6-thioguanine
- Thiotepa
- Vinblastine
- Vinorelbine

* Most commonly indicated

Note. Based on information from Wilkes, 1998.

apy usually lasts for about one week and heals approximately 21 days after infusion of chemotherapy (Scully et al., 2006).

Stem Cell Transplantation

OM in hematopoietic stem cell transplant (HSCT) recipients is a significant problem and usually is caused by the much higher doses of chemotherapy used in these conditioning regimens. Allogeneic transplants are associated with higher levels of OM than autologous transplants (Sonis et al., 2001). Approximately 80% of patients who undergo HSCT experience some level of OM (NCI, 2008). McGuire et al. (1993) reported that approximately 89% of patients receiving either an allogeneic or autologous transplant had OM, and 36% of the same sample reported OM-associated pain. In a longitudinal study of 59 transplant recipients undergoing HSCT, 76% of participants had ulcerative lesions that developed approximately five days after conditioning with a duration of approximately six days (Woo, Sonis, Monopoli, & Sonis, 1993). Wardley et al. (2000) found that of those patients undergoing some form of HSCT, 99% reported some level of OM and 67% reported grade III or IV OM. Patients who undergo HSCT are at an even higher risk for OM when total body irradiation is given concurrently with consolidating chemotherapy. Sonis et al. (2004) reported that when patients receive total body irradiation as part of the conditioning regimen for HSCT, the incidence of grades III and IV OM exceeded 60%. Conversely, the same researchers reported lower levels (30%–50%) of OM without total body irradiation.

Pathophysiology

Historically, the primary cause of OM was believed to be epithelial damage to the oral mucosa. Therapies, such as chemotherapy and radiation, meant to destroy quickly replicating cancer cells also damaged the healthy epithelial cells of the mucosa. As the epithelial cells were damaged, the epithelium thinned, allowing ulceration to develop. Those ulcerated lesions created an entranceway for infection from bacteria and other microorganisms, creating significant life-threatening problems such as systemic infection. Although it is true that damage to the epithelial cells as previously discussed is part of the overall cause of mucositis, there is much more to this complex problem.

According to Sonis (2004), OM is more than a result of epithelial injury, and the existence of other mediators and circumstances must be taken into account. Sonis (2004) proposed a pathophysiologic model (see Figure 16-3) for mucositis, which encompasses five distinct phases: (a) initiation, (b) primary damage response, (c) signaling and amplification, (d) ulceration, and (e) healing. Each of these phases will now be discussed.

Initiation

The first phase of the process is the initiation phase, which occurs very quickly after administration of chemotherapy or radiation therapy. During the initiation phase, DNA and non-DNA damage occurs, ensuing injury of the basal and epithelial cells in the submucosa. Additionally, this dilemma is mediated by the generation of reactive oxygen species, which can create further biologic problems later. According to Denham and Hauer-Jensen (2002), although the mucosa appears completely normal, the death of the submucosal cells contributes to the greatest overall destruction.

Primary Damage Response

Following initiation, a series of individual biologic events happen that create further damage. Chemotherapy and radiation treatment cause DNA damage and consequent cell death in the epithelium of the mucosa. The transcription factor NF-κB is activated, which then is capable of controlling nearly 200 genes connected with mucositis (Sonis, 2004). Amplification of injury occurs as these genes, present in the endothelium, fibroblasts, macrophages, and epithelium, become activated. At this point, proinflammatory cytokines, including tumor necrosis factor alpha, interleukin (IL)-1 beta, and IL-6, are activated and cause damage. Patients are not likely to feel the effects of damage during this phase.

Signal Amplification

The third phase is signal amplification. Via a positive feedback loop, proteins and cytokines continue to damage tissue as well as increase the primary damage from chemotherapy or radiation therapy. The continued bombardment of positive signals accelerates and ampli-

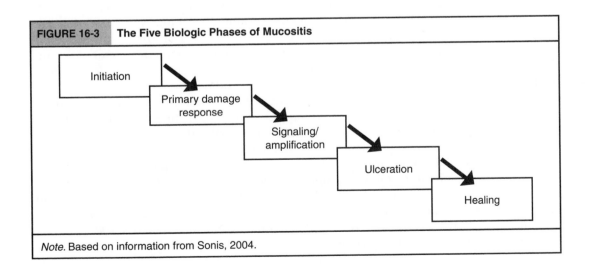

FIGURE 16-3   The Five Biologic Phases of Mucositis

Initiation

Primary damage response

Signaling/ amplification

Ulceration

Healing

Note. Based on information from Sonis, 2004.

fies the biologic effect of a dose of chemotherapy, thus causing continuous injury to the oral mucosa. In this phase, patients still may not feel the effects of the ongoing mucosal damage (Sonis, 2004).

Ulceration

Ulceration is the fourth phase of the model and is considered the most complex and symptomatic for patients and caregivers (Sonis, 2004). As the biologic barrage begins to take its harmful toll on the mucosa, injury is manifested in the form of ulceration. Fibrinous exudates may cover the oral lesions, which become inundated with high levels of bacteria. In patients who are already neutropenic, this accumulation of bacteria may put patients at significant risk for invasion of microorganisms that may lead to bacteremia and sepsis (Sonis, 2004). Interestingly, it is during the ulcerative phase that OM greatly affects the patient's well-being by causing very painful lesions (Sonis, 1998). Patients may begin to experience considerable pain and have difficulty swallowing, leading to a decrease in nutritional intake, coupled with decreased talking and an increased potential for bleeding.

Healing

The final phase of the pathobiology model is healing. Fortunately, eventual healing of the oral mucosa takes place, which happens when treatments such as chemotherapy or radiation are terminated. New messenger molecules direct the epithelium to heal through regeneration. During the healing phase, an augmented creation of white bloods cells occurs, which helps to fight and disable infection from bacteria and other harmful microorganisms. However, it is essential to understand that cells and tissue of the mucosa may not immediately return to their original state. In instances where several cycles of chemotherapy or radiation are delivered, complete healing may not have time to occur, which often leads the patient to have more severe OM in future cycles of treatment.

Assessment

Thorough and systematic assessment of the oral cavity has significant importance in the treatment and prevention of OM. In fact, Jaroneski (2006) noted that for oncology nurses caring for patients with OM, assessment is the paramount clinical intervention. A systematic assessment conducted by the oncology nurse should include a pretreatment assessment that considers the patient- and treatment-related risk factors presented in Figure 16-1 and Table 16-1. Additionally, during the pretreatment assessment, nurses should inquire about the patients' usual daily oral care techniques (brushing and flossing) and ability to conduct oral care during their respective cancer treatment (Eilers & Million, 2007). If time permits, patients who are about to initiate chemotherapy or radiation treatment are recommended to obtain a complete oral assessment by a dental professional with the goal of alleviating any dental caries or other dental problems before treatment.

Numerous assessment tools are available to oncology nurses to help record the extent and severity of OM, including the Oral Assessment Guide (Eilers, Berger, & Petersen, 1988), the Oral Mucositis Index (McGuire et al., 2002; Schubert, Williams, Lloyd, Donaldson, & Chapko, 1992), the Oral Mucositis Assessment Scale (Sonis et al., 1999), the Western Consortium for Cancer Nursing Research tool (Western Consortium for Nursing Research, 1987), and the World Health Organization (WHO) Oral Toxicity Scale (WHO, 1979). Each of these respec-

tive assessment tools has both benefits and weaknesses related to ease of
use and reliability. The WHO scale for
OM is presented in Table 16-2 and is
considered a simple, easy-to-use scale
that is suitable for daily clinical practice (Lalla et al., 2008).

Beck (2004) recommended that
all patients with cancer receive a systematic assessment of the oral cavity.
Nurses should ask patients if they are
experiencing any rubbing or tissue
damage from an ill-fitting appliance.
Nurses should ask about current oral
pain, changes in saliva and swallow-

TABLE 16-2	World Health Organization Scale for Oral Mucositis
Grade	**Indication**
0	No oral mucositis
1	Erythema and soreness
2	Ulcers, able to eat solids
3	Ulcers, requires liquid diet (due to mucositis)
4	Ulcers, alimentation not possible (due to mucositis)

Note. Based on information from World Health Organization, 1979.

ing, obvious lesions, or any other changes to the oral mucosa. Patients usually are very aware
of any alterations or differences in their own oral cavity and should be considered an excellent source for determining overall change.

The oral assessment should be conducted in a room or area with a good source of natural light. Before the assessment, nurses should ask patients to remove any dental appliances
such as partial or full dentures. Nurses should gather the equipment needed to conduct the
oral assessment, including nonsterile gloves, tongue blade, dental mirror, and gauze. Nurses should wash their hands and put on gloves prior to the assessment. During the visual inspection, nurses will want to look at the outer lips, teeth, gums, tongue, inside cheek area,
and hard and soft palate. Wrapping the tongue in a piece of gauze may be important to help
move the tongue for inspection of the floor of the oral cavity under the tongue. Additionally, nurses should gently pull the upper and lower cheeks away to inspect the tissue close to
the gums. The oral assessment will likely take only a few minutes, and patients should be referred to a dentist or hygienist if a more thorough examination is warranted.

The oral cavity in a healthy individual is usually moist, clean, pink, and intact. Abnormal
assessment findings in the oral mucosa include changes in color (pallor, erythema, white
patches), changes in moisture (dryness, decreased amounts of saliva), changes in cleanliness
(accumulation of debris, odor), changes in integrity (ulcers, cracks, lesions), and changes in
perception (hoarseness, difficulty swallowing, pain) (Beck, 2004). Following an oral assessment, nurses should document findings in the patient record. Nurses would then use both
the patient report and physical findings from the oral examination to develop or guide interventions, especially for patients who are experiencing OM.

Interventions

To date, the management of OM has been primarily palliative in nature (Lalla et al.,
2008). However, numerous preventive therapeutic interventions are currently being developed (Lalla & Peterson, 2006). In 2004, the Mucositis Study Group of the Multinational Association of Supportive Care in Cancer and the International Society for Oral Oncology, two multidisciplinary groups, published evidence-based clinical practice guidelines
for the prevention and treatment of OM (Rubenstein et al., 2004). More recent guidelines from the same organizations were reviewed, and an update was published in *Cancer*
in 2007 (Keefe et al., 2007). Additionally, two Cochrane reviews focused on interventions

for the treatment and prevention of OM (Clarkson, Worthington, & Eden, 2004; Worthington, Clarkson, & Eden, 2007).

More recently and from a more nursing-focused approach, the Oncology Nursing Society (ONS) Putting Evidence Into Practice (PEP) resource for OM presented evidence-based practice recommendations for OM (Harris, Eilers, Cashavelly, Maxwell, & Harriman, 2007). The ONS PEP resource presented the research in several categories, including *Recommended for Practice, Likely to Be Effective, Benefits Balanced With Harms, Not Recommended for Practice,* and *Expert Opinion.* This chapter will now focus on these interventions, as oncology nurses need to be knowledgeable of those interventions both supported and not supported for use in patients with OM.

Recommended for Practice

Interventions are placed in the *Recommended for Practice* category when they have strong evidence of support from rigorously designed studies. Of all the interventions that have been developed to either lessen or prevent OM, oral care is widely considered to be the foundation of mucosal health (Harris, Eilers, Harriman, Cashavelly, & Maxwell, 2008). Oral care is hypothesized to reduce pain, bleeding, and high levels of microbial flora, prevent infection, and reduce the risk of dental complications (Cawley & Benson, 2005; Harris et al., 2008; Rubenstein et al., 2004). Thus, the ONS PEP resource places oral care protocols, or formalized and standardized plans that have been developed by multidisciplinary teams, in the *Recommended for Practice* category. According to Harris et al. (2008), basic components of an oral care protocol include assessment, patient education, tooth brushing, flossing, and use of an oral rinse.

It is recommended that clinicians (a) collaborate with a multidisciplinary team in all phases of treatment; (b) conduct a systematic oral assessment at least daily or upon each patient visit; (c) teach patients when to report self-assessment findings to the clinician; and (d) provide written instructions and education to patients regarding oral care and verify patient understanding with return demonstration and explanation (Harris et al., 2007).

The ONS PEP resource for OM also presented recommendations specifically for patients. Patients are recommended to (a) brush all tooth surfaces for at least 90 seconds twice daily using a soft toothbrush; (b) allow the toothbrush to air dry before storing and replace the toothbrush on a regular basis; (c) floss at least once daily or as advised by the clinician; (d) rinse the mouth four times daily (with a bland mouth rinse like normal saline) or as advised by the clinician; (e) avoid tobacco, alcohol, and irritating foods; (f) use water-based moisturizers to protect lips; and (g) maintain adequate hydration (Harris et al., 2007).

Likely to Be Effective

Cryotherapy

Cryotherapy is the use of ice chips during chemotherapy administration to prevent OM. Sucking on ice chips during the administration of chemotherapy is hypothesized to cause local vasoconstriction and reduce blood flow to the tissue of the oral mucosa, thus resulting in a decreased delivery of chemotherapy to the area (Lalla et al., 2008). Studies have suggested that cryotherapy actually reduces the severity of oral mucositis in patients receiving bolus doses of certain chemotherapy agents (fluorouracil, melphalan) (Cascinu, Fedeli, Fedeli, & Catalano, 1994; Mahood et al., 1991). The ONS PEP resource for OM recommends the use of cryotherapy during rapid infusion of fluorouracil and melphalan. Specifically, patients are encouraged to hold ice or ice-cold water in their mouth for 5 minutes before and 30 minutes after chemotherapy infusion. This recommendation only applies to these two specific chemotherapies and is not recommended with other medications, such as capecitabine or oxaliplatin (Harris et al., 2007).

Palifermin

Palifermin, a recombinant human keratinocyte growth factor that stimulates epithelial cells of the oral mucosa, has been shown to reduce the severity and duration of OM in patients receiving high-dose chemotherapy and total body irradiation with autologous stem cell transplantation (Spielberger et al., 2004). It is recommended that this drug be given at 60 mcg/kg/day IV for three days prior to beginning the conditioning regimen and for three days after the transplantation to prevent OM (Harris et al., 2007). An important note is that palifermin administration is associated with mild rash and taste changes.

Effectiveness Not Established

The ONS PEP resource for OM recognized numerous medications and interventions for which effectiveness has not been established by research. This recommendation does not mean that these interventions are not effective, but rather that they need more thorough, well-conducted randomized clinical trials to establish effectiveness. Figure 16-4 presents interventions placed in the category of *Effectiveness Not Established.*

Not Recommended for Practice

Discussing the interventions for the prevention or management of OM that are categorized as *Not Recommended for Practice* is just as important as recognizing interventions that are effective. This classification is defined as an intervention for which ineffectiveness or harm clearly has been demonstrated or for which the cost burden exceeds the potential benefit (Harris et al., 2007). Interventions placed in this category will now be discussed.

- Chlorhexidine used as a mouthwash is not effective in reducing chemotherapy- or radiation-induced OM. Other researchers have reported that chlorhexidine might be responsible for induced discomfort, taste alterations, and teeth staining (Dodd et al., 2000; Eilers, 2004).
- Granulocyte macrophage–colony-stimulating factor mouthwash is another intervention that is not recommend for practice in the prevention of OM in patients undergoing HSCT (Harris et al., 2007). Valcarcel et al. (2002) demonstrated no positive effects of this intervention on the severity or duration of OM.

FIGURE 16-4	Interventions Placed in the *Effectiveness Not Established* Category

- Allopurinol
- Amifostine
- Anti-inflammatory rinses
- Antimicrobial agents
- Benzydamine HCl
- Flurbiprofen tooth patch
- Granulocyte–colony-stimulating factor (subcutaneous)
- Granulocyte macrophage–colony-stimulating factor (subcutaneous)
- Immunoglobulin
- L-alanyl-L-glutamine
- Low-level laser therapy
- Multiagent ("magic" or "miracle") mouthwashes
- Oral aloe vera
- Pilocarpine
- Povidone-iodine (oral)
- Tetracaine
- Zinc supplementation

Note. Based on information from Harris et al., 2007.

• Sucralfate, a mucosal coating agent, has not been recommended for use in patients to prevent radiation-induced OM (Harris et al., 2007). Sucralfate showed a lack of tolerability related to nausea and vomiting in patients. Furthermore, some patients who received sucralfate also experienced rectal bleeding.

Patient Teaching Points

Perhaps the most significant intervention that oncology nurses can provide for patients who will potentially experience OM is an oral care protocol. In this author's experience, patients receiving chemotherapy or radiation treatment want to help with their individual care in some way. Teaching patients to assess and perform self-care for their own oral cavity is an excellent intervention that likely lessens the experience of OM and involves patients in their own care.

Oral Self-Assessment

Patients can be taught to assess their own oral cavity for any erythema, edema, white lesions, bleeding, or feelings of pain, soreness, or anything that "feels" different. The self-assessment should be conducted once daily. This assessment is particularly important for patients receiving outpatient chemotherapy, who might only see their healthcare provider every two to three weeks between cycles of chemotherapy. Patients conducting their own oral assessment should wash their hands prior to the inspection and should use good lighting to help them to see all areas of the oral mucosa.

Oral Care

As presented previously, the ONS PEP resource (Harris et al., 2007) recommends that patients utilize an oral care protocol that focuses on proper tooth brushing, flossing, and rinsing of the oral cavity. Patients should be taught to brush all the surfaces of their teeth with a soft-bristled toothbrush for 90 seconds at least two times per day. If patients cannot tolerate a toothbrush, a sponge or "toothette" can be used, or patients can even clean the teeth with a piece of gauze wrapped around their finger. To deter growth of microorganisms, toothbrushes should be allowed to dry before being stored. Patients should floss their teeth once daily or as advised by a clinician. Additionally, patients should rinse their mouth four times a day with a bland mouth rinse such as normal saline, sodium bicarbonate, or a saline and sodium bicarbonate mixture. This rinsing is thought to help remove loose debris as well as moisturize the oral cavity. Many over-the-counter mouthwashes should be avoided because they contain alcohol, which can irritate the oral cavity or lesions if they are present. The patient should moisturize the lips with a water-based product.

Patient teaching should include avoiding tobacco products, which may exacerbate OM. Patients are encouraged to avoid alcohol and certain foods and liquids (e.g., those that are spicy, acidic, rough, or hot). Patients need to maintain adequate oral hydration (nonalcoholic) to help keep the oral mucosa moist. Finally, patients should be taught when to report adverse findings or oral pain to their healthcare provider.

Expected Outcomes

The clinical burden of OM is evident, and a serious need exists for interventions to alleviate or reduce this burden. As previously discussed, OM can be so severe that patients may experience modifications of anticancer therapy, such as breaks in the treatment regimen or dose reduction of chemotherapy (Scully et al., 2006). In some instances, this dose reduction or complete termination is necessary. Oncology nurses are in a great position to assist in controlling the symptom of OM so that patients can obtain the ultimate outcomes. These outcomes include (a) controlling symptoms during treatment so that patients have a tolerable quality of life and (b) controlling symptoms so that every patient can receive the best treatment, absent of dose reduction, delay, or termination of treatment, in hopes of receiving a complete cure of their cancer.

Need for Future Research

Because OM is such a debilitating and detrimental side effect associated with cancer treatment, it is frustrating that only a few interventions are approved for use. Numerous interventions were placed in the *Effectiveness Not Established* category of the ONS PEP resource for OM. This categorization does not mean that the intervention is ineffective, but that more randomized clinical trials are needed to test their effectiveness. Further research should evaluate whether agents can be used in combination for clinical effectiveness (Lalla et al., 2008). An important need exists for research to determine whether portions of oral care protocols (for example, brushing and flossing) truly decrease the severity and duration of OM. Finally, it would be very beneficial to test an algorithm that could be used to predict an individual's risk for development of clinically significant OM so that patients at highest risk could receive needed prevention interventions.

Conclusion of Case Study

Recall that G.B. is a patient who is scheduled to begin chemotherapy treatment of leucovorin and 5-FU the following week for a diagnosis of colon cancer. Because he will receive a bolus therapy of 5-FU daily for five days, it might be beneficial for him to suck on ice 5 minutes prior to and 30 minutes after chemotherapy infusion during each day of treatment. Prior to beginning the first chemotherapy treatment, it is advisable for G.B. to see his dentist for a thorough oral assessment.

Because G.B. is likely to experience some level of OM, the patient should be taught how to conduct his own oral assessment and be encouraged to report any pain or other findings to his healthcare team. He should be taught a particular oral care protocol, which includes brushing, flossing, and rinsing his mouth daily (see Patient Teaching Points). Finally, because his wife was also present for chemotherapy teaching, the nurse should take the opportunity to teach not only the patient but also family members who may be called upon to assist the patient with oral care during his treatment.

Conclusion

OM is a clinically significant side effect that can cause pain, infection, dysfunction, and detriment to quality of life and can place patients who are receiving treatment for cancer at high risk for infection. Progress in the understanding of oral mucosal pathobiology coupled with new preventive interventions and oral care protocols have improved the care of patients with OM. However, interventions are still needed that can lessen or preferably eliminate this debilitating clinical problem. Recall that some patients with unmanaged OM request a decrease in their treatment dosage or terminate their cancer therapy altogether. Oncology nurses are in an excellent position to assist patients in the management of OM so that patients can have an opportunity to receive the ultimate treatment for their respective cancer.

References

American Cancer Society. (1999, July). *Mouth sores painful for patients: New scoring system to aid in treating mouth sores*. Retrieved June 15, 2008, from http://www.cancer.org/docroot/NWS/content/NWS_1_1x_Mouth_Sores_Painful_for_Patients.asp

Avritscher, E.B., Cooksley, C.D., & Elting, L.S. (2004). Scope and epidemiology of cancer therapy-induced oral and gastrointestinal mucositis. *Seminars in Oncology Nursing, 20*(1), 3–10.

Barasch, A., & Peterson, D.E. (2003). Risk factors for ulcerative oral mucositis in cancer patients: Unanswered questions. *Oral Oncology, 39*(2), 91–100.

Beck, S.L. (2004). Mucositis. In C.H. Yarbro, M.H. Frogge, & M. Goodman (Eds.), *Cancer symptom management* (3rd ed., pp. 276–291). Sudbury, MA: Jones and Bartlett.

Cascinu, S., Fedeli, A., Fedeli, S.L., & Catalano, G. (1994). Oral cooling (cryotherapy), an effective treatment for the prevention of 5-fluorouracil-induced stomatitis. *European Journal of Cancer. Part B, Oral Oncology, 30B*(4), 234–236.

Cawley, M.M., & Benson, L.M. (2005). Current trends in managing oral mucositis. *Clinical Journal of Oncology Nursing, 9*(5), 584–595.

Clarkson, J.E., Worthington, H.V., & Eden, T.O.B. (2007). Interventions for treating oral mucositis for patients with cancer receiving treatment. *Cochrane Database of Systematic Reviews* 2007, Issue 2. Art. No.: CD001973. DOI: 10.1002/14651858.CD001973.pub3.

Denham, J.W., & Hauer-Jensen, M. (2002). The radiotherapeutic injury—a complex 'wound'. *Radiotherapy and Oncology, 63*(2), 129–145.

Dodd, M.J., Dibble, S.L., Miaskowski, C., MacPhail, L., Greenspan, D., Paul, S., et al. (2000). Randomized clinical trial of the effectiveness of 3 commonly used mouthwashes to treat chemotherapy-induced mucositis. *Oral Surgery, Oral Medicine, Oral Pathology, Oral Radiology, and Endodontology, 90*(1), 39–47.

Eilers, J. (2004). Nursing interventions and supportive care for the prevention and treatment of oral mucositis associated with cancer treatment. *Oncology Nursing Forum, 31*(Suppl. 4), 13–23.

Eilers, J., Berger, A.M., & Petersen, M.C. (1988). Development, testing, and application of the oral assessment guide. *Oncology Nursing Forum, 15*(3), 325–330.

Eilers, J., & Million, R. (2007). Prevention and management of oral mucositis in patients with cancer. *Seminars in Oncology Nursing, 23*(3), 201–212.

Elting, L.S., Cooksley, C., Chambers, M., Cantor, S.B., Manzullo, E., & Rubenstein, E.B. (2003). The burdens of cancer therapy. Clinical and economic outcomes of chemotherapy-induced mucositis. *Cancer, 98*(7), 1531–1539.

Harris, D.J., Eilers, J.G., Cashavelly, B.J., Maxwell, C.L., & Harriman, A. (2007). *Putting evidence into practice: Mucositis*. Pittsburgh, PA: Oncology Nursing Society.

Harris, D.J., Eilers, J., Harriman, A., Cashavelly, B.J., & Maxwell, C. (2008). Putting evidence into practice: Evidence-based interventions for the management of oral mucositis. *Clinical Journal of Oncology Nursing, 12*(1), 141–142.

Jaroneski, L.A. (2006). The importance of assessment rating scales for chemotherapy-induced oral mucositis. *Oncology Nursing Forum, 33*(6), 1085–1090.

Keefe, D.M., Peterson, D.E., & Schubert, M.M. (2006). Developing evidence-based guidelines for management of alimentary mucositis: Process and pitfalls. *Supportive Care in Cancer, 14*(6), 492–498.

Keefe, D.M., Schubert, M.M., Elting, L.S., Sonis, S.T., Epstein, J.B., Raber-Durlacher, J.E., et al. (2007). Updated clinical practice guidelines for the prevention and treatment of mucositis. *Cancer, 109*(5), 820–831.

Lalla, R.V., & Peterson, D.E. (2006). Treatment of mucositis, including new medications. *Cancer Journal, 12*(5), 348–354.

Lalla, R.V., Sonis, S.T., & Peterson, D.E. (2008). Management of oral mucositis in patients who have cancer. *Dental Clinics of North America, 52*(1), 61–77, viii.

Mahood, D.J., Dose, A.M., Loprinzi, C.L., Veeder, M.H., Athmann, L.M., Therneau, T.M., et al. (1991). Inhibition of fluorouracil-induced stomatitis by oral cryotherapy. *Journal of Clinical Oncology, 9*(3), 449–452.

McGuire, D.B., Altomonte, V., Peterson, D.E., Wingard, J.R., Jones, R.J., & Grochow, L.B. (1993). Patterns of mucositis and pain in patients receiving preparative chemotherapy and bone marrow transplantation. *Oncology Nursing Forum, 20*(10), 1493–1502.

McGuire, D.B., Peterson, D.E., Muller, S., Owen, D.C., Slemmons, M.F., & Schubert, M.M. (2002). The 20 item oral mucositis index: Reliability and validity in bone marrow and stem cell transplant patients. *Cancer Investigation, 20*(7–8), 893–903.

National Cancer Institute. (2008). *Oral complications of chemotherapy and head and neck radiation (PDQ®)*. Retrieved June 13, 2008, from http://www.cancer.gov/cancertopics/pdq/supportivecare/oralcomplications/ HealthProfessional/page2

Peterman, A., Cella, D., Glandon, G., Dobrez, D., & Yount, S. (2001). Mucositis in head and neck cancer: Economic and quality of life outcome. *Journal of the National Cancer Institute Monographs, 2001*(29), 45–51.

Peterson, D.E., & Cariello, A. (2004). Mucosal damage: A major risk factor for severe complications after cytotoxic therapy. *Seminars in Oncology, 31*(3, Suppl. 8), 35–44.

Raber-Durlacher, J.E., Weijl, N.I., Abu Saris, M., de Koning, B., Zwinderman, A.H., & Osanto, S. (2000). Oral mucositis in patients treated with chemotherapy for solid tumors: A retrospective analysis of 150 cases. *Supportive Care in Cancer, 8*(5), 366–371.

Rose-Ped, A.M., Bellm, L.A., Epstein, J.B., Trotti, A., Gwede, C., & Fuchs, H.J. (2002). Complications of radiation therapy for head and neck cancers. The patient's perspective. *Cancer Nursing, 25*(6), 461–467.

Rubenstein, E.B., Peterson, D.E., Schubert, M., Keefe, D., McGuire, D., Epstein, J., et al. (2004). Clinical practice guidelines for the prevention and treatment of cancer therapy-induced oral and gastrointestinal mucositis. *Cancer, 100*(Suppl. 9), 2026–2046.

Schubert, M.M., Williams, B.E., Lloyd, M.E., Donaldson, G., & Chapko, M.K. (1992). Clinical assessment scale for the rating of oral mucosal changes associated with bone marrow transplantation. *Cancer, 69*(10), 2469–2477.

Scully, C., Sonis, S., & Diz, P.D. (2006). Oral mucositis. *Oral Diseases, 12*(3), 229–241.

Shih, A., Miaskowski, C., Dodd, M.J., Stotts, N.A., & MacPhail, L. (2003). Mechanisms for radiation-induced oral mucositis and the consequences. *Cancer Nursing, 26*(3), 222–229.

Sonis, S.T. (1998). Mucositis as a biological process: A new hypothesis for the development of chemotherapy-induced stomatotoxicity. *Oral Oncology, 34*(1), 39–43.

Sonis, S.T. (2004). The pathobiology of mucositis. *Nature Reviews Cancer, 4*(4), 277–284.

Sonis, S.T., Eilers, J.P., Epstein, J.B., LeVeque, F.G., Liggett, W.H., Jr., Mulagha, M.T., et al. (1999). Validation of a new scoring system for the assessment of clinical trial research of oral mucositis induced by radiation or chemotherapy. *Cancer, 85*(10), 2103–2113.

Sonis, S.T., Elting, L.S., Keefe, D., Peterson, D.E., Schubert, M., Hauer-Jensen, M., et al. (2004). Perspectives on cancer therapy-induced mucosal injury: Pathogenesis, measurement, epidemiology, and consequences for patients. *Cancer, 100*(Suppl. 9), 1995–2025.

Sonis, S.T., Oster, G., Fuchs, H., Bellm, L., Bradford, W.Z., Edelsberg, J., et al. (2001). Oral mucositis and the clinical and economic outcomes of hematopoietic stem-cell transplantation. *Journal of Clinical Oncology, 19*(8), 2201–2205.

Spielberger, R., Stiff, P., Bensinger, W., Gentile, T., Weisdorf, D., Kewalramani, T., et al. (2004). Palifermin for oral mucositis after intensive therapy for hematologic cancers. *New England Journal of Medicine, 351*(25), 2590–2598.

Valcarcel, D., Sanz, M.A., Jr., Sureda, A., Sala, M., Munoz, L., Subira, M., et al. (2002). Mouth washing with recombinant human granulocyte-macrophage colony stimulating factor (rhGM-CSF) do not improve grade III-IV oropharyngeal mucositis (OM) in patients with hematological malignancies undergoing stem cell transplantation. Results of a randomized double-blind placebo controlled study. *Bone Marrow Transplantation, 29*(9), 783–787.

Vokurka, S., Bystricka, E., Koza, V., Scudlova, J., Pavlicova, V., Valentova, D., et al. (2006). Higher incidence of chemotherapy induced oral mucositis in females: A supplement of multivariate analysis to a randomized multicentre study. *Supportive Care in Cancer, 14*(9), 974–976.

Wardley, A.M., Jayson, G.C., Swindell, R., Morgenstern, G.R., Chang, J., Bloor, J., et al. (2000). Prospective evaluation of oral mucositis in patients receiving myeloablative conditioning regimens and haemopoietic progenitor rescue. *British Journal of Haematology, 110*(2), 292–299.

Western Consortium for Cancer Nursing Research. (1987). Priorities for cancer nursing research. A Canadian replication. *Cancer Nursing, 10*(6), 319–326.

Wilkes, J.D. (1998). Prevention and treatment of oral mucositis following cancer chemotherapy. *Seminars in Oncology, 25*(5), 538–551.

Woo, S.B., Sonis, S.T., Monopoli, M.M., & Sonis, A.L. (1993). A longitudinal study of oral ulcerative mucositis in bone marrow transplant recipients. *Cancer, 72*(5), 1612–1617.

World Health Organization. (1979). *WHO handbook for reporting results from cancer treatment* (pp. 15–22). Geneva, Switzerland: Author.

Worthington, H.V., Clarkson, J.E., & Eden, T.O.B. (2007). Interventions for preventing oral mucositis for patients with cancer receiving treatment. *Cochrane Database of Systematic Reviews* 2007, Issue 4. Art. No.: CD000978. DOI: 10.1002/14651858.CD000978.pub3.

CHAPTER 17

Neutropenia and Infection

Colleen O'Leary, RN, MSN, AOCNS®

Case Study

R.M., a 68-year-old woman with lung cancer, is admitted for her third cycle of docetaxel and cisplatin. Her past medical history includes hypertension, coronary artery disease, and hyperlipidemia. After her first cycle of chemotherapy, she experienced neutropenia with an absolute neutrophil count (ANC) of 100 cells/mm³ for two weeks. During this period of time she also had oral candidiasis. She is currently feeling well and ready to start her treatment. The nurse recognizes that the patient is at increased risk for neutropenia with this cycle because of her sex, age, comorbidities, and previous fungal infection and neutropenia. The nurse verifies that colony-stimulating factors (CSFs) are ordered as part of the chemotherapy regimen. The patient's neutrophils begin to drop during her therapy, and at the conclusion of her treatment cycle her ANC is 600 cells/mm³. Based on her ANC, neutropenic precautions are initiated.

Overview

Neutropenia is a decrease in circulating neutrophils that can be caused by problems with neutrophil production or distribution, infection, treatment, or drugs (Lynch & Rogers, 2000). Despite the etiology, neutropenia has significant negative clinical outcomes for patients with cancer, including being one of the greatest predictors of life-threatening infection in patients. Other serious patient outcomes of neutropenia include hospitalization, increased IV antibiotic use, effect on quality of life for patients and caregivers, loss of productivity, economic costs to patients, families, and the healthcare system, and suboptimal delivery of treatment regimens (Nirenberg et al., 2006). Chemotherapy-induced neutropenia (CIN) is the major dose-limiting toxicity of systemic cancer chemotherapy and is associated with significant morbidity, mortality, and costs (Lyman, Lyman, & Agboola, 2005).

Definitions

ANC is an essential tool used to determine potential risk for neutropenia. The ANC represents the number of mature white blood cells (WBCs) in circulation. The Infectious Diseases Society of America (IDSA) defines neutropenia as an ANC less than 500 cells/mm³ or an ANC of 500–1,000 cells/mm³ in patients with whom further decline is anticipated (Hughes et

FIGURE 17-1	Calculating Absolute Neutrophil Count

The absolute neutrophil count (ANC) is calculated as follows.

$$ANC = \frac{\text{Segmented neutrophils + bands}}{100} \times \frac{\text{white blood cell}}{\text{(WBC) count}}$$

An example of calculating the ANC of a patient with the counts of:

> Segmented neutrophils = 50
> Bands = 4
> WBC = 2700

ANC = (50 + 4) ÷ 100 = 0.54
     = 0.54 × 2700 = 1458
     = 1458

al., 2002). ANC is calculated by multiplying the WBC count by the percentage of bands and segmented neutrophils (see Figure 17-1).

The degree and duration of neutropenia can help to determine the risk of infection. Short-term neutropenia is defined as lasting less than 10 days, whereas long-term neutropenia exceeds 10–14 days (Wujcik, 2004). Following administration, each chemotherapy agent has a relatively predictable period of neutropenia. The nadir, which is the point of lowest WBCs following treatment, frequently, but not always, occurs 7–10 days after therapy. Cell-cycle–specific drugs produce rapid nadirs in 7–14 days, and cell-cycle–nonspecific drugs cause nadirs in 10–14 days (Polovich, White, & Kelleher, 2005; Scott, 2004). Some cell-cycle–nonspecific drugs, such as nitrosoureas, produce a delayed and prolonged neutropenia. For adults, the nadir associated with nitrosoureas can occur at 26–63 days, whereas in children, the nadir occurs at 21–35 days (Scott). Figure 17-2 depicts a general overview of nadir length. A greater degree and longer duration of neutrope-

FIGURE 17-2	Specific Drug Nadirs

Cell Cycle Specific	Cell Cycle Nonspecific	Cell Cycle Nonspecific
Rapid nadir of 7–10 days Recovery of 7–21 days	Moderate nadir of 10–14 days Recovery of 21–24 days	Prolonged or delayed nadir of • 26–63 days for adults • 21–35 days for children Recovery of • 35–89 days for adults • 40–50 days for children
Antimetabolites • Azacitidine • Capecitabine • Cytarabine • Fludarabine • Fluorouracil • Gemcitabine • Methotrexate • Pentostatin	**Alkylating Agents** • Busulfan • Carboplatin • Cisplatin • Cyclophosphamide • Dacarbazine • Ifosfamide • Melphalan • Oxaliplatin • Temozolomide • Thiotepa	**Nitrosoureas** • Lomustine • Streptozocin
Plant Alkaloids • Docetaxel • Etoposide • Irinotecan • Paclitaxel • Topotecan • Vinblastine • Vincristine • Vinorelbine	**Antitumor Antibiotics** • Bleomycin • Daunorubicin • Doxorubicin • Epirubicin • Idarubicin • Mitomycin • Mitoxantrone • Valrubicin	

Note. Based on information from Polovich et al., 2005.

nia can put patients at a greater risk for complications. A commonly used scale for grading the severity of neutropenia associated with cancer chemotherapy is the Common Terminology Criteria for Adverse Events (CTCAE) from the National Cancer Institute Cancer Therapy Evaluation Program (NCI CTEP, 2009). This scale categorizes neutropenia from grade 1 through 4 (see Table 17-1). However, the grade of toxicity does not always correlate directly

TABLE 17-1	Common Terminology Criteria for Adverse Events
Grade	Absolute Neutrophil Count (cells/mm³)
1	> 1,500
2	< 1,500–1,000
3	< 1,000–500
4	< 500

Note. Based on information from National Cancer Institute Cancer Therapy Evaluation Program, 2009.

with the incidence of infection. Although the CTCAE is used most often for grading the response to chemotherapy in clinical trials, it also can prove to be a valuable tool for practitioners when describing the degree of neutropenia.

Risk Factors

Despite the thought that the longer a patient is receiving chemotherapy, the greater the risk for developing neutropenia, it is those patients undergoing their first cycle of chemotherapy who are at greater risk for developing neutropenia. The National Comprehensive Cancer Network (NCCN, 2008) identifies risk factors for neutropenia that can be classified as patient-specific, disease-specific, or treatment-specific. Figure 17-3 shows examples of each of these types of risk factors.

Patient-Specific Risk Factors

Patient-specific risk factors include advanced age, female sex, poor performance status, poor nutritional status, comorbid conditions, and poor pretreatment health. In a study of 18 published risk models developed to assess neutropenia, advanced age (> 65 years) and poor performance status were validated in at least two of the models chosen. Furthermore, 10 studies found older age to be a general risk factor for the development of severe neutropenia (Lyman et al., 2005). Older patients often are treated with lower chemotherapy doses to minimize the occurrence of neutropenic complications (Wujcik, 2004). However, because older patients with cancer can obtain the same benefit from aggressive chemotherapy as younger patients, effective management of the risk of neutropenia is crucial in order to administer full-dose chemotherapy to this population of patients. Studies have shown that poor performance status is a significant risk for neutropenia and that in older adults, physiologic age or frailty may be a more accurate predictor of risk than chronologic age. Several tools can be used to measure a patient's performance status. One such tool is the Eastern Cooperative Oncology Group (ECOG) scale (Oken et al., 1982) (see Table 17-2). Once the patient's performance status is graded, the grade can be used to help to identify whether he or she is at greater risk for neutropenia.

The presence of comorbid conditions also increases the risk of neutropenia in patients with cancer. Renal disease and cardiovascular disease increase the risk for developing febrile neutropenia (FN) in patients with non-Hodgkin lymphoma (Lyman et al., 2005). The presence of liver disease, renal disease, and cardiovascular disease increases the risk of neutro-

FIGURE 17-3	Risk Factors for Neutropenia

Patient-Related Factors
- Age > 65
- Female
- Poor performance status
- Albumin < 35 g/L
- Comorbid conditions
  - With non-Hodgkin lymphoma
    * Renal disease
    * Cardiovascular disease
  - With breast cancer
    * Liver disease
    * Renal disease
    * Cardiovascular disease
  - Sepsis
  - Pneumonia
  - Hypertension
  - Prior fungal infections
  - Chronic obstructive pulmonary disease
- Previous neutropenia
- Decreased white blood cell count
- Hemoglobin < 12 g/dl
- Open wounds
- Active tissue infections

Disease-Related Factors
- Hematologic malignancies
- Advanced disease
- Uncontrolled cancer
- Lung cancer
- Elevated lactate dehydrogenase in lymphoma
- Leukemia
- Diabetes

Treatment-Related Factors
- Chemotherapy regimen
- High-dose cyclophosphamide
- Etoposide
- High-dose anthracyclines
- Relative dose intensity > 80%
- Extensive prior chemotherapy
- Concurrent or prior radiation therapy
- Previous history of severe neutropenia with similar chemotherapy

Note. From "Bone Marrow Suppression" (p. 489), by B.H. Gobel and C. O'Leary in M.E. Langhorne, J.S. Fulton, and S.E. Otto (Eds.), *Oncology Nursing* (5th ed.), 2007, St. Louis, MO: Elsevier Mosby. Copyright 2007 by Elsevier. Adapted with permission.

penia in patients with breast cancer. Comorbid conditions such as sepsis, pneumonia, hypertension, prior fungal infections, and chronic obstructive pulmonary disease have been shown to increase the risk for serious neutropenic complications, including prolonged hospitalizations for FN and death. NCCN (2007) also identified the presence of diabetes mellitus as increasing the risk for developing FN.

Other patient-specific predictors of neutropenia include previous neutropenia, decreased WBC count, hemoglobin levels less than 12 g/dl and serum albumin concentrations of 3.5 g/L or less, open wounds, and active tissue infections.

Disease-Specific Factors

Patients with hematologic malignancies are at a greater risk for the development of CIN than patients with solid tumors. This is most likely because of bone marrow involvement of the tumor as well as the intensity of treatment required for hematologic diseases. Because of this involvement of bone marrow, neutropenia may be the initial presenting symptom in patients with hematologic malignancies. In all cancer types, both advanced disease and uncontrolled cancer are significant predictors of hospitalization for neutropenia and serious complications, including death. NCCN also identified patients with lung cancer and elevated lactate dehydrogenase, such as in lymphoma and leukemia, at a higher risk for neutropenia.

Treatment-Related Risk Factors

Some chemotherapy regimens are more myelosuppressive than others, which puts the patient at a higher risk for neutropenia. High-dose cyclophosphamide, the use of etoposide, and high doses of anthracyclines have all been identified as significant predictors of severe neutropenia. Other treatment-related predictors include relative dose intensity greater than

TABLE 17-2	Eastern Cooperative Oncology Group (ECOG) Performance Status
Grade	**ECOG Performance Status**
0	Fully active, able to carry on all predisease performance without restriction.
1	Restricted in physically strenuous activity but ambulatory and able to carry out work of a light or sedentary nature (e.g., light house work, office work).
2	Ambulatory and capable of all self-care but unable to carry out any work activities. Up and about more than 50% of waking hours.
3	Capable of only limited self-care, confined to bed or chair more than 50% of waking hours.
4	Completely disabled. Cannot carry on any self-care. Totally confined to bed or chair.
5	Dead

Note. From "Toxicity and Response Criteria of the Eastern Cooperative Oncology Group," by M.M. Oken, R.H. Creech, D.C. Tormey, J. Horton, T.E. Davis, E.T. McFadden, et al., 1982, *American Journal of Clinical Oncology, 5*(6), p. 654. Table courtesy of the Eastern Cooperative Oncology Group, Robert Comis, MD, Group Chair.

80%, extensive prior chemotherapy, concurrent or prior radiation therapy, and previous history of severe neutropenia with similar chemotherapy.

Pathophysiology

A number of WBC subtypes are referred to as granulocytes. The foremost are neutrophils, also called polymorphonuclear segmented cells or segs or polys. The neutrophils account for 60% of circulating WBCs and are the first responders to infection by bacteria, viruses, and other pathogens.

Production of mature neutrophils in the bone marrow takes 10–14 days, but once released into the circulation, they live for only four to eight hours. Because the life span of circulating neutrophils is so short, the bone marrow must continually produce neutrophils. This continuous replenishing supply of neutrophils moves from the marrow space through the blood to sites of infection. Neutrophils are drawn to pathogens by either random movement through the circulation or via chemotaxis. When chemotherapy is administered, the bone marrow is suppressed and stem cells may be damaged. The neutrophil count is lowered as the mature cells die and are not replaced, which in turn impairs the body's ability to fight infection.

The risk of death related to infection is paramount when the body's ability to fight infection is impaired. Approximately 70%–75% of the deaths from acute leukemia and 50% of the deaths in patients with solid tumors are related to infection secondary to neutropenia (Larson & Nirenberg, 2004). At least half of the neutropenic patients who become febrile have an established or occult infection, and at least one-fifth of the patients with neutrophil counts less than 100 cells/mm^3 have bacteremia (Hughes et al., 2002).

Assessment

Nurses are ideally positioned and qualified to conduct appropriate risk assessments and play an integral role in directing the quality of patient care by implementing guidelines for the consistent management of neutropenic complications. A thorough patient history is important in assessing for the presence or risk of neutropenia. This history should include a review of previous cancer therapy. Previous chemotherapy, biotherapy, radiation therapy, or multimodal therapies can put a patient at increased risk for neutropenia. A patient's medication regimen, including hematopoietic growth factors, also should be reviewed. Common medications that may cause neutropenia include procainamide, phenytoin, amoxicillin, cimetidine, captopril, enalapril, ibuprofen, levamisole, and ranitidine (Godwin & Shin, 2007). Continued use of these medications will need to be addressed, especially in light of any additional comorbid conditions. The use of agents such as trimethoprim-sulfamethoxazole or amphotericin B can decrease the neutrophil count (Barber, 2001). Therefore, antibiotic use also should be reviewed.

Physical examination of patients should focus on assessing for signs of infection. With infection, neutrophils are sent to the site of infection to produce the common signs of redness, swelling, and pus formation. However, in patients with decreased neutrophils, the number of mature neutrophils may not be sufficient to mount this response. Therefore, the usual objective signs of infection may not be present with a decreased neutrophil count. In neutropenic patients, fever is the most common and perhaps the only response to infection. Fever can be defined by three oral temperatures above 38.5°C (101.3°F) (Wujcik, 2004). Fever can be a significant finding in patients with an ANC less than 500 cells/mm^3 because of the high risk of sepsis in these individuals.

The most common sites of infection in patients with neutropenia are the respiratory tract, gastrointestinal (GI) tract, genitourinary (GU) tract including the perineum and anus, skin, and mucous membranes (see Table 17-3). The respiratory tract should be assessed for abnormal breath sounds, cough, and characteristics of expectorations. Abdominal tenderness, stiffness, guarding, and diarrhea should be evaluated as potential infections of the GI tract. Subtle signs of infection, including any breaks in integrity in the perineum and anus, should be noted. All catheter exit sites should be assessed for edema, drainage, erythema, and tenderness. Tenderness and erythema along the subcutaneous tunnel of an indwelling catheter may indicate a tunnel infection. Tenderness and ulceration of the mucous membranes should be noted, and the oral cavity should be inspected for thrush and plaques. Oral cultures for fungus and virus should be obtained because mucositis can easily progress to secondary infections (Wujcik, 2004). (For more information on mucositis, see Chapter 16.) Assessment for changes in mental status and nutritional status should be included. Protein-calorie malnutrition can cause decreased lymphocytes, diminished levels of the com-

TABLE 17-3 Common Sites of Infection

System	Assess For
Respiratory tract	Abnormal breath sounds Cough Color, amount, and viscosity of expectorations
Gastrointestinal tract	Abdominal tenderness Stiffness Guarding Diarrhea
Genitourinary tract	Breaks in integrity of perineum and/or anus Subtle signs of infection
Skin (including catheter sites)	Edema Drainage Erythema Tenderness
Mucous membranes	Redness Tenderness Ulceration

Note. From "Bone Marrow Suppression" (p. 490), by B.H. Gobel and C. O'Leary in M.E. Langhorne, J.S. Fulton, and S.E. Otto (Eds.), *Oncology Nursing* (5th ed.), 2007, St. Louis, MO: Elsevier Mosby. Copyright 2007 by Elsevier. Adapted with permission.

plement system, and a decrease of immunoglobulins (Ig) IgA, IgE, IgG, and IgM (Camp-Sorrell, 2005; Rust, Simpson, & Lister, 2000).

Important diagnostic tools for assessing neutropenia include obtaining a complete blood count with differential and the respective ANC. To diagnose bloodstream infections, though, blood cultures should be taken before administration of antibiotics. Blood cultures should be obtained at the first fever and may continue daily as long as the patient remains febrile, until the source of infection is identified and antibiotic sensitivity is determined, or the neutrophil count returns to normal. The current standard for obtaining blood cultures requires a minimum of 20 ml/culture set and two sets per episode of fever. The IDSA recommends using two sites for blood cultures (Hughes et al., 2002); however, NCCN advises that obtaining an adequate volume of blood is more important and therefore recommends the use of a central venous catheter (CVC) when available (NCCN, 2008). It is common practice to use the CVC until a positive culture is received. Then cultures can be drawn from both the peripheral blood and the CVC to differentiate bacteremia from an infected catheter (Wujcik, 2004). Clearly, additional research is needed to develop a practice consensus on this issue.

Another diagnostic tool used in the assessment of neutropenia is the chest radiograph (CXR), which may reveal widespread infiltrates or darkened areas on the lung. Serial CXRs have been useful in showing subtle changes in patients with prolonged neutropenia. However, no studies have been completed on the risks or effects of the use of serial CXRs or on how long they should be done. Additionally, computed tomography has determined pneumonia in up to 60% of cases of neutropenic patients with fevers of unknown origin lasting 48 hours despite normal CXR (Wujcik, 2004). To determine lower respiratory infections, invasive bronchoscopic procedures often are used.

In patients with diarrhea, testing for *Clostridium difficile* is indicated. *Clostridium difficile* is a bacterium that causes toxin release and is treated with an antifungal medication. Also, patients with prolonged neutropenia are at risk for typhlitis, an inflammation of the small intestine or colon that can progress to bowel perforation.

Interventions

A focus of nursing care for neutropenic patients is the prevention of complications and the maintenance of optimal functioning. The Oncology Nursing Society (ONS) has described nursing-sensitive patient outcomes (NSPOs) as those outcomes affecting patients and their health problems that are directly affected by nursing interventions (Given et al., 2004). NSPOs must be within the scope of nursing practice and evidence-based. The results of nursing interventions within NSPOs include changes in patients' functional status, symptom experience, safety, psychological distress, and/or costs (Given et al.). ONS, NCCN, NCI, IDSA, and the American Society of Clinical Oncology (ASCO) have current guidelines regarding NSPOs and other recommended interventions to protect neutropenic patients from negative outcomes. These guidelines address interventions related to infection control, CSFs, vaccinations, antimicrobial therapies, oxygen and respiratory care, and oral care.

Infection Control

One of the simplest and most effective interventions for reducing the risk of infection is hand hygiene and is rated as recommended for practice by the ONS Putting Evidence Into Practice (PEP) resource on prevention of infection. Hand hygiene has been shown to decrease the risk of transmitting infection from person to person (Boyce & Pittet, 2002; Hilburn, Hammond, Fendler, & Groziak, 2003; Mank & van der Leslie, 2003; Sehulster & Chinn, 2003; Shelton, 2003; Tablan, Anderson, Besser, Bridges, & Hajjeh, 2004; Wilson, 2002). As early as 1861, physician Ignaz Semmelweis discussed the importance of hand hygiene for healthcare workers. He was the first person to demonstrate the role of hand hygiene in the prevention of person-to-person transmission of infection (Larson, 1999). Studies continued throughout the 1960s when a group of investigators studied the transmission of *Staphylococcus (S.) aureus* to infants in an intensive care unit. *S. aureus* resides in the normal flora of the anterior nares and is rarely airborne. It usually is transmitted by direct contact. In these early studies, Mortimer, Lipsitz, Wolinsky, Gonzaga, and Rammelkamp (1962) found that *S. aureus* was transmitted by the airborne route only 6%–10% of the time. However, 54% of the babies handled by nurses with unwashed hands were colonized with *S. aureus*. When noncarrier nurses handled a baby colonized with *S. aureus* and then handled another baby without hand washing, the transmission rate from the nurses' hands was 43%. Hand washing subsequently reduced the transmission rate to 14%. This study provided clear evidence that when compared to no hand washing, cleansing of hands between patient contacts reduces the transmission of healthcare-associated pathogens. Larson and Nirenberg (2004) also looked at the effectiveness of various types of antiseptic hand hygiene. They defined effective hand hygiene as including washing hands with soap and water or the use of antiseptic hand rub if hands are not visibly contaminated.

Historically, neutropenic patients were isolated in private reverse-flow rooms when hospitalized. The practice of placing a neutropenic patient in strict isolation is beginning to decrease. Strict protective isolation has not been shown to decrease infections, febrile episodes, or antibiotic use for neutropenic patients (Mank & van der Leslie, 2003; Nauseef & Maki, 1981). However, these studies were small and should be interpreted with caution. Because of this lack of high-level evidence, the ONS PEP resource on prevention of infection designates protective isolation as being in the category *Effectiveness Not Established* (Zitella et al., 2006).

Many practitioners and institutions still have strict dietary restrictions for patients with neutropenia (Nirenberg et al., 2006). However, no recent studies have shown that the use of dietary restrictions reduces the risk of infection in general in neutropenic patients (Larson & Nirenberg, 2004; Moody, Charlson, & Finlay, 2002; Nauseef & Maki, 1981; Wilson, 2002). The ONS PEP resource lists dietary restrictions in the *Effectiveness Not Established* category (Zitella et al., 2006). Common-sense efforts when preparing and consuming food still need to be taken. The Centers for Disease Control and Prevention, IDSA, and the American Society for Blood and Marrow Transplantation (2000) guidelines recommend that all foods be well cooked and all raw foods, including seafood, mayonnaise, and raw eggs, be avoided during the neutropenic period in patients following hematopoietic stem cell transplantation (HSCT). General dietary restrictions for patients with neutropenia have not shown to be any more effective than the U.S. Food and Drug Administration's (FDA's) safe food-handling practices (DeMille, Deming, Lupinacci, & Jacobs, 2006; FDA, 2008; Nirenberg et al., 2006).

Colony-Stimulating Factors

The prophylactic use of CSFs can reduce the risk, severity, and duration of both severe neutropenia and FN in adult and pediatric patients. Rather than stimulating the immune system to produce increased neutrophils, CSFs accelerate the maturation of immature neutrophils that are already present. The use of CSFs does not reduce infection-related mortality or overall survival (Bohlius, Herbst, Reiser, Schwarzer, & Engert, 2004; Lyman, Kuderer, & Djulbegovic, 2002; Sung, Nathan, Lange, Beyene, & Buchanan, 2004). The

TABLE 17-4	Guidelines for Prophylactic Use of Colony-Stimulating Factors for Febrile Neutropenia		
	Chemotherapy Treatment Intent		
Risk for Febrile Neutropenia*	**Curative/Adjuvant**	**Prolong Survival/ Quality of Life**	**Symptom Management/ Quality of Life**
High (> 20%)	CSF (category 1 for G-CSF)	CSF (category 1 for G-CSF)	CSF
Intermediate (10%–20%)	Consider CSF	Consider CSF	Consider CSF
Low (< 10%)	No CSF	No CSF	No CSF

* Following chemotherapy in adult patients with solid tumors and nonmyeloid malignancies.
CSF—colony-stimulating factors; G-CSF—granulocyte–colony-stimulating factor

Note. Reproduced with permission from *The NCCN (1.2009) Myeloid Growth Factors Clinical Practice Guidelines in Oncology.* © National Comprehensive Cancer Network, 2008. Available at http://www.nccn.org. Accessed December 14, 2008. To view the most recent and complete version of the guideline, go online to www.nccn.org.

These Guidelines are a work in progress that will be refined as often as new significant data becomes available. The NCCN Guidelines are a statement of consensus of its authors regarding their views of currently accepted approaches to treatment. Any clinician seeking to apply or consult any NCCN guideline is expected to use independent medical judgment in the context of individual circumstances to determine any patient's care or treatment. The National Comprehensive Cancer Network makes no warranties of any kind whatsoever regarding their content, use, or application and disclaims any responsibility for their application or use in any way.

These Guidelines are copyrighted by the National Comprehensive Cancer Network. All rights reserved. These Guidelines and illustrations herein may not be reproduced in any form for any purpose without the express written permission of the NCCN.

NCCN guidelines address the use of CSFs based on the risk for FN (see Table 17-4). Both ASCO and NCCN guidelines recommend the use of CSFs for all patients undergoing chemotherapy who have a greater than 20% risk for FN (NCCN; Smith et al., 2006). In addition, the ONS PEP resource designates the use of CSFs for patients with cancer who are undergoing chemotherapy with greater than 20% risk of FN as recommended for practice (Zitella et al., 2006).

Vaccination

Annual influenza vaccination of all people who are at high risk for complications from influenza, including patients with cancer, is recommended beginning in September and throughout the influenza season (Tablan et al., 2004). People who are at risk for transmitting influenza to high-risk individuals, including healthcare workers and family members of high-risk individuals, also should be vaccinated. Patients who are not receiving chemotherapy have a superior response to vaccination compared to those patients who are receiving chemotherapy (Ring, Marx, Steer, & Harper, 2002). Therefore, patients with cancer should be vaccinated before beginning chemotherapy treatments. The ONS PEP resource lists annual influenza vaccine in the *Recommended for Practice* category (Zitella et al., 2006).

Vaccination for pneumococcal disease is recommended for most patients with cancer (Tablan et al., 2004). Patients with cancer who should be vaccinated include all patients 65 years old and older, patients living in long-term care facilities, and patients ages 5–64 who are receiving immunosuppressive therapy or who have generalized malignancies, multiple myeloma, leukemia, lymphoma, or chronic conditions. The patient should receive the vaccination once every five years. Another formulation of a pneumococcal vaccination exists for children younger than the age of two. It is recommended that this vaccination is administered to all children younger than two and children ages 24–59 months who are at an increased risk for pneumococcal disease, including those with cancer (Tablan et al.). The ONS PEP resource on prevention of infection designates pneumococcal vaccination as recommended for practice (Zitella et al., 2006).

Antimicrobial Therapy

Table 17-5 depicts the IDSA guidelines for the use of antimicrobial agents in neutropenic patients with cancer. Because a variety of microorganisms are responsible for infection in patients with neutropenia, a discussion of antimicrobial therapies is imperative. The prophylactic use of trimethoprim-sulfamethoxazole to prevent *Pneumocystis carinii* pneumonia is recommended for patients with acute lymphocytic leukemia, patients receiving fludarabine therapy, patients receiving prolonged corticosteroid treatments, and allogeneic or autologous HSCT recipients (Hughes et al., 2002; NCCN, 2008; Smith et al., 2006). Because of the lack of efficacy in preventing gram-negative infections, an increased risk of adverse side effects including skin rashes (Stevens-Johnson syndrome), hematuria, agranulocytosis, and liver or lung damage, and the potential for antibacterial resistance, trimethoprim-sulfamethoxazole is not recommended for prophylaxis in afebrile neutropenic patients (Cruciani et al., 2003; Engels, Lau, & Barza, 1998; Gafter-Gvili, Fraser, Paul, & Leibovici, 2005; Hughes et al., 2002).

Because of a lack of evidence for effectiveness, antifungal prophylaxis is not recommended for all patients with cancer. However, it is recommended for patients who are at high risk, including those with acute leukemia or those undergoing HSCT (Bow et al., 2002; Cornely, Ullmann, & Karthaus, 2003; Glasmacher et al., 2003; Gotzsche & Johansen, 2002; Hughes et al., 2002; Johansen & Gotzsche, 2000; Kanda et al., 2000; NCCN, 2008).

The use of antifungal therapy for the prevention of oral candidiasis is common (Pappas et al., 2004). It is important to note that antifungal drugs that are absorbed or partially absorbed from the GI tract, such as fluconazole, ketoconazole, itraconazole, miconazole, and clotrimazole, have been shown to be effective in preventing oral candidiasis. However, antifungal drugs that are not absorbed from the GI tract, such as amphotericin B, nystatin, thymostimulin, polyenes, natamycin, and norfloxacin, did not prevent oral candidiasis (Clarkson, Worthington, & Eden, 2007; Worthington & Clarkson, 2002).

The use of antibacterial prophylaxis with quinolones such as ciprofloxacin (Cipro®, Bayer Pharmaceuticals) or levofloxacin (Levaquin®, Ortho-McNeil-Janssen Pharmaceuticals, Inc.) for high-risk patients undergoing chemotherapy is recommended (Bucaneve et al., 2005; Cruciani et al., 1996; Cullen et al., 2005; Engels et al., 1998; Gafter-Gvili et al., 2005; NCCN, 2006; Shelton, 2003).

Patients who have had a prior active herpes infection that required treatment are more susceptible to a recurrence of the active infection while their immune system is compromised. The preferred treatment for an active herpes infection includes the use of acyclovir or valacyclovir. Because of this, the use of acyclovir or valacyclovir for herpes prophylaxis is recommended during CIN in patients who have had prior active herpes infections that required treatment (NCCN, 2008). NCCN also recommends herpes prophylaxis for patients receiving T-cell–depleting agents such as fludarabine during HSCT until 30 days after transplantation and during induction or reinduction therapy for acute leukemia through the neutropenic period.

TABLE 17-5	2002 Infectious Diseases Society of America Guidelines for Use of Antimicrobial Agents in Neutropenic Patients With Cancer	

Treatment Characteristic	Patient Characteristics	Intervention
Initial antibiotic therapy	Low-risk adults	Oral ciprofloxacin plus amoxicillin-clavulanate
	Moderate-risk adults	Cefepime, ceftazidime, imipenem, or meropenem
	High-risk adults	Aminoglycosides plus penicillin, cephalosporin (cefepime or ceftazidime), or carbapenem if vancomycin criteria *not* met If vancomycin criteria are met: Vancomycin *plus* one or two antibiotics. Choose cefepime, ceftazidime, or carbapenem with or without aminoglycoside; or penicillin plus aminoglycoside and vancomycin.
First week of therapy	Afebrile for 3–5 days	Etiologic agent identified: Adjust therapy to appropriate drug. No etiologic agent identified: Continue use of same drug. Low-risk patient on oral therapy: Continue use of same drug. Low-risk patient on IV therapy: Change to oral ciprofloxacin after 48 hours plus amoxicillin-clavulanate for adults or cefixime for children. High-risk patient: Continue use of same drug.
	Persistent fever throughout first 3–5 days	No clinical worsening: Continue same antibiotic. Stop vancomycin if cultures do not yield organism. Disease progression: Change antibiotic.
	Febrile after 5 days	Consider adding antifungal with or without change in antibiotic.
Duration of antibiotic therapy	Afebrile by day 3	Absolute neutrophil count (ANC) is > 500 cells/mm^3 for two consecutive days, no definite site of infection, and cultures do not yield positive results: Stop antibiotic therapy when patient is afebrile for > 48 hours. ANC < 500 cells/mm^3 by day 7, the patient was low risk, and no subsequent complications occur: Stop therapy when the patient is afebrile for 5–7 days.
	Persistent fever on day 3	ANC is > 500 cells/mm^3: Stop antibiotic therapy 4–5 days after the ANC is > 500 cells/mm^3. ANC < 500 cells/mm^3: Reassess and continue antibiotic therapy for 2 weeks; reassess and consider stopping therapy if no disease site is found.
Use of antiviral drugs		Antiviral drugs are not recommended for routine use unless clinical or laboratory evidence of viral infection is evident.
Granulocyte transfusion		Granulocyte transfusions are not recommended for routine use.

Note. Based on information from Hughes et al., 2002.

The ONS PEP resource on prevention of infection addresses the use of antimicrobial therapy also. It lists under *Recommended for Practice* the use of antifungal drug prophylaxis for severely neutropenic, afebrile patients, prophylaxis with quinolones for high-risk, afebrile, neutropenic patients with cancer undergoing chemotherapy, and herpes viral prophylaxis for selected seropositive patients with cancer (Zitella et al., 2006).

Oxygen and Respiratory Care

People with symptoms of respiratory infections should be restricted from visiting immunosuppressed patients (Tablan et al., 2004). Patients with documented or suspected airborne respiratory infections should be placed in a negative airflow room with an anteroom to maintain proper air balance. If an anteroom is not available, then a high-efficiency particulate air (HEPA) filter should be utilized. The ONS PEP resource on prevention of infection lists both restriction of visitors with symptoms of respiratory infections and environmental interventions, including negative airflow rooms and HEPA filter utilization, under *Recommended for Practice* (Zitella et al., 2006). Those patients who utilize oxygen or other respiratory medications need to be diligent in the care of their equipment in order to prevent infection. Oxygen humidifier tubing, nasal prongs, and masks should be changed when they malfunction or become visibly contaminated, and medication nebulizers should be cleaned and disinfected between uses on the same patient.

Oral Care

Oral care is an important aspect of caring for patients with neutropenia. Refer to Chapter 16 on oral mucositis for information on this topic.

Patient Teaching Points

Many NSPOs have been studied and identified. One of the most important aspects of NSPOs is teaching patients what they can do to effect positive outcomes as well. A vital role of oncology nurses is teaching patients and their caregivers about the side effects of the cancer treatment. This education should include the potential for and consequences of neutropenia, interventions to decrease the risk of infection, signs and symptoms of infection, and what to do if the patient experiences any of the signs and symptoms of infection. Patients should be taught to report signs of infection including fever, chills and sweating, sore throat, shortness of breath, difficulty urinating, diarrhea, mouth sores, rectal discomfort, abdominal pain, sinus tenderness, and redness or swelling at the site of any catheter or injury. Instructions on what constitutes a fever, a temperature greater than 38°C (100.4°F), and how often to monitor temperature should also be included in teaching (Nirenberg et al., 2006). Neutropenia is the single most significant risk factor in the development of sepsis and septic shock in patients with cancer (Camp-Sorrell, 2005). Failure to recognize the possible signs of infection and obtain prompt effective treatment puts the patient at risk for severe infection, which if left untreated may lead to bacteremia, sepsis, end-organ damage, and death.

Sepsis is a constellation of symptoms that represent a systemic response to infection. It presents with symptoms such as hypotension, fever, oliguria, increased lactate production, hypoxemia, and altered mental status. All of these represent signs of organ hypoperfusion, which if left untreated leads to end-organ damage and death. In the United States, more than 751,000 patients (3 per 1,000 people) per year develop sepsis with a mortality rate of 30%–35% (Martens et al., 2007). Families' relationships with nurses can become more significant during periods of neutropenia (Eggenberger, Krumwiede, Meiers, Mliesmer, & Earle, 2004). Nurses can support family caring throughout the neutropenic experience. Providing patients and caregivers with interventions to reduce the risk of infection is critical to achieving positive patient outcomes.

Need for Future Research

Research in cancer and cancer therapies is ever-changing and evolving. Research efforts will continue to include the area of neutropenia and infection. Although established guidelines exist for the use of CSFs, the use of CSFs as a preventive measure should continue to be studied. Risk factors for neutropenia are well documented. Risk assessment tools have been developed. However, it appears that no standard risk assessment tool exists that is commonly used by nurses. Developing such a tool that addresses issues within the realm of nursing will help nurses to identify interventions to employ to protect patients from developing potentially life-threatening infections.

Conclusion of Case Study

The doctor orders vital signs every four hours and a diet without any fresh fruits or vegetables, and starts R.M. on nystatin three times a day. Because the patient is currently afebrile, no antibiotics are initiated. The nurse discusses the use of nystatin with the doctor, and they decide to change the medication to fluconazole. In addition, the nurse reviews the literature to find that no indications exist for preventing R.M. from eating fruits and vegetables as long as they are cleaned well. The nurse is diligent in her physical assessment of R.M., paying special attention to breath sounds, abdominal discomfort, skin, and mucous membranes. After three days, R.M.'s ANC is 1,200 cells/mm³. She remains afebrile during her hospitalization and is being discharged home. The nurse prepares discharge instructions. She reviews with R.M. and her family the importance of hand washing. She instructs R.M. on the importance of good oral care and proper nutrition. She cautions against eating any raw or undercooked foods and emphasizes that fruits and vegetables should be cleaned thoroughly. She reviews potential signs of infection, including fever, that R.M. should report to the physician. Although R.M. experienced CIN with this chemotherapy cycle, she was discharged home without complications.

Conclusion

Neutropenia has the potential for significant negative clinical outcomes for patients with cancer, including infection, increased hospitalizations, and decreased quality of life. Preventing infection in patients with cancer is crucial. Nurses are critical in implementing infection prevention strategies themselves, as well as teaching these strategies to patients and families. Understanding the risk factors for developing neutropenia along with the recommended treatments allows healthcare providers to offer the most effective care to patients, thus preventing possible negative outcomes for the patients.

References

Barber, F.D. (2001). Management of fever in neutropenic patients with cancer. *Nursing Clinics of North America, 36*(4), 631–644.

Bohlius, J., Herbst, C., Reiser, M., Schwarzer, G., & Engert, A. (2008). Granulopoiesis-stimulating factors to prevent adverse effects in the treatment of malignant lymphoma. *Cochrane Database of Systematic Reviews* 2008, Issue 4. Art. No.: CD003189. DOI: 10.1002/14651858.CD003189.pub4.

Bow, E.J., Laverdiere, M., Lussier, N., Rotstein, C., Cheang, M.S., & Ioannou, S. (2002). Antifungal prophylaxis for severely neutropenic chemotherapy recipients: A meta analysis of randomized-controlled clinical trials. *Cancer, 94*(12), 3230–3246.

Boyce, J.M., & Pittet, D. (2002). Guidelines for hand hygiene in health-care settings: Recommendations of the Healthcare Infection Control Practices Advisory Committee and the HICPAC/SHEA/APIC/IDSA Hand Hygiene Task Force. *Infection Control and Hospital Epidemiology, 23*(Suppl. 12), S3–S40.

Bucaneve, G., Micozzi, A., Menichetti, F., Martino, P., Dionisi, M.S., Martinelli, G., et al. (2005). Levofloxacin to prevent bacterial infection in patients with cancer and neutropenia. *New England Journal of Medicine, 353*(10), 977–987.

Camp-Sorrell, D. (2005). Myelosuppression. In J.K. Itano & K.N. Taoka (Eds.), *Core curriculum for oncology nursing* (4th ed., pp. 259–274). St. Louis, MO: Elsevier Saunders.

Centers for Disease Control and Prevention, Infectious Diseases Society of America, & American Society for Blood and Marrow Transplantation. (2000). Guidelines for preventing opportunistic infections among hematopoietic stem cell transplant recipients. *Recommendations and Reports: Morbidity and Mortality Weekly Report, 49*(RR-10), 1–128.

Clarkson, J.E., Worthington, H.V., & Eden, T.O.B. (2007). Interventions for preventing oral candidiasis for patients with cancer receiving treatment. *Cochrane Database of Systematic Reviews* 2007, Issue 1. Art. No.: CD003807. DOI: 10.1002/14651858.CD003807.pub3.

Cornely, O.A., Ullmann, A.J., & Karthaus, M. (2003). Evidence-based assessment of primary antifungal prophylaxis in patients with hematologic malignancies. *Blood, 101*(9), 3365–3372.

Cruciani, M., Malena, M., Bosco, O., Nardi, S., Serpelloni, G., & Mengoli, C. (2003). Reappraisal with meta-analysis of the addition of gram-positive prophylaxis to fluoroquinolone in neutropenic patients. *Journal of Clinical Oncology, 21*(22), 4127–4137.

Cruciani, M., Rampazzo, R., Malena, M., Lazzarini, L., Todeschini, G., Messori, A., et al. (1996). Prophylaxis with fluoroquinolones for bacterial infections in neutropenic patients: A meta-analysis. *Clinical Infectious Diseases, 23*(4), 795–805.

Cullen, M., Steven, N., Billingham, L., Gaunt, C., Hastings, M., Simmonds, P., et al. (2005). Antibacterial prophylaxis after chemotherapy for solid tumors and lymphomas. *New England Journal of Medicine, 353*(10), 988–998.

DeMille, D., Deming, P., Lupinacci, P., & Jacobs, L.A. (2006). The effect of the neutropenic diet in the outpatient setting: A pilot study. *Oncology Nursing Forum, 33*(2), 337–343.

Eggenberger, S.K., Krumwiede, N., Meiers, S.J., Mliesmer, M., & Earle, P. (2004). Family caring strategies in neutropenia. *Clinical Journal of Oncology Nursing, 8*(6), 617–621.

Engels, E.A., Lau, J., & Barza, M. (1998). Efficacy of quinolone prophylaxis in neutropenic cancer patients: A meta analysis. *Journal of Clinical Oncology, 16*(3), 1179–1187.

Gafter-Gvili, A., Fraser, A., Paul, M., & Leibovici, L. (2005). Meta-analysis: Antibiotic prophylaxis reduces mortality in neutropenic patients. *Annals of Internal Medicine, 142*(12, Pt. 1), 979–995.

Given, B., Beck, S., Etland, C., Gobel, B.H., Lamken, L., & Marsee, V.D. (2004, July). *Nursing-sensitive patient outcomes.* Retrieved August 18, 2007, from http://www.ons.org/ourcomes/measures/outcomes.shtml

Glasmacher, A., Prentice, A., Gorschluter, M., Engelhart, S., Hahn, C., Djulbegovic, B., et al. (2003). Itraconazole prevents invasive fungal infections in neutropenic patients treated for hematologic malignancies: Evidence from a meta-analysis of 3,597 patients. *Journal of Clinical Oncology, 21*(24), 4615–4626.

Godwin, J.E., & Shin, P.D. (2007, August). *Neutropenia.* Retrieved August 9, 2007, from http://www.emedicine.com/med/topic1640.htm

Gotzsche, P.E., & Johansen, H.K. (2002). Routine versus selective antifungal administration for control of fungal infections in patients with cancer. *Cochrane Database of Systematic Reviews* 2002, Issue 2. Art. No.: CD000026. DOI: 10.1002/14651858.CD000026.

Hilburn, J., Hammond, B.S., Fendler, E.J., & Groziak, P.A. (2003). Use of alcohol hand sanitizer as an infection control strategy in an acute care facility. *American Journal of Infection Control, 31*(2), 109–116.

Hughes, W.T., Armstrong, D., Bodey, G.P., Bow, E.J., Brown, A.E., Calandra, T., et al. (2002). 2002 guidelines for the use of antimicrobial agents in neutropenic patients with cancer. *Clinical Infectious Diseases, 34*(6), 730–751.

Johansen, H.K., & Gotzsche, P.C. (2000). Amphotericin B lipid soluble formulations versus amphotericin B in cancer patients with neutropenia. *Cochrane Database of Systematic Reviews* 2000, Issue 3. Art. No.: CD000969. DOI: 10.1002/14651858.CD000969.

Kanda, Y., Yamamoto, R., Chizuka, A., Hamaki, T., Suguro, M., Arai, C., et al. (2000). Prophylactic action of oral fluconazole against fungal infection in neutropenic patients. A meta-analysis of 16 randomized, controlled trials. *Cancer, 89*(7), 1611–1625.

Larson, E. (1999). Skin hygiene and infection prevention: More of the same or different approaches? *Clinical Infectious Diseases, 29*(5), 1287–1294.

Larson, E., & Nirenberg, A. (2004). Evidence-based nursing practice to prevent infection in hospitalized neutropenic patients with cancer. *Oncology Nursing Forum, 31*(4), 717–723.

Lyman, G.H., Kuderer, N.M., & Djulbegovic, B. (2002). Prophylactic granulocyte colony-stimulating factors in patients receiving dose-intensive cancer chemotherapy: A meta-analysis. *American Journal of Medicine, 112*(5), 406–411.

Lyman, G.H., Lyman, C.H., & Agboola, O. (2005). Risk models for predicting chemotherapy-induced neutropenia. *Oncologist, 10*(6), 427–437.

Lynch, M.P., & Rogers, B.B. (2006). Neutropenia. In D. Camp-Sorrell & R. Hawkins (Eds.), *Clinical manual for the oncology advanced practice nurse* (2nd ed., pp. 845–851). Pittsburgh, PA: Oncology Nursing Society.

Mank, A., & van der Leslie, H. (2003). Is there still an indication for nursing patients with prolonged neutropenia in protective isolation? An evidence-based nursing and medical study of 4 years experience for nursing patients with neutropenia without isolation. *European Journal of Oncology Nursing, 7*(1), 17–23.

Martens, M., Kumar, M.M., Kumar, S., Goldberg, M., Kawata, M., Pennycooke, O., et al. (2007). Quantitative analysis of organ tissue damage after septic shock. *American Surgeon, 73*(3), 243–248.

Moody, K., Charlson, M.E., & Finlay, J. (2002). The neutropenic diet: What's the evidence? *Journal of Pediatric Hematology/Oncology, 24*(9), 717–721.

Mortimer, E.A., Jr., Lipstiz, P.J., Wolinsky, E., Gonzaga, A.J., & Rammelkamp, C.H., Jr. (1962). Transmission of staphylococci between newborns. Importance of the hands to personnel. *American Journal of Diseases of Children, 104,* 289–295.

National Cancer Institute Cancer Therapy Evaluation Program. (2009). *Common terminology for adverse events* (version 4.0). Retrieved July 29, 2009, from http://ctep.cancer.gov/protocoldevelopment/electronic_applications/docs/ctcaev4.pdf

National Comprehensive Cancer Network. (2008). *NCCN Clinical Practice Guidelines in Oncology™: Myeloid growth factors* [v.1.2009]. Retrieved December 14, 2008, from http://www.nccn.org/professionals/physician_gls/PDF/myeloid_growth.pdf

Nauseef, W.M., & Maki, D.G. (1981). A study of the value of simple protective isolation in patients with granulocytopenia. *New England Journal of Medicine, 304*(8), 448–453.

Nirenberg, A., Bush, A.P., Davis, A., Friese, C.R., Gillespie, T.W., & Rice, R.D. (2006). Neutropenia: State of the knowledge part 1 [Oncology Nursing Society white paper]. *Oncology Nursing Forum, 33*(6), 1193–1201.

Oken, M.M., Creech, R.H., Tormey, D.C., Horton, J., Davis, T.E., McFadden, E.T., et al. (1982). Toxicity and response criteria of the Eastern Cooperative Oncology Group. *American Journal of Clinical Oncology, 5*(6), 649–655.

Pappas, P.G., Rex, J.H., Sobel, J.D., Fuller, S.G., Dismikes, W.E., Walsh, T.J., et al. (2004). Guidelines for the treatment of candidiasis. *Clinical Infectious Diseases, 38*(2), 161–189.

Polovich, M., White, J.M., & Kelleher, L.O. (Eds.). (2005). *Chemotherapy and biotherapy guidelines and recommendations for practice* (2nd ed.). Pittsburgh, PA: Oncology Nursing Society.

Ring, A., Marx, G., Steer, C., & Harper, P. (2002). Influenza vaccination and chemotherapy: A shot in the dark? *Supportive Care in Cancer, 10*(6), 462–465.

Rust, D.M., Simpson, J.K., & Lister, J. (2000). Nutritional issues in patients with severe neutropenia. *Seminars in Oncology Nursing, 16*(2), 152–162.

Scott, T.E. (2004). Neutropenia. In N.E. Kline (Ed.), *Essentials of pediatric oncology nursing: A core curriculum* (2nd ed., pp. 67–69). Glenview, IL: Association of Pediatric Oncology Nurses.

Sehulster, L., & Chinn, R.Y. (2003). Guidelines for environmental infection control in health-care facilities: Recommendations of CDC and the Healthcare Infection Control Practices Advisory Committee (HICPAC). *Recommendations and Reports: Morbidity and Mortality Weekly Report, 52*(RR-10), 1–42.

Shelton, B.K. (2003). Evidence-based care for the neutropenic patient with leukemia. *Seminars in Oncology Nursing, 19*(2), 133–141.

Smith, T.J., Khatcheressian, J., Lyman, G.H., Ozer, H., Armitage, J.O., Balducci, L., et al. (2006). 2006 update of recommendations for the use of white blood cell growth factors: An evidence-based clinical practice guideline. *Journal of Clinical Oncology, 24*(19), 3187–3205.

Sung, L., Nathan, P.C., Lange, B., Beyene, J., & Buchanan, G.R. (2004). Prophylactic granulocyte colony-stimulating factor and granulocyte-macrophage colony-stimulating factor decrease febrile neutropenia after chemotherapy in children with cancer: A meta-analysis of randomized controlled trials. *Journal of Clinical Oncology, 22*(16), 3350–3356.

Tablan, O.C., Anderson, L.J., Besser, R., Bridges, C., & Hajjeh, R. (2004). Guidelines for preventing health-care associated pneumonia, 2003: Recommendations of CDC and the Healthcare Infection Control Practices Advisory Committee. *Recommendations and Reports: Morbidity and Mortality Weekly Report, 53*(RR-3), 1–36.

U.S. Food and Drug Administration. (2008). *Be food safe: Harmful bacteria can make people sick.* Retrieved December 14, 2008, from http://www.foodsafety.gov/~fsg/f08steps.html

Wilson, B.J. (2002). Dietary recommendations for neutropenic patients. *Seminars in Oncology Nursing, 18*(1), 44–49.

Worthington, H.V., & Clarkson, J.E. (2002). Prevention of oral mucositis and oral candidiasis for patients with cancer treated with chemotherapy: Cochrane systematic review. *Journal of Dental Education, 66*(8), 903–911.

Wujcik, D. (2004). Infection. In C.H. Yarbro, M.H. Frogge, & M. Goodman (Eds.), *Cancer symptom management* (3rd ed., pp. 252–275). Sudbury, MA: Jones and Bartlett.

Zitella, L., Friese, C., Gobel, B.H., Woolery-Antill, M., O'Leary, C., Hauser, J., et al. (2006). *Putting evidence into practice: Prevention of infection.* Pittsburgh, PA: Oncology Nursing Society.

CHAPTER 18

Osteoporosis and Bone Health

Carrie Tompkins Stricker, PhD, CRNP, AOCN®

Case Study

G.P. is a 62-year-old postmenopausal woman with stage II invasive breast cancer who recently completed four cycles of docetaxel and cyclophosphamide chemotherapy. Her tumor was both estrogen and progesterone receptor positive, and she was prescribed five years of adjuvant hormonal therapy with anastrozole. Anastrozole is an aromatase inhibitor (AI), and treatment with AIs results in loss of bone mineral density (BMD) in breast cancer survivors. G.P.'s case will be revisited throughout this chapter to illustrate principles of prevention, diagnosis, and management of osteoporosis in individuals with cancer.

Overview

Maintenance of bone health is a growing concern for men and women with cancer, as the number of individuals who are at increased risk for developing osteopenia, osteoporosis, and related fractures continues to grow. The risk for bone complications in cancer survivors is increasing because of the evolution of antineoplastic therapy and its associated effects, combined with demographic trends such as the aging of the U.S. population. Direct effects of cancer (i.e., bony infiltration) and treatment exposures converge with preexisting risk factors such as age, comorbidities, heredity, and lifestyle factors to elevate the risk for bone morbidity in individuals with cancer. For example, postmenopausal women with breast cancer are vulnerable to long-term effects on bone health as a result of therapies such as AIs, as well as declining BMD related to age, other comorbidities, and declining physical activity. Hormonal changes resulting from cancer diagnosis and treatment play a major role. Premature menopause is one of the strongest predictors of osteoporosis in women, and hypogonadism is a major risk factor in men (Gilbert & McKiernan, 2005; Richelson, Wahner, Melton, & Riggs, 1984; World Health Organization [WHO], 2003). Cancer treatments can lead to hypogonadism in both men and women, sometimes in addition to direct effects of certain antineoplastic therapies on bone demineralization. Given the tremendous impact on quality of life and the functional and economic cost of osteoporosis and related fractures, it is imperative that oncology nurses proactively screen for, assess, prevent, and manage osteoporosis and related complications in patients and cancer survivors.

Epidemiology: Prevalence and Impact

General Population

Osteoporosis is defined as a systemic skeletal disease characterized by low bone mass, deterioration of bone microarchitecture, and increased bone fragility and susceptibility to fracture (van der Sluis & van den Heuvel-Eibrink, 2008). Osteoporosis is characterized by decreased bone strength, with vertebral, hip, and other bone fractures as chief clinical manifestations (Bringhurst, Demay, Krane, & Kronenberg, 2005). Although more than 10 million individuals in the United States (approximately 8 million women and 2 million men) are estimated to have osteoporosis, a much smaller proportion are actually diagnosed and receive subsequent treatment (Bringhurst et al.). In the general population of women in the United States, osteoporosis is a prevalent condition with significant health and economic consequences. The onset of menopause precipitates rapid bone loss in women, and most women will meet the diagnostic criteria for osteoporosis by ages 70–80 (Bringhurst et al.). Osteoporosis is less prevalent in men for several physiologic reasons, including the lack of a midlife menopause. In addition, men accumulate more bone mass during growth and have larger bone sizes, slower rates of bone loss, and a shorter life expectancy (Amin & Felson, 2001). Nonetheless, men age 50 years and older have an estimated 20% lifetime risk of developing osteoporosis and a 13% risk of fragility fracture, and these risks increase with treatments such as androgen deprivation therapy (ADT) (Brown & Guise, 2007).

The development of fractures is the most significant consequence of osteoporosis. In the United States, a Caucasian woman's lifetime risk of having a fracture in a common osteoporosis-related site is 30%–45% (WHO, 2003), and approximately 300,000 hip fractures occur in the United States each year (Bringhurst et al., 2005). The incidence rate for all fractures in men is about half that of women, and hip fractures in men account for about one-third of all hip fractures per year (Adler, 2006). Mortality rates following hip fracture are higher, approximately double, in men than in women (Smith, 2006). The costs of hip fractures are great, as most require hospitalization, surgical intervention, and extended rehabilitation, notwithstanding the elevated risk of deep vein thrombosis and pulmonary embolism of approximately 20%–50% (Bringhurst et al.). In women ages 75–84, annual mortality rates rise from a baseline of approximately 5% up to 17% following hip fracture, and the increased risk of mortality is even more dramatic in men, rising from 8% to 34% per year (Adler). Even more prevalent are vertebral fractures, with an incidence of approximately 700,000 per year. Although vertebral fractures rarely require hospitalization, they often are associated with long-term morbidity including pain and loss of height, and multiple fractures may result in kyphosis (Bringhurst et al.). Osteoporotic fractures also may lead to decreased quality of life and increased mortality, specifically in cancer survivors (Gilbert & McKiernan, 2005). Avoidance of fracture is a primary goal of osteoporosis prevention and therapy.

Individuals With Cancer

The prevalence of osteoporosis in individuals with cancer is not well described, but many individuals have a higher risk for developing osteoporosis and related bone complications because of cancer and cancer treatment. Few studies have compared rates of osteoporosis and fracture between individuals with and without cancer, but available data support an elevated risk in specific populations, such as men undergoing ADT as hormonal treatment of prostate cancer (Morote et al., 2007; Planas et al., 2007). Even without direct comparisons, however, certain groups of cancer survivors clearly are at increased risk. In addition to men with prostate cancer receiving ADT (Smith, 2006), these include women with breast cancer (Hillner et al., 2003), individuals receiving long-term glucocorticoids as part of cancer therapy (Van Staa, Leufkens, Abenhaim, Zhang, & Cooper, 2000), and certain survivors of childhood and adolescent cancers, particularly those who receive hematopoietic stem cell transplantation (HSCT), extensive methotrexate or glucocorticoid therapy, or who experience premature menopause because of cancer treatment (Sala & Barr, 2007; Taskinen, Saarinen-Pihkala, Hovi, Vettenranta, & Makitie, 2007).

Prevalence estimates are available for some groups of individuals with cancer. Between 23% and 80.6% of men with prostate cancer have osteoporosis, depending on which groups of men are being studied and treatment-related factors such as the receipt and duration of hormonal therapy (Malcolm et al., 2007; Morote et al., 2007; Planas et al., 2007). Prevalence rates of fracture range from 4% to nearly 20% in men receiving ADT, and the risk of fracture increases as does treatment duration (Hatano, Oishi, Furuta, Iwamuro, & Tashiro, 2000; Malcolm et al.; Oefelein et al., 2001; Shahinian, Kuo, Freeman, & Goodwin, 2005; Townsend, Sanders, Northway, & Graham, 1997). In adults who have undergone HSCT, more than half may experience osteopenia or osteoporosis within one to two years following transplantation (Schulte, Beelen, Schaefer, & Mann, 2000; Valimaki et al., 1999). More than a quarter of pediatric acute lymphoblastic leukemia (ALL) survivors may develop fractures (Sala & Barr, 2007).

Risk Factors

Risk Factors in the General Population

Osteoporosis risk factors for the general population are shown in Figure 18-1. The U.S. Preventive Services Task Force (USPSTF) considers a body weight of less than 70 kg to be the single best predictor of low BMD (USPSTF, 2002). In addition, a personal history of fragility fracture in adulthood is one of the most significant risk factors for subsequent osteoporotic fracture (Hamdy et al., 2005). A fragility fracture is defined as a low trauma fracture at typical sites such as the vertebrae, hip, or radius. African Americans and Latinos have higher BMDs than Caucasians (Cummings, Bates, & Black, 2002). Specific osteoporosis risk factors in men include secondary causes of low BMD such as alcohol abuse, hypogonadism, and long-term glucocorticoid use (Brown & Guise, 2007). Finally, the National Osteoporosis Foundation (NOF) recognizes a number of medical conditions and certain medications as risk factors for osteoporosis, with hypogonadism, amenorrhea, cytotoxic drugs,

FIGURE 18-1	Risk Factors for Osteoporosis in the General Population
Endogenous	**Exogenous**
• Age	• Premature menopause
• Female sex	• Primary or secondary amenorrhea
• Slight body build	• Primary and secondary hypogonadism in men
• Asian or Caucasian race	• Previous fragility fracture
	• Glucocorticoid therapy
	• Maternal history of hip fracture
	• Low body weight
	• Cigarette smoking
	• Excessive alcohol consumption
	• Prolonged immobilization
	• Low dietary calcium intake
	• Vitamin D deficiency

Note. From *Prevention and Management of Osteoporosis: Report of a WHO Scientific Group* (p. 69), by World Health Organization, 2003, Geneva, Switzerland: Author. Retrieved from http://whqlibdoc.who.int/trs/WHO_TRS_921.pdf. Copyright 2003 by World Health Organization. Reprinted with permission.

tamoxifen, and gonadotropin-releasing hormone agonists being of particular concern for individuals with cancer (Pfeilschifter & Diel, 2000).

Risk Factors in Individuals With Cancer

A number of risk factors for osteoporosis and fracture have been identified for individuals with cancer (see Figure 18-2). Endogenous factors are those internal characteristics that are typically not modifiable (e.g., age, race), and exogenous risk factors are external, modifiable factors. Premature menopause and hypogonadism resulting from cancer diagnosis and treatment is the primary risk factor for osteopenia and osteoporosis in cancer survivors (Brown et al., 2006; Pfeilschifter & Diel, 2000). Premature menopause resulting from chemotherapy is most commonly observed in premenopausal women with breast cancer, but it is a risk for any premenopausal female treated with gonadotoxic chemotherapy, particularly alkylating agents, or with pelvic radiotherapy (Pfeilschifter & Diel). Men at greatest risk for hypogonadism are those receiving ADT, such as leuprolide, for prostate cancer (Smith, 2006). Survivors of childhood and adolescent cancers are also at risk for bone morbidity related to hypogonadism, particularly those who are treated with gonadotoxic chemotherapy, although growth hormone deficiency and hypogonadotropic hypogonadism resulting from cranial radiotherapy also pose significant risk (Sala & Barr, 2007). Although hypogonadism plays the most predominant role in the pathogenesis of cancer- and treatment-related bone loss, other risk factors include prolonged treatment with glucocorticoids, radiotherapy, and a childhood or adolescent diagnosis of ALL, lymphomas, malignant bone tumors, rhabdomyosarcoma, or a malignant brain tumor confers an increased risk for osteopenia, osteoporosis, and fracture (Pfeilschifter & Diel; Sala & Barr). Although concern exists that chemotherapy may have direct negative effects on bone, pronounced and/or persistent effects appear to be limited to a few agents, such as ifosfamide and methotrexate, particularly when used for treatment of cancer in children and adolescents (Sala & Barr). A recent case-control study in 217 adult survivors of lymphoma and testicular cancer showed no difference in BMD and osteoporosis in male survivors treated with chemotherapy compared to those who received only surgery and/or radiotherapy (Brown et al.). In contrast, certain hormonal therapies, such as tamoxifen in premenopausal women and AIs in postmenopausal women with breast cancer, directly contribute to bone loss in these populations (Stricker, 2007). Long-term detrimental skeletal effects are a significant risk for growing numbers of cancer survivors, and an awareness of subpopulations who are at increased risk is critical to minimizing morbidity and mortality resulting from bone complications.

FIGURE 18-2   Risk Factors for Osteoporosis in Individuals With Cancer

- Premature menopause (commonly due to chemotherapy, pelvic radiotherapy, cranial radiotherapy in children)
- Hypogonadism (commonly due to hormonal therapy such as androgen deprivation therapy, pelvic radiotherapy)
- Growth hormone deficiency
- Prolonged treatment with glucocorticoids
- Methotrexate or ifosfamide chemotherapy
- Childhood/adolescent diagnosis of certain cancers (i.e., acute lymphoblastic leukemia, malignant bone tumors, rhabdomyosarcoma, brain tumors)
- Other risk factors in survivors of pediatric/adolescent cancers
  - Treatment with cranial irradiation
  - Chemotherapy with ifosfamide or methotrexate
  - Hematopoietic stem cell transplantation
  - Prolonged glucocorticoid therapy

Note. Based on information from Brown et al., 2006; Pfeilschifter & Diel, 2000; Sala & Barr, 2007.

Risk Factors in Women With Breast Cancer

Women with breast cancer are a population that is at particular risk for problems with bone health. Risk factors for bone loss in women with breast cancer vary by menopausal status, given the importance of estrogen in the pathogenesis of osteoporosis in women. For premenopausal women with breast cancer, chemotherapy-related amenorrhea (CRA) and premature menopause are the greatest risk factors for osteopenia and osteoporosis, although the use of hormonal therapies, such as tamoxifen and luteinizing hormone-releasing hormone (LHRH) agonists, also induces negative effects. In postmenopausal women with breast cancer, the movement toward the use of AIs as first-line adjuvant hormonal treatment (Winer et al., 2004) is predominantly responsible for the increased risk of bone loss in these women, given that postmenopausal women taking AIs have lower BMD and a higher incidence of fractures than those on tamoxifen or placebo (Baum et al., 2003; Coleman et al., 2004; Coombes et al., 2004; Goss et al., 2005; Howell, 2003; Lonning et al., 2005).

Amenorrhea Caused by Chemotherapy and Hormonal Therapy

In premenopausal women, including women diagnosed with breast cancer, the development of CRA is the greatest risk factor for bone loss (Bruning et al., 1990; Saarto et al., 1997; Shapiro, Manola, & Leboff, 2001; Vehmanen, Elomaa, Blomqvist, & Saarto, 2006; Vehmanen et al., 2004). Estrogen is protective against bone loss, and, therefore, CRA precipitates rapid bone loss caused by a marked and sudden reduction in circulating estradiol concomitant with a rise in follicle-stimulating hormone (Saarto et al.). Age is the biggest risk factor for CRA, and women 40 years old and older are at much greater risk than their younger counterparts (Bines, Oleske, & Cobleigh, 1996). Premenopausal women who stop menstruating during adjuvant chemotherapy have reductions in lumbar spine BMD as high as 7.7% during the first year following chemotherapy (Saarto et al.; Shapiro et al.), approximately double the rate of loss that occurs over the first two years of natural menopause (Filipponi et al., 1995) and more than seven times the annual rate of 1% that occurs in established menopause (Cummings et al., 2002; Love et al., 1992).

Some premenopausal women with breast cancer are treated with ovarian ablation as hormonal therapy, either by surgical oophorectomy or by medical castration using LHRH agonists, such as leuprolide. Ovarian ablation also induces amenorrhea and causes rapid and substantial bone loss (Genant, Cann, Ettinger, & Gordon, 1982; Sverrisdottir, Fornander, Jacobsson, von Schoultz, & Rutqvist, 2004). Ovarian ablation is also a concern for women with other cancers treated with pelvic radiotherapy.

Hormonal Therapy: Tamoxifen

Other hormonal treatments for breast cancer also affect bone metabolism. Tamoxifen can have both positive and negative effects on BMD. Tamoxifen has protective effects on bone in postmenopausal women but is associated with loss of BMD in premenopausal women (Vehmanen et al., 2006). Premenopausal women taking tamoxifen experience average declines in BMD of about 1.5% per year (Fisher et al., 1998; Sverrisdottir et al., 2004; Vehmanen et al., 2006).

Hormonal Therapy: Aromatase Inhibitors

AIs are used as hormonal therapy in postmenopausal women with hormone-dependent breast cancer, and their deleterious effects on bone are well established (Eastell & Hannon, 2005). Adjuvant use of AIs for two to five years is associated with both higher fracture rates

(Baum et al., 2003; Coombes et al., 2004; Goss et al., 2003) and greater bone loss (Coleman et al., 2004; Eastell et al., 2008; Howell, 2003; Lonning et al., 2005; Perez et al., 2004) compared to tamoxifen or placebo (as high as 7.2% over five years on anastrozole), although the fracture rate was not statistically significantly higher in two studies (Goss et al., 2003; Lonning et al.). In one study, no women who had normal BMD at baseline developed osteoporosis while taking anastrozole for five years (Eastell et al.).

Risk Factors in Men With Prostate Cancer

Osteoporosis and related fractures are prevalent among men with prostate cancer, largely because of the increasingly diverse application of ADT for treatment (Hatano et al., 2000; Malcolm et al., 2007; Morote et al., 2007; Oefelein et al., 2001; Planas et al., 2007; Shahinian et al., 2005; Townsend et al., 1997). ADT accelerates bone loss and is associated with a higher risk of fracture (Morote et al., 2003; Smith, 2006). ADT is accomplished by either surgical castration with orchiectomy or chemical castration with gonadotropins (LHRH analogs). Rates of bone loss and osteoporosis increase over time with ADT, although the most rapid bone loss appears to occur in the first year following initiation of hormonal therapy (Morote et al., 2003, 2006, 2007). Rates of bone loss average 2%–3% during initial use of ADT (Morote et al., 2007; Smith).

Although men receiving ADT are at highest risk, men with prostate cancer not treated with hormonal therapy also appear to have lower BMD and higher rates of osteoporosis than men without prostate cancer, although the underlying mechanism is not clear (Morote et al., 2007; Planas et al., 2007). About one-quarter to one-third of men diagnosed with prostate cancer and not receiving ADT had osteoporosis (Malcolm et al., 2007; Morote et al., 2007). Other risk factors include age older than 70 years and low dietary intake of calcium (Malcolm et al.; Planas et al.). Despite these risks, adherence to screening guidelines is poor in men with prostate cancer. For example, only 14%–26% of men without bony metastases receiving ADT were screened or treated for osteoporosis, including only half of men who were at even greater risk because of a history of previous fracture (Tanvetyanon, 2005; Yee, White, Murata, Handanos, & Hoffman, 2007).

Hematopoietic Stem Cell Transplantation

Individuals who undergo HSCT for cancer treatment are at elevated risk for bone loss and fracture. A pattern of early bone loss of 6%–10% during the first six months of therapy is typical in adult HSCT survivors (Schulte et al., 2000; Valimaki et al., 1999). Bone complications are also a concern in survivors of HSCT during childhood or adolescence, about one-third of whom develop osteopenia or osteoporosis (Bhatia, Ramsay, Weisdorf, Griffiths, & Robison, 1998; Taskinen et al., 2006, 2007). In one study of 44 allogeneic HSCT survivors, 35% had osteopenia or osteoporosis, 11% experienced nonvertebral fractures, and 20% had vertebral compression fractures detected by dual-energy x-ray absorptiometry (DEXA) scanning, the latter being an especially alarming finding in this young sample of survivors with a mean age of 10 years old (Taskinen et al., 2007). Risk factors for bone complications in HSCT survivors include presence of graft-versus-host disease (GVHD), gonadal hormone insufficiency including testosterone, and delayed pubertal growth and being prepubertal at the time of HSCT (Bhatia et al.; Schulte et al.; Taskinen et al., 2006, 2007). One study identified female sex as a risk factor (Bhatia et al.). Cumulative steroid dose is weakly associated with bone mineral loss during and after HSCT (Schulte et al.).

Risk Factors in Survivors of Childhood and Adolescent Cancers

Given that the achievement of a satisfactory peak bone mass by the end of adolescence is the best protection against bone demineralization and osteoporosis later in life, cancer and cancer therapies that affect bone formation and growth prior to adulthood have both immediate and long-term detrimental effects on bone health for survivors of childhood and adolescent cancers (Sala & Barr, 2007). A comprehensive review of adverse skeletal effects of pediatric cancer and cancer therapy is beyond the scope of this chapter, and excellent reviews are available elsewhere (Sala & Barr; van der Sluis & van den Heuvel-Eibrink, 2008). However, as increasing numbers of childhood and adolescent cancer survivors may be seen in adult oncology settings, all oncology nurses need to be aware of groups who are at particular risk (see Figure 18-2) (Sala & Barr; Taskinen et al., 2007). For example, in a sample of pediatric brain tumor survivors, two-thirds of those who received cranial radiotherapy had osteopenia, but nearly one-third of those who were not irradiated still developed osteopenia (Odame et al., 2006). Survivors of malignant sarcoma may experience deficits in BMD for as long as 10 or more years following therapy, and 65% of such long-term survivors had osteopenia or osteoporosis (Holzer et al., 2003). Identifying survivors of childhood and adolescent cancers who are at high risk for developing osteopenia, osteoporosis, and related fractures is the first step toward preventing these complications in this population of cancer survivors.

Glucocorticoid Treatment

The most common cause of secondary osteoporosis is glucocorticoid-induced osteoporosis (Adler, 2006). Use of doses as low as 5–7.5 mg daily for only three months resulted in a doubling or tripling of fracture risk (Adler). Many chemotherapy and other cancer treatment regimens incorporate glucocorticoids, especially for the treatment of hematologic malignancies—for example, cyclophosphamide, doxorubicin, vincristine, and prednisone (CHOP regimen) for lymphoma. Glucocorticoid drugs adversely affect the normal balance between bone formation and resorption in a number of ways, but the predominant mechanism appears to be by decreasing the formation of new bone cells (Adler).

Pathophysiology

Normal Bone Physiology and Overview of Pathophysiology of Osteoporosis

The skeleton serves the essential functions of providing support and structure for the human body and is highly vascular. Bone, which composes the skeleton, also serves as a reservoir for essential vitamins, minerals, and other ions necessary for homeostasis, including calcium, phosphorus, and vitamin D. Bone is a dynamic tissue that undergoes continuous remodeling throughout life, and approximately 18% of the total skeletal calcium is deposited and resorbed each year (Bringhurst et al., 2005). This remodeling serves two purposes: (a) to restore bone microdamage in order to maintain skeletal strength, and (b) to release skeletal calcium in order to maintain adequate serum calcium levels (Bringhurst et al.). The skeleton contains 99% of the body's calcium stores; when the exogenous supply is inadequate, bone tissue is reabsorbed from the skeleton to maintain serum calcium at a constant level (NOF, 2008a).

The bone microenvironment comprises osteoclasts, which are responsible for the breakdown of bone, osteoblasts (which form new bone), and mature, resting bone cells called osteocytes (Bringhurst et al., 2005). A complex interaction between the breakdown of old bone and formation of new bone is responsible for maintaining adequate BMD. Osteocytes are believed to sense mechanical and other stress signals and, in response, to send signals to osteoblasts to induce new bone formation. Osteoblasts typically move into areas where old bone has been resorbed and then secrete a substance called osteoid, which eventually is mineralized into new bone. Old bone is broken down by osteoclasts, which secrete acidic and proteolytic substances to resorb the bone matrix and form bone resorption pits. Bone formation and resorption is a complex and dynamic process that is regulated by circulating hormones such as parathyroid hormone (PTH), estrogen and androgens, and vitamin D, as well as locally produced growth factors. Many other factors, including exogenous influences such as nutrition, certain medications, and mechanical stresses such as physical activity, also influence bone remodeling.

The sex hormones play an important role in bone metabolism. In men, testosterone is believed to influence BMD predominantly through its conversion to estradiol, an estrogen, by the aromatase enzymes (Adler, 2006). Estrogen deficiency plays a key role in the development of postmenopausal osteoporosis in women and also influences bone density in men (Adler; Amin & Felson, 2001; Boonen, Laan, Barton, & Watts, 2005; Smith, 2006). Estrogen protects against bone loss and reduces bone turnover in both men and women, although the responsible mechanisms are not entirely clear (Adler; Ramaswamy & Shapiro, 2003; Smith). Estrogen receptors have been identified on cells within the bone microenvironment, including osteoblasts, but the complex interplay between these factors has not yet been elucidated (WHO, 2003). As estrogen wanes as a result of increasing age and declining ovarian function, as well as secondary to hypogonadism in men, bone homeostasis becomes disrupted. Bone resorption exceeds new bone formation, leading to bone loss (Bringhurst et al., 2005). During natural menopause, bone is lost at approximate rates of 1%–2% per year (Ahlborg, Johnell, Turner, Rannevik, & Karlsson, 2003; Love et al., 1992). Through a variety of different mechanisms, cancer treatments may interfere with the positive effects of estrogen on bone metabolism and consequently accelerate bone loss.

When bone loss is caused by estrogen deprivation resulting from CRA, it occurs more rapidly and to a more substantial degree in the lumbar spine as opposed to the femoral neck because of the type of bone that composes these sites (Vehmanen et al., 2006). The appendicular skeleton, such as the hip, is composed of cortical bone, which has a slower metabolic rate than does cancellous bone. Cancellous bone, also called trabecular bone, composes the axial skeleton (the spine) and manifests more rapid bone turnover (Watts, 1999).

Hormonal Therapy for Breast Cancer

Because estrogen plays a pivotal role in bone metabolism, cancer treatments that lead to estrogen deficiency play a key role in the development of cancer treatment–induced bone loss (CTIBL). Tamoxifen, ovarian ablation, and AIs all can have this effect. Tamoxifen is a selective estrogen receptor modulator (SERM), meaning that it acts upon estrogen receptors in various target tissues throughout the body. It has estrogenic effects in some tissues, such as in the endometrium, and antagonist effects in others, such as in the breast and bone (Ellmen, Hakulinen, Partanen, & Hayes, 2003). In postmenopausal women, who have low circulating levels of estrogen, the estrogen-agonist properties help to prevent bone resorption (Love et al., 1992; Vehmanen et al., 2006). The opposite effects in premenopausal women may result because of its weaker agonist effect in the bone compared to estrogen, with which it competes for binding to bone-specific estrogen receptors (Sverrisdottir et al., 2004). AIs lead to bone loss in postmenopausal women by a different mechanism. Although bioavailable levels of estrogen are approximately 90% lower following menopause, residual estrogen is believed to influence bone metabolism in postmenopausal women. AIs deplete postmenopausal estrogen levels by an additional 90% because of their interference with the aromatase enzyme, which converts adrenal androgens to estrogen (Eastell & Hannon, 2005), often precipitating CTIBL.

Androgen Deprivation Therapy for Prostate Cancer

Estrogens also play a critical role in bone metabolism in men (Greendale, Edelstein, & Barrett-Connor, 1997; Khosla et al., 1998; Slemenda et al., 1997). Although men with prostate cancer undergoing ADT with LHRH analogs experience reductions in BMD, treatment with estrogens to achieve medical castration does not accelerate bone turnover nor decrease BMD (Eriksson, Eriksson, Stege, & Carlstrom, 1995; Scherr, Pitts, & Vaughn, 2002). ADT induces declines in testosterone levels, precipitating bone loss. In addition, for men receiving ADT for prostate cancer, skeletal sensitivity to PTH may play an important role in the pathogenesis of osteoporosis, given that treatment with gonadotropins increases PTH-mediated activation of osteoclasts in men with prostate cancer (Leder, Smith, Fallon, Lee, & Finkelstein, 2001).

Bone Loss and Hematopoietic Stem Cell Transplantation

Bone loss in HSCT survivors is thought to be multifactorial. Hypogonadism and premature menopause caused by high-dose chemotherapy certainly may play a role. In allogeneic transplant recipients, chronic GVHD may elevate the risk for osteopenia, osteoporosis, and fracture both directly and indirectly through necessary pharmacologic treatments (Taskinen et al., 2007). Cytokines implicated in GVHD processes may have negative effects on bone metabolism by disrupting the normal balance between bone formation and bone resorption, and cyclosporin and corticosteroids, both used to treat GVHD, are known risk factors for osteoporosis (NOF, 2008a). Other potential mechanisms of bone loss include vitamin D deficiency and secondary hyperparathyroidism, as well as an acute catabolic reaction to increased toxins associated with high-dose antineoplastic treatment (Schulte et al., 2000).

Bone Loss in Survivors of Pediatric and Adolescent Cancers

The pathophysiology of bone loss in survivors of pediatric and adolescent cancers is similarly complex (Sala & Barr, 2007; van der Sluis & van den Heuvel-Eibrink, 2008). Hypogonadism caused by gonadal toxicity of chemotherapy and radiotherapy is a common risk factor. Direct effects on bone metabolism of chemotherapies such as methotrexate and ifosfamide are a concern for some individuals. Glucocorticoid effects lead to bone loss in certain individuals, including ALL survivors. Cranial irradiation can lead to hypogonadotropic hypogonadism, growth hormone deficiency, and resultant bone loss. Finally, certain groups of childhood cancer survivors, such as those with ALL, are at increased risk for physical inactivity and resultant bone loss.

Screening

As the number of cancer survivors continues to grow, now approaching 12 million in the United States alone (National Cancer Institute, 2008), osteopenia and osteoporosis are becoming more prevalent, heightening the importance of early detection and treatment. Various clinical practice guidelines address screening for osteopenia and osteoporosis (see Table 18-1), including those of NOF, USPSTF, and the American Society of Clinical Oncology (ASCO), the latter specifically for women with breast cancer (Hillner et al., 2003; NOF, 2008a; USPSTF, 2006). Each recommends screening with BMD testing for all women 65 years of age and older, as well as for younger postmenopausal women with one or more risk factors for osteoporosis. ASCO guidelines recommend annual BMD measurement, which is more aggressive than the two-year interval recommended for monitoring healthy postmenopausal women by other organizations (USPSTF, 2002; WHO, 2003). In general, the closer the BMD value is to the threshold at which treatment would be initiated, the sooner BMD testing should be repeated (Cummings et al., 2002). No evidence-based screening guidelines exist for men, but the International Society for Clinical Densitometry (ISCD) now recommends that all men older than age 70 have a baseline BMD evaluation (Adler, 2006). Furthermore, expert panels recommend that men undergoing surgical or chemical castration, such as ADT for prostate cancer, should have BMD measured at baseline (National Comprehensive Cancer Network, 2008), and some recommend annual measurement thereafter (Brown & Guise, 2007). Men with other risk factors for osteoporosis should be evaluated at a younger age, although risk factors for osteoporosis and related fracture are less understood for men than for women (Adler). Older age and lower weight clearly predict a higher risk of fracture in men as well as in women. Low calcium intake, smoking, height loss, prior history of fracture, and family history of osteoporosis also may predict an increased risk of fracture, but these require further validation.

Recommendations for screening survivors of pediatric and adolescent cancers vary, but the Children's Oncology Group survivorship guidelines recommend screening at baseline in certain pediatric survivors (see Table 18-1) (Children's Oncology Group, 2006). Others have recommended that survivors of sarcoma have baseline BMD measurement taken upon completion of chemotherapy, and then every two years in those with low BMD (Holzer et al., 2003). In the setting of HSCT, some have recommended routine assessment of the spine, even in individuals with normal BMD, given the high incidence of vertebral compression fractures in even young survivors (Taskinen et al., 2007).

Assessment

The gold standard for osteoporosis screening is the DEXA scan, a highly accurate x-ray technique that can measure BMD at any bony site (Cummings et al., 2002). BMD is defined as the average concentration of mineral in a two- or three-dimensional image or in a defined section of bone, and BMD testing commonly is used to estimate overall bone strength (Cummings et al.). Bone strength is determined principally by BMD and bone size (Cummings et al.), with 75%–85% of variance in bone strength accounted for by BMD (Sala & Barr, 2007). DEXA scanning is painless, takes only a few minutes to complete, and exposes the individual to approximately one-tenth the radiation of a chest x-ray (Cummings et al.; NOF, 2008a). Testing typically is performed at the hip, spine, or wrist, as these are the most common sites for osteoporotic fracture. Central testing of the hip or spine is the preferred measurement. Hip BMD is the best predictor of hip frac-

TABLE 18-1	Selected Guidelines for Bone Mineral Density Screening	
Guideline	**Population**	**Frequency/Timing**
American Society of Clinical Oncology (Hillner et al., 2003)	Women with breast cancer • Postmenopausal women receiving aromatase inhibitors • Premenopausal women undergoing premature menopause	Every 1–2 years
Children's Oncology Group, 2006	Pediatric cancer survivors Individuals with a history of • Hematopoietic stem cell transplant • Methotrexate chemotherapy ≥ 40 g/m^2 • Corticosteroids (cumulative dose ≥ 9 g/m^2 prednisone)	Baseline at entry into follow-up, and thereafter as clinically indicated
National Osteoporosis Foundation, 2008a	Postmenopausal women and men ages 50 and older • Women ages 65 and older, or postmenopausal with risk factors • Men ages 70 and older, or 50–70 years old with risk factors • Individuals with fracture	Every 2 or more years
U.S. Preventive Services Task Force, 2006	Postmenopausal women	Starting at age 65, or at age 60 with risk factors: Every 2 or more years

tures and also predicts the risk of fractures at other skeletal sites. Hip BMD often preferentially guides clinical decision making when results are discrepant between the hip and spine (Bringhurst et al., 2005). Unfortunately, hip DEXA is not as effective for men as it is for women at identifying one's risk for fracture (Adler, 2006). Testing at the spine appears to be the most sensitive for detecting early signs of both bone loss and gain, but BMD can be falsely elevated because of degenerative arthritis (Bringhurst et al.; Cummings et al.). Peripheral DEXA scans of the heel, finger, or forearm also can be performed but are not as predictive of the risk of major fracture. However, in men, forearm BMD or prior forearm fracture is useful in identifying their risk for osteoporosis and future fractures (Adler; Radiological Society of North America, 2006).

Alternative methods of determining BMD include qualitative computed tomography (QCT) and ultrasound. In addition to measuring bone density and volume, QCT can distinguish trabecular from cortical bone (NOF, 2008a). DEXA scanning generally is preferred over QCT because it is less expensive, is associated with less radiation exposure, and is more reliable (Lindsay & Cosman, 2005). Ultrasound densitometry also can be used to assess BMD of the heel, tibia, patella, and other peripheral sites but is not as precise as DEXA (Bringhurst et al., 2005).

Diagnosis

A diagnosis of osteoporosis typically is made based on DEXA scan results, but individuals who sustain a fragility fracture also can be diagnosed with osteoporosis regardless

TABLE 18-2	Interpreting Dual Energy X-Ray Absorptiometry Scans
Variable	**Clinical Significance**
Bone mineral density (BMD) (g/cm²)	Absolute measure of BMD
Percent change from prior study	Quantifies rate of bone loss Aids in decision making about frequency of BMD monitoring as well as initiation of therapy
T-score	Compares BMD to young adult (age 25–45) of same sex Used to guide decision making about monitoring and treatment in adults
Z-score	Compares BMD to adult of same sex and same age Used to guide decision making about monitoring and treatment in children and adolescents

Note. Based on information from Cummings et al., 2002; Lindsay & Cosman, 2005.

of BMD (Brown & Guise, 2007). DEXA scans report an individual's BMD in grams per centimeter squared (g/cm²) as well as in T- and Z-scores (see Table 18-2), which are more clinically useful and characterize the difference between the patient's score and reference norms. The T-score compares an individual's BMD score to that of a healthy young (age 24–45) adult of the same sex, whereas the Z-score compares an individual's BMD to that of individuals of the same age and sex (Cummings et al., 2002). T- and Z-scores are expressed in standard deviations (SDs) above or below the mean and are highly predictive of fracture risk. One SD is approximately equal to 10%–15% of the mean value for young adults (Cummings et al.), and the risk of fracture approximately doubles for each one SD drop in BMD (Lindsay & Cosman, 2005; Marshall, Johnell, & Wedel, 1996).

WHO defines osteopenia and osteoporosis based on BMD at the spine, hip, or wrist in white postmenopausal women (see Table 18-3) (WHO, 2003). Some experts and guidelines recommend use of the hip T-score as the gold standard for the diagnosis of osteoporosis, whereas others consider a T-score of –2.5 or less at either the hip or the spine to be diagnostic (Cummings et al.). The clinical usefulness of the term *osteopenia* is debatable, as more than half of all postmenopausal women will have a T-score of less than –1, and therefore this classification encompasses a group of women at widely variable risk of fracture (Cummings et al.).

When interpreting DEXA scan results in men, the appropriate reference norm (young men or young women) has been debated, particularly because some data have shown that men fracture at a higher absolute BMD (Adler, 2006). ISCD (2006) now recommends that a male database be used to define osteoporosis in men. Although controversy exists as to whether the same definitions of osteoporosis and osteopenia should apply to men as to women, nonetheless, the same defining scores typically are used (Adler).

Diagnosis in Children

In children, the Z-score, rather than the T-score, is used to diagnose osteopenia and osteoporosis (Saggese, Baroncelli, & Bertelloni, 2001). Osteopenia is defined as a BMD Z-score between –1 and –2, and osteoporosis as a BMD Z-score of less than –2. Others use the terminology of "low bone density for chronologic age" as preferred terminology (Writing Group for the ISCD Position Development Conference, 2004).

Differential Diagnosis

Once a diagnosis of osteopenia or osteoporosis has been made, additional evaluation should be considered to identify any treatable causes of bone loss (Lindsay & Cosman,

2005). The best approach is not clear, as the chance of finding a secondary cause in patients with low BMD is unknown (Cummings et al., 2002). Laboratory work should include a complete blood count and serum calcium, and a thyroid-stimulating hormone can be drawn if clinical signs and symptoms of hyperthyroidism are present (Bringhurst et al., 2005). Elevated serum calcium may indicate hyperparathyroidism, and thus a serum PTH level should be drawn. Low serum calcium may reflect malnutrition or osteomalacia, which is a condition of impaired bone mineralization most commonly arising because of vitamin D deficiency (Bringhurst et al.). The most specific screening test for vitamin D deficiency is a serum 25-hydroxyvitamin D level (Lindsay & Cosman). WHO recommends vitamin D repletion below a level of 50 nmol/L (20 mcg/L) (WHO, 2003).

TABLE 18-3	World Health Organization Definitions
Bone Mineral Density (BMD) Category	**BMD Score**
Normal	BMD is within 1 standard deviation (SD) of a "young normal" adult (T-score of –1 and above).
Osteopenia	BMD is between 1 and 2.5 SD below that of a "young normal" adult (T-score between –1 and –2.5).
Osteoporosis	BMD is 2.5 SD or more below that of a "young normal" adult (T-score at or below –2.5). • Women in this group who have already experienced one or more fractures are deemed to have severe or "established" osteoporosis.

Note. Based on information from World Health Organization, 2003.

Case Study (Part 2)

G.P., a breast cancer survivor, is clearly at risk for bone loss because she has been prescribed a planned five years of adjuvant hormonal therapy with anastrozole, an AI. Her oncologist recognizes this risk and orders a baseline DEXA scan prior to initiating anastrozole. G.P.'s baseline DEXA scan shows the following values, both consistent with osteopenia.
- Right total femur: T-score = –1.4 (0.689 g/cm^2)
- Lumbar spine: T-score = –1.8

G.P.'s oncologist does not prescribe pharmacologic therapy for osteoporosis at this time but asks the nurse to meet with the patient to discuss bone health, including preventive strategies. The nurse explains to G.P. that she has osteopenia, which is a weakening of the bone that could lead to osteoporosis and increased risk for fracture if not addressed. The patient asks why she was not told to begin medication at this time, and the nurse asks her about other potential risk factors for osteoporosis. The nurse determines that G.P. weighs 130 pounds and has never had a prior hip or vertebral fracture, but has an older sister who has sustained a hip fracture. The nurse then explains that she has two possible risk factors for osteoporosis (low weight and a first-degree relative with a fragility fracture), in addition to the risk related to AI therapy, and therefore preventive strategies are imperative. However, because she has early osteopenia of the hip (T-score = –1.4), pharmacologic treatment is not yet indicated.

Prevention and Treatment

The primary goal for both prevention and treatment of osteoporosis is fracture prevention by enhancing bone strength and minimizing skeletal trauma (Lindsay & Cosman, 2005; WHO, 2003). Nutritional and behavioral strategies are recommended for all men and women, including adequate calcium and vitamin D intake, avoidance of smoking or excessive alcohol intake, and either weight-bearing or muscle resistance training exercises (NOF, 2008a). A consensus regarding the threshold for initiation of pharmacologic treatment does not exist, because fracture risk continuously increases as BMD declines (Kanis et al., 2001). An international collaborative effort recently validated models for predicting fracture risk based on BMD in addition to clinical risk factors (Kanis et al., 2007). At present, clinical practice guidelines recommend therapy initiation based on BMD in combination with other risk factors, and rapid bone loss should lower the threshold for initiation of treatment. Several organizations recommend initiation of pharmacologic therapy once BMD falls to 2.5 or more SDs below the mean value for young adults (T-score ≤ -2.5) (Hillner et al., 2003; NOF, 2008a; WHO). Both the NOF and the USPSTF recommend initiation of treatment for all women who have a prior history of a fragility fracture, regardless of BMD (NOF, 2008a; USPSTF, 2002), and individuals with vertebral fractures have a particularly high risk of subsequent fracture (Bringhurst et al., 2005; Cummings et al., 2002). Table 18-4 summarizes recommendations for initiation of treatment.

TABLE 18-4	Recommendations for Initiating Pharmacologic Therapy for Osteoporosis
Recommendation	**Endorsing Organizations**
Bone mineral density T-scores below –2.5	World Health Organization (2003) American Society of Clinical Oncology breast cancer guidelines (Hillner et al., 2003) National Osteoporosis Foundation (2008a)
Prior hip or vertebral fracture (i.e., fragility fracture)	National Osteoporosis Foundation (2008a) U.S. Preventive Services Task Force (2006)

Prevention: Calcium and Vitamin D Supplementation

All individuals at risk for osteoporosis should ensure adequate daily intake of calcium and vitamin D through diet and/or supplementation. NOF recently updated its age-based guidelines for calcium and vitamin D intake (see Table 18-5) based on growing evidence of widespread calcium and vitamin D deficiency in the United States and throughout the world, particularly in adults age 50 and older (NOF, 2008a, 2008c). ASCO guidelines are similar and recommend that all women with a history of breast cancer take 1,200 mg/day of calcium and 400–600 IU/day of vitamin D (Hillner et al., 2003). Calcium and vitamin D prophylaxis has been recommended during and after chemotherapy treatment for sarcoma (Holzer et al., 2003), but calcium was not effective in preventing bone loss during

TABLE 18-5	National Osteoporosis Foundation Recommendations for Calcium and Vitamin D Intake	
Age	**Calcium**	**Vitamin D***
< 50 years	1,000 mg/day	400–800 IU/day
≥ 50 years	1,200 mg/day	800–1,000 IU/day

* Vitamin D3 is the best form of vitamin D for bone health and can be obtained from supplements as well as dietary sources such as fortified milk, egg yolks, and saltwater fish.

IU—international units

Note. Based on information from National Osteoporosis Foundation, 2008b.

the first six months following allo-geneic HSCT in adults, even when given with vitamin D and/or calci-tonin (Schulte et al., 2000; Taskinen et al., 2006). Although calcium and vitamin D supplementation alone is insufficient for the prevention of fractures (Jackson et al., 2006; Shea et al., 2002), adequate calcium and vitamin D intake from diet and/or supplementation remains an impor-tant core approach for bone health maintenance in both men and wom-en (NOF, 2008a, 2008c).

Multiple resources provide direc-tion for obtaining adequate dietary intake of calcium and vitamin D through dietary sources, supplemen-tation, and direct exposure to sun-light (National Institutes of Health Office of Dietary Supplements, 2005, 2007; NOF, 2008a, 2008c). Figure 18-3 provides a summary of key di-etary and other sources. Caffeine in-terferes with calcium absorption, as do other foods such as wheat bran. The safe upper limit for vitamin D intake is 2,000 IU/day, and vitamin D toxicity usually is only observed with doses greater than 40,000 IU/day (Bringhurst et al., 2005). The

FIGURE 18-3	Key Dietary and Environmental Sources of Vitamin D and Calcium
Calcium*	**Vitamin D**
Yogurt, plain, 8 oz = 400 mg	Salmon, cooked, 3.5 oz = 360 IU
Yogurt, fruit, 8 oz = 250 to 400 mg	Mackerel, cooked, 3.5 oz = 345 IU
Milk, 8 oz = 300 mg	Tuna fish, canned in oil, 3 oz = 200 IU
Calcium-fortified orange juice, 8 oz = 300 mg	Fortified ready-to-eat cereal (fortified with 10% of the daily value), 3/4 cup to 1
Canned salmon, solids, 3 oz = 200 mg	cup = 40 IU
Cheese, 1 oz = 200 mg	Egg, 1 yolk = 20 IU
Ice cream, 1 cup = 200 mg	Direct exposure to sunlight for 10–15 minutes at least 2
Tofu, 1/2 cup = 200 mg	times weekly
Cottage cheese, 1 cup = 100 mg	
Cooked greens, 1/2 cup = 100 mg	
Cooked/dried beans/peas, 1 cup = 100 mg	
Nonfat powdered milk, 1 tablespoon = 50 mg (add to puddings, homemade baked goods, casseroles)	

* Calcium amounts (in mg) are rounded to the nearest 50 or 100 mg unit.

IU—international units; oz—ounces

Note. Based on information from National Institutes of Health Office of Dietary Supplements, 2005, 2007.

safe upper limit for calcium intake is 2,500 mg daily. Calcium and vitamin D supplemen-tation is underutilized by many cancer survivors, and one study of men with prostate can-cer receiving ADT documented inadequate calcium intake in up to 93% of men (Planas et al., 2007).

Lifestyle Strategies

Lifestyle strategies for promoting bone health should be discussed with all men and wom-en who are at risk for bone loss. In addition to adequate dietary and supplemental calcium and vitamin D intake, lifestyle strategies include performing lifelong weight-bearing and aer-obic exercise, avoiding smoking and excessive alcohol intake, and addressing other risk fac-tors such as impaired vision or increased fall risk (NOF, 2008a). Weight-bearing exercises use bones and muscles to work against gravity as the feet and legs bear the body's weight, such as walking, jogging, Tai Chi, stair climbing, dancing, and tennis. Muscle-strengthening exer-cises include weight lifting and other resistive exercises. According to a Cochrane systematic review, aerobic, weight-bearing, and resistance exercises are all effective at improving BMD of the spine in postmenopausal women, and walking also is effective at improving BMD of the hip (Bonaiuti et al., 2002).

Case Study (Part 3)

Given G.P.'s risk factors (low body weight, family history, AI therapy), she will be closely monitored, and the nurse works with G.P.'s oncologist to arrange for repeat DEXA scanning in one year, consistent with ASCO recommendations for breast cancer survivors. The nurse counsels G.P. to increase her weight-bearing exercise from 15 minutes twice weekly to 30 minutes four times weekly. The nurse determines that G.P.'s dietary calcium intake is only about 400 mg/day and her dietary vitamin D intake is less than 100 IU/day, but she takes a multivitamin that includes 500 IU of vitamin D and 200 mg of calcium daily. So that the patient can meet the daily requirements of 800–1,000 IU of vitamin D and 1,200 mg of calcium, the nurse instructs the patient to start a calcium citrate supplement that includes 630 mg of calcium and 400 IU of vitamin D, taken as one tablet twice daily.

Pharmacologic Treatment

A number of pharmacologic options exist for the treatment of osteoporosis and prevention of related fractures. The Osteoporosis Research Advisory Group performed a meta-analysis of randomized trials evaluating these treatments and concluded that vitamin D, calcitonin, raloxifene, and bisphosphonates all reduce the risk of vertebral fractures (Cranney, Guyatt, et al., 2002), and 1-34 PTH also was deemed to be effective by a recent systematic review (MacLean et al., 2008). In these and another meta-analysis (Boonen et al., 2005), only alendronate and risedronate reduced the risk of nonvertebral fractures, including hip fractures. Studies of pharmacologic treatments have primarily been conducted in postmenopausal women, and most pharmacologic agents are only indicated in postmenopausal women. However, several agents have been tested in other populations at risk, including bisphosphonates for management of osteoporosis in men, women with breast cancer, and children and adolescents undergoing treatment for ALL (Brown & Guise, 2007; Lethaby et al., 2007). PTH (teriparatide) has also been shown to improve bone mass in men at high risk for fracture (Eli Lilly and Company, 2007b). Limited clinical trial data and resulting lack of evidence-based guidelines may be significant barriers to optimal pharmacologic management of osteoporosis in special populations such as men (Lethaby et al.).

Bisphosphonates

Bisphosphonates currently are the most effective inhibitors of bone resorption (Tauchmanova et al., 2006). They work by directly inhibiting the bone-resorbing activity of osteoclasts, resulting in fewer bone resorption pits, as well as by causing osteoclast cell death and reduction in the development of precursors (Reszka, Halasy-Nagy, Masarachia, & Rodan, 1999; Selandar, Lehenkari, & Vaananen, 1994). Bisphosphonates consistently decrease overall bone turnover (Brown & Guise, 2007). Bisphosphonates also improve bone mass, in part by enabling resorption pits to be filled in by osteoblasts (Brown & Guise). Four bisphosphonates currently are approved for the prevention and treatment of osteoporosis, including three oral agents: alendronate (Fosamax®, Merck and Co., Inc.), ibandronate (Boniva®, Roche Laboratories), and risedronate (Actonel®, Procter & Gamble Pharmaceuticals & Sanofi-Aventis) (Stricker, 2007). Most recently, the once-yearly IV bisphosphonate zoledronic acid (Reclast®, Novartis Pharmaceuticals Corp.) has been approved for the treatment of osteoporosis in postmenopausal women (Novartis Pharmaceuticals Corporation, 2007b). In addition to myriad studies documenting their efficacy in postmenopausal women, bisphosphonates also prevent bone loss in men, including those with nonmetastatic prostate cancer who are receiving ADT (Brown & Guise; Greenspan, Nelson, Trump, & Resnick, 2007; Lethaby et al., 2007; Smith et al., 2003). Bisphosphonates are recommended for the management of osteoporosis in men with prostate cancer who are receiving ADT (Planas et al., 2007), and alendronate and risedronate are approved for the treatment of osteoporosis in men based on their efficacy in improving BMD and reducing fracture risk (Brown & Guise).

Bisphosphonates generally are well tolerated, and no increased risk of serious gastrointestinal effects occurs with oral bisphosphonates if administration instructions are followed closely (see Figure 18-4) and if they are not administered to individuals with known esophageal disease (Bone et al., 2004; Brown & Guise, 2007). Transient flu-like symptoms (arthralgias/myalgias, bone pain, low-grade fever) may occur following initial doses of IV preparations, and reversible mild cases of hypocalcemia and hypomagnesemia can occur (Brown & Guise). Osteonecrosis of the jaw, a rare but clinically significant adverse event involving exposure of the mandible or maxilla, has been described as a potential complication of pamidronate, zoledronic acid, and alendronate (Farrugia et al., 2006; Marx, Sawatari, Fortin, & Broumand, 2005).The incidence appears to be quite low, with most cases attributable to dental extractions in patients receiving IV bisphosphonates as therapy for metastatic cancer. Patients being treated with IV bisphosphonates should undergo a baseline dental evaluation and avoid invasive procedures if possible while on therapy, and should discuss with their dentist whether they should take a one- to two-month drug holiday prior to any invasive procedures (Brown & Guise; NOF, 2006). Finally, although it is much less problematic with today's dosing and administration guidelines, renal toxicity is the biggest potential safety concern with IV preparations (Brown & Guise). Serum creatinine should be measured before each dose, and doses reduced or withheld according to package insert instructions.

FIGURE 18-4	**Instructions for Taking Oral Bisphosphonates**
• Take drug on an empty stomach with approximately 1 cup (8 oz) of water. • Remain upright for 30 minutes after taking pill.	
Note. Based on information from Merck & Co., Inc., 2008.	

Selective Estrogen Receptor Modulators

Raloxifene (Evista®, Eli Lilly and Co.), a 60 mg daily pill, is indicated for the treatment of osteoporosis in postmenopausal women and also reduces the risk of invasive breast cancer (Eli Lilly and Company, 2007a). Raloxifene is a SERM that inhibits bone resorption by binding to and stimulating estrogen receptors, thereby improving BMD and reducing vertebral, but not hip, fractures in postmenopausal women (Cranney, Tugwell, et al., 2002). Side effects include an increased risk for venous thromboembolism. Raloxifene should be used with caution in breast cancer survivors, particularly those with hormone receptor–positive disease who are taking tamoxifen, because preclinical data support cross-resistance between these two drugs (Van Poznak & Sauter, 2005).

Calcitonin

Salmon calcitonin (Miacalcin®, Novartis Pharmaceuticals Corp.) nasal spray 200 IU/day is approved for the treatment of osteoporosis in postmenopausal women (Novartis Pharmaceuticals Corporation, 2007a). Calcitonin nasal spray reduces the risk of vertebral, but not hip, fractures in postmenopausal women with established osteoporosis (Chesnut et al., 2000). Rhinitis is a frequent but mild to moderate side effect. Miacalcin is dosed at 200 IU/day intranasally in alternating nostrils to reduce the risk of nasal irritation.

Other Agents

Hormone replacement therapy (HRT) is no longer recommended for the prevention or treatment of osteoporosis in postmenopausal women, based largely on the results of the Women's Health Initiative trials, which showed an increased risk of breast cancer (Anderson et al., 2004; Rossouw et al., 2002). HRT improved BMD, but other health risks, such as breast and colorectal cancer and cardiovascular disease, exceeded benefits (Anderson et al.; Rossouw et al.).

PTH (teriparatide; PTH[1-34]; Forteo®, Eli Lilly and Co.) is an anabolic agent approved by the U.S. Food and Drug Administration (FDA) to treat osteoporosis in postmenopausal women at high risk for fracture and to increase bone mass in men at high risk for fracture (Eli Lilly and Company, 2007b). Teriparatide is an anabolic (bone-building) agent administered at a dose of 20 mcg daily subcutaneous injection and should not be used for first-line treatment of osteoporosis because of its adverse risk profile. The safety and efficacy of PTH(1-34) have not been demonstrated beyond two years of treatment, and it is not recommended for use in individuals with cancer because of the association in animal studies between its use and the development of osteosarcoma (Hillner et al., 2003).

Tibolone is a synthetic steroid that improves BMD. It has been used in Europe for nearly two decades but has not yet been approved by the FDA for use in the United States. Its safety in survivors of breast cancer and other neoplasms is not yet known (Hickey, Saunders, & Stuckey, 2005).

General Principles of Treatment

Although few studies have addressed the treatment of bone loss and osteoporosis specifically in individuals with cancer, effects of bone-building therapies in this setting have been consistent with those expected in non-oncologic populations of men and postmenopausal women (Saarto et al., 1997, 2001; Vehmanen et al., 2001, 2004). Therefore, management strategies for patients with cancer and survivors typically are extrapolated from studies of postmenopausal women and general populations of men.

The optimum length of treatment for osteopenia and osteoporosis is currently unknown. Data from both clinical trials and cost-effectiveness analyses generally support treatment durations of three to five years (Kanis et al., 2001). Safety has been demonstrated for up to 10 years (Bone et al., 2004). The benefit of treatment may persist beyond treatment cessation, although this is less true for calcium, vitamin D, and fluorides than it is for HRT and bisphosphonates (Kanis et al., 2001). BMD should be monitored every one to two years (Hillner et al., 2003; NOF, 2008a; USPSTF, 2002; WHO, 2003). Pharmacologic treatment may decrease a patient's risk of fracture even when no increase in BMD is apparent, and evidence of BMD loss may not indicate lack of response, as patients could have lost more bone mass without treatment. Changes in BMD of less than 2%–4% in the vertebrae and 3%–6% at the hip between tests can be caused by the precision error of the method and should not necessarily prompt change in therapy (Cummings et al., 2002; NOF, 2008a). Treatment should not be changed after the first period of monitoring, as subsequent gains can be observed following initial declines (Cummings et al.). Careful monitoring of BMD every one to two years is essential to optimal osteoporosis and fracture prevention and treatment.

Patient Teaching Points

An important first step in patient education is to help individuals understand their risk for bone loss, osteoporosis, and fracture. Oncology nurses should assess the risk profile of every individual with cancer based on age, cancer diagnosis and treatments, and side effects of treatment, such as CRA. It is imperative to counsel all individuals about their risk, appropriate BMD monitoring schedules, and lifestyle strategies, including adequate calcium and vitamin D intake, avoidance of smoking, and regular physical activity. For individuals who require pharmacologic treatment for osteoporosis, patient education should center on appropriate dosing and administration, prevention and management of potential side effects, and the importance of adherence to therapy.

A variety of resources are available to assist with patient education about calcium and vitamin D intake. NOF has designed a simple method for estimating calcium intake from dietary sources, which is available in its *Clinician's Guide to Prevention and Treatment of Osteoporosis* on its Web site at www.nof.org (NOF, 2008a). Individuals should also be taught how to read food labels. The percentage of daily calcium listed on food labels is based on a total daily requirement of 1,000 mg; therefore, individuals can multiply percent values by 10 to calculate milligrams (for example, 30% = 300 mg). Individuals whose total daily dietary calcium intake is less than the recommended amount should be counseled regarding calcium supplementation. Calcium supplements come in a variety of formulations. Gastric acid is necessary for optimal calcium absorption, particularly for calcium carbonate. Individuals with low production of gastric acid, including those on medications that reduce its production, should take calcium citrate (Bringhurst et al., 2005).

Oncology nurses also should help individuals with cancer to ascertain their typical daily intake of vitamin D because most individuals do not have enough daily sun exposure to maintain adequate vitamin D production, particularly during the wintertime (WHO, 2003). Chief dietary sources include milk fortified with vitamin D (400 IU per quart) and cereals (40–50 IU per serving), egg yolks, saltwater fish, and liver (NOF, 2008a). Most individuals will need supplemental vitamin D to ensure adequate intake (WHO). Many calcium supplements and most multivitamins contain vitamin D.

Conclusion of Case Study

G.P. returns one year after starting anastrozole and after undergoing a follow-up DEXA scan. She is now 63 years old. Over the past year, she has had difficulty keeping up with weight-bearing exercise and still only engages in 15–20 minutes two to three times per week. She has been taking her calcium plus vitamin D caplets twice daily. Her repeat DEXA scan shows the following values.

- Right femur: T-score = –1.9, a 5% drop in BMD compared to prior study
- Lumbar spine: T-score = –2.3, a 3% drop compared to prior study

Although G.P.'s values are still in the range of osteopenia, her oncologist wishes to prescribe pharmacologic therapy, given the significant drop in G.P.'s BMD levels over the past year, combined with her hip T-score of less than –1.5 combined with three pertinent risk factors (low weight, AI therapy, and first-degree relative with fragility fracture). After a discussion of options, therapy with a bisphosphonate is recommended. G.P. voices her desire to take a pill as infrequently as possible, and she feels that remembering to take medicine one day per month will be easiest for her to remember. She therefore starts on ibandronate 150 mg per month, with a plan to recheck her DEXA scan in one to two years. To prevent further bone loss, she most likely will remain on bisphosphonate therapy for the duration of her AI hormonal therapy. The nurse meets with G.P. to review instructions for taking ibandronate, reinforce calcium and vitamin D intake, and discuss barriers to exercise. The nurse also refers her to a strength-training exercise program at her local YMCA, which G.P. thinks will help her to better adhere to an exercise routine.

Conclusion

Patients with cancer and cancer survivors are at increased risk for bone loss, osteoporosis, and fracture because of a variety of demographic and disease- and treatment-related factors. Unfortunately, focus on bone health in these individuals often is overshadowed by cancer and other health-related concerns, and many cancer survivors do not benefit from osteoporosis prevention and treatment strategies. Adherence to osteoporosis screening guidelines is poor in many individuals with cancer. Oncology nurses can play a critical role in identifying patients with cancer and survivors who are at risk for bone loss, educating individuals about preventive and treatment strategies, and working with other healthcare providers to ensure prescription of necessary pharmacologic therapies. By promoting bone health in cancer survivors, oncology nurses can help to ameliorate the negative health and economic consequences of osteoporosis and related fracture in the nearly 12 million cancer survivors living in the United States.

References

Adler, R.A. (2006). Epidemiology and pathophysiology of osteoporosis in men. *Current Osteoporosis Reports, 4*(3), 110–115.

Ahlborg, H.G., Johnell, O., Turner, C.H., Rannevik, G., & Karlsson, M.K. (2003). Bone loss and bone size after menopause. *New England Journal of Medicine, 349*(4), 327–334.

Amin, S., & Felson, D.T. (2001). Osteoporosis in men. *Rheumatic Diseases Clinics of North America, 27*(1), 19–47.

Anderson, G.L., Limacher, M., Assaf, A.R., Bassford, T., Beresford, S.A., Black, H., et al. (2004). Effects of conjugated equine estrogen in postmenopausal women with hysterectomy: The Women's Health Initiative randomized controlled trial. *JAMA, 291*(14), 1701–1712.

Baum, M., Buzdar, A., Cuzick, J., Forbes, J., Houghton, J., Howell, A., et al. (2003). Anastrozole alone or in combination with tamoxifen versus tamoxifen alone for adjuvant treatment of postmenopausal women with early-stage breast cancer: Results of the ATAC (Arimidex, Tamoxifen Alone or in Combination) trial efficacy and safety update analyses. *Cancer, 98*(9), 1802–1810.

Bhatia, S., Ramsay, N.K., Weisdorf, D., Griffiths, H., & Robison, L.L. (1998). Bone mineral density in patients undergoing bone marrow transplantation for myeloid malignancies. *Bone Marrow Transplantation, 22*(1), 87–90.

Bines, J., Oleske, D.M., & Cobleigh, M.A. (1996). Ovarian function in premenopausal women treated with adjuvant chemotherapy for breast cancer. *Journal of Clinical Oncology, 14*(5), 1718–1729.

Bonaiuti, D., Shea, B., Iovine, R., Negrini, S., Robinson, V., Kemper, H.C., et al. (2002). Exercise for preventing and treating osteoporosis in postmenopausal women. *Cochrane Database of Systematic Reviews* 2002, Issue 2. Art. No.: CD000333. DOI: 10.1002/14651858.CD000333.

Bone, H.G., Hosking, D., Devogelaer, J.P., Tucci, J.R., Emkey, R.D., Tonino, R.P., et al. (2004). Ten years' experience with alendronate for osteoporosis in postmenopausal women. *New England Journal of Medicine, 350*(12), 1189–1199.

Boonen, S., Laan, R.F., Barton, I.P., & Watts, N.B. (2005). Effect of osteoporosis treatments on risk of non-vertebral fractures: Review and meta-analysis of intention-to-treat studies. *Osteoporosis International, 16*(10), 1291–1298.

Bringhurst, F.R., Demay, M.B., Krane, S.M., & Kronenberg, H.M. (2005). Bone and mineral metabolism in health and disease. In D.L. Kasper, E. Braunwald, A.S. Fauci, S.L. Hauser, D.L. Longo, & J.L. Jameson (Eds.), *Harrison's internal medicine* (16th ed., pp. 2238–2249). New York: McGraw-Hill.

Brown, J.E., Ellis, S.P., Silcocks, P., Blumsohn, A., Gutcher, S.A., Radstone, C., et al. (2006). Effect of chemotherapy on skeletal health in male survivors from testicular cancer and lymphoma. *Clinical Cancer Research, 12*(21), 6480–6486.

Brown, S.A., & Guise, T.A. (2007). Drug insight: The use of bisphosphonates for the prevention and treatment of osteoporosis in men. *Nature Clinical Practice: Urology, 4*(6), 310–319.

Bruning, P.F., Pit, M.J., de Jong-Bakker, M., van den Ende, A., Hart, A., & van Enk, A. (1990). Bone mineral density after adjuvant chemotherapy for premenopausal breast cancer. *British Journal of Cancer, 61*(2), 308–310.

Chesnut, C.H., 3rd, Silverman, S., Andriano, K., Genant, H., Gimona, A., Harris, S., et al. (2000). A randomized trial of nasal spray salmon calcitonin in postmenopausal women with established osteoporosis: The prevent recurrence of osteoporotic fractures study. PROOF Study Group. *American Journal of Medicine, 109*(4), 267–276.

Children's Oncology Group. (2006, March). *Long-term follow-up guidelines for survivors of childhood, adolescent, and young adult cancers* (Version 2.0). Retrieved January 18, 2008, from http://www.survivorshipguidelines. org

Coleman, R.E., Banks, R.M., Hall, E., Price, D., Girgis, S., Bliss, J.M., et al. (2004, December). *Intergroup Exemestane Study: 1 year results of the bone sub-protocol.* Paper presented at the 27th Annual San Antonio Breast Cancer Symposium, San Antonio, TX.

Coombes, R.C., Hall, E., Gibson, L.J., Paridaens, R., Jassem, J., Delozier, T., et al. (2004). A randomized trial of exemestane after two to three years of tamoxifen therapy in postmenopausal women with primary breast cancer. *New England Journal of Medicine, 350*(11), 1081–1092.

Cranney, A., Guyatt, G., Griffith, L., Wells, G., Tugwell, P., Rosen, C., et al. (2002). Meta-analyses of therapies for postmenopausal osteoporosis. IX: Summary of meta-analyses of therapies for postmenopausal osteoporosis. *Endocrine Reviews, 23*(4), 570–578.

Cranney, A., Tugwell, P., Zytaruk, N., Robinson, V., Weaver, B., Adachi, J., et al. (2002). Meta-analyses of therapies for postmenopausal osteoporosis. IV. Meta-analysis of raloxifene for the prevention and treatment of postmenopausal osteoporosis. *Endocrine Reviews, 23*(4), 524–528.

Cummings, S.R., Bates, D., & Black, D.M. (2002). Clinical use of bone densitometry: Scientific review. *JAMA, 288*(15), 1889–1897.

Eastell, R., Adams, J.E., Coleman, R.E., Howell, A., Hannon, R.A., Cuzick, J., et al. (2008). Effect of anastrozole on bone mineral density: 5-year results from the anastrozole, tamoxifen, alone or in combination trial 18233230. *Journal of Clinical Oncology, 26*(7), 1051–1057.

Eastell, R., & Hannon, R. (2005). Long-term effects of aromatase inhibitors on bone. *Journal of Steroid Biochemistry and Molecular Biology, 95*(1–5), 151–154.

Eli Lilly and Company. (2007a). *Evista.* Retrieved December 27, 2007, from http://www.evista.com/hcp/index.jsp

Eli Lilly and Company. (2007b). *Forteo.* Retrieved December 27, 2007, from http://www.forteo.com

Ellmen, J., Hakulinen, P., Partanen, A., & Hayes, D.F. (2003). Estrogenic effects of toremifene and tamoxifen in postmenopausal breast cancer patients. *Breast Cancer Research and Treatment, 82*(2), 103–111.

Eriksson, S., Eriksson, A., Stege, R., & Carlstrom, K. (1995). Bone mineral density in patients with prostatic cancer treated with orchidectomy and with estrogens. *Calcified Tissue International, 57*(2), 97–99.

Farrugia, M.C., Summerlin, D.J., Krowiak, E., Huntley, T., Freeman, S., Borrowdale, R., et al. (2006). Osteonecrosis of the mandible or maxilla associated with the use of new generation bisphosphonates. *Laryngoscope, 116*(1), 115–120.

Filipponi, P., Pedetti, M., Fedeli, L., Cini, L., Palumbo, R., Boldrini, S., et al. (1995). Cyclical clodronate is effective in preventing postmenopausal bone loss: A comparative study with transcutaneous hormone replacement therapy. *Journal of Bone and Mineral Research, 10*(5), 697–703.

Fisher, B., Costantino, J.P., Wickerham, D.L., Redmond, C.K., Kavanah, M., Cronin, W.M., et al. (1998). Tamoxifen for prevention of breast cancer: Report of the National Surgical Adjuvant Breast and Bowel Project P-1 Study. *Journal of the National Cancer Institute, 90*(18), 1371–1388.

Genant, H.K., Cann, C.E., Ettinger, B., & Gordon, G.S. (1982). Quantitative computed tomography of vertebral spongiosa: A sensitive method for detecting early bone loss after oophorectomy. *Annals of Internal Medicine, 97*(5), 699–705.

Gilbert, S.M., & McKiernan, J.M. (2005). Epidemiology of male osteoporosis and prostate cancer. *Current Opinion in Urology, 15*(1), 23–27.

Goss, P.E., Ingle, J.N., Martino, S., Robert, N.J., Muss, H.B., Piccart, M.J., et al. (2003). A randomized trial of letrozole in postmenopausal women after five years of tamoxifen therapy for early-stage breast cancer. *New England Journal of Medicine, 349*(19), 1793–1802.

Goss, P.E., Ingle, J.N., Martino, S., Robert, N.J., Muss, H.B., Piccart, M.J., et al. (2005). Randomized trial of letrozole following tamoxifen as extended adjuvant therapy in receptor-positive breast cancer: Updated findings from NCIC CTG MA.17. *Journal of the National Cancer Institute, 97*(17), 1262–1271.

Greendale, G.A., Edelstein, S., & Barrett-Connor, E. (1997). Endogenous sex steroids and bone mineral density in older women and men: The Rancho Bernardo Study. *Journal of Bone and Mineral Research, 12*(11), 1833–1843.

Greenspan, S.L., Nelson, J.B., Trump, D.L., & Resnick, N.M. (2007). Effect of once-weekly alendronate on bone loss in men receiving androgen deprivation therapy for prostate cancer: A randomized controlled trial. *Annals of Internal Medicine, 146*(6), 416–424.

Hamdy, R.C., Chesnut, C.H., 3rd, Gass, M.L., Holick, M.F., Leib, E.S., Lewiecki, M.E., et al. (2005). Review of treatment modalities for postmenopausal osteoporosis. *Southern Medical Journal, 98*(10), 1000–1014.

Hatano, T., Oishi, Y., Furuta, A., Iwamuro, S., & Tashiro, K. (2000). Incidence of bone fracture in patients receiving luteinizing hormone-releasing hormone agonists for prostate cancer. *BJU International, 86*(4), 449–452.

Hickey, M., Saunders, C.M., & Stuckey, B.G. (2005). Management of menopausal symptoms in patients with breast cancer: An evidence-based approach. *Lancet Oncology, 6*(9), 687–695.

Hillner, B.E., Ingle, J.N., Chlebowski, R.T., Gralow, J., Yee, G.C., Janjan, N.A., et al. (2003). American Society of Clinical Oncology 2003 update on the role of bisphosphonates and bone health issues in women with breast cancer. *Journal of Clinical Oncology, 21*(21), 4042–4057.

Holzer, G., Krepler, P., Koschat, M.A., Grampp, S., Dominkus, M., & Kotz, R. (2003). Bone mineral density in long-term survivors of highly malignant osteosarcoma. *Journal of Bone and Joint Surgery (British Volume), 85*(2), 231–237.

Howell, A. (2003, December). *Effect of anastrozole on bone mineral density: 2-year results of the 'Arimidex' (anastrazole), tamoxifen, alone or in combination (ATAC) trial.* Paper presented at the 26th Annual San Antonio Breast Cancer Symposium, San Antonio, TX.

International Society for Clinical Densitometry. (2006). *ICSD official positions.* Retrieved June 20, 2006, from http://www.iscd.org/visitors/positions/OfficialPositionsText.cfm

Jackson, R.D., LaCroix, A.Z., Gass, M., Wallace, R.B., Robbins, J., Lewis, C.E., et al. (2006). Calcium plus vitamin D supplementation and the risk of fractures. *New England Journal of Medicine, 354*(7), 669–683.

Kanis, J.A., Johnell, O., Oden, A., Dawson, A., De Laet, C., & Jonsson, B. (2001). Ten year probabilities of osteoporotic fractures according to BMD and diagnostic thresholds. *Osteoporosis International, 12*(12), 989–995.

Kanis, J.A., Oden, A., Johnell, O., Johansson, H., De Laet, C., Brown, J., et al. (2007). The use of clinical risk factors enhances the performance of BMD in the prediction of hip and osteoporotic fractures in men and women. *Osteoporosis International, 18*(8), 1033–1046.

Khosla, S., Melton, L.J., 3rd, Atkinson, E.J., O'Fallon, W.M., Klee, G.G., & Riggs, B.L. (1998). Relationship of serum sex steroid levels and bone turnover markers with bone mineral density in men and women: A key role for bioavailable estrogen. *Journal of Clinical Endocrinology and Metabolism, 83*(7), 2266–2274.

Leder, B.Z., Smith, M.R., Fallon, M.A., Lee, M.L., & Finkelstein, J.S. (2001). Effects of gonadal steroid suppression on skeletal sensitivity to parathyroid hormone in men. *Journal of Clinical Endocrinology and Metabolism, 86*(2), 511–516.

Lethaby, C., Wiernikowski, J., Sala, A., Naronha, M., Webber, C., & Barr, R.D. (2007). Bisphosphonate therapy for reduced bone mineral density during treatment of acute lymphoblastic leukemia in childhood and adolescence: A report of preliminary experience. *Journal of Pediatric Hematology/Oncology, 29*(9), 613–616.

Lindsay, R., & Cosman, F. (2005). Osteoporosis. In D.L. Kasper, E. Braunwald, A.S. Fauci, S.L. Hauser, D.L. Longo, & J.L. Jameson (Eds.), *Harrison's internal medicine* (16th ed., pp. 2268–2278). New York: McGraw-Hill.

Lonning, P.E., Geisler, J., Krag, L.E., Erikstein, B., Bremnes, Y., Hagen, A.I., et al. (2005). Effects of exemestane administered for 2 years versus placebo on bone mineral density, bone biomarkers, and plasma lipids in patients with surgically resected early breast cancer. *Journal of Clinical Oncology, 23*(22), 5126–5137.

Love, R.R., Mazess, R.B., Barden, H.S., Epstein, S., Newcomb, P.A., Jordan, V.C., et al. (1992). Effects of tamoxifen on bone mineral density in postmenopausal women with breast cancer. *New England Journal of Medicine, 326*(13), 852–856.

MacLean, C., Newberry, S., Maglione, M., McMahon, M., Ranganath, V., Suttorp, M., et al. (2008). Systematic review: Comparative effectiveness of treatments to prevent fractures in men and women with low bone density or osteoporosis. *Annals of Internal Medicine, 148*(3), 197–213.

Malcolm, J.B., Derweesh, I.H., Kincade, M.C., DiBlasio, C.J., Lamar, K.D., Wake, R.W., et al. (2007). Osteoporosis and fractures after androgen deprivation initiation for prostate cancer. *Canadian Journal of Urology, 14*(3), 3551–3559.

Marshall, D., Johnell, O., & Wedel, H. (1996). Meta-analysis of how well measures of bone mineral density predict occurrence of osteoporotic fractures. *BMJ, 312*(7041), 1254–1259.

Marx, R.E., Sawatari, Y., Fortin, M., & Broumand, V. (2005). Bisphosphonate-induced exposed bone (osteonecrosis/osteopetrosis) of the jaws: Risk factors, recognition, prevention, and treatment. *Journal of Oral and Maxillofacial Surgery, 63*(11), 1567–1575.

Merck & Co., Inc. (2008, February). *Fosamax* [Package insert]. Retrieved June 8, 2008, from http://www.merck.com/product/usa/pi_circulars/f/fosamax/fosamax_pi.pdf

Morote, J., Martinez, E., Trilla, E., Esquena, S., Abascal, J.M., Encabo, G., et al. (2003). Osteoporosis during continuous androgen deprivation: Influence of the modality and length of treatment. *European Urology, 44*(6), 661–665.

Morote, J., Morin, J.P., Orsola, A., Abascal, J.M., Salvador, C., Trilla, E., et al. (2007). Prevalence of osteoporosis during long-term androgen deprivation therapy in patients with prostate cancer. *Urology, 69*(3), 500–504.

Morote, J., Orsola, A., Abascal, J.M., Planas, J., Trilla, E., Raventos, C.X., et al. (2006). Bone mineral density changes in patients with prostate cancer during the first 2 years of androgen suppression. *Journal of Urology, 175*(5), 1679–1683.

National Cancer Institute. (2008). *Estimated U.S. cancer prevalence.* Retrieved January 15, 2008, from http://cancercontrol.cancer.gov/ocs/prevalence/prevalence.html

National Comprehensive Cancer Network. (2008, November 12). *NCCN Clinical Practice Guidelines in Oncology™: Prostate cancer* [v.1.2009]. Retrieved January 15, 2009, from http://www.nccn.org/professionals/physician_gls/PDF/prostate.pdf

National Institutes of Health Office of Dietary Supplements. (2005, September 23). *Dietary supplement fact sheet: Calcium.* Retrieved January 20, 2007, from http://dietary-supplements.info.nih.gov/factsheets/vitamind.asp

National Institutes of Health Office of Dietary Supplements. (2007, August 30). *Dietary supplement fact sheet: Vitamin D.* Retrieved January 20, 2007, from http://dietary-supplements.info.nih.gov/factsheets/vitamind.asp

National Osteoporosis Foundation. (2006, June 14). *Osteonecrosis of the jaw (ONJ).* Retrieved June 18, 2008, from http://www.nof.org/patientinfo/osteonecrosis.htm

National Osteoporosis Foundation. (2008a). *Clinician's guide to prevention and treatment of osteoporosis.* Retrieved May 28, 2008, from http://www.nof.org/professionals/NOF_Clinicians_Guide.pdf

National Osteoporosis Foundation. (2008b). *National Osteoporosis Foundation's updated recommendations for calcium and vitamin D intake.* Retrieved January 15, 2008, from http://www.nof.org/prevention/calcium_and_VitaminD.htm

National Osteoporosis Foundation. (2008c). *What you should know about calcium.* Retrieved January 15, 2009, from http://www.nof.org/prevention/calcium2.htm

Novartis Pharmaceuticals Corporation. (2007a). *Miacalcin* [Package insert]. Retrieved December 27, 2007, from http://www.miacalcin.com/hcp/pi.jsp

Novartis Pharmaceuticals Corporation. (2007b). *Reclast* [Package insert]. Retrieved November 25, 2007, from http://www.reclast.com

Odame, I., Duckworth, J., Talsma, D., Beaumont, L., Furlong, W., Webber, C., et al. (2006). Osteopenia, physical activity and health-related quality of life in survivors of brain tumors treated in childhood. *Pediatric Blood and Cancer, 46*(3), 357–362.

Oefelein, M.G., Ricchuiti, V., Conrad, W., Seftel, A., Bodner, D., Goldman, H., et al. (2001). Skeletal fracture associated with androgen suppression induced osteoporosis: The clinical incidence and risk factors for patients with prostate cancer. *Journal of Urology, 166*(5), 1724–1728.

Perez, E.A., Josse, R.G., Pritchard, K.I., Ingle, J.N., Martino, S., Findlay, B.P., et al. (2004). Effect of letrozole versus placebo on bone mineral density in women completing ≥ 5 years of adjuvant tamoxifen: NCIC CTG MA-17B [Abstract]. *Breast Cancer Research and Treatment, 88*(Suppl. 1), S36.

Pfeilschifter, J., & Diel, I.J. (2000). Osteoporosis due to cancer treatment: Pathogenesis and management. *Journal of Clinical Oncology, 18*(7), 1570–1593.

Planas, J., Morote, J., Orsola, A., Salvador, C., Trilla, E., Cecchini, L., et al. (2007). The relationship between daily calcium intake and bone mineral density in men with prostate cancer. *BJU International, 99*(4), 812–815.

Radiological Society of North America. (2006). *Bone density scan.* Retrieved April 20, 2006, from http://www.radiologyinfo.org/content/dexa.htm

Ramaswamy, B., & Shapiro, C.L. (2003). Osteopenia and osteoporosis in women with breast cancer. *Seminars in Oncology, 30*(6), 763–775.

Reszka, A.A., Halasy-Nagy, J.M., Masarachia, P.J., & Rodan, G.A. (1999). Bisphosphonates act directly on the osteoclast to induce caspase cleavage of mst1 kinase during apoptosis. A link between inhibition of the mevalonate pathway and regulation of an apoptosis-promoting kinase. *Journal of Biological Chemistry, 274*(49), 34967–34973.

Richelson, L., Wahner, H., Melton, L.I., & Riggs, B.L. (1984). Relative contributions of aging and estrogen deficiency to postmenopausal bone loss. *New England Journal of Medicine, 311*(20), 1273–1275.

Rossouw, J.E., Anderson, G.L., Prentice, R.L., LaCroix, A.Z., Kooperberg, C., Stefanick, M.L., et al. (2002). Risks and benefits of estrogen plus progestin in healthy postmenopausal women: Principal results from the Women's Health Initiative randomized controlled trial. *JAMA, 288*(3), 321–333.

Saarto, T., Blomquist, C., Valimaki, M., Makela, P., Sarna, S., & Elomaa, I. (1997). Chemical castration induced by adjuvant cyclophosphamide, methotrexate, and fluorouracil chemotherapy causes rapid bone loss that is reduced by clodronate: A randomized study in premenopausal breast cancer patients. *Journal of Clinical Oncology, 15*(4), 1341–1347.

Saarto, T., Vehmanen, L., Elomaa, I., Valimaki, M., Makela, P., & Blomqvist, C. (2001). The effect of clodronate and antioestrogens on bone loss associated with oestrogen withdrawal in postmenopausal women with breast cancer. *British Journal of Cancer, 84*(8), 1047–1051.

Saggese, G., Baroncelli, G.I., & Bertelloni, S. (2001). Osteoporosis in children and adolescents: Diagnosis, risk factors, and prevention. *Journal of Pediatric Endocrinology and Metabolism, 14*(7), 833–859.

Sala, A., & Barr, R.D. (2007). Osteopenia and cancer in children and adolescents: The fragility of success. *Cancer, 109*(7), 1420–1431.

Scherr, D., Pitts, W.R., Jr., & Vaughn, E.D., Jr. (2002). Diethylstilbesterol revisited: Androgen deprivation, osteoporosis and prostate cancer. *Journal of Urology, 167*(2, Pt. 1), 535–538.

Schulte, C., Beelen, D.W., Schaefer, U.W., & Mann, K. (2000). Bone loss in long-term survivors after transplantation of hematopoietic stem cells: A prospective study. *Osteoporosis International, 11*(4), 344–353.

Selandar, K., Lehenkari, P., & Vaananen, H.K. (1994). The effects of bisphosphonates on the resorption cycle of isolated osteoclasts. *Calcified Tissue International, 55*(5), 368–375.

Shahinian, V.B., Kuo, Y.F., Freeman, J.L., & Goodwin, J.S. (2005). Risk of fracture after androgen deprivation for prostate cancer. *New England Journal of Medicine, 352*(2), 154–164.

Shapiro, C.L., Manola, J., & Leboff, M. (2001). Ovarian failure after adjuvant chemotherapy is associated with rapid bone loss in women with early-stage breast cancer. *Journal of Clinical Oncology, 19*(14), 3306–3311.

Shea, B., Wells, G., Cranney, A., Zytaruk, N., Robinson, V., Griffith, L., et al. (2002). Meta-analyses of therapies for postmenopausal osteoporosis. VII. Meta-analysis of calcium supplementation for the prevention of postmenopausal osteoporosis. *Endocrine Reviews, 23*(4), 552–559.

Slemenda, C.W., Longcope, C., Zhou, L., Hui, S.L., Peacock, M., & Johnston, C.C. (1997). Sex steroids and bone mass in older men. Positive associations with serum estrogens and negative associations with androgens. *Journal of Clinical Investigation, 100*(7), 1755–1759.

Smith, M.R. (2006). Treatment-related osteoporosis in men with prostate cancer. *Clinical Cancer Research, 12*(20, Pt. 2), 6315s–6319s.

Smith, M.R., Eastham, J., Gleason, D.M., Shasha, D., Tchekmedyian, S., & Zinner, N. (2003). Randomized controlled trial of zoledronic acid to prevent bone loss in men receiving androgen deprivation therapy for nonmetastatic prostate cancer. *Journal of Urology, 169*(6), 2008–2012.

Stricker, C.T. (2007). Endocrine effects of breast cancer treatment. *Seminars in Oncology Nursing, 23*(1), 55–70.

Sverrisdottir, A., Fornander, T., Jacobsson, H., von Schoultz, E., & Rutqvist, L.E. (2004). Bone mineral density among premenopausal women with early breast cancer in a randomized trial of adjuvant endocrine therapy. *Journal of Clinical Oncology, 22*(18), 3694–3699.

Tanvetyanon, T. (2005). Physician practices of bone density testing and drug prescribing to prevent or treat osteoporosis during androgen deprivation therapy. *Cancer, 103*(2), 237–241.

Taskinen, M., Kananen, K., Valimaki, M., Loyttyniemi, E., Hovi, L., Saarinen-Pihkala, U., et al. (2006). Risk factors for reduced areal bone mineral density in young adults with stem cell transplantation in childhood. *Pediatric Transplantation, 10*(1), 90–97.

Taskinen, M., Saarinen-Pihkala, U.M., Hovi, L., Vettenranta, K., & Makitie, O. (2007). Bone health in children and adolescents after allogeneic stem cell transplantation: High prevalence of vertebral compression fractures. *Cancer, 110*(2), 442–451.

Tauchmanova, L., De Simone, G., Musella, T., Orio, F., Ricci, P., Nappi, C., et al. (2006). Effects of various antireabsorptive treatments on bone mineral density in hypogonadal young women after allogeneic stem cell transplantation. *Bone Marrow Transplantation, 37*(1), 81–88.

Townsend, M.F., Sanders, W.H., Northway, R.O., & Graham, S.D., Jr. (1997). Bone fractures associated with luteinizing hormone-releasing hormone agonists used in the treatment of prostate carcinoma. *Cancer, 79*(3), 545–550.

U.S. Preventive Services Task Force. (2002). Screening for osteoporosis in postmenopausal women: Recommendations and rationale. *Annals of Internal Medicine, 137*(6), 526–528.

U.S. Preventive Services Task Force. (2006). *The guide to clinical preventive services: Recommendations of the U.S. Preventive Services Tack Force* [AHRQ Pub. No. 06-0588]. Washington, DC: Agency for Healthcare Research and Quality.

Valimaki, M.J., Kinnunen, K., Volin, L., Tahtela, R., Loyttyniemi, E., Laitinen, K., et al. (1999). A prospective study of bone loss and turnover after allogeneic bone marrow transplantation: Effect of calcium supplementation with or without calcitonin. *Bone Marrow Transplantation, 23*(4), 355–361.

van der Sluis, I.M., & van den Heuvel-Eibrink, M.M. (2008). Osteoporosis in children with cancer. *Pediatric Blood and Cancer, 50*(Suppl. 2), 474–478.

Van Poznak, C., & Sauter, N. (2005). Clinical management of osteoporosis in women with a history of breast carcinoma. *Cancer, 104*(3), 443–456.

Van Staa, T.P., Leufkens, H.G., Abenhaim, L., Zhang, B., & Cooper C. (2000). Use of oral corticosteroids and risk of fractures. *Journal of Bone and Mineral Research, 15*(6), 993–1000.

Vehmanen, L., Elomaa, I., Blomqvist, C., & Saarto, T. (2006). Tamoxifen treatment after adjuvant chemotherapy has opposite effects on bone mineral density in premenopausal patients depending on menstrual status. *Journal of Clinical Oncology, 24*(4), 675–680.

Vehmanen, L., Saarto, T., Elomaa, I., Makela, P., Valimaki, M., & Blomqvist, C. (2001). Long-term impact of chemotherapy-induced ovarian failure on bone mineral density (BMD) in premenopausal breast cancer patients: The effect of adjuvant clodronate treatment. *European Journal of Cancer, 37*(18), 2373–2378.

Vehmanen, L., Saarto, T., Risteli, J., Risteli, L., Blomqvist, C., & Elomaa, I. (2004). Short-term intermittent intravenous clodronate in the prevention of bone loss related to chemotherapy-induced ovarian failure. *Breast Cancer Research and Treatment, 87*(2), 181–188.

Watts, N.B. (1999). Clinical utility of biochemical markers of bone remodeling. *Clinical Chemistry, 45*(8, Pt. 2), 1359–1368.

Winer, E.P., Hudis, C., Burstein, H.J., Wolff, A.C., Pritchard, K.I., Ingle, J.N., et al. (2004). *Use of aromatase inhibitors as adjuvant therapy for postmenopausal women with hormone receptor-positive breast cancer: Status Report 2004.* Retrieved December 16, 2004, from http://www.asco.org/ac/1,1003,_12-002033-00_18-0036744-00_19-0036745-00_20-001,00.asp

World Health Organization. (2003). *Prevention and management of osteoporosis: Report of a WHO Scientific Group.* Geneva, Switzerland: Author. Retrieved November 30, 2007, from http://whqlibdoc.who.int/trs/WHO_TRS_921.pdf

Writing Group for the ISCD Position Development Conference. (2004). Diagnosis of osteoporosis in men, premenopausal women, and children. *Journal of Clinical Densitometry, 7*(1), 17–26.

Yee, E.F., White, R.E., Murata, G.H., Handanos, C., & Hoffman, R.M. (2007). Osteoporosis management in prostate cancer patients treated with androgen deprivation therapy. *Journal of General Internal Medicine, 22*(9), 1305–1310.

CHAPTER 19

Cancer Pain

Christine Miaskowski, RN, PhD, FAAN

Case Study

S.S. is a 66-year-old African American woman who had a modified radical mastectomy for breast cancer six years ago. Two months after her surgery, she described a burning, dysesthetic pain in her breast and axillary incisions that she rated as 8 out of 10. She stated that although the incision had healed, she could not wear her prosthesis or a bra because it exacerbated the pain at the incision site. She stated that at times she experienced shock-like pain in the incision sites. In addition, she had stopped using her arm because the pain was so severe. At the time, S.S. was diagnosed as having postmastectomy pain, which is a neuropathic pain problem that can occur in women following breast cancer surgery (Poleshuck et al., 2006; Stevens, Dibble, & Miaskowski, 1995). She was treated with gabapentin, which was slowly titrated to a dose of 3,600 mg/day. In addition, she received physical therapy to improve her range of motion and shoulder mobility. She continues to take the gabapentin, and her neuropathic pain is well controlled.

Today, she presents to the outpatient clinic with severe pain in both hips that has persisted for two months. She rates the pain as 7 on a 0–10 scale. She indicates that the pain is exacerbated with movement and that it interferes with her ability to sleep, engage in her routine household activities, and go to church. She tells the nurse that the pain is "wearing her down" and that she finds herself crying spontaneously several times a day. A careful neurologic examination is essentially negative. However, a bone scan reveals metastatic disease to both hips. While the medical oncologist is consulting with the radiation oncologist about a treatment plan for the metastatic disease, the development of a pain management plan is a priority.

Overview

Pain is a common experience for patients with cancer. At the time of diagnosis, approximately 20%–75% of patients have pain. In addition, 17%–57% of patients undergoing active cancer treatment (Caraceni & Portenoy, 1999; Goudas, Bloch, Gialeli-Goudas, Lau, & Carr, 2005; Stevens et al., 1995; Valeberg et al., 2008) and 23%–100% of patients in the terminal stages of their disease report moderate to severe pain (Gomez-Batiste et al., 2007; Zeppetella, O'Doherty, & Collins, 2000; Zeppetella & Ribeiro, 2002). Finally, 23%–90% of patients with cancer experience episodic breakthrough pain (BTP) (Caraceni & Portenoy; Zeppetella & Ribeiro, 2002). Unfortunately, over the past 30 years, the epidemiology of cancer pain has remained relatively constant, and numerous studies continue to document the significant undertreatment of cancer pain (Miaskowski et al., 2005).

Risk factors for the undertreatment of cancer pain include belonging to a minority group (Anderson et al., 2002), being female (Cleeland et al., 1994), and being an older adult (Bernabei et al., 1998). In addition, patients with cancer who have a current or previous history of substance abuse need to be evaluated to determine the optimal approaches to management of their cancer pain (Kushel & Miaskowski, 2006). Finally, chronic pain syndromes associated with cancer or cancer treatment may persist in cancer survivors (Burton, Fanciullo, Beasley, & Fisch, 2007; Deimling, Bowman, & Wagner, 2007; Mao et al., 2007; Mols, Coebergh, & van de Poll-Franse, 2007; Rannestad & Skjeldestad, 2007). The undertreatment of cancer pain has profound negative effects on patients' mood, functional status, and quality of life (Burrows, Dibble, & Miaskowski, 1998). Therefore, assessment and aggressive management of cancer pain are priorities for all oncology nurses.

Pathophysiology

Acute Cancer Pain Problems

Patients can experience acute and chronic pain from cancer, diagnostic procedures, treatments, or preexisting painful conditions (e.g., osteoarthritis, painful diabetic peripheral neuropathy, lower back pain). Oncology nurses need to recognize the most common pain conditions and syndromes that are associated with cancer and its treatment.

The most common types of acute pain that are associated with cancer treatment are postoperative pain and oral mucositis (Miaskowski et al., 2005). Because surgery is the most common initial treatment for most cancers, patients with cancer will experience postoperative pain. In most cases, acute postoperative pain decreases over time as healing occurs. Refer to Chapter 16 for more discussion of acute oral pain.

Chronic Cancer Pain Problems

The most common cause of chronic pain associated with cancer is bone metastasis. Patients at high risk for the development of bone metastasis are those with breast, prostate, or lung cancer or multiple myeloma. The most common sites of metastasis are the vertebrae, pelvis, femur, and skull. Patients usually describe this pain as severe and localized to the metastatic site. Patients may experience BTP associated with activity. In addition, bone metastasis may cause fractures, hypercalcemia, and spinal cord compression (Miaskowski et al., 2005).

Neuropathic pain can occur in patients with cancer following surgery, chemotherapy, or varicella zoster virus infections (shingles). The surgical procedures that are associated with the development of neuropathic pain include radical neck dissection, mastectomy, thoracotomy, nephrectomy, and limb amputation. Patients often describe burning, tingling, and dysesthetic sensations with or without the loss of sensation at the site of the surgical incision. The pain may be exacerbated with movement (Miaskowski et al., 2005). The most common classes of drugs associated with chemotherapy-induced neuropathy include vinca alkaloids, taxanes, platinum compounds, and thalidomide. Usually, the severity and duration of the neuropathy are dose-related. The specific symptoms that the patient experiences may be related to the specific drug administered as well as its dose. Dose-related neuropathies associated with chemotherapy are characterized by dysesthesias in the feet and hands and may be associated with hyporeflexia (Kannarkat, Lasher, & Schiff, 2007; Visovsky, Collins, Abbott, Aschenbrenner, & Hart, 2007). Patients with cancer, particularly during times of immunosuppression, may experience an acute varicella zoster infection. Approximately 25%–50% of these patients, subsequent to the acute infection, develop postherpetic neuralgia. This chronic pain condition is characterized by burning and aching pain sensations. In addition, lancinating or shock-like pain may be superimposed on the persistent pain (Dworkin et al., 2007).

Assessment

As noted in the cancer pain guideline published by the American Pain Society (APS) (Miaskowski et al., 2005), assessment of cancer pain is a continuous process that includes universal screening for pain, comprehensive pain assessments, and ongoing reassessments of the patient's pain. All patients with cancer should be screened for the presence of pain at each outpatient visit or hospital admission. If pain is present, a comprehensive pain assessment should be performed.

Figure 19-1 outlines the four components of a comprehensive pain assessment (Miaskowski et al., 2005). The detailed pain history should focus on the differentiation of persistent pain from BTP. Persistent cancer pain is pain that is continuous throughout most of the day and usually is managed with around-the-clock medication. BTP is a transitory exacerbation or flare of moderate to severe pain that occurs in patients who are on chronic opioid therapy with otherwise stable persistent pain. BTP can be sudden and severe, and it comes and goes (Portenoy, Payne, & Jacobsen, 1999; Zeppetella, 2008). Figure 19-2 outlines an interview guide that oncology nurses can use to obtain a comprehensive assessment of persistent cancer pain and BTP. With the increasing emphasis on quality of life as an outcome of cancer treatment, oncology nurses need to obtain information on the effects of pain on patients' ability to function. Nurses can use this outcome measure to evaluate the effectiveness of the pain management plan.

Cancer pain is a multidimensional experience. Therefore, as part of any comprehensive pain assessment, the impact of pain on the psychosocial aspects of a patient's life requires systematic investigation. Specific areas to assess include the meaning of the pain to patients and their family caregivers; significant past experiences with pain and pain management; how patients and family caregivers have coped with pain in the past, as well as their current level of coping; any concerns about the use of opioid analgesics; and the economic impact of the pain on the patients and family caregivers. This portion of the assessment may provide information on barriers to cancer pain management (Ward et al., 1993). Specific interventions can be designed to overcome many of these barriers. In addition, the oncology nurse may determine that patients and family caregivers need referrals to psychologists or social workers to assist with some of the identified problems or barriers.

The physical examination and diagnostic tests focus on determining the cause of the pain and the extent of the patient's disease. Pain may be the first indication of tumor recurrence or progression. Therefore, new complaints of pain require an appropriate and comprehensive evaluation.

FIGURE 19-1	Components of a Comprehensive Pain Assessment

1. Obtain a detailed pain history.
   a. Determine the presence of persistent pain.
   b. Determine the presence of breakthrough pain.
   c. Determine the impact of pain on the patient's functional status.
2. Perform a psychosocial assessment.
3. Perform a physical examination.
   a. Examine the site of the pain.
   b. Perform a detailed neurologic and musculoskeletal examination.
4. Perform a diagnostic evaluation for signs and symptoms associated with the most common cancer pain presentations and syndromes.

FIGURE 19-2   **Components of a Detailed History of Persistent Cancer Pain and Breakthrough Pain**

Persistent Pain
1. Onset—When did the pain start?
2. Description—What does the pain feel like? What words would you use to describe your pain?
3. Location—Where is your pain? Show me where it hurts.
4. Intensity/severity—On a scale of 0 to 10 with 0 being no pain and 10 being the worst pain you can imagine, how much does it hurt right now? How much does it hurt at its worst? OR Using the following scale (none, mild, moderate, severe, very severe, intolerable), tell me how much your pain hurts right now and at its worst.
5. Aggravating and relieving factors—What makes your pain better? What makes your pain worse?
6. Previous and current pharmacologic and nonpharmacologic treatments and their effectiveness
7. Effects of pain on function—How does your pain interfere with your mood, ability to engage in normal activities, ability to sleep, ability to participate in social activities, and ability to participate in sexual activities?

Breakthrough Pain (BTP)
1. Define BTP for the patient as sudden flare-ups of pain that come and go. These flare-ups are called BTP because the pain "breaks through" the patient's treatment for persistent cancer pain.
2. Do you have BTP?
3. Frequency and duration of BTP—How many episodes of BTP do you have each day? How long does each episode of BTP last?
4. Intensity/severity of BTP—see number 4 under persistent pain.
5. Occurrence of BTP—Does your BTP occur with movement or activity? Does your BTP occur spontaneously?
6. Previous and current pharmacologic and nonpharmacologic treatments and their effectiveness
7. Effects of BTP on function—How does your pain interfere with your mood, ability to engage in normal activities, ability to sleep, ability to participate in social activities, and ability to participate in sexual activities?

Evidence-Based Interventions

The effective management of cancer pain should include both pharmacologic and nonpharmacologic interventions (Miaskowski et al., 2005). APS (Miaskowski et al.) and the National Comprehensive Cancer Network (NCCN) (Swarm et al., 2007) have published clinical practice guidelines on the management of cancer pain. In addition, the Oncology Nursing Society (ONS) Putting Evidence Into Practice (PEP) team has published recommendations on pharmacologic interventions for nociceptive and neuropathic pain in adults (Aiello-Laws, Delzer, Peterson, & Reynolds, 2007). The recommendations within these documents are similar and are summarized in the next sections of this chapter.

Principles of Cancer Pain Management

The effective management of cancer pain requires that oncology nurses work with patients and family caregivers to ensure that pain is assessed; that a treatment plan is initiated; that the effectiveness of the treatment plan is reassessed on an ongoing basis; and that appropriate modifications occur to the treatment plan whenever they are needed. Pain management requires that patients and family caregivers be incorporated as essential participants in the development and implementation of the pain management plan. Without ongoing patient assessment and education, the optimal management of cancer pain will not occur.

Both the APS and NCCN guidelines on cancer pain management contain algorithm-based approaches that can guide the initial and ongoing management of cancer pain (Miaskowski et al., 2005; Swarm et al., 2007). Factors to consider when initiating an analgesic regimen for cancer pain are the severity of the patient's pain, the etiology of the pain, the setting in which the regimen is initiated (e.g., hospital, clinician's office, patient's home), whether the patient is opioid naïve or currently taking an opioid analgesic, and the patient's previous experience with analgesic medications, including their efficacy and side effects. In general, mild pain (i.e., worst pain intensity between 1 and 4) usually is relieved with a nonopioid analgesic or a combination of a nonopioid and an opioid analgesic (e.g., codeine and acetaminophen, hydrocodone and acetaminophen). Moderate (i.e., worst pain intensity between 5 and 6) and severe (i.e., worst pain intensity between 7 and 10) pain usually require an opioid analgesic.

A worst pain score of 7–10 should be considered a pain emergency. This level of pain warrants rapid titration of a short-acting, immediate-release opioid analgesic. Rapid titration can be done with either oral or IV opioids. The advantages of IV administration are that the peak analgesic effect is achieved within 15 minutes; repeated doses can be administered more frequently; analgesia may be achieved more rapidly; and adverse effects can be monitored more easily. However, this approach requires that patients be monitored carefully either in an emergency department, inpatient setting, or in a chemotherapy infusion unit with appropriate emergency equipment.

The starting dose of an opioid analgesic will depend on whether the patient is taking an opioid analgesic. For IV titration, if a patient is not taking an opioid analgesic, the dose of IV morphine can range from 2–5 mg. If the patient is taking an opioid analgesic, then the IV dose of morphine (or an equianalgesic dose equivalent of another opioid agonist with a short half-life) can be equivalent to 10%–20% of the total daily dose of the current opioid regimen. (For example, if a patient is taking 60 mg of oxycodone daily, the patient can receive 6–12 mg of IV morphine.) For oral titration, if a patient is not taking an opioid analgesic, an appropriate starting dose is 5–10 mg of immediate-release oral morphine or another pure mu-opioid agonist with a short half-life (e.g., hydromorphone, oxymorphone, oxycodone). If the patient is taking an opioid analgesic, an immediate-release dose of morphine (or its equivalent) that is 10%–20% of the person's total daily dose can be administered. The effectiveness of the analgesic should be reassessed using the same 0–10 numeric rating scale every 15 minutes after IV administration or every 60 minutes after oral administration. If the pain rating is unchanged, then the dose of the analgesic medication should be titrated until effective pain control is achieved.

Less aggressive approaches can be used to titrate analgesic medications for worst pain intensity ratings in the moderate range. Because many patients with chronic cancer pain (i.e., pain with a duration of greater than three months) will have persistent pain as well as BTP, the pain management plan needs to address both types of pain. The optimal analgesic regimen for a patient with both persistent pain and BTP is one that contains a controlled-release opioid (e.g., controlled-release morphine, oxycodone, or oxymorphone; transdermal fentanyl) that is administered around the clock *and* an immediate-release (e.g., morphine, hydromorphone, oxycodone, oxymorphone) or rapid-onset (e.g., oral transmucosal fentanyl citrate, fentanyl buccal tablet) opioid analgesic. A critical step in the initiation and ongoing use of opioid analgesics is the development of effective approaches to assess and manage opioid-induced side effects. Patients and family caregivers need education and written instructions on the reasons for the two types of analgesic medications, on how to optimize the titration and use of the controlled- and immediate-release preparations, and on how to effectively manage opioid-induced side effects.

Pharmacologic Cancer Pain Management

Effective cancer pain management requires the use of nonopioid analgesics, opioid analgesics, and coanalgesics. The choice of analgesic medication most often is based on the cause and severity of pain. For example, if the patient has neuropathic pain, a coanalgesic (e.g., gabapentin, nortriptyline) may be a more effective treatment. In many cases, patients with chronic cancer pain will require combinations of analgesics to achieve optimal analgesia. The specific analgesic medications used should be based on their mechanisms of action and the etiology of the patient's pain.

Nonopioid Analgesics

Nonopioid analgesics, which include acetaminophen, aspirin, and nonsteroidal anti-inflammatory drugs (NSAIDs), are the most commonly used analgesics for the management of mild to moderate pain. These drugs exert their analgesic effects primarily within the peripheral nervous system. A large amount of interindividual variability exists in response to nonopioid analgesics. In addition, this class of drugs exhibits the pharmacologic property of a ceiling effect (i.e., a maximum therapeutic dose exists, above which no additional analgesic effect occurs and an increased risk of toxicity results if the dose is escalated).

Acetaminophen is an analgesic and antipyretic that does not have an anti-inflammatory effect (Smith, 2009). The addition of acetaminophen to an opioid analgesic may allow for a reduction in the dose of the opioid analgesic. Chronic daily dosing with more than 4 g/day of acetaminophen is not recommended because of the increased risk of hepatotoxicity. Oncology nurses need to assess the amount of acetaminophen the patient is taking on a daily basis. To avoid hepatotoxicity, this assessment needs to include all combination products containing acetaminophen (e.g., over-the-counter analgesics and cold preparations, combination products of an opioid with acetaminophen) (McNicol, Strassels, Goudas, Lau, & Carr, 2005; Miaskowski et al., 2005; Potter, 2005).

NSAIDs are effective for the treatment of mild pain and have an opioid-sparing effect in the treatment of moderate to severe pain. As a class of analgesics, NSAIDs inhibit the enzyme cyclooxygenase. This enzyme catalyzes the synthesis of endoperoxides from arachidonic acid to produce proinflammatory and other types of prostaglandins. Inhibition of this enzyme by nonselective NSAIDs results in analgesia. In addition, inhibition of this enzyme results in decreased production of prostaglandins that protect the gastric mucosa and renal parenchyma, which can result in dyspepsia, gastrointestinal bleeding, and renal failure. NSAIDs are most useful in the treatment of cancer pain when the pain is associated with inflammation (e.g., patients with pain from bone metastasis). However, this class of analgesic may need to be used with caution in patients with cancer who have neutropenia or thrombocytopenia (McNicol et al., 2005; Miaskowski et al., 2005).

Opioid Analgesics

Opioid analgesics are the mainstay of chronic cancer pain management. This class of analgesic medications is effective for moderate to severe pain. Opioids produce analgesia by binding to opioid receptors within and outside the central nervous system. Most of the opioid analgesics that are available for clinical use (e.g., morphine, hydromorphone, oxycodone, oxymorphone) bind to the mu-opioid receptor to exert their analgesic effects. The recommended starting doses and equianalgesic doses of commonly used opioid analgesics for the management of cancer pain are listed in Table 19-1.

TABLE 19-1	Commonly Used Opioid Analgesics for the Management of Cancer Pain		
Opioid Analgesic	**Usual Starting Doses and Dose Equivalents**		**Comments**
	Oral	**Parenteral**	
Morphine	15–30 mg q 3–4 hrs	10 mg q 3–4 hrs	Prototypical mu agonist Available in multiple formulations Half-life = 2–3 hrs
Morphine controlled-release formulations			Controlled-release formulations release their contents when the tablet is crushed.
• MS Contin® (Purdue Pharma L.P.)	15–30 mg q 12 hrs	Not available	Half-life = 2–3 hrs
• Oramorph® SR (Xanodyne Pharmaceuticals, Inc.)	15–30 mg q 12 hrs	Not available	Kadian and Avinza are extended-release formulations of morphine in capsules that can be opened and sprinkled on food or placed in nasogastric tube feedings.
• Kadian® (Alpharma Inc.)	20 mg q 24 hrs	Not available	
• Avinza® (King Pharmaceuticals)	30 mg q 24 hrs	Not available	
Hydromorphone	4–8 mg q 3–4 hrs	1.5 mg q 3–4 hrs	Significantly more potent than morphine Half-life = 2–3 hrs
Levorphanol	2–4 mg q 6–8 hrs	2 mg q 6–8 hrs	Opioid with a long half-life Half-life = 12–15 hrs
Oxymorphone	10–15 mg q 3–4 hrs	1 mg q 3–4 hrs	Oxymorphone has a short half-life and is both a potent congener of morphine and an active metabolite of oxycodone. Oxymorphone does not affect the CYP2D6 or CYP3A4 enzymes.
Oxymorphone controlled release	10–15 mg q 12 hrs	Not available	–
Oxycodone	10–30 mg q 4 hrs	Not available	Half-life = 2–3 hrs
Oxycodone controlled release	10 mg q 12 hrs	Not available	–
Transdermal fentanyl	25 mcg/hr patch q 72 hrs	Not available	Patch allows for slow absorption through the skin. Half-life = not applicable
Combination Opioid-Nonopioid Preparations			
Codeine (with aspirin or acetaminophen)	30–60 mg q 3–4 hrs	Not available	Half-life = 2–4 hrs
Hydrocodone with acetaminophen	5–10 mg q 3–4 hrs	Not available	Half-life = 2–4 hrs
Oxycodone with aspirin or acetaminophen	5–10 mg q 3–4 hrs	Not available	Half-life = 2–3 hrs
Tramadol	50–100 mg q 6 hrs	Not available	Half-life = 2–4 hrs

Note. Based on information from Jacox et al., 1994; Miaskowski et al., 2005.

As noted in the cancer pain guideline published by APS (Miaskowski et al., 2005), based on ongoing reassessments of the pain, opioid doses should be adjusted for each patient to achieve pain relief with an acceptable level of side effects. Because many patients with cancer have persistent pain as well as BTP, they will need to take their analgesic medications on a regular schedule (i.e., around the clock). One of the easiest and most effective ways to achieve around-the-clock dosing is to use a controlled-release opioid preparation (i.e., controlled-release morphine, controlled-release oxycodone, controlled-release oxymorphone, transdermal fentanyl) because these formulations are administered on a fixed schedule that is dependent on the formulation of the drug. In addition, patients will require an immediate-release (e.g., morphine, hydromorphone, oxycodone, oxymorphone) or a rapid-onset (e.g., oral transmucosal fentanyl citrate, fentanyl buccal tablet) opioid analgesic for the management of BTP.

A brief note regarding methadone is warranted here. Methadone should be used only by clinicians who understand its unique pharmacology. It is recommended that a switch to methadone from another opioid be accompanied by a large (75%–90%) decrease in the calculated equianalgesic dose to account for its potential high potency. Because the plasma concentration of methadone slowly rises to steady-state levels over four to five half-lives (i.e., almost one week in most patients), titration should be done slowly with close patient monitoring (Fine & Portenoy, 2007) (see Table 19-2 for considerations with methadone use).

If the persistent component of the patient's pain is not well controlled, the dose of the controlled-release opioid can be increased by 30%–50% or to a dose equal to the amount of supplemental medication the patient is taking for BTP. Larger dose increases can be considered if the patient is in severe pain and is able to tolerate the increase. Dose increases are safest if performed after steady-state levels of the analgesic medication are achieved (i.e., usually in five to six half-lives) (Fine & Portenoy, 2007; Mercadante, 2007).

If patients experience inadequate pain relief or an unacceptable level of side effects from a specific opioid analgesic, they can be switched to a different opioid analgesic (i.e., opioid rotation) (Mercadante & Bruera, 2006; Mercadante, Villari, Ferrera, & Casuccio, 2006; Ross, Riley, Quigley, & Welsh, 2006). When switching from one opioid to another, equianalgesic doses of the new drug are calculated (refer to Table 19-1) and used as a starting point. The dose of the new drug must be adjusted to reflect the possibility of incomplete cross-tolerance to opioid analgesics; individual variation in response to different opioid analgesics;

TABLE 19-2	Considerations With the Use of Methadone
Consideration	**Comments**
Mechanisms of action of methadone	Mu opioid agonist Antagonist at the N-methyl-D-aspartate receptor Blocks the reuptake of serotonin and norepinephrine
Properties of methadone	Long and variable half-life—typically around 24 hours, but varies from 12–150 hours. The long half-life of methadone does not match its duration of analgesia (i.e., 6–12 hours). Methadone's long half-life can lead to increased risk for sedation and respiratory depression.
Adverse effects	Prolongation of the QTc interval Reports that patients on very high doses were at increased risk for torsades de pointes (i.e., serious ventricular arrhythmia)

Note. Based on information from De Conno et al., 1996.

and the impact of uncontrolled pain and comorbidities on the patient's response to the new drug (Fine & Portenoy, 2007).

Opioid analgesics are used to manage BTP. If the patient experiences incident pain (i.e., pain is most often associated with movement or activity), the most effective approach to decrease this type of BTP is to premedicate with an immediate-release opioid analgesic approximately 45 minutes before the planned activity. Management of the spontaneous type of BTP (i.e., pain that occurs spontaneously, often without warning) requires an opioid preparation that can be absorbed quickly. Two rapid-onset opioid preparations (oral transmucosal fentanyl citrate and fentanyl buccal tablet) are approved by the U.S. Food and Drug Administration for the management of BTP in patients with cancer who are opioid tolerant (i.e., taking at least 60 mg of morphine equivalents every day for one week). Oral transmucosal fentanyl citrate and fentanyl buccal tablets are distinct formulations with distinct pharmacokinetics. In clinical studies with patients with cancer, both preparations provided pain relief within 15 minutes of administration (Gordon, 2006; Zeppetella & Ribeiro, 2006).

Side effects of opioid analgesics need to be anticipated and treated either prophylactically or as they occur. Constipation and sedation are the most common side effects associated with opioid analgesics. Other side effects include nausea and vomiting, dry mouth, urinary retention, pruritus, myoclonus, altered cognitive function, dysphoria, euphoria, sleep disturbances, respiratory depression, sexual dysfunction, and inappropriate secretion of antidiuretic hormone (Cherny et al., 2001; McNicol et al., 2003; Miaskowski et al., 2005). Great interindividual variability exists in the side effects that patients experience. Oncology nurses need to perform systematic assessments to determine which side effects the patient is experiencing and proceed to develop an appropriate management plan.

Constipation is the most common side effect and is estimated to occur in 40%–70% of patients on oral opioid analgesics (McNicol et al., 2003). Patients do not develop tolerance to opioid-induced constipation. At the time that the opioid prescription is written, patients should be started on a bowel regimen that includes a stool softener and a stimulant laxative to increase bowel motility. A useful laxative regimen includes docusate sodium (100–300 mg/day) with senna (2–6 tablets twice a day), laxative suppositories, or lactulose (Miaskowski et al., 2005).

Patients will develop tolerance to the side effects of sedation and nausea and vomiting in about five to seven days if the opioid dose is not escalated. Sedation may not require treatment once the dose of the opioid analgesic is stabilized. Central nervous system stimulants (e.g., caffeine, methylphenidate) may be used to reduce opioid-induced sedation. Antiemetics may be required until the patient develops tolerance to nausea and vomiting.

Usually, respiratory depression is not a significant clinical problem in patients with cancer who are on chronic opioid therapy. Caution is advised when opioid antagonists (e.g., naloxone) are given to patients who have received opioids for more than one week. In these cases, symptomatic respiratory depression should be treated with a dilute solution of naloxone (0.4 mg in 10 ml of saline) administered in 0.5 ml (0.02 mg) boluses by IV push every two minutes. The dose should be titrated to avoid precipitating profound withdrawal symptoms, seizures, and severe pain (Miaskowski et al., 2005).

Coanalgesics

This class of analgesic medications is composed of drugs that have pain-relieving effects in certain conditions, but whose primary or initial indication is not for the treatment of pain. The most common drugs in this class are anticonvulsants, antidepressants, and corticosteroids. Most of these medications are used in the management of neuropathic pain. Much of the data on the safety and efficacy of these medications come from studies of postherpetic neuralgia and diabetic neuropathy rather than cancer pain.

Recently, an expert panel from the International Association for the Study of Pain published evidence-based recommendations on the use of these medications in the treatment of neuropathic pain (Dworkin et al., 2007). As with other analgesic medications, a large amount of interindividual variability exists in the effectiveness of the various coanalgesics. In addition, pain relief may take several weeks to occur. Most of these medications need to be titrated slowly to achieve the optimal dose. Slow titration is required to reduce the occurrence of intolerable side effects. Patients with neuropathic pain need to receive nonopioid or opioid analgesics to control their pain while the coanalgesic medication is titrated to an effective dose.

Anticonvulsants are used frequently to treat neuropathic pain (Backonja, 2002, 2003). In fact, gabapentin was recommended as first-line treatment for neuropathic pain (Dworkin et al., 2007). Gabapentin and pregabalin are two anticonvulsants used in the management of neuropathic pain. These two drugs modulate cellular calcium influx into nociceptive neurons by binding to voltage-gated calcium channels and decrease the release of glutamate, norepinephrine, and substance P (Matthews & Dickenson, 2001). Compared to other coanalgesics, gabapentin produces fewer intolerable side effects. The most common side effects are sedation and dizziness. Gabapentin is started at doses of 100–300 mg at bedtime and can be titrated every three days until an effective dose of 1,800–3,600 mg/day is reached. Dose titration may take several weeks.

Pregabalin is a relatively new anticonvulsant that has shown efficacy in a variety of neuropathic pain conditions. The side effects of pregabalin are similar to those of gabapentin. Pregabalin is started at doses of 75–150 mg/day (in either two or three divided doses). The maximum dose ranges from 300–600 mg/day (Dworkin et al., 2007).

Antidepressants are the best-studied coanalgesics for the management of neuropathic pain. These medications block the presynaptic reuptake of serotonin and/or norepinephrine in the central nervous system. Several systematic reviews and meta-analyses concluded that tricyclic antidepressants are effective for multiple types of neuropathic pain (e.g., postherpetic neuralgia, diabetic neuropathy) whether patients do or do not have concurrent depression (Saarto & Wiffen, 2007; Sindrup, Otto, Finnerup, & Jensen, 2005).

Because tricyclic antidepressants are effective, inexpensive, and usually given once daily, they may be used as initial treatment for neuropathic pain in patients who do not have conditions that would contraindicate their use (e.g., ischemic heart disease, heart failure, conduction disorders, arrhythmias). In addition, patients who receive tricyclic antidepressants need to be monitored for adverse events (e.g., cardiotoxicity, confusion, urinary retention, orthostatic hypotension, nightmares, weight gain, drowsiness, dry mouth, constipation). Secondary amine tricyclic antidepressants (e.g., nortriptyline, desipramine) are preferred because they are better tolerated than the tertiary amine tricyclic antidepressants (e.g., amitriptyline, imipramine) but have comparable analgesic efficacy. The initial doses of antidepressants can range from 10–25 mg/day and can be titrated to 100–150 mg every three days (Dworkin et al., 2007).

Corticosteroids (e.g., prednisone, dexamethasone, methylprednisolone) can be used to reduce edema around neural tissues. Corticosteroids are used routinely in the treatment of malignant spinal cord compression. In addition, corticosteroids can be useful in the treatment of pain caused by malignant lesions of the brachial or lumbar plexus. They can be used to treat the pain associated with bone metastasis, bowel obstruction, and lymphedema (Knotkova & Pappagallo, 2007).

Nonpharmacologic Cancer Pain Management

In most cases, effective management of chronic cancer pain requires the use of analgesic medications. Nonpharmacologic interventions often are used as adjuncts to pharmacologic approaches. Cognitive and behavioral approaches (e.g., distraction, relaxation, cognitive restructuring and reframing, music therapy) are designed to reduce the cognitive and affective components of pain. They give patients assistance and direction with how to interpret painful sensations and associated events. In addition, physical strategies (e.g., heat, cold, massage) can improve pain management.

Oncology nurses can teach patients and their family caregivers how to use techniques such as relaxation and breathing exercises or music to reduce the anxiety and distress associated with cancer pain. These techniques may be useful in decreasing muscle tension. In addition, they may serve to distract patients from their pain. Family members can learn these techniques and assist patients in implementing these techniques on an as-needed basis to achieve optimal pain management.

Expected Outcomes

Chronic cancer pain is a multidimensional experience that affects patients' physical, psychological, and social well-being (McGuire, 1992). Therefore, the goals of cancer pain management are to reduce pain and improve patients' level of function. In addition, the achievement of optimal pain control with minimal side effects should improve patients' mood as well as their ability to interact with individuals who are important to their psychological well-being.

Oncology nurses need to remember that unrelieved pain in patients can have deleterious effects on family caregivers (Miaskowski, Kragness, Dibble, & Wallhagen, 1997; Miaskowski, Zimmer, Barrett, Dibble, & Wallhagen, 1997). For example, family caregivers who cared for patients with cancer who had pain reported higher levels of anxiety, depression, fatigue, and caregiver strain, as well as decreased quality of life, compared to family caregivers who cared for pain-free patients with cancer. Nurses need to encourage family caregivers to speak with patients about their pain experience and to work with them to achieve optimal pain management.

Patient Teaching Points

Patient and family caregiver education is the cornerstone of effective cancer pain management (de Wit et al., 2001; West et al., 2003). As noted in the APS and ONS PEP cancer pain guidelines, patients and family caregivers should be given accurate and understandable information about the importance of effective cancer pain management, the use of analgesic medications, other methods of pain relief, and how to communicate effectively with clinicians about unrelieved pain (Miaskowski et al., 2005).

Several studies have shown that patients and family caregivers have numerous myths and misconceptions about cancer pain and its management (de Wit et al., 1997; Yeager, Miaskowski, Dibble, & Wallhagen, 1995, 1997). Patient and family education should clarify myths and misconceptions. In particular, patients and family caregivers should be taught the differences between physical dependence, tolerance, and psychological addiction. They should understand that tolerance and physical dependence are expected to occur with long-term opioid treatment. The presence of tolerance and physical dependence does not equate with psychological addiction.

A pain management diary may be a useful tool to assist patients and family caregivers in evaluating the effectiveness of their pain management plan (Schumacher et al., 2002). Patients and family caregivers can be taught to use the diary data to adjust and titrate their dose of analgesic medication when changes in pain intensity occur. In addition, patients and family caregivers should be taught how to communicate with their clinicians about unrelieved pain. Some patients may benefit from using a script to communicate with their clinician about pain management (Miaskowski et al., 2004; West et al., 2003). Patients and family caregivers should receive a written pain management plan that includes all of the information listed in Figure 19-3.

FIGURE 19-3	**Topics to Include in a Written Pain Management Plan**

1. Information on the cause(s) of the patient's pain
2. Information on the types of analgesic medications prescribed and the purpose of each analgesic medication
3. Instructions for having the analgesic prescriptions filled
4. Specific instructions for how to dose and titrate the analgesic medications and when to expect relief from the analgesic medications
5. Specific instructions for how to manage constipation and other side effects of analgesic medications
6. Instructions on how to store and safely handle analgesic medications
7. Name and phone number of a person to call if pain is not relieved or increases or side effects become intolerable
8. Instructions for how to use nonpharmacologic approaches for pain management

Need for Future Research

Most of the research studies on cancer pain have focused on the epidemiology of persistent pain and BTP and on barriers to effective cancer pain management. In most cases, these studies were descriptive and cross-sectional in nature. Only a limited amount of information is available on the impact of unrelieved pain on patients and family caregivers, as well as on changes in cancer pain over time. Additional longitudinal studies are warranted that document the natural history of chronic cancer pain and the use of analgesic medications.

Most of the pharmacologic management of cancer pain is inferred from studies of other chronic pain conditions (e.g., diabetic neuropathy, postherpetic neuralgia) or is based on clinical experience. Little is known about the factors that predict interindividual differences in responses to specific analgesic medications. Additional research is warranted on optimal approaches to manage opioid-induced side effects. In addition, research is needed to determine the optimal approaches to provide patient and family caregiver education about cancer pain management.

Conclusion of Case Study

A pain score of 7 on a 0–10 scale is considered a pain emergency. S.S. is transferred to the chemotherapy infusion unit to receive IV morphine. In this setting, the nursing staff can monitor S.S., and the patient can have rapid titration of an IV opioid. An initial dose of 5 mg of morphine is administered intravenously. After 15 minutes, the patient rates her pain at 7 and the dose is repeated. In another 15 minutes, the patient states that her pain is at 5, and she receives one additional dose of 5 mg of IV morphine. Fifteen minutes following the third dose of morphine, she rates her pain at 3.

Based on the 15 mg of IV morphine that was required to achieve adequate pain control, the physician prescribes 20 mg of controlled-release morphine twice a day with a dose of 5 mg of immediate-release morphine every one to two hours for BTP. In addition, the patient receives prescriptions for a bowel regimen. The oncology nurse makes a follow-up phone call in 24 hours. The patient reports that her pain is under control and that she slept through the night. The oncology nurse tells her to complete her pain management diary and to return to the outpatient setting in one week to evaluate her analgesic regimen.

Conclusion

Oncology nurses play a central role in helping patients to achieve optimal pain management. The cornerstone of cancer pain management is a comprehensive initial assessment and ongoing assessments that evaluate the effectiveness of the pain management plan in terms of patients' ability to function, their mood, and their quality of life. Patients with cancer and their family caregivers require education on how to titrate their analgesics to achieve optimal pain control and how to manage the side effects of analgesic medications. Finally, oncology nurses need to encourage patients to incorporate nonpharmacologic interventions into their pain management plan.

References

Aiello-Laws, L.B., Delzer, N.A., Peterson, M.E., & Reynolds, J.K. (2007). *Putting evidence into practice: Pain.* Pittsburgh, PA: Oncology Nursing Society.

Anderson, K.O., Richman, S.P., Hurley, J., Palos, G., Valero, V., Mendoza, T.R., et al. (2002). Cancer pain management among underserved minority outpatients: Perceived needs and barriers to optimal control. *Cancer, 94*(8), 2295–2304.

Backonja, M. (2003). Anticonvulsants for the treatment of neuropathic pain syndromes. *Current Pain and Headache Reports, 7*(1), 39–42.

Backonja, M.M. (2002). Use of anticonvulsants for treatment of neuropathic pain. *Neurology, 59*(5, Suppl. 2), S14–S17.

Bernabei, R., Gambassi, G., Lapane, K., Landi, F., Gatsonis, C., Dunlop, R., et al. (1998). Management of pain in elderly patients with cancer. SAGE Study Group. Systematic Assessment of Geriatric Drug Use via Epidemiology. *JAMA, 279*(23), 1877–1882.

Burrows, M., Dibble, S.L., & Miaskowski, C. (1998). Differences in outcomes among patients experiencing different types of cancer-related pain. *Oncology Nursing Forum, 25*(4), 735–741.

Burton, A.W., Fanciullo, G.J., Beasley, R.D., & Fisch, M.J. (2007). Chronic pain in the cancer survivor: A new frontier. *Pain Medicine, 8*(2), 189–198.

Caraceni, A., & Portenoy, R.K. (1999). An international survey of cancer pain characteristics and syndromes. IASP Task Force on Cancer Pain. International Association for the Study of Pain. *Pain, 82*(3), 263–274.

Cherny, N., Ripamonti, C., Pereira, J., Davis, C., Fallon, M., McQuay, H., et al. (2001). Strategies to manage the adverse effects of oral morphine: An evidence-based report. *Journal of Clinical Oncology, 19*(9), 2542–2554.

Cleeland, C.S., Gonin, R., Hatfield, A.K., Edmonson, J.H., Blum, R.H., Stewart, J.A., et al. (1994). Pain and its treatment in outpatients with metastatic cancer. *New England Journal of Medicine, 330*(9), 592–596.

De Conno, F., Groff, L., Brunelli, C., Zecca, E., Ventafridda, V., & Ripamonti, C. (1996). Clinical experience with oral methadone administration in the treatment of pain in 196 advanced cancer patients. *Journal of Clinical Oncology, 14*(10), 2836–2842.

Deimling, G.T., Bowman, K.F., & Wagner, L.J. (2007). The effects of cancer-related pain and fatigue on functioning of older adult, long-term cancer survivors. *Cancer Nursing, 30*(6), 421–433.

de Wit, R., van Dam, F., Loonstra, S., Zandbelt, L., van Buuren, A., van der Heijden, K., et al. (2001). Improving the quality of pain treatment by a tailored pain education programme for cancer patients in chronic pain. *European Journal of Pain, 5*(3), 241–256.

de Wit, R., van Dam, F., Zandbelt, L., van Buuren, A., van der Heijden, K., Leenhouts, G., et al. (1997). A pain education program for chronic cancer pain patients: Follow-up results from a randomized controlled trial. *Pain, 73*(1), 55–69.

Dworkin, R.H., O'Connor, A.B., Backonja, M., Farrar, J.T., Finnerup, N.B., Jensen, T.S., et al. (2007). Pharmacologic management of neuropathic pain: Evidence-based recommendations. *Pain, 132*(3), 237–251.

Fine, P.G., & Portenoy, R.K. (2007). *A clinical guide to opioid analgesia.* New York: Vendome Group, LLC.

Gomez-Batiste, X., Porta-Sales, J., Pascual, A., Nabal, M., Espinosa, J., Paz, S., et al. (2007). Catalonia WHO palliative care demonstration project at 15 years (2005). *Journal of Pain and Symptom Management, 33*(5), 584–590.

Gordon, D.B. (2006). Oral transmucosal fentanyl citrate for cancer breakthrough pain: A review. *Oncology Nursing Forum, 33*(2), 257–264.

Goudas, L.C., Bloch, R., Gialeli-Goudas, M., Lau, J., & Carr, D.B. (2005). The epidemiology of cancer pain. *Cancer Investigation, 23*(2), 182–190.

Jacox, A., Carr, D.B., Payne, R., Berde, C.B., Breitbart, W., Cain, J.M., et al. (1994). *Management of cancer pain* [Clinical Practice Guideline No. 9. AHCPR Publication No. 94-0592]. Rockville, MD: Agency for Health Care Policy and Research, U.S. Department of Health and Human Services, Public Health Service.

Kannarkat, G., Lasher, E.E., & Schiff, D. (2007). Neurologic complications of chemotherapy agents. *Current Opinion in Neurology, 20*(6), 719–725.

Knotkova, H., & Pappagallo, M. (2007). Adjuvant analgesics. *Anesthesiology Clinics, 25*(4), 775–786.

Kushel, M.B., & Miaskowski, C. (2006). End-of-life care for homeless patients: "She says she is there to help me in any situation". *JAMA, 296*(24), 2959–2966.

Mao, J.J., Armstrong, K., Bowman, M.A., Xie, S.X., Kadakia, R., & Farrar, J.T. (2007). Symptom burden among cancer survivors: Impact of age and comorbidity. *Journal of American Board of Family Medicine, 20*(5), 434–443.

Matthews, E.A., & Dickenson, A.H. (2001). Effects of spinally delivered N- and P-type voltage-dependent calcium channel antagonists on dorsal horn neuronal responses in a rat model of neuropathy. *Pain, 92*(1–2), 235–246.

McGuire, D.B. (1992). Comprehensive and multidimensional assessment and measurement of pain. *Journal of Pain and Symptom Management, 7*(5), 312–319.

McNicol, E., Horowicz-Mehler, N., Fisk, R.A., Bennett, K., Gialeli-Goudas, M., Chew, P.W., et al. (2003). Management of opioid side effects in cancer-related and chronic noncancer pain: A systematic review. *Journal of Pain, 4*(5), 231–256.

McNicol, E.D., Strassels, S.A., Goudas, L., Lau, J., & Carr, D.B. (2005). NSAIDS or paracetamol, alone or combined with opioids, for cancer pain. *Cochrane Database of Systematic Reviews* 2005, Issue 2. Art. No.: CD005180. DOI: 10.1002/14651858.CD005180.

Mercadante, S. (2007). Opioid titration in cancer pain: A critical review. *European Journal of Pain, 11*(8), 823–830.

Mercadante, S., & Bruera, E. (2006). Opioid switching: A systematic and critical review. *Cancer Treatment Reviews, 32*(4), 304–315.

Mercadante, S., Villari, P., Ferrera, P., & Casuccio, A. (2006). Opioid-induced or pain relief-reduced symptoms in advanced cancer patients? *European Journal of Pain, 10*(2), 153–159.

Miaskowski, C., Cleary, J., Burney, R., Coyne, P., Finley, R., Foster, R., et al. (2005). *Guideline for the management of cancer pain in adults and children* (APS Clinical Practice Guidelines Series, No. 3). Glenview, IL: American Pain Society.

Miaskowski, C., Dodd, M., West, C., Schumacher, K., Paul, S.M., Tripathy, D., et al. (2004). Randomized clinical trial of the effectiveness of a self-care intervention to improve cancer pain management. *Journal of Clinical Oncology, 22*(9), 1713–1720.

Miaskowski, C., Kragness, L., Dibble, S., & Wallhagen, M. (1997). Differences in mood states, health status, and caregiver strain between family caregivers of oncology outpatients with and without cancer-related pain. *Journal of Pain and Symptom Management, 13*(3), 138–147.

Miaskowski, C., Zimmer, E.F., Barrett, K.M., Dibble, S.L., & Wallhagen, M. (1997). Differences in patients' and family caregivers' perceptions of the pain experience influence patient and caregiver outcomes. *Pain, 72*(1–2), 217–226.

Mols, F., Coebergh, J.W., & van de Poll-Franse, L.V. (2007). Health-related quality of life and health care utilisation among older long-term cancer survivors: A population-based study. *European Journal of Cancer, 43*(15), 2211–2221.

Poleshuck, E.L., Katz, J., Andrus, C.H., Hogan, L.A., Jung, B.F., Kulick, D.I., et al. (2006). Risk factors for chronic pain following breast cancer surgery: A prospective study. *Journal of Pain, 7*(9), 626–634.

Portenoy, R.K., Payne, D., & Jacobsen, P. (1999). Breakthrough pain: Characteristics and impact in patients with cancer pain. *Pain, 81*(1–2), 129–134.

Potter, M.B. (2005). NSAIDs alone or with opioids as therapy for cancer pain. *American Family Physician, 72*(3), 436–437.

Rannestad, T., & Skjeldestad, F.E. (2007). Pain and quality of life among long-term gynecological cancer survivors: A population-based case-control study. *Acta Obstetricia et Gynecologica Scandinavica, 86*(12), 1510–1516.

Ross, J.R., Riley, J., Quigley, C., & Welsh, K.I. (2006). Clinical pharmacology and pharmacotherapy of opioid switching in cancer patients. *Oncologist, 11*(7), 765–773.

Saarto, T., & Wiffen, P.J. (2007). Antidepressants for neuropathic pain. *Cochrane Database of Systematic Reviews* 2007, Issue 4. Art. No.: CD005454. DOI: 10.1002/14651858.CD005454.pub2.

Schumacher, K.L., Koresawa, S., West, C., Dodd, M., Paul, S.M., Tripathy, D., et al. (2002). The usefulness of a daily pain management diary for outpatients with cancer-related pain. *Oncology Nursing Forum, 29*(9), 1304–1313.

Sindrup, S.H., Otto, M., Finnerup, N.B., & Jensen, T.S. (2005). Antidepressants in the treatment of neuropathic pain. *Basic Clinical and Pharmacologic Toxicology, 96*(6), 399–409.

Smith, H.S. (2009). Potential analgesic mechanisms of acetaminophen. *Pain Physician, 12*(1), 269–280.

Stevens, P.E., Dibble, S.L., & Miaskowski, C. (1995). Prevalence, characteristics, and impact of postmastectomy pain syndrome: An investigation of women's experiences. *Pain, 61*(1), 61–68.

Swarm, R., Anghelescu, D.L., Benedetti, C., Boston, B., Cleeland, C., Coyle, N., et al. (2007). Adult cancer pain. *Journal of the National Comprehensive Cancer Network, 5*(8), 726–751.

Valeberg, B.T., Rustoen, T., Bjordal, K., Hanestad, B.R., Paul, S., & Miaskowski, C. (2008). Self-reported prevalence, etiology, and characteristics of pain in oncology outpatients. *European Journal of Pain, 12*(5), 582–590.

Visovsky, C., Collins, M., Abbott, L., Aschenbrenner, J., & Hart, C. (2007). Putting evidence into practice: Evidence-based interventions for chemotherapy-induced peripheral neuropathy. *Clinical Journal of Oncology Nursing, 11*(6), 901–913.

Ward, S.E., Goldberg, N., Miller-McCauley, V., Mueller, C., Nolan, A., Pawlik-Plank, D., et al. (1993). Patient-related barriers to management of cancer pain. *Pain, 52*(3), 319–324.

West, C.M., Dodd, M.J., Paul, S.M., Schumacher, K., Tripathy, D., Koo, P., et al. (2003). The PRO-SELF©: Pain Control Program—An effective approach for cancer pain management. *Oncology Nursing Forum, 30*(1), 65–73.

Yeager, K.A., Miaskowski, C., Dibble, S.L., & Wallhagen, M. (1995). Differences in pain knowledge and perception of the pain experience between outpatients with cancer and their family caregivers. *Oncology Nursing Forum, 22*(8), 1235–1241.

Yeager, K.A., Miaskowski, C., Dibble, S., & Wallhagen, M. (1997). Differences in pain knowledge in cancer patients with and without pain. *Cancer Practice, 5*(1), 39–45.

Zeppetella, G. (2008). Opioids for cancer breakthrough pain: A pilot study reporting patient assessment of time to meaningful pain relief. *Journal of Pain and Symptom Management, 35*(5), 563–567.

Zeppetella, G., O'Doherty, C.A., & Collins, S. (2000). Prevalence and characteristics of breakthrough pain in cancer patients admitted to a hospice. *Journal of Pain and Symptom Management, 20*(2), 87–92.

Zeppetella, G., & Ribeiro, M.D. (2002). Episodic pain in patients with advanced cancer. *American Journal of Hospice and Palliative Care, 19*(4), 267–276.

Zeppetella, G., & Ribeiro, M.D. (2006). Opioids for the management of breakthrough (episodic) pain in cancer patients. *Cochrane Database of Systematic Reviews* 2006, Issue 1. Art. No.: CD004311. DOI: 10.1002/14651858.CD004311.pub2.

CHAPTER 20

Peripheral Neuropathy

Barbara A. Biedrzycki, MSN, CRNP, AOCNP®

Case Study

A.M. is a 55-year-old woman who was diagnosed with multiple myeloma last year. During first-line therapy with vincristine, doxorubicin, and dexamethasone, she became partially disabled. A.M. was unable to work outside the home, mainly because of significant disease- and treatment-related fatigue. Although she was too fatigued for strenuous work, she was able to continue to help raise her three school-aged grandchildren. In addition to the fatigue, she had developed mild peripheral neuropathy. She considered the peripheral neuropathy to be more of a minimal nuisance than a side effect of therapy. In fact, she never mentioned the numbness and tingling in her feet to her oncologist, and he never asked. A.M. did not tell her oncology nurse about the peripheral neuropathy because it did not seem as important as learning effective strategies to manage the fatigue. A.M. wanted to get the most out of her limited time with her oncology nurse.

A.M.'s oncologist recommended a clinical trial using a combination of thalidomide and an investigational product. When the oncology research nurse met with A.M. during the consenting process, A.M. realized for the first time what a devastating symptom peripheral neuropathy could be. The oncology research nurse explained what peripheral neuropathy was. She educated A.M. on how participating in the clinical trial could worsen the mild existing numbness and tingling in her feet and may even cause new presentations of peripheral neuropathy. The oncology research nurse explained that the research product dose may need to be reduced or stopped if the peripheral neuropathy worsens.

Overview

Peripheral neuropathy is a collective term used to name neurologic dysfunctions that occur outside of the brain and spinal cord. These peripheral neuropathies can have different etiologies, symptoms, and prognoses. Some may mistakenly consider peripheral neuropathy to refer only to abnormalities affecting the fingers and toes. Although numbness and tingling of the fingers and toes is the most common peripheral neuropathy, the term *peripheral neuropathy* refers to many symptoms that can affect any body part that is innervated by peripheral nerves. Peripheral neuropathy is a complex symptom because it can have so many different etiologies and manifestations.

Patients with cancer are at risk for the development of peripheral neuropathy caused by the cancer, the treatment, or both. For example, lytic lesions and amyloid deposits, common manifestations of multiple myeloma, may cause people to be more susceptible to developing peripheral neuropathy. In other cancers, solid tumors may cause neuropathic pain by pressing on nearby nerves. The anticancer treatments administered may compound the increased risk of developing peripheral neuropathy from the cancer itself. Research and clinical experience have identified the anticancer treatments that cause peripheral neuropathy. The categories of anticancer drugs that can cause peripheral neuropathy include the following (Rosson, 2006; Wickham, 2007).

- Epothilones
- Platinum analogs
- Proteasome inhibitors
- Sedative hypnotics
- Taxanes
- Vinca alkaloids

Ten percent to 100% of patients treated with anticancer therapies known to confer an increased risk for peripheral neuropathy develop the condition (Bakitas, 2007).

Peripheral neuropathy can cause pain, as well as changes in dexterity, ambulation, and bodily functions, which can lead to safety issues and a diminished quality of life. For example, individuals with peripheral disease may have an increased risk of falling because of altered perception of the location and movement of their feet. Peripheral neuropathy can affect patients' abilities to independently care for personal needs such as dressing and hygiene.

Definition

Peripheral neuropathy literally means disease of the nerves outside of the brain and spinal cord, the two components of the central nervous system. Figure 20-1 lists characteristics of chemotherapy-induced peripheral neuropathy. Peripheral neuropathy can be inherited or acquired. Inherited peripheral neuropathy is the result of genetic miscoding or mutations. The most common inherited neurology disorder is Charcot-Marie-Tooth disease, named after the three physicians who discovered the disease in 1886. Charcot-Marie-Tooth disorders progress slowly, deteriorating peripheral nerves and causing a loss of muscle and sensory function in the extremities (Charcot-Marie-Tooth Association, n.d.; Shy et al., 2008). The literature has not demonstrated an association between inherited peripheral neuropathy and cancer.

FIGURE 20-1	Characteristics of Chemotherapy-Induced Peripheral Neuropathy

Sensory Symptoms
- Paresthesia
- Hyperesthesia
- Hypoesthesia
- Dysesthesia
- Pain
- Numbness and tingling
- Hyporeflexia or areflexia
- Diminished or absent proprioception
- Diminished or absent vibratory sensation
- Diminished or absent cutaneous sensation
- Diminished or absent sense of discrimination between sharp and dull

Motor Symptoms
- Weakness
- Gait disturbance
- Balance disturbance
- Difficulty with fine motor skills

Autonomic Symptoms
- Constipation
- Urinary retention
- Sexual dysfunction
- Blood pressure alterations

Note. From "Putting Evidence Into Practice®: Evidence-Based Interventions for Chemotherapy-Induced Peripheral Neuropathy," by C. Visovsky, M. Collins, L. Abbott, J. Aschenbrenner, and C. Hart, 2007, *Clinical Journal of Oncology Nursing, 11*(6), p. 902. Copyright 2007 by Oncology Nursing Society. Reprinted with permission.

Common causes of acquired peripheral neuropathy include trauma caused by environmental, human, or chemical injury; bacterial and viral infections, such as the bacterium *Borrelia burgdorferi* that causes Lyme disease, and the herpes viruses that cause herpes zoster and herpes simplex infections; autoimmune disorders such as acquired immunodeficiency; systemic diseases, including diabetes, kidney disease, alcoholism, vitamin deficiencies, vascular damage, and blood diseases; and cancer and anticancer treatments (National Institute of Neurological Disorders and Stroke, 2008). Sometimes the etiology of peripheral neuropathy is idiopathic in that no cause can be determined. Peripheral neuropathy may be acute or chronic, transient or persistent, mild to severe in intensity, hardly noticeable to disabling. Painful neuropathy may be worse at night, causing disrupted sleep and resulting in daytime fatigue and dysphoric mood (Bakitas, 2007).

Incidence

An analysis of adults aged 40 and older, excluding those with a history of cerebrovascular attacks or strokes, found that 9% of the sample without diabetes, 21.5% of those with undiagnosed diabetes, and 19.2% of the patients diagnosed with diabetes had a positive sign of peripheral neuropathy (Koopman et al., 2006). Patients who have cancer may be more prone than the general population to the development of peripheral neuropathy because of their disease or their cancer treatment. Unfortunately, some cancers, such as multiple myeloma, and their specific treatments, such as bortezomib, thalidomide, and vincristine, all can cause peripheral neuropathy (Blade & Rosinol, 2007; Richardson et al., 2006). More than 80% of patients with multiple myeloma had baseline peripheral neuropathy by clinical examination (83%) and by self-report via surveys (81%) before treatment (Richardson et al.). Peripheral neuropathy at baseline usually is not clinically relevant (Blade & Rosinol). The key term here is *clinically relevant*, meaning the peripheral neuropathy was not severe and did not warrant a clinical action or change in the treatment plan. In Blade and Rosinol's research, those with baseline peripheral neuropathy had a higher incidence of severe peripheral neuropathy when treated with bortezomib compared to those without peripheral neuropathy at baseline. Richardson et al. (2006) found that severe peripheral neuropathy resulted in bortezomib dose reduction in 12% of those affected and in termination of treatment in 5%. Peripheral neuropathy is a devastating symptom to people with cancer, not only because of the disabling sensations and abnormal motor function, but also because peripheral neuropathy may result in reduction, delay, or termination of treatments (Visovsky, Collins, Abbott, Aschenbrenner, & Hart, 2007).

Within the population of people affected by cancer, data regarding the incidence rate of chemotherapy-induced peripheral neuropathy are available and usually are specific for the neurotoxic anticancer agent that is administered. For example, severe peripheral neuropathy (National Cancer Institute Cancer Therapy Evaluation Program [2009] Common Terminology Criteria for Adverse Events [CTCAE] grade 3 or 4) occurs in 30% of patients treated with microtubule-stabilizing agents, such as taxanes and epothilones (Lee & Swain, 2006). Examples of taxanes are docetaxel, paclitaxel, and nab-paclitaxel, and an example of an epothilone is ixabepilone.

Bakitas' (2007) review of 45 clinical trials that conducted clinical research on neurotoxic chemotherapeutic agents found that the incidence rate of peripheral neuropathy was 10%–100%. The wide variance in the incidence rates may be explained by (a) the reporting methods used, (b) dosage and means of delivery, (c) patient factors, including comorbid conditions and age, and (d) the measurement tool used. Standardization of measurement tools and reporting methods may decrease variance for future research.

In the general population, 2 out of every 10 people will develop a type of peripheral neuropathy from varicella zoster (shingles) (National Institute of Allergy and Infectious Diseases [NIAID], 2007). Shingles is caused by the same virus that causes chicken pox. After the acute illness of chicken pox, the virus lies dormant in the nerves until it is reactivated, possibly by a combination of age and immune deficiencies (U.S. Food and Drug Administration [FDA], 2006). A live vaccine, Zostavax® (Merck & Co., Inc.), was recently approved for the prevention, but not the treatment, of herpes zoster. The vaccine is indicated for people older than 60 years of age, because of the increased risk of developing herpes zoster with older age. The vaccine should not be given to people with lymphoma, leukemia, or other cancers that affect the bone marrow or lymphatic systems (Merck & Co., Inc., 2008). Cancer treatment, stress, and the cancer itself, in addition to increased age, may weaken the immune system, thus promoting an increased risk for an outbreak of the herpes-varicella zoster infection.

Risk Factors

Risk factors for cancer treatment–associated peripheral neuropathy include comorbid conditions such as diabetes, alcohol overuse, metabolic imbalances, vitamin B_{12} deficiency, cachexia, HIV, or paraneoplastic syndrome; cancer; older age; and medications. Some anticancer agents are more likely to cause peripheral neuropathy than others (Rosson, 2006; Wickham, 2007). A summary of anticancer agents known to cause peripheral neuropathy and the frequency of the sensory, motor, and autonomic effects can be found in Table 20-1. Factors associated with drug administration also may have an impact on the risk of develop-

TABLE 20-1	**Neurotoxic Anticancer Agents**			
		Effects (+ indicates frequency)		
Class	**Agent**	**Sensory**	**Motor**	**Autonomic**
Epothilones	Ixabepilone			
Platinum analogs	Cisplatin	++		+
	Carboplatin	+		
	Oxaliplatin	+++	+	
Proteasome inhibitors	Bortezomib			
Sedative hypnotics	Thalidomide	++		
Taxanes	Docetaxel	++		
	Nab-paclitaxel	+		
	Paclitaxel	+++	+	++
Vinca alkaloids	Vinblastine	+		
	Vincristine	+++	+	++

Note. Based on information from Abraxis BioScience, 2007; Rosson, 2006; Wickham, 2007; Wilkes & Barton-Burke, 2008.

ing peripheral neuropathy (i.e., cumulative doses, length of infusion, and treatment schedule may affect the onset, duration, or intensity of peripheral neuropathy).

Ixabepilone, an epothilone B analog, is a microtubule stabilizing agent that has a safety profile similar to paclitaxel, yet is 3–20 times more potent (Wilkes & Barton-Burke, 2008). Sensory neuropathy increases with dosing of ixabepilone and resolves when it is no longer administered. In clinical trials, by the fifth cycle, more than half of the patients treated with ixabepilone develop sensory neuropathy, with 3% being moderate to severe (Vahdat, 2008). Cisplatin, carboplatin, and oxaliplatin are examples of first-, second-, and third-generation platinum analogs. These drugs are known for the characteristic distribution of sensory impairment. Numbness and tingling typically occur in the areas that would be covered with gloves and stockings. Prolonged therapy may increase the risk of this chronic sensory impairment, which may resolve months after treatment has stopped. The potential for acute sensory neuropathy also exists with oxaliplatin. Within hours of administration and up to 14 days after administration, an exposure to cold may cause transient abnormal sensations in the hands, feet, throat, and around the mouth (Wilkes & Barton-Burke).

Bortezomib is a proteasome inhibitor that is indicated as treatment for multiple myeloma. In the safety and efficacy studies for Velcade® (Millennium Pharmaceuticals, Inc., 2003), the majority of bortezomib research participants (80%) had mild, preexisting peripheral neuropathy. However, 14% of the research participants developed peripheral neuropathy that affected daily living while receiving bortezomib treatment. When bortezomib was reduced or stopped, the peripheral neuropathy improved or resolved completely in most research participants. Specific guidelines exist regarding bortezomib dosing in the presence of peripheral neuropathy (Millennium Pharmaceuticals, Inc., 2007).

Thalidomide, a hypnotic sedative, had a devastating product development history. From 1956 to 1962, women who took thalidomide to prevent morning sickness and to aid in sleeping gave birth to children with a unique physical deformity known as *phocomelia*. Because of thalidomide, children were born with shortened or absent long bones of the arms, and some had flipper-like hands or feet. Many years later, this tragic side effect was further investigated for its impact on cancer as an antiangiogenesis agent. This side effect did not directly lead to its consideration as an anticancer treatment, but rather thalidomide was reinvestigated while exploring options for anticancer treatment. The same mechanism that prevented adequate growth of the extremities of the fetuses now is used to inhibit new growth of blood vessels in tumors. The peripheral neuropathy associated with thalidomide is reversible if treatment is stopped when the symptom of numbness in the toes or feet is first experienced. However, if treatment continues. Peripheral neuropathy is more likely to be permanent and may progress up the legs.

About half of the people treated with taxanes, such as paclitaxel and docetaxel, can expect transient peripheral neuropathy. Numbness and paresthesias with a glove-and-stocking distribution may be present. A loss of sensation to the positioning of the fingers and toes, known as proprioception, also may occur. The risk for peripheral neuropathy increases if both docetaxel and cisplatin are administered together.

Two vinca alkaloids are extracted from the periwinkle plant: vinblastine and vincristine, and vinorelbine tartrate is a semisynthetic derivative of vinblastine. In addition to progressive peripheral neuropathy from numbness, weakness, and loss of deep tendon reflexes to motor dysfunction, vinblastine and vincristine also may cause central nervous system dysfunction. This may include depression, double vision (diplopia), jaw pain, metallic taste, and vocal cord paralysis (Wilkes & Barton-Burke, 2008). Exogenous and endogenous cytokines associated with cancer therapy (even therapy not typically associated with peripheral neuropathy) may induce peripheral nerve damage when diabetes mellitus is also present (Visovsky, Meyer, Roller, & Poppas, 2008).

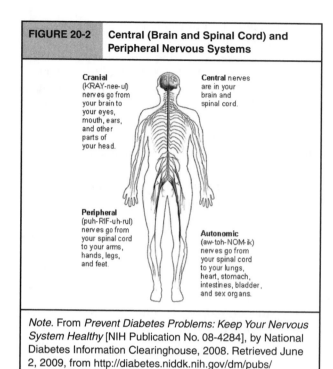

FIGURE 20-2	Central (Brain and Spinal Cord) and Peripheral Nervous Systems

Cranial (KRAY-nee-ul) nerves go from your brain to your eyes, mouth, ears, and other parts of your head.

Central nerves are in your brain and spinal cord.

Peripheral (puh-RIF-uh-rul) nerves go from your spinal cord to your arms, hands, legs, and feet.

Autonomic (aw-toh-NOM-ik) nerves go from your spinal cord to your lungs, heart, stomach, intestines, bladder, and sex organs.

Note. From *Prevent Diabetes Problems: Keep Your Nervous System Healthy* [NIH Publication No. 08-4284], by National Diabetes Information Clearinghouse, 2008. Retrieved June 2, 2009, from http://diabetes.niddk.nih.gov/dm/pubs/complications_nerves.

Pathophysiology

The nervous system is composed of a central (brain and spinal cord) and peripheral nervous system (see Figure 20-2). The peripheral nervous system consists of nerves that are connected to the brain or spinal cord. The peripheral nervous system is composed of (a) 12 pairs of cranial nerves: olfactory, optic, oculomotor, trochlear, trigeminal, abducens, facial, auditory, glossopharyngeal, vagus, spinal accessory, and hypoglossal; (b) a total of 31 spinal nerves: 8 cervical, 12 thoracic, 5 lumbar, 5 sacral, and 1 coccygeal; and (c) the corresponding dermatomes. The three types of peripheral nerves are sensory, motor, and autonomic. When the nerve impulses leave the spinal column and brain, they can innervate or activate various functions, including sensory (normal or abnormal sensations of pain, spatial positioning, temperature, responses to vibration and touch); motor or muscle (hyperactive, hypoactive, or absent activity, responses, or reflexes); or autonomic (involuntary and semivoluntary activities such as heart rate, blood pressure, sweating, urinary retention, pupil size, constipation, or diarrhea).

The nervous system is complex in its normal physiology. It involves a closed loop system of processing data from the afferent (the sensory component) and efferent (the motor component) nerves through the central nervous system back to the motor, sensory, and autonomic neurons that cause sensations, movement, and bodily functions. Although the nervous system is complicated under normal conditions, it is even more challenging when the effects of chemotherapy, disease, or other factors alter normal neurologic function. Peripheral nerves carry essential sensory and motor information back and forth from the brain and spinal cord to every part of the body (National Institute of Neurological Disorders and Stroke, 2008). The pathophysiology of peripheral neuropathy is not well understood (Rosson, 2006). Chemotherapy can damage the peripheral nerve fibers and, therefore, diminish or ablate completely the motor and sensory function associated with peripheral nerves because, in part, the electrical message does not travel well over damaged nerve fibers.

Exactly how chemotherapy nerve damage occurs is not well understood. It is thought that chemotherapy may first damage sensory axons that, in turn, cause the destruction of other axons and their myelin sheaths. The distal ends of the longest axons, those that are in the toes, often are the first affected by chemotherapy-induced peripheral neuropathy. However, peripheral neuropathy can start for some patients in their hands first. Typically, as peripheral neuropathy worsens, the dysfunction proceeds from the toes through the feet and up the legs; similar reactions can occur in the fingers, hands, and arms. In most cases, the damaged axons may be repaired if the offending agent, the chemotherapy, is stopped. This process is not well understood either but may be related to a substance called nerve growth factor (Wickham, 2007).

Characteristics of Peripheral Neuropathy

The diversity within the pathology of peripheral neuropathy leads to multiple symptoms or characteristics (see Figure 20-1). For example, the patient may have a diminished sensation (hypesthesia), increased sensation (hyperesthesia), or abnormal response to a temperature change (dysesthesia) or a touch sensation in response to a stimulus within the fingers, hands, toes, or feet. These sensations also may be experienced without an external stimulus such as touch or temperature changes.

Occasionally, people with peripheral neuropathy experience a loss of the sense of position of their feet and hands (proprioception). To compensate, patients may frequently watch their feet as they are walking. Although this compensation method works well for most, oncology nurses should advise patients to look up frequently to avoid accidents.

Bakitas' (2007) qualitative research study described the experience of peripheral neuropathy as a "constant drone." Half of the research participants did not recall being told to expect peripheral neuropathy as a side effect of the cancer treatment. The researchers also found that patients sometimes confused peripheral neuropathy with other symptoms.

Autonomic symptoms of constipation, urinary retention, sexual dysfunction, and blood pressure alterations also are manifestations of peripheral neuropathy. It is important to ask the patient about bowel and bladder problems in the recent past. See the section on history taking for further information.

Knowing the location and details of specific characteristics may lead to identifying the etiology of the peripheral neuropathy (see Table 20-2). In addition, knowing that a patient has been treated with certain neurotoxic drugs can guide the patient education plan to prepare the patient for potential treatment-related reactions. This proactive education could divert social withdrawal and a diminished quality of life. Lack of knowledge regarding peripheral neuropathy may result in disproportionate fear of the symptom.

Assessment

A three-prong approach to assessment consisting of using measurement tools, obtaining a thorough health history review, and performing a clinical examination, including a full neu-

TABLE 20-2	Characteristics of Various Types of Peripheral Neuropathy		
Type	**Pathology**	**Signs and Symptoms**	**Example**
Mononeuropathy	Individual peripheral nerve	Located at individual nerve distribution	Carpal tunnel syndrome that affects the median nerve
Radiopathy	Peripheral nerve root	Occurs at nerve dermatome and myotome	Varicella herpes zoster
Axonal neuropathy	Longest axons affected first, progresses proximally	Stocking-glove sensory loss of lower or upper extremities	Chemotherapy, paraneoplastic syndrome, diabetes
Sensory neuropathy	Dorsal root ganglion	Disabling, asymmetrical sensory abnormalities	Paraneoplastic syndrome associated with small cell lung cancer, cisplatin

Note. Based on information from Briemberg & Amato, 2007.

rologic assessment, may be the most efficient method to assess baseline peripheral neuropathy and to monitor changes.

During the history, the nurse should inquire about the following.
- Diabetes, alcohol use, vitamin B$_{12}$ deficiency, paraneoplastic syndrome, HIV infections, atherosclerosis, and vascular insufficiency
- Hereditary diseases
- Nutritional status
- Change in vision or hearing
- Gait stability, falls, and tripping
- Dropping things, trouble dressing, difficulty picking up coins
- Pain
- Numbness, tingling, and abnormal sensations in extremities
- Bowel and bladder habits
- Medications, including prescription and over-the-counter medications, herbs, vitamins, and alternative therapies
- Previous cancer therapies
- Daily activities and performance status
- Employment characteristics, such as current status, type of work, and occupational exposures to hazards

While conducting a physical assessment, the nurse should pay particular attention to
- Vital signs—orthostatic changes in heart rate and blood pressure
- Gait evaluation—instability and hugging the wall while walking
- Muscle strength—unequal strength and muscle weakness
- Coordination—speed and accuracy of rapidly alternating hands and touching the nose with finger
- Movement—tremors and spasms
- Deep tendon reflexes (DTRs)—diminished or absent DTRs; the Achilles reflex may be the first DTR to be lost.
- Sensations—abnormal responses to sharp and dull pain, vibration, position, temperature, and touch.

Tests

Neurophysiologic testing, such as nerve conduction tests, electromyography, skin and nerve biopsies, quantitative sudomotor axon reflex tests, and tilt table tests, is available but not widely used in clinical practice to assess peripheral neuropathies (see Table 20-3). These tests, usually conducted by a neurologist, are mainly used in clinical research when determining the critical data for an anticancer agent's safety profile. Because peripheral neuropathy is an expected side effect, and strategies to reduce or minimize the effects of peripheral neuropathy are

TABLE 20-3	Neurologic Tests
Test	**Evaluates**
Nerve conduction studies	Nerve transmission of electric stimuli
Electromyography	Electric activity within muscle
Skin biopsy	Loss of epidermal nerve fibers (small fiber neuropathy)
Quantitative sudomotor axon reflex test	Autonomic nerve fibers that stimulate sweating
Tilt table test	Autonomic nerve involvement; changes in blood pressure and pulse
Nerve biopsy	Vasculitis; inflammation; demyelination; amyloid deposits

well known, most patients with peripheral neuropathy in the clinic setting are not evaluated by a neurologist. Early peripheral neuropathy is not likely to be detected with an electromyogram or nerve conduction tests (Rosson, 2006).

Oncology nurses can use simple tools, such as a paperclip, reflex hammer, tuning fork, pencil, cotton ball, and filament, to obtain objective measurements of peripheral neuropathy. Table 20-4 provides details regarding how to perform objective measurements and what type of nerve fibers are being tested (Visovsky et al., 2008). An opened paperclip also can be used for the sharp-versus-dull discrimination test. The end of the paperclip is the sharp end, and the bend of the paperclip is the dull tool.

TABLE 20-4   Objective Measures of Neuropathy

Assessment	Nerve Fibers Tested	Procedure	Tool(s)
Semmes-Weinstein monofilaments	Small	With the patient's eyes closed, apply the finest filament perpendicularly to specified locations on each hand and foot in a three-second sequence. Instruct the patient to note when the filament is felt. If the filament is not felt at a specific location after two attempts, the next-largest monofilament is used for testing.	
Vibration sensation	Large	Strike a 128 Hz tuning fork with the heel of the hand and hold stem to a bony surface of the index finger or great toe moving from distal to proximal areas if no vibration is felt.	
Sharp-versus-dull sensation	Large	Two objects are used, one sharp and the other dull or soft. As each object is randomly applied to different areas on the extremities, the patient states whether the sensation felt is sharp or dull.	
Deep tendon reflexes	Large	A reflex hammer is used to strike the Achilles and patellar tendon. After the strike of the hammer, a quick reflex resulting in plantar flexion of the foot and extension of the leg results. Reflexes are graded from 0 (absent) to 4 (enhanced).	
Proprioception	Large	Testing of proprioception can include several tests that relate to balance and coordination. Such tests include the Romberg test, up/down test, finger-to-nose test, and thumb-to-finger test.	

Note. From "Evaluation and Management of Peripheral Neuropathy in Diabetic Patients With Cancer," by C. Visovsky, R. Meyer, J. Roller, and M. Poppas, 2008, *Clinical Journal of Oncology Nursing, 12*(2), p. 245. Copyright 2008 by Oncology Nursing Society. Reprinted with permission.

Grading

Several grading systems are available to assess peripheral neuropathy. These include the Eastern Cooperative Oncology Group (ECOG) system, NCI CTCAE, and the Total Neuropathy Score (TNS) (see Table 20-5). Having a plethora of assessment tools can be a challenge rather than an advantage. Grades are not equivalent across the various tools, and because the grading categories are not clearly defined, different clinicians may have different assessments of the same patient. For example, a small study of two neurologists who assessed 37 patients using four measurement tools demonstrated that they were not grading similarly

TABLE 20-5	Comparison of Three Grading Tools for Peripheral Neuropathy			
Tool	**Grade 1**	**Grade 2**	**Grade 3**	**Grade 4**
Eastern Cooperative Oncology Group				
Motor	Subjective weakness; no objective findings	Mild objective weakness without significant impairment of function	Objective weakness with impairment of function	Paralysis
Sensory	Mild paresthesias; loss of deep tendon reflexes	Mild or moderate objective sensory loss; moderate paresthesias	Severe objective sensory loss or paresthesias that interfere with function	–
National Cancer Institute Common Terminology Criteria for Adverse Events				
Motor	Asymptomatic; clinical or diagnostic observations only; intervention not indicated	Moderate symptoms; limiting instrumental ADL	Severe symptoms; limiting self-care ADL; assistive device indicated	Life threatening consequences; urgent intervention indicated
Sensory	Asymptomatic; loss of deep tendon reflexes or paresthesia	Moderate symptoms; limiting instrumental ADL	Severe symptoms; limiting self-care ADL	Life-threatening consequences; urgent intervention indicated
Total Neuropathy Score				
Motor	Slightly difficult	Moderate difficulty	Requires help/assistance	Paralysis
Sensory	Symptoms limited to fingers or toes	Symptoms extend to ankle or wrist	Symptoms extend to knee or elbow	Symptoms above knees or elbows or functionally disabling
Number of autonomic symptoms	1	2	3	4 or 5

ADL—activities of daily living
Note. Based on information from Cavaletti et al., 2007; Eastern Cooperative Oncology Group, n.d.; National Cancer Institute Cancer Therapy Evaluation Program, 2009.

(known as interobserver disagreement) (Posta et al., 1998). Experts critique the most commonly used assessment tools as being too vague, in that the distinctions between the grades are not well defined.

The TNS includes signs and symptoms of peripheral neuropathy, as well as nerve conduction tests. It is critiqued for not including pain severity and for being too burdensome for clinical practice (Smith, Beck, & Cohen, 2008). A reduced version of the TNS (TNSr) omits the neurophysiologic testing of the amplitudes of the sural nerve sensory action potential and peroneal nerve compound muscle action potential. These tests usually are performed by neurologists. Psychometric testing of TNSr indicated that it correlated well with NCI CTCAE and ECOG scores (Cavaletti et al., 2006). Advocates for the TNS stress that the extra time needed to conduct the TNS is offset by the additional knowledge gained (Cavaletti et al., 2006).

Many clinicians feel that having the patient complete the self-reported tools enhances the evaluation. A major concern of self-reported tools is patient burden. The Functional Assessment of Cancer Therapy/Gynecologic Oncology Group–Neurotoxicity (FACT/GOG-Ntx) questionnaire is a 38-item survey that measures quality of life and includes an 11-item neurotoxicity subscale (FACT/GOG-Ntx subscale) that measures the domains of sensory, hearing, and motor function and dysfunction. It was designed to measure platinum/paclitaxel-induced neurologic symptoms in women with breast cancer on clinical trials. Huang, Brady, Cella, and Fleming (2007) were able to condense the evaluation to a four-item scale that is as reliable as and more efficient than the 11-item scale (see Figure 20-3). Reducing the number of items by 64% while maintaining the quality measurement of platinum/paclitaxel-induced neurotoxicity made the tool more user-friendly.

Although a variety of assessment tools are available, they are underutilized. Many healthcare providers may assess only whether peripheral neuropathy is present or absent. Sweeney (2002) suggested that nurses evaluate patients who are at risk for peripheral neuropathy at every treatment and follow-up visit. An assessment should include a history of risk factors, a review of symptoms, and an assessment of large- and small-fiber peripheral nerve function (Wampler, Hamolsky, Hamel, Melisko, & Topp, 2005). A simple evaluation for adequate large-fiber peripheral nerve function can be accomplished by assessing for a sense of vibration when a vibrating tuning fork is placed over a bony prominence on an extremity, such as a knuckle, and evaluation for a sense of touch by assessing the feeling of a cotton swab lightly brushed against the fingers or toes when the patient's eyes are closed. Small-fiber peripheral nerve function can be assessed by two-point discrimination using a paperclip. The curved end and the tip can provide smooth and sharp sensations. Table 20-4 contains more details on the components of a neurologic examination. Brief noninvasive neurosensitivity testing (two-point discrimination and static and moving pressure thresholds) may be adequate to follow chemotherapy-induced peripheral neuropathy (Rosson, 2006). The extent of vibration reduction from fingers and toes to above the elbows and knees and reduction in or absence of DTRs (ankle reflex was lost first) were early predictors of peripheral neuropathy in a moderately sized study of patients treated with paclitaxel, cisplatin, and ifosfamide (Cavaletti et al., 2004).

FIGURE 20-3	**Four Sensory-Focused Items of the FACT/GOG-Ntx* Subscale**

1. I have numbness or tingling in my hands.
2. I have numbness or tingling in my feet.
3. I feel discomfort in my hands.
4. I feel discomfort in my feet.

* Functional Assessment of Cancer Therapy/Gynecologic Oncology Group–Neurotoxicity

Note. Based on information from Huang et al., 2007.

Shingles is well known for its characteristic sharp, burning pain that may persist for months as painful postherpetic neuralgia (FDA, 2006; NIAID, 2007). Typically an uncomfortable sensation may begin days before the development of the characteristic rash with depressed centers that occur along a dermatome. The prodrome of a sudden unexplained intense discomfort may be a warning symptom that shingles will be appearing in a few days.

Evidence-Based Interventions

The Oncology Nursing Society (ONS) Putting Evidence Into Practice (PEP) Chemotherapy-Induced Peripheral Neuropathy Team conducted an extensive review of the literature of interventions to prevent or reduce the effects of peripheral neuropathy for people with cancer. The project team then provided a critical analysis of the data based on their scientific merit as being evidence-based. Evidence-based analyses enhance real-time application of scientifically sound research, when available, and guide oncology nursing care with expert opinion when research evidence is not available.

The ONS PEP Chemotherapy-Induced Peripheral Neuropathy Team was not able to recommend any intervention to prevent or reduce peripheral neuropathy, nor was it able to provide recommendations that are likely to be effective for nursing practice (Visovsky, Collins, Abbott, et al., 2007). These conclusions were based on the fact that strong evidence to support prophylactic or therapeutic intervention is lacking. The team provided expert opinion on five low-risk interventions that are appropriate quality oncology nursing care (see Figure 20-4).

FIGURE 20-4	Expert Opinion on Peripheral Neuropathy
Educate about and encourage early disclosure of signs and symptoms. Provide personal safety strategies. Teach proper foot care. Teach strategies to prevent autonomic dysfunction.	
Note. Based on information from Visovsky, Collins, Abbott, et al., 2007.	

Expected Outcomes

Neurotoxic drugs impair daily activities and quality of life (Boehmke & Dickerson, 2005). Peripheral neuropathy is not only a daily nuisance that interferes with a person's full enjoyment of life; it may also affect safety. A comprehensive evidence-based review indicated that people with peripheral neuropathy are probably at an increased risk of falling (Thurman, Stevens, & Rao, 2008). However, strong evidence exists to support that a fall within the past year predicts an increased fall risk (Thurman et al.).

Physical therapy may be helpful to alleviate the discomfort associated with peripheral neuropathy and to overcome disabling symptoms. For example, physical therapy may include (a) neurostimulation, (b) muscle strengthening, (c) low-impact exercise, (d) massage, (e) whirlpool therapy, (f) foot-drop prevention, (g) hand exercises, and (h) acupuncture (Armstrong, Almadrones, & Gilbert, 2005; Wickham, 2007). An occupational therapist may offer helpful strategies to maintain or improve functional disabilities. For example, an occupational therapist may provide instructions on the proper use of orthopedic devices to facilitate self-care hygiene. Oncology nurses, through their knowledge of the etiology, symptoms, and treatment options for patients with peripheral neuropathy, have the opportunity to affect the quality of life of patients (Marrs & Newton, 2003).

Patient Teaching Points

Patient education is an important intervention for peripheral neuropathy. In fact, although no strong evidence is available to support any nursing practice interventions, the expert opinion reported in the ONS PEP resource indicates that education and support to preserve patient safety may prevent or reduce the effects of peripheral neuropathy for people with cancer (Visovsky, Collins, Abbott, et al., 2007). Although limited scientific evidence exists to support these interventions, these low-risk interventions were recommended based on clinical practice and experts' recommendations in peer-reviewed publications. Five areas for teaching are recommended for the oncology nurse to provide to the patient (Visovsky, Collins, Abbott, et al., 2007).

1. Promptly report signs and symptoms of peripheral neuropathy.
2. Practice safety by removing trip hazards, using visual guidance to accompany movement, using skid-free mats while bathing and showering, and using assistive mobility devices.
3. Provide good foot care by inspecting the feet and wearing properly fitting shoes.
4. Prevent ischemic and thermal burns by lowering hot water heater temperature, testing water with a thermometer before beginning personal hygiene, and looking at the feet and hands for signs of injury.
5. Prevent autonomic dysfunction like postural hypotension, constipation, and urinary retention by dangling legs before standing, eating a high-fiber diet, and drinking adequate fluids.

Patients are more knowledgeable than ever. Those who are treated with neurotoxic anticancer drugs may be aware that cancer therapies may be reduced, delayed, or completely stopped as a result of peripheral neuropathy. This may cause patients to be reluctant to disclose symptoms that are not readily apparent. Nurturing a trusting, therapeutic relationship will promote self-disclosure of symptoms and optimize oncology nursing care.

Peripheral neuropathy is quite different than many of the side effects of cancer treatments. Many of the other side effects have visual confirmations that the patient is experiencing toxicity, whereas peripheral neuropathy is more subtle. Markman (2006) suggested that the sharp contrast between the abrupt treatment-induced emesis and bone marrow suppression and the subtle onset of peripheral neuropathy contributes to peripheral neuropathy being underappreciated and underreported.

Need for Future Research

Although tremendous need exists for all aspects of cancer research, research is especially needed for symptom management. Data outcomes from randomized, controlled clinical trials on symptom management will provide the strongest evidence to support evidence-based practice. As demonstrated by the thorough work of the ONS PEP Chemotherapy-Induced Peripheral Neuropathy Team, a startling lack of adequate evidence exists upon which to base clinical practice for the management of peripheral neuropathy (Visovsky, Collins, Hart, Abbott, & Aschenbrenner, 2007). Without sufficient clinical trials to provide data to support evidence-based practice, the quality of oncology care cannot be ascertained. ClinicalTrials.gov, the most-used cancer registry and search engine to locate federally and privately funded research studies, indicated that as of June 2008, more than 184 clinical trials were open that were studying peripheral neuropathy, and 37 were currently enrolling people with cancer

(National Institutes of Health, n.d.). Clearly, research is ongoing to determine ways to prevent or lessen peripheral neuropathy in patients with cancer, but tremendous need exists for research to help patients to alleviate this debilitating symptom of cancer treatment.

Conclusion of Case Study

Prior to the third cycle of A.M.'s therapy, her oncology nurse notes a change from her previous assessments that were conducted before each treatment. A.M. previously had denied having trouble picking up coins, buttoning her clothes, and tying her shoes, but now she hesitates with her responses and gazes down at her untied shoe. A.M. was reluctant to disclose the changes because she did not want anything to interfere with the proposed treatment plan. A.M. recalled her oncology nurse previously advising her that sometimes the medication needs to be reduced or stopped completely when peripheral neuropathy worsens. A.M.'s oncology nurse senses her anxiety and notes a change in her physical appearance. In addition to the untied shoe, a button on her blouse was not fastened. The oncology nurse provides reassurance that disclosing the signs and symptoms of peripheral neuropathy is very important for A.M.'s overall treatment plan and may prevent severe and permanent complications. A thorough assessment including the protocol-specified peripheral neuropathy assessment tool, a thorough health history review, and a comprehensive physical examination would determine whether it would be safe to continue on the same treatment dose. A.M.'s baseline grade 1 peripheral neuropathy increases, and according to the protocol, the treatment drug is reduced by 25%.

The oncology nurse is aware that education and support to preserve the client's safety are the only recommended nursing practice interventions (Visovsky, Collins, Abbott, et al., 2007). In addition to stressing the importance of promptly sharing signs and symptoms of peripheral neuropathy, she teaches A.M. what she can do to ensure her safety. This includes strategies to prevent falls and protect her extremities. Because A.M. may not be able to sense the position of her feet, she should watch her feet as she walks. The oncology nurse stresses that A.M. should practice this skill in a level area that is free of hazards. She advises that it may take some time for A.M. to become accustomed to looking down at her feet as she also gazes forward. Other safety tips to prevent falls include (a) keeping walkways well lighted, (b) removing scatter rugs, (c) installing hand rails as needed, (d) using assistive mobility devices, and (e) consulting with a physical therapist.

A.M. can adapt strategies used by people with diabetes who have peripheral neuropathy to care for her extremities. She should avoid restrictive shoes and clothing. She should inspect her feet and hands for injuries that may result from pressure, penetrating objects, irritants, and temperature changes. These injuries may occur even without A.M. being aware of them.

Recalling that peripheral neuropathy can cause autonomic dysfunction, in addition to sensory and motor dysfunction, the oncology nurse teaches A.M. how to manage postural hypotension, constipation, and urinary retention. She should dangle her feet before standing, change positions slowly, especially when moving from lying to standing, maintain a high-fiber diet, and drink adequate amounts of fluids. A.M. should report vertigo and imbalance, which could be symptoms of postural hypotension, as well as changes in her bowel and bladder habits, which could be symptoms of constipation and urinary retention.

A.M. understands that the treatment dose reduction is necessary to prevent worsening and permanent peripheral neuropathy. She realizes the importance of reporting the signs and symptoms of peripheral neuropathy. A.M. feels empowered through the education provided to help with the assessment and management of peripheral neuropathy.

Conclusion

Patients may underreport symptoms and minimize the severity of disability associated with peripheral neuropathy. Therapy that is prone to the development or worsening of peripheral neuropathy may be delayed, dose reduced, or stopped completely as a result of reporting of peripheral neuropathy. Patients may stretch their comfort zone and safety limits beyond normal capacities in order to continue with therapy as originally scheduled. Oncology nurses have an essential role to educate patients about peripheral neuropathy and the expectations and value in reporting symptoms. Peripheral neuropathy can be a distressing symptom, causing pain and limiting function. An additional rationale for encouraging full disclosure from patients is to be sure that they understand the expected outcome of their peripheral neuropathy. Some peripheral neuropathy can diminish with treatment modifications or resolve completely after therapy has stopped.

As indicated by the lack of strong scientific evidence supporting interventions to prevent or reduce the effects of peripheral neuropathy for people with cancer, additional research is needed to provide strong evidence for practice. The ONS PEP Chemotherapy-Induced Peripheral Neuropathy Team clearly demonstrated this need. Oncology nurses can help to provide evidence for practice by becoming more involved with scientifically sound clinical research and encouraging patients to participate.

References

Abraxis BioScience. (2007). Abraxane (paclitaxel protein-bound particles for injectable suspension) [Package insert]. Los Angeles: Author.

Armstrong, T., Almadrones, L., & Gilbert, M.R. (2005). Chemotherapy-induced peripheral neuropathy. *Oncology Nursing Forum, 32*(2), 305–311.

Bakitas, M.A. (2007). Background noise: The experience of chemotherapy-induced peripheral neuropathy. *Nursing Research, 56*(5), 323–331.

Blade, J., & Rosinol, L. (2007). Complications of multiple myeloma. *Hematology/Oncology Clinics of North America, 21*(6), 1231–1246.

Boehmke, M.M., & Dickerson, S.S. (2005). Symptom, symptom experiences, and symptom distress encountered by women with breast cancer undergoing current treatment modalities. *Cancer Nursing, 28*(5), 382–389.

Briemberg, H.R., & Amato, A.A. (2007). *Approach to the patient with sensory loss* [UpToDate]. Retrieved June 8, 2008, from http://www.uptodate.com/patients/content/topic.do?topicKey=genneuro/5436&title=Diabetes

Cavaletti, G., Bogliun, G., Marzorati, L., Zincone, A., Piatti, M., Colombo, N., et al. (2004). Early predictors of peripheral neurotoxicity in cisplatin and paclitaxel combination therapy. *Annals of Oncology, 15*(9), 1439–1442.

Cavaletti, G., Frigeni, B., Lanzani, F., Piatti, M., Rota, S., Briani, C., et al. (2007). The Total Neuropathy Score as an assessment tool for grading the course of chemotherapy-induced peripheral neurotoxicity: Comparison with the National Cancer Institute-Common Toxicity Scale. *Journal of the Peripheral Nervous System, 12*(3), 210–215.

Cavaletti, G., Jann, S., Pace, A., Plasmati, R., Siciliano, G., Briani, C., et al. (2006). Multi-center assessment of the Total Neuropathy Score for chemotherapy-induced peripheral neurotoxicity. *Journal of the Peripheral Nervous System, 11*(2), 135–141.

Charcot-Marie-Tooth Association. (n.d.). *An overview of Charcot-Marie-Tooth disorders.* Retrieved May 20, 2008, from http://www.charcot-marie-tooth.org/about_cmt/overview.php

Eastern Cooperative Oncology Group. (n.d.). *ECOG: Common toxicity criteria.* Retrieved June 8, 2008, from http://www.ecog.org/general/ctc.pdf

Huang, H.Q., Brady, M.F., Cella, D., & Fleming, G. (2007). Validation and reduction of FACT/GOG-Ntx subscale for platinum/paclitaxel-induced neurologic symptoms: A Gynecologic Oncology Group study. *International Journal of Gynecological Cancer, 17*(2), 387–393.

Koopman, R.J., Mainous, A.G., Liszka, H.A., Colwell, J.A., Slate, E.H., Carnemolla, M.A., et al. (2006). Evidence of nephropathy and peripheral neuropathy in US adults with undiagnosed diabetes. *Annals of Family Medicine, 4*(5), 427–432.

Lee, J.J., & Swain, S.M. (2006). Peripheral neuropathy induced by microtubule-stabilizing agents. *Journal of Clinical Oncology, 24*(10), 1633–1642.

Markman, M. (2006). Chemotherapy-induced peripheral neuropathy: Underreported and underappreciated. *Current Pain and Headache Reports, 10*(4), 275–278.

Marrs, J., & Newton, S. (2003). Updating your peripheral neuropathy "know-how." *Clinical Journal of Oncology Nursing, 7*(3), 299–303.

Merck & Co., Inc. (2008). Zostavax [Package insert]. Whitehouse Station, NJ: Author.

Millennium Pharmaceuticals, Inc. (2003). Velcade [Package insert]. Retrieved February 6, 2009, from http://www.fda.gov/cder/foi/label/2003/021602lbl.pdf

Millennium Pharmaceuticals, Inc. (2007). Velcade [Package insert]. Cambridge, MA: Author.

National Cancer Institute Cancer Therapy Evaluation Program. (2009). *Common terminology criteria for adverse events* (version 4.0). Retrieved July 29, 2009, from http://ctep.cancer.gov/protocoldevelopment/electronic_applications/docs/ctcaev4.pdf

National Institute of Allergy and Infectious Diseases. (2007, October). *Shingles.* Retrieved May 20, 2008, from http://www3.niaid.nih.gov/topics/shingles/default.htm

National Institute of Neurological Disorders and Stroke. (2008). *NIH peripheral neuropathy conference report.* Retrieved May 20, 2008, from http://www.ninds.nih.gov/news_and_events/proceedings/10_2006_NIH_Peripheral_Neuropathy_Conference.htm#Prelude

National Institutes of Health. (n.d.). *Clinicaltrials.gov.* Retrieved June 8, 2008, from http://clinicaltrials.gov

Posta, T.J., Heimans, J.J., Muller, M.J., Ossenkoppele, G.J., Vermorken, J.B., & Aaronson, N.K. (1998). Pitfalls in grading severity of chemotherapy-induced peripheral neuropathy. *Annals of Oncology, 9*(7), 739–744.

Richardson, P.G., Breimberg, H., Jagganath, S., Wen, P.Y., Ralogie, B., Berenson, J., et al. (2006). Frequency, characteristics, and reversibility of peripheral neuropathy during treatment of advanced multiple myeloma. *Journal of Clinical Oncology, 24*(19), 3113–3120.

Rosson, G.D. (2006). Chemotherapy-induced neuropathy. *Clinics in Podiatric Medicine and Surgery, 23*(3), 637–649.

Shy, M.E., Chen, L., Swan, E.R., Taube, R., Krajewski, K.M., Herrmann, D., et al. (2008). Neuropathy progression in Charcot-Marie-Tooth disease type 1A. *Neurology, 70*(5), 378–383.

Smith, E.M.L., Beck, S.L., & Cohen, J. (2008). The Total Neuropathy Score: A tool for measuring chemotherapy-induced peripheral neuropathy. *Oncology Nursing Forum, 35*(1), 96–102.

Sweeney, C.W. (2002). Understanding peripheral neuropathy in patients with cancer: Background and patient assessment. *Clinical Journal of Oncology Nursing, 6*(3), 163–166.

Thurman, D.J., Stevens, J.A., & Rao, J.K. (2008). Practice parameter: Assessing patients in a neurology practice for risk of falls (an evidence-based review): Report of the Quality Standards Subcommittee of the American Academy of Neurology. *Neurology, 70*(6), 473–479.

U.S. Food and Drug Administration Center for Biologics Evaluation and Research. (2006). *Product approval information—Licensing action: Zostavax questions and answers.* Retrieved May 20, 2008, from http://www.fda.gov/CBER/products/zosmer052506qa.htm

Vahdat, L.T. (2008). Clinical studies with epothilones for the treatment of metastatic breast cancer. *Seminars in Oncology, 35*(2, Suppl. 2), S22–S30.

Visovsky, C., Collins, M., Abbott, L., Aschenbrenner, J., & Hart, C. (2007). Putting evidence into practice®: Evidence-based interventions for chemotherapy-induced peripheral neuropathy. *Clinical Journal of Oncology Nursing, 11*(6), 901–913.

Visovsky, C., Collins, M.L., Hart, C., Abbott, L.I., & Aschenbrenner, J.A. (2007). *Putting evidence into practice: Peripheral neuropathy.* Retrieved June 8, 2008, from http://www.ons.org/outcomes/volume2/peripheral/pdf/ShortCard_peripheral.pdf

Visovsky, C., Meyer, R.R., Roller, J., & Poppas, M. (2008). Evaluation and management of peripheral neuropathy in diabetic patients with cancer. *Clinical Journal of Oncology Nursing, 12*(2), 243–247.

Wampler, M.A., Hamolsky, D., Hamel, K., Melisko, M., & Topp, K.S. (2005). Case report: Painful peripheral neuropathy following treatment with docetaxel for breast cancer. *Clinical Journal of Oncology Nursing, 9*(2), 189–193.

Wickham, R. (2007). Chemotherapy-induced peripheral neuropathy: A review and implications for oncology nursing practice. *Clinical Journal of Oncology Nursing, 11*(3), 361–376.

Wilkes, G.M., & Barton-Burke, M. (2008). *2008 oncology nursing drug handbook.* Sudbury, MA: Jones and Bartlett.

CHAPTER 21

Altered Sexuality Patterns

Patricia W. Nishimoto, RN, DNS, FAAN, and
Debra D. Mark, RN, PhD

Case Study

J.N., a 27-year-old man with stage II testicular cancer, is meeting with the nurse today to receive chemotherapy teaching. J.N. says, "I know that I'm a career man and I'm not going to get married; that's not in my plans. Definitely, I'm not going to have children. This cancer is just a small blip on the radar screen of my life. Besides, the doctor told me that I only need a little surgery and a little chemotherapy and then can go back to my life." The nurse discusses the drugs J.N. is going to receive and the possible side effects, which include infertility. Does the nurse discuss sperm banking, and if so, what is the best way to discuss that option?

Overview

Thirty years ago, cancer was commonly a terminal diagnosis. Today, survivorship is at the forefront of oncology care with an emphasis on quality of life (QOL) (Sideris et al., 2005)—"treating cancer alone is no longer enough" (Alfano & Rowland, 2006, p. 439). According to Hewitt, Greenfield, and Stovall (2006), three of seven essential components identified for successful survivorship care relate to aspects of sexuality: (a) assessment of medical and psychosocial late effects, (b) intervention for consequences of cancer and its treatment, such as sexual dysfunction, and (c) intervention for psychological distress experienced by cancer survivors and their caregivers. More than 45% of patients treated for cancer report changes in sexual function (Baker, Denniston, Smith, & West, 2005), and these changes affect not only the patient but also the partner (Galbraith, Arechiga, Ramirez, & Pedro, 2005; Kadmon, Ganz, Rom, & Woloski-Wruble, 2008). Although sexual dysfunction during cancer treatment can occur and have a negative effect on QOL (Galbraith et al.; Kendirci, Bejma, & Hellstrom, 2006), it does not happen to all who are diagnosed with cancer (Hendren et al., 2005). To more fully realize the nursing role and facilitate patients' QOL, the nurse has the professional responsibility to complete a comprehensive, thorough assessment and to be aware of effective interventions.

To meet the evidence-based challenge of this chapter, the first thought was to include only sexuality-related concerns that have strong evidence-based interventions: erectile dysfunction (ED) and infertility. This approach would have left out three commonly identified concerns of patients—dyspareunia, body image, and changes in libido—as these concerns do not have solid research findings surrounding treatment. Typically, patients ask their nurses about all five concerns; hence, they are all included in this chapter. To avoid repetition, expected outcomes and teaching points common to all five may be found at the end of the chapter.

Erectile Dysfunction

Overview of Symptom

Busy oncology nurses may be tempted to focus on helping men to understand their new diagnosis of cancer and ignore issues of ED. Yet, it is at the moment of diagnosis that many men begin to question how the diagnosis and treatment might affect their sexual function. If sexuality is not directly discussed, nurses may later learn that because of unspoken fears or misunderstanding, their patients selected less-than-optimal treatment (Donatucci & Greenfield, 2006). When men are hesitant to discuss sexual issues with their healthcare team, they may try home remedies to regain erectile function, and those "remedies" can ultimately endanger their health. Selection of less-than-optimal treatment and possible risks of home remedies are two reasons why oncology nurses need to address ED with their patients.

Definition

ED is defined as "consistent or recurring inability of a man to achieve and/or maintain an erection sufficient for satisfactory sexual performance or intercourse" (Kendirci et al., 2006, p. 186). ED is not unique to men diagnosed with cancer. The American Urological Association (2006) estimated that 15–30 million men in the United States have ED. However, it can occur as a result of the diagnosis of or treatments for cancer; therefore, oncology nurses need to have information about ED in order to address patient concerns.

Risk Factors

When a patient complains of ED, the nurse should not automatically assume it is caused by cancer. Non-cancer-related risk factors may affect ED. These risk factors include age; medications (see Figure 21-1); diseases such as diabetes, hypertension, hypogonadism, heart disease, atherosclerosis, and hypercholesterolemia; use of alcohol, tobacco, or recreational drugs; depression; pain; anxiety; fatigue; nerve damage; and cultural or religious beliefs such as the belief that the cancer was caused by past sexual misbehavior and that ED is punishment. Commonly overlooked risk factors for ED concern the health of the partner and/or the partner's interest in sexual activity.

Often, it is not the specific cancer diagnosis that directly affects ED but rather the symptoms surrounding cancer, such as fatigue. Treatment modalities such as radiation therapy, hormone therapy, chemotherapy, or surgery can affect the risk of ED. For example, some surgeries (e.g., retroperitoneal lymph node dissec-

FIGURE 21-1	Medications That Increase Risk of Erectile Dysfunction

- Anticonvulsants
- Antidepressants
- Antihypertensives
- Antipsychotics
- Chemotherapy
- Diuretics
- Hormone therapy
- Lipid regulators
- Opioids
- Tranquilizers

Note. Based on information from American Association of Clinical Endocrinologists, 2003; Ralph & McNicholas, 2000.

tion; rectal, bladder, penile, or prostate surgery) increase the risk of ED. Predictors of erectile function following prostatectomy include the patient's age; the grade, stage, and localization of disease; degree of nerve preservation; preoperative erectile function; and if or when penile rehabilitation is started (Donatucci & Greenfield, 2006; Gonzalgo & Eastham, 2007; Kendirci et al., 2006).

Pathophysiology of Symptom

Why It Happens

To understand ED, knowledge about erection physiology is helpful. The penis is innervated by autonomic nerves. When there is a stimulus, smooth muscle relaxation takes place and blood begins to fill the penis. Erection occurs as blood accumulates in the penis.

ED can occur as a result of physical or psychological reasons. Physiologic reasons include changes because of aging, damage to nerves or venous blood flow, and response to diagnosis or treatment side effects. The pathophysiology of ED caused by aging is morphologic deterioration of the corpus cavernosa, which is the penile tissue that fills with blood during erection. ED may be a consequence of autonomic nerve damage causing less vasocongestion. When nerve-sparing surgery is performed, the cause of immediate post-surgery ED is *neurapraxia*, or surgical trauma to the neurovascular system (Kendirci et al., 2006).

Unlike surgical ED, which can be immediate, ED caused by external radiation therapy (XRT) tends to have a delayed onset because of progressive damage to the cavernosal tissue of the penis. Men seem to better adapt to erection changes following XRT than changes occurring postoperatively because the changes occur progressively over years rather than immediately (Kendirci et al., 2006). The risk of developing ED following XRT is correlated to the dosage received by the bulb of the penis (Ponholzer et al., 2005). Palladium implants have less risk of causing ED, but it is not correlated to the amount of radiation delivered (Ponholzer et al.; Wahlgren, Nilsson, Ryberg, Lennernas, & Brandberg, 2005).

Psychological factors such as anxiety, pain, stress, relationship problems with a partner, decreased sexual self-confidence, or concerns of masculinity can have a dramatic impact on ED. A stigma seems to exist for some men if they think ED is caused by psychological factors. It often is helpful to remind patients that the brain is the most important sexual organ. Using the analogy of how anxiety can increase pain sensation may decrease the man's perceived stigma of psychological reasons causing physiologic effects.

What Causes It

Prostate surgery technique can affect erection. Open surgical techniques versus closed techniques for prostate cancer have different postsurgical recovery consequences on erectile function (e.g., venous leakage following prostatectomy or nerve damage) (Kendirci et al., 2006). Recent research indicates that ED occurring after prostate surgery may not be caused by just damage to nerves or blood flow. Investigators have done penile biopsies and found physiologic changes in the muscle fibers and collagen content that contribute to deterioration of the penile tissue. In addition to postsurgical-induced ED arising from nerve damage or venous leakage, postprostatectomy and penile biopsy indicate changes in the trabecular elastic, smooth muscle fibers, and collagen content, which may be contributing factors in the process of cavernosal fibrosis (deterioration) (Iacono et al., 2005).

In the case of surgical treatment of rectal cancer and risk of erection dysfunction, a total mesorectal excision improves the cure rate, but the pelvic autonomic nerves are at risk (Dyer-Smith, Woodcock, & Hartley, 2006; Matsumoto et al., 2005). In contrast, no relationship has been found between neoadjuvant radiotherapy and increased risk of male sexual dysfunction following surgery for rectal cancer (Dyer-Smith et al.). Surgical treatment such as a radical cystectomy removes the bladder, prostate, seminal vesicles, and proximal urethra, which causes consequent nerve damage and erection dysfunction. Besides surgical causes, hormone and androgen deprivation therapy can cause ED by dramatically reducing testosterone levels.

Psychological factors of anxiety, sleep deprivation, or changes in body image can affect libido and result in lack of blood engorgement of the penis. Psychological or physiologic factors can cause ED; therefore, assessment is vital to determine appropriate treatment options.

Assessment

Subjective Assessment

The most important aspect of assessment of ED is the subjective assessment of the patient himself and the meaning of the ED to him. Figure 21-2 lists questions that the provider can ask the patient when assessing ED.

Laboratory Tests

Testosterone level is often the first consideration by providers. Although testosterone level affects libido and sleep-related erections, no direct correlation is present between testosterone level and erection (Fahmy, Mitra, Blacklock, & Desai, 1999). Controversy exists as to whether testosterone should be tested and, if so, which of the three forms of testosterone to measure. Other tests that are performed include fasting blood sugar, if diabetes is suspected to be causing the ED, and ultrasound to check penile blood flow. Possible tests that may be done but are not routine include nocturnal penile tumescence, cavernosometry to check penile vascular pressure, or cavernosography, in which dye is injected to assess blood flow to the penis. The nurse's role, as with all parts of oncology care, is to help explain the tests and ensure that patients do not have misunderstandings about the tests.

Physical Examination

Providers should conduct the following as part of the physical examination of men who have ED: (a) blood pressure, (b) assessment of femoral and popliteal pulses to ascertain atherosclerotic disease, (c) abdominal examination, (d) examination of genitals for testicular size

FIGURE 21-2	**Areas to Address During Assessment of Erectile Dysfunction (ED)**

1. When was the onset of ED?
2. Did the onset of ED occur in conjunction with a recent death, new medication, job change, or surgery?
3. Is there a pattern to ED (e.g., self-pleasuring, time of day, with a certain partner)?
4. Have the patient describe how the character of erections have changed from a year ago.
5. How is ED affecting the patient's relationship with his partner?
6. Inquire about medical and psychiatric history, looking at possible comorbidities.
7. Ask about patterns of drug use, including prescription medication, alcohol, tobacco, herbal products, and recreational drugs.
8. What things has the patient already tried to improve ED?
9. What is the score on the International Index of Erectile Function Survey or whichever instrument you are using to do an assessment?

Note. Based on information from Ralph & McNicholas, 2000; Rosen et al., 1997; Spark, 2008.

and consistency, (e) penile shaft fibrosis, and (f) foreskin retractability (Ralph & McNicholas, 2000). A neurologic examination is indicated for some depending on their medical history (see Figure 21-3).

Evidence-Based Practice Recommendations

Support of interventions for ED is based on several systematic reviews and synthesis of the literature (American Urological Association, 2006; European Association of Urology, 2006; Ralph & McNicholas, 2000). These guidelines and recent supporting studies are the basis for the recommendations (see Figure 21-4). Six interventions are recommended for practice, and three interventions are considered likely to be effective. The other interventions do not have established effectiveness or are unlikely to work. The national and international guidelines specifically do not include interventions that are not recommended for practice (American Urological Association; European Association of Urology), so these were considered to be not recommended for practice by the chapter authors. The authors recommend that nurses consider it not recommended for practice for patients to discontinue any prescribed medication that they feel may be causing ED or to take any "herbal/folk" treatment unless they have discussed those options with their providers.

When working with patients who have ED, not all nurses will feel comfortable discussing the topic or treatment options. Each nurse should work within his or her comfort level and range of expertise when discussing questions about ED. What is vital is that nurses be aware that these are serious concerns that negatively affect QOL of their patients and need to be addressed. If this is not the nurse's area of comfort, each nurse has the responsibility to validate if it is an important concern and, if so, to refer the patient to the appropriate member of the team who can address the concerns.

FIGURE 21-3	Objective Assessments for Erectile Dysfunction
Physical Examination	**Laboratory/Radiology Tests**
• Genital examination: Testicular size, penile shaft fibrosis, and foreskin retractability • Blood pressure; femoral and popliteal pulses • Abdominal examination • Neurologic examination if indicated by history	• Nocturnal penile tumescence • Fasting blood sugar • Serum testosterone level • Prolactin • Thyroid function

Note. Based on information from Ralph & McNicholas, 2000; Spark, 2008.

Expected Outcomes Specific to Erectile Dysfunction

The patient will be provided with enough information to make an informed decision about optimal treatment options for him. The goal is that the patient will feel comfortable with his decision and will learn to live with the changes in sexual function.

Patient Teaching Points Specific to Erectile Dysfunction

Patient and partner education should include a discussion about the fact that the lack of erection does not mean loss of desire for the partner. It is helpful when both the patient and partner are interested in exploring various options. Because several options are available, nurses need to discuss the pros and cons of each so that the couple can make decisions that best fit their values and lifestyle. Of greater importance is the necessity to assess patients for ED and encourage early intervention to prevent complications such as scarring and fibrosis of erectile tissue.

FIGURE 21-4	Evidence-Based Practice Interventions for Erectile Dysfunction

Recommended for Practice*
- Inform patient and partner of treatment options and associated risks and benefits (American Urological Association [AUA], 2006).
- Oral phosphodiesterase-5 (PDE5) inhibitors are contraindicated in patients taking organic nitrates (AUA, 2006; European Association of Urology [EAU], 2006; Ralph & McNicholas, 2000; Rosen et al., 2007; Stephenson et al., 2005).
- Intraurethral alprostadil (AUA, 2006; EAU, 2006; Ralph & McNicholas, 2000)
- Intracavernous vasoactive drug injection (AUA, 2006; EAU, 2006; Ralph & McNicholas, 2000; Stephenson et al., 2005)
- Vacuum constriction devices (AUA, 2006; EAU, 2006; Ralph & McNicholas, 2000; Raina, Agarwal, et al., 2005; Stephenson et al., 2005)
- Penile prosthesis implantation (Akin-Olugbade et al., 2006; AUA, 2006; EAU, 2006; Ralph & McNicholas, 2000; Ramsawh et al., 2005; Stephenson et al., 2005)

Likely to Be Effective
- Combination therapy (Burnett, 2005; Cavallini et al., 2005; Mydlo et al., 2005; Nandipati et al., 2006; Raina, Agarwal, et al., 2005; Raina, Nandipati, et al., 2005)
- Penile rehabilitation (Kendirci et al., 2006; Madsen & Ganey-Code, 2006; Mulhall et al., 2005)
- Testosterone replacement (American Association of Clinical Endocrinologists, 2003)

Benefits Balanced With Harms
- No interventions at the time of publication

Effectiveness Not Established
- Trazodone hydrochloride (AUA, 2006)
- Testosterone therapy for patients with normal serum testosterone levels (AUA, 2006)
- Yohimbine (AUA, 2006)
- Venous surgery (AUA, 2006; Gontero et al., 2005)
- Psychosexual therapy (AUA, 2006; EAU, 2006; Ralph & McNicholas, 2000)
- Neuroprotective agents (Madsen & Ganey-Code, 2006)

Effectiveness Unlikely
- Arterial surgery (AUA, 2006)

Not Recommended for Practice
- No interventions at the time of publication

*Should be applied in a stepwise fashion (AUA, 2006)

Patient and partner education should include emphasis of certain points as applicable to the individual situation.
- All men following radical prostate surgery will have ED (Madsen & Ganey-Code, 2006).
- Urinary continence occurs before erectile function returns (Kendirci et al., 2006).
- Return of erectile function following surgery takes an average of 18 months to 2 years (Burnett, 2005; Kendirci et al., 2006).
- Combination therapy may be an effective treatment approach (Burnett, 2005; Cavallini, Modenini, Vitali, & Koverech, 2005; Mydlo, Viterbo, & Crispen, 2005; Nandipati, Raina, Agarwal, & Zippe, 2006; Raina, Agarwal, Allamaneni, Lakin, & Zippe, 2005).
- Brachytherapy has less risk for ED, but long-term results are not known (Katz, 2007; Wahlgren et al., 2005).
- Brachytherapy may cause burning with ejaculation; semen may be bloody (Witt, Haas, Marrinan, & Brown, 2003).

- Condoms should be used for four weeks after brachytherapy because radiation seeds could be expelled with ejaculation (Colella & Scrofine, 2004).
- Medications and devices are intended to help with erections, not orgasms, as orgasms are possible without an erection. Medications such as phosphodiesterase-5 (PDE-5) inhibitors can cause priapism, an erection lasting longer than four hours. Priapism may result in permanent damage and requires immediate medical attention when it occurs.
- Open communication about the effectiveness of therapy is key, so that staff can potentially offer other options.
- Discuss safety concerns associated with purchasing medication over the Internet (e.g., PDE-5 inhibitors), taking a pill from a friend, or cutting pills in half, which may result in unequal distribution of the active ingredient.
- Offer suggestions for how to deal with loss of spontaneity when there are interruptions in sexual activity associated with use of an external device (e.g., a vacuum device or an erection ring to trap blood in the penis).
- Describe the safety issues for patients with diabetes or those with circulatory and sensory compromise of using herbal treatments, vacuum devices, "splints," or erection rings that keep blood in the penis to maintain erection.
- Provide written information that may be shared with partners and help to ensure consistency of treatment expectations, as well as where and how to obtain treatments.

Need for Future Research Specific to Erectile Dysfunction

Future studies are needed with respect to physical issues, such as an investigation about the changes that couples make in sexual activity when using an erection aid and the success of such changes (Heiman et al., 2007), as well as psychosocial and QOL issues. Of interest are how men weigh possible sexual outcomes and what factors they consider when making decisions about treatment options (Rosen, Fisher, Beneke, Homering, & Evers, 2007).

Dyspareunia

Definition

For women, *dyspareunia* is the pain experienced during vaginal entry or intercourse. For men, *dyspareunia* is penile pain with vaginal or rectal intercourse.

Risk Factors

The risk of experiencing dyspareunia increases with the types of surgical procedures, such as neovagina creation (surgery to construct a vaginal canal), hysterectomy, cystectomy, or penile or rectal surgery; with aging or menopausal symptoms that result in a decrease of vaginal lubrication; with the use of certain medications (see Figure 21-5); with vaginal ulcers resulting from treatment;

FIGURE 21-5	Medications That Decrease Vaginal Lubrication

- Antidepressants
- Antihistamines
- Antihypertensives
- Birth control pills
- Cancer treatments (e.g., hormone therapy, chemotherapy, aromatase inhibitors)
- Medications to treat urinary tract infection (e.g., antibiotics)
- Medications to treat vaginal infection
- Tranquilizers
- Nicotine

Note. Based on information from Nishimoto, 2008.

or with radiation therapy or laser treatment for penile carcinoma (Windahl, Skeppner, Andersson, & Fugl-Meyer, 2004).

Pathophysiology of Symptom

Why It Happens

The causes of dyspareunia are numerous. Surgery can damage pelvic nerves (e.g., with hysterectomy). Surgical damage to autonomic nerves may lead to less vasocongestion, less lubrication, enlargement of the vagina, and less feeling of the sensation of heat or vibration in the vagina. Blood flow to the vulva, clitoris, and vagina is mediated by nerve roots S2/S3 and the hypogastric plexus autonomic fibers (Styles, MacLean, Reid, & Sultana, 2006). In the case of rectal cancer surgery, the likelihood is 100% that a patient will experience dyspareunia (Hendren et al., 2005).

What Causes It

The physiologic reason for female dyspareunia is vaginal atrophy occurring when the vaginal epithelium thins from decreased estrogen levels. Surgery, aging, or medications may contribute to female gonadal failure, causing vaginal dryness. In the case of aging, approximately 17%–30% of menopausal women have decreased vaginal lubrication. Cancer-related drugs that increase dyspareunia are aromatase inhibitors, chemotherapy, and hormonal manipulation. Aromatase inhibitors have been found to affect vaginal lubrication and libido more than tamoxifen (Mok, Juraskova, & Friedlander, 2008; Morales et al., 2004). If the cancer or its treatments cause weight loss, women may suffer pain because of loss of the fat pad around the mons pubis.

Dyspareunia may be associated with certain types of cancer. Women with advanced, recurrent, or persistent cervical cancer have a greater incidence of decreased vaginal lubrication (Stead, 2004) and are more likely to experience dyspareunia. In addition to cervical cancer, other gynecologic malignancies (e.g., vulvar, uterine, or ovarian cancers) can cause dyspareunia. Men with penile carcinoma are at risk for dyspareunia (Windahl et al., 2004) resulting from the cancer or the side effects of treatment, such as thinning of penile skin from radiation therapy.

Physical causes of dyspareunia include shortened vagina after radiation therapy, surgery that affects innervation to the vagina or vaginal lubrication, scar tissue (contractures), radiation-induced urethral irritation or stenosis, increased sensitivity to vaginal barrel distention, muscle tension, genital infections or ulcers, or treatments that cause thinning of the skin of the penis or vagina. Inflammation, thrush, sexually transmitted diseases, and infections can cause male dyspareunia.

Assessment

Laboratory Tests

Laboratory tests that may help to identify possible causes of dyspareunia include vaginal alkalinity (pH greater than 5); predominance of basal cells in the vaginal wall; fasting blood sugar (diabetes can cause dyspareunia, and treatments that include steroids will affect glucose control); follicle-stimulating hormone (FSH) and luteinizing hormone (LH) to ascertain menopausal status; prolactin, which affects testosterone production; and thyroid function, which can affect energy level. A urinalysis may help to identify if the pain is caused by cystitis or renal calculi rather than dyspareunia. Vaginal blood flow may be measured by vaginal photoplethysmography, oxygenation temperature method, or laser Doppler perfusion imaging (Styles et al., 2006).

Physical Examination

For women, the gynecologic examination should focus on the loss of vaginal rugae; pale, dry vaginal tissue; vaginal ulcers or lesions; submucosal petechial hemorrhages; loss of vaginal elasticity; and shortening of the vaginal barrel (Katz, 2007). Patients receiving steroids or antibiotics are at increased risk for vaginal or penile fungal infections, and immunosuppressive therapy increases the risk of recurrent genital herpes and thinning of vaginal or penile tissue. Examination of the external genitalia includes labia majora, labia minora, and the mons pubis. A rectal examination should be performed because hemorrhoids, anal fissures, and stool impaction may cause dyspareunia. For men, the physical examination should note any lesions or thinning of the penile skin.

Evidence-Based Practice Interventions

Support for interventions for dyspareunia is based on a synthesis of the literature (Amsterdam & Krychman, 2006; Champion et al., 2007; Hendren et al., 2005; Katz, 2007; McCorkle, Siefert, Dowd, Robinson, & Pickett, 2007). See Figure 21-6 for these suggested interventions.

Expected Outcomes Specific to Dyspareunia

The patient will be provided with enough information to make informed decisions about optimal treatment options for dyspareunia. The goal is that the patient will feel comfortable in discussing sexual functioning with the nurse so that interventions can be suggested.

The goals of intervention are that the patient will have either no dyspareunia or reduced dyspareunia. This is intended to increase the patient's perception of QOL. Decreasing or eliminating dyspareunia will decrease the risk of negative changes in body image, sexual satisfaction, and libido. When providing suggestions about interventions for dyspareunia, nurses should ensure that suggestions are presented in a culturally sensitive manner.

Patient Teaching Points Specific to Dyspareunia

Patient and partner education should include a discussion that dyspareunia does not have to be tolerated and may not be permanent. Communication is important not only between partners but also between the patient and the provider so that interventions can be evaluated and changes can be made.

Patients with dyspareunia should be educated about the causes and treatments for dyspareunia, motivated to try the interventions, and taught behavioral skills about using vaginal lubricants, performing Kegel exercises, accessing Web sites, and using vaginal dilators. Discuss the differences between vaginal lubricants and vaginal moisturizers and the rationale for avoiding scented lubricants.

FIGURE 21-6	Evidence-Based Practice Interventions for Dyspareunia

Recommended for Practice
• No interventions at the time of publication

Likely to Be Effective
• Vaginal moisturizers (Barclay & Vega, 2007; Herbenick et al., 2008)
• Vaginal lubricants (Barclay & Vega, 2007; Herbenick et al., 2008)

Benefits Balanced With Harms
• Nerve-sparing surgery[a]
• Nonpharmacologic intervention[b]

Effectiveness Not Established
• Low-dose hormone replacement therapy—local[c]
• Sex therapy (Champion et al., 2007; McCorkle et al., 2007; Sublett, 2007)
• Multimodal therapy that uses medication, sex counseling, and exercises[d]

Effectiveness Unlikely
• Herbals, black cohosh, dietary soy (Reed et al., 2008)

Not Recommended for Practice
• Hormone replacement therapy—systemic[e]
• Topical estrogen[f]

[a] Interventions include nerve-sparing surgery of the hypogastric, splanchnic, and pelvic autonomic nerves (Hendren et al., 2005).
[b] These include changing sexual practices, including positioning, self-pleasuring, and oral or manual stimulation (Katz, 2007); performing Kegel exercises to strengthen the pubococcygeal muscle to relax vaginal muscles; and stopping smoking.
[c] Contraindicated if patient is on aromatase inhibitors because potential for enhanced vaginal absorption of estrogen (Katz, 2007).
[d] Replication studies are needed (Amsterdam & Krychman, 2006).
[e] Not proven safe for women with hormone-dependent tumors (Amsterdam & Krychman, 2006).
[f] Topical estrogen is effective in decreasing vaginal dryness, but safety of use in women with hormone-dependent tumors is not established (Hickey et al., 2008).

Provide specific instructions on the use of a vaginal dilator: Start using dilators within four weeks after completion of therapy; begin with a narrow diameter and increase to a maximum of 1.5 inches; use the dilator daily if possible, but if not, then use it a minimum of three times a week; and use dilators for a minimum of three years (Lancaster, 2004).

Need for Future Research Specific to Dyspareunia

Two areas that require future research include: How does local estrogen therapy affect women after six months of use (Katz, 2007); and what are the typical coping strategies that women with dyspareunia use? Little is known about the risk of cancer caused by continued local estrogen therapy, how it affects the vaginal mucosa, or if it increases the risk of infection. Similarly, little is known about how women cope with dyspareunia, and yet that information is important to nurses who work with these women. Questions about how women cope with dyspareunia would include: Do they avoid sexual situations that affect their relationships? Do they change positions? Do they have decreased libido? How does dyspareunia coping style affect their body image or sexual function?

Altered Body Image

Definition

Altered body image is the discrepancy between the way someone formerly perceived himself or herself and how that individual now sees himself or herself (Pelusi, 2006). Body image affects psychosocial adjustment (Alfano & Rowland, 2006), influences a person's self-worth (Pelusi), and is an important component of QOL (DeFrank, Mehta, Stein, & Baker, 2007).

Risk Factors

People who have poor self-esteem or who are unsatisfied with their body image prior to diagnosis are at risk for experiencing further alterations in body image following a diagnosis of cancer. Body image assessment usually is not performed at the time of diagnosis because the focus is on cancer diagnosis and determination of appropriate treatment. After treatment, a resulting poor body image may be attributed solely to cancer treatment, when it may have been present prior to diagnosis. The significance of body image is indicated by the finding that 47% of healthy women without a diagnosis of cancer were dissatisfied with their body image (Pelusi, 2006; Rosen, Taylor, Leiblum, & Bachmann, 1993). Although body image dissatisfaction may reflect societal and cultural beliefs about beauty and myths about body image and age, healthcare providers need to be aware of these beliefs and myths and their effect on the patient. Studies of male athletes and body image indicate that body image is a concern of healthy men, with the specific finding that men do not feel their body is "muscular enough" (Baum, 2006; Esco, Olson, & Williford, 2006).

The reaction of partners and others also can affect body image (Sheppard & Ely, 2008). People whose partners did not react negatively during the first sexual encounter after surgery had fewer concerns about changes in their body image (Huber, Ramnarace, & McCaffrey, 2006). The lack of understanding of body changes related to aging can further contribute to altered body image and confound patient perceptions and treatments. As adults age, they lose muscle mass and experience changes in skin elasticity (wrinkles, sagging breasts), and pubic hair becomes more sparse. Age, maturity, and developmental stage of the patient affect how the changes are perceived. McCaffrey's (2006) work with children reinforces the value of staff assessing body image and initiation of interventions to prevent or decrease the attendant depressive symptoms and social anxiety that can occur.

Pathophysiology of Symptom

Why It Happens

Multiple factors can cause changes in body image, which is a multidimensional concept (Boehmer, Linde, & Freund, 2007). They include type of cancer diagnosis, precocious puberty (the onset of puberty before age 8 in girls and age 9 in boys), delayed development of secondary sex characteristics, weight changes, alopecia, surgical changes, lymphedema, and scars. It is not necessarily the changes themselves that cause alterations in body image, but how the patient perceives the changes.

What Causes It

The type of cancer and the corresponding treatments have been found to affect body image (Dixon & Dixon, 2006). Specifically, men diagnosed with melanoma, bladder, or colon cancer had less body image satisfaction than did men with prostate cancer (DeFrank et al., 2007).

Chemotherapy, radiation therapy, and hormone therapy may cause delayed development of secondary sex characteristics, delay in menarche, or alopecia (Ng, Kristjanson, & Medigovich, 2006). Weight changes, either a decrease or increase, that affect body image can occur because of anorexia from malignancy, side effects of treatment, and the use of steroids or hormones. Hormone therapy can cause loss of muscle bulk or gynecomastia, affect penis size, and cause fatigue, which can interfere with the image of oneself as a strong, self-sufficient individual (Ng et al.). The incidence of gynecomastia (male breast enlargement) occurs in 8% of men who have had orchiectomy; 3%–15% of men treated with luteinizing hormone-releasing hormone (LHRH) agonists; and 19% of men treated with a combination of LHRH agonists and flutamide (Ng et al.).

Side effects of chemotherapy affect body image. Alopecia (see Chapter 2) can affect body image more than surgical removal of a breast for some; the change in cognitive function can affect how a person views himself or herself; and the change in body smell while receiving chemotherapy can affect body image in ways that staff often forget to assess (Browall, Gaston-Johansson, & Danielson, 2006).

Surgical causes of body image changes can happen after stomal surgery, breast surgery, orchiectomy (Kaufman & Chang, 2007), or genital surgery. The loss of a body part or change in shape of a body part can affect body image, and the impact is magnified depending on the meaning of the body part to the patient. How surgical changes influence the fitting of clothes and appearance when dressed has an impact on body image (Geiger et al., 2006). Cultural factors may affect the meaning and significance of the loss of the body part (Sideris et al., 2005). Penile size can decrease after surgery for penile cancer (Ralph, Garaffa, & Garcia, 2006) or after radical prostatectomy (Kendirci et al., 2006). To help with body image from penile surgery, a penile graft may be done, but graft overgrowth or poor graft take of penile-preserving surgery can occur and further damage body image (Ralph et al.).

Body image alterations from XRT include concern about the permanent tattoos, skin color and texture changes, and thinning or loss of hair in the radiated field. Daily XRT to breasts or sexual organs that have to be exposed during treatment can lead patients to see that body part as "diseased" and not pleasurable, causing almost a dissociative effect. Precocious puberty that alters body image can be caused by high-dose cranial radiation therapy (greater than 50 gray [Gy]) causing gonadotropin deficiency. Doses of 18–47 Gy increase the risk of precocious puberty (Alvarez et al., 2007).

The incidence of lymphedema following breast cancer treatment has decreased (from 40%–50% of patients to 1%–4%) because of earlier detection, sentinel lymph node dissection, and changes in XRT technique ("Fertility and Pregnancy After Cancer Treatment," 2006). Although lymphedema in patients with breast cancer is declining, awareness is still needed (see Chapter 15). Research about sexual function and body image often focuses on patients with curable disease, although the body image of terminally ill patients with lower limb lymphedema (Frid, Strang, Friedrichsen, & Johansson, 2006) or cancer anorexia-cachexia syndrome (McClement, 2005) can be greatly affected. Thus, a patient's prognosis should not stop the nurse from assessing body image.

Assessment

Assessment is much more than the traditional laboratory tests and physical examinations. Baseline body image assessment (Huber et al., 2006; Pelusi, 2006) includes performance status, partner availability, health status, depression, anxiety, and the meaning of the cause of cancer. Assessment includes asking if the alterations in body image have caused concern or distress.

Laboratory Tests

No traditional laboratory tests are done to diagnose body image alterations. Multiple body image surveys are available for clinical use and assessment (see Table 21-1).

Physical Examination

Multiple physical factors, such as a stoma, change in muscle mass, loss of body part, hair distribution on the body

TABLE 21-1	Surveys for Body Image Assessment
Instrument	**Instrument Psychometrics**
Amputee Body Image Scale	14 items Reliability: Cronbach's alpha = 0.87 (Gallagher et al., 2007)
Multidimensional Body Self-Relations Questionnaire	7 scale items with a 5-point response format Reliability: Cronbach's alpha = 0.981 for men; 0.994 for women (DeFrank et al., 2007)
Body Image Score	10 items with a 4-point response format Reliability: Cronbach's alpha = 0.93 (Hopwood et al., 2001)

(usually involves loss of hair, but sometimes treatment can cause hair growth, which also affects hair distribution), surgical scars, delayed development of secondary sex characteristics, precocious puberty, lymphedema, and acne, can affect body image. It is not the physical factors that cause the changed body image but rather how the person perceives the changes. Thus, nurses cannot automatically assume that the stoma has affected the person's body image. Instead of assuming, nurses should ask if having a stoma has affected how that person sees himself or herself. Because it is the perception that affects body image, there can be "invisible" changes not evident to others and a diagnosis that is not visible to others, and yet body image is affected (Shell, Carolan, Zhang, & Meneses, 2008).

Evidence-Based Practice Recommendations

Support for altered body image interventions is based on synthesis of the literature (Alfano & Rowland, 2006; Davis, 2006; Huber et al., 2006; Katz, 2007; Ralph et al., 2006; Roberts, Livingston, White, & Gibbs, 2003; Sandel et al., 2005; Windahl et al., 2004). See Figure 21-7 for suggested interventions.

Expected Outcomes Specific to Altered Body Image

Because body image changes are common for patients of both sexes and of all ages, nurses should address this aspect of care with all patients. Expected outcomes include staff members feeling comfortable to discuss body image changes and sexuality with patients. When body image changes or sexuality issues are present, they will be addressed in a culturally sensitive manner. Consultations for body image changes and sexual counseling will be made available to the patient if he or she so desires. Body image changes and sexuality will be discussed with patients despite their age, sex, ethnicity, sexual orientation, marital status, or prognosis.

Patient Teaching Points Specific to Altered Body Image

Cultural background, response of others, age, developmental stage, sex, and belief systems can each affect how an individual will respond to changes in body image. Nurses should not assume that a particular type of surgery or treatment will automatically create an altered body image. Instead, the nurse should be aware of possible changes that might occur with specific treatments.

- Be aware that the need for rapid treatment initiation may prevent pretreatment discussion about options to help decrease negative body image. For example, testicular cancer can require rapid treatment initiation without time for discussion about the option of a testicular prosthesis, safety, or possible complications (Chapple & McPherson, 2004).
- Be able to provide in-depth teaching points for patients commonly seen by each nurse. For example, if the nurse works often with people who have ostomy surgery, suggestions can be offered to the patient prior to the first experience of engaging in sex. These include using a belt, cummerbund, or picture-frame taping to keep the appliance from dislocating during sexual activity; emptying the appliance to reduce weight and decrease the risk of appliance slipping during sex; using crotchless underwear, wearing an attractive teddy or T-shirt, or using a pouch cover; using pouch deodorants and avoiding gassy food or drinks to avoid embarrassing odors; and using a smaller stoma appliance to reduce bulk or changing positioning to avoid lying directly on the stoma (Junkin & Beitz, 2005).
- Inform patients about resources for changes in body image such as the American Cancer Society's *Look Good . . . Feel Better* program and Internet support groups (Sheppard & Ely, 2008), and offer a bibliography of suggested readings.

Need for Future Research Specific to Altered Body Image

Studies need to be conducted on a patient's reaction to cancer, scarring, or a stoma (Hendren et al., 2005) and to examine how ethnicity, age, and sex affect the reaction. Intervention studies are needed to investigate how to facilitate a healthy body image during and after treatment for cancer (Pelusi, 2006).

FIGURE 21-7	Evidence-Based Practice Interventions for Altered Body Image

Recommended for Practice
- No interventions at the time of publication

Likely to Be Effective
- Breast conservation surgery (Alfano & Rowland, 2006)
- Nursing interventions to improve body image (Alfano & Rowland, 2006; Katz, 2007; Sandel et al., 2005)
- Couple-based interventions (Scott et al., 2004; Scott & Kayser, 2009)

Benefits Balanced With Harms
- Hormone therapy for adolescent females (Davis, 2006)
- Type of surgery for penile cancer (Akin-Olugbade et al., 2006; Ralph et al., 2006; Windahl et al., 2004)

Effectiveness Not Established
- Plastic surgery (Akin-Olugbade et al., 2006; Alfano & Rowland, 2006; Boehmer et al., 2007; Chapple & McPherson, 2004; Ralph et al., 2006; Ramsawh et al., 2005; Sandam & Harcourt, 2007)

Effectiveness Unlikely
- No interventions at the time of publication

Not Recommended for Practice
- No interventions at the time of publication

Changes in Libido

Overview of Symptom

Changes in libido can be one of the more discouraging and distressing symptoms resulting from the diagnosis or treatment of cancer. Loss of libido is the sexual side effect that often is most disturbing to patients and can remain upsetting to them for long periods of time (Burwell, Case, Kaelin, & Avis, 2006). Yet, it is a hidden problem often shrouded in shame or embarrassment. Patients often ask, "How does a person whose life has been 'saved' due to medical technology complain over the loss of libido without feeling ungrateful?" and "Is the loss of libido not a small price to pay?" And so, the symptom often remains silent in the clinic office.

Changes in libido can herald the onset of certain malignancies (e.g., a primary brain tumor, testicular cancer). The *Diagnostic and Statistical Manual of Mental Disorders* (American Psychiatric Association, 2000) lists changes in libido, one of four types of female sexual dysfunction, as the most common sexual problem, reported by 33% of women.

Definition

Libido is made up of four factors: (a) erotic desire or interest to engage in sex, (b) purpose or object of desire, (c) willingness, and (d) actual behavior. Although *libido* is a term often used interchangeably with sexual appetite, sexual desire, or "life force," there is a difference, although a close relationship exists between *arousal* and *libido*. Arousal is the physiologic response (i.e., erection or vaginal lubrication), whereas libido is the desire. A person can be aroused and be able to have an erection or vaginal lubrication but have a loss of libido and have no desire to engage in sexual activity.

Risk Factors

Risk factors for changes in libido include medical conditions such as a diagnosis of cancer; medications and their side effects; and other treatments such as surgery. Psychological risk factors include anxiety and depression. The aging process or fatigue alone may be a risk factor for changes in libido.

Pathophysiology of Symptom

Why It Happens

Changes in libido are multifactorial and include psychological and physiologic reasons. When working with patients who have changes in libido, nurses need to remember to ask if the changes cause concern for the patients. Decreased libido may not be perceived as a problem by everyone who experiences it.

What Causes It

Psychological factors include depression (Shell et al., 2008), invasive surgery that provokes a post-traumatic stress disorder of past sexual abuse, concern that sex may cause recurrence or metastasis of disease (Kritcharoen, Suwan, & Jirojwong, 2005), and stress that decreases androgen, thus resulting in decreased desire. The two greatest psychological predictors for lowered libido following surgical menopause for benign reasons include preoperative depression and preoperative sexual problems (Shifren & Avis, 2007).

Physiologic factors include surgery, drugs, treatment side effects, type of cancer diagnosis, and non-cancer-related causes. Surgery may cause a decrease in libido. For example, in one study, 73% of patients suffered a decrease in libido after rectal surgery (Hendren et al., 2005). In another study, 25% of men who had an orchiectomy indicated a loss of libido, but it was undetermined whether the cause was physical or psychological, because testosterone levels remained stable after removal of one testicle. Libido can be affected by side effects from the surgical procedure, such as urine leakage after prostate surgery or creation of a neobladder. Loss of libido also can occur because of an intentional reduction in sexual hormones via chemicals or surgery called gonadal ablation.

Multiple drugs (antidepressants, antihistamines, antihypertensives, narcotics, oral contraceptives, and long-term use of sedatives), alcohol, and chronic use of cocaine and marijuana can affect libido. Many people being treated for cancer utilize drugs, and therefore a complete medication history is needed. Medications taken specifically to treat cancer can affect libido, but it is not always a clear cause and effect. For example, a selective estrogen receptor modulator, such as tamoxifen, can affect libido, but the effects are not caused by just taking the drug; it is multifactorial (e.g., grief about a cancer diagnosis, fatigue from chemotherapy or radiation therapy that was done prior to the start of tamoxifen, reaction of a partner to include the partner being so upset about the patient having a diagnosis of cancer that the partner leaves the relationship). Hormone ablation therapy also can cause loss of libido (Ng et al., 2006).

Treatment side effects can affect sexual desire. Nausea, either from treatment or from abdominal pressure caused by a sexual position; fatigue (i.e., if the person is very tired and therefore may not have desire and vaginal lubrication, thus causing dyspareunia); or dyspareunia, secondary to treatment, can cause a decrease in libido because of pain with intercourse. The type of cancer affects libido. Women with advanced, recurrent, or persistent cervical cancer have a greater incidence of decreased libido (Stead, 2004). Frontal lobe brain tumors can result in disinhibition, or a lack of socially appropriate sexual restraint, and can influence how a person responds to increased libido. Prostate cancer has the potential to affect libido indirectly. Symptoms of prostate cancer can include pain with erection or ejaculation. The fear of pain may decrease libido.

Non-cancer-related reasons for loss of libido include age and medical conditions. Serum total and free testosterone concentrations decrease with age (Shah & Montoya, 2007). Known medical conditions that affect libido are diabetes, hypertension, myxedema, hyperthyroidism, Addison disease, acromegaly, chronic renal failure, multiple sclerosis, chronic respiratory conditions, and cardiac disease.

Assessment

Taking a history is imperative and should include the following: (a) past history of libido; (b) patient's current partner status, and if there is a partner, what is the partner's health status; (c) past sexual abuse; (d) past sexual experiences; (e) whether the change in libido is a concern to the patient or partner; and (f) cultural or religious values or beliefs that may affect the change in libido. The use of the ACS Desire Diary can help to evaluate patients' concerns (ACS, 2006). Nurses can instruct patients to

- Use the Desire Diary for one week.
- Evaluate their Desire Diary to see if any patterns, such as settings, people, or times of the day, result in an increased sense of desire. Once they have noted some patterns, they can begin putting themselves in the situations that spark a sexual mood, such as exercising, planning a relaxed evening out with their partner, making a special effort to look and feel sexy, reading a steamy story with sex, watching a movie with a romantic or sexual plot, or fantasizing about a sexual encounter.
- Get their partner's input, and discuss any fears either of them has about their sexual relationship. If the patients or partners have questions about medical risks, they should discuss them with their doctor (ACS, 2006).

Laboratory Tests

A low serum testosterone level, less than 300 ng/dl, can be helpful in identifying a possible cause for a decreased libido (Rosen, 2007). The testosterone level alone is not an absolute cause of low libido; however, an association exists between the two even in patients without cancer (Travison, Morley, Araujo, O'Donnell, & McKinlay, 2006). This helps to explain why testosterone replacement is not 100% effective and may diminish over treatment time (Travison et al.).

A second laboratory test that can be done is prolactin level. Hyperprolactinemia, which inhibits gonadotropin-releasing hormone, is relatively common after transplantation and can decrease libido in men (Katz, 2007).

History and Physical Examination

No specific physical examination is done for evaluation of decreased libido. A "well-person" examination would provide physical conditions such as pulmonary or cardiac conditions that could affect libido. What is more important for a patient with a diagnosis of cancer and who has decreased libido is that is a good history is taken. Inquire about nausea, pain, fatigue, or a patient's concerns about scars or body changes that would affect libido. Use the physical examination as a time to focus on the history and the patient's perception/meaning of any changes.

Evidence-Based Practice Recommendations for Changes in Libido

The literature revealed few recommendations for practice that would improve libido. Currently, the therapy most likely to be effective is the treatment of underlying symptoms. For example, if the patient is depressed, the use of an antidepressant is likely to improve libido. Even with women in healthy relationships who are not depressed, the antidepressant bupropion (Wellbutrin SR®, GlaxoSmithKline) doubled the amount of sexual interest in 33% of the patients (Segraves et al., 2001). If nausea is an underlying cause of decreased libido, using an antiemetic before sexual activity or simply changing body positions to relieve abdominal pressure may be effective. Because exercise intolerance may decrease libido, improving aerobic capacity and reducing symptoms of fatigue are likely to be effective.

Interventions for treatment of changes in libido that may be beneficial but have side effects are testosterone patches and intermittent androgen therapy. The testosterone patch has been found to increase sexual desire for some women (Braunstein et al., 2005; Buster et al., 2005) but produces side effects of a deeper voice, hair loss, and an enlarged clitoris. The result of increased libido with the use of testosterone patches does not hold true for all women (Barton et al., 2007). The American Association of Clinical Endocrinologists (2003) recommended against the routine use of testosterone or androgen therapy in patients with breast cancer, prostate cancer, palpable prostate nodules, a prostate-specific antigen level higher than 3 ng/ml that has not been evaluated, erythrocytosis, hyperviscosity, untreated obstructive sleep apnea, severe lower urinary tract symptoms with an International Prostate Symptom Score greater than 19, or class III or IV heart failure. If a patient has hypogonadism, testosterone therapy is advised if there is no diagnosis of prostate or breast cancer, but the patient requires frequent monitoring (Rosen, 2007; Shah & Montoya, 2007). If a patient requires intermittent androgen therapy, libido will decrease during therapy but will return during the break from therapy (Ng et al., 2006).

The effectiveness of drug therapies besides the ones already described has not been clearly established in the literature, and the therapies have yet to be approved by the U.S. Food and Drug Administration.

Expected Outcomes Specific to Changes in Libido

An opportunity for patients to discuss concerns about changes in libido is the overall outcome. Patients should feel that their concerns are being taken seriously and that options will be discussed with them. Refer to the common expected outcomes presented at the end of this chapter.

Patient Teaching Points Specific to Changes in Libido

Teaching points include addressing how depression, medications, fatigue, constipation, nausea, vomiting, body image changes, and partner availability can affect libido. Nurses should be sensitive to counseling patients on the partner's possible reaction to the diagnosis and body image changes, as patients may worry that their partner will be repulsed by these changes. Suggestions may include the use of the ACS Desire Diary, which is useful for looking at patterns so that interventions can be planned (ACS, 2006).

Need for Future Research Specific to Changes in Libido

Continued research is needed regarding changes in libido for patients with a cancer diagnosis. Examples include (a) How can studies of libido be incorporated into clinical trials of new therapies being tested? (b) What are the cultural questions regarding the importance of libido to different cultural belief groups (age, sex, sexual orientation, ethnicity, marital status, socioeconomic status, and educational level)? (c) Does the potential impact on libido affect decisions about cancer treatment options? (d) Is libido included in treatment discussions? and (e) How does the reaction of a partner to a cancer diagnosis or treatment affect the libido of the patient?

Infertility

Overview of Symptom

Although cancer often is seen as a disease of older adults, more than 140,000 Americans of child-bearing age are diagnosed with cancer each year (Bruce, 2007). In addition, cancer survivors of pediatric and adolescent malignancies make up 1 out of every 900 Americans aged 15–44 years old (Leonard, 2006). Therefore, many adult patients with cancer, as well as parents of children with cancer, are concerned about the risks to fertility (Lee et al., 2006). Fertility preservation strategies have been shown to improve emotional coping, whereas infertility increases the risk of emotional distress. Many people do not pursue the available options of surrogacy, gamete donation, or adoption because of religious beliefs, personal beliefs, or adoption agency criteria (Nieman et al., 2006). Reproductive concerns affect sexual functioning (Champion et al., 2007; Nieman et al.), which is why infertility is included in the chapter on sexual dysfunction.

Definition

In the general population, *infertility* is defined as the inability to conceive after one year of unprotected intercourse (Lambert & Fisch, 2007). For a patient who has had a bilateral orchiectomy, bilateral oophorectomy, or treatment that yields the same effect, infertility is immediate.

Risk Factors

Risk factors for infertility in a patient with cancer include decreased fertility present before diagnosis, age of the patient, type of malignancy, stage of disease, type of surgery performed, and other treatments used, such as radiation therapy, chemotherapy, or hormonal manipulation.

Many patients undergoing cancer treatment have a lack of information about how to preserve fertility. One role of the healthcare provider is to inform patients and partners about options to preserve fertility. Healthcare providers may not discuss fertility preservation with patients for numerous reasons: (a) lack of knowledge of fertility preservation; (b) concerns that the patient is not able to afford fertility preservation; (c) personal judgment that the patient would not want to engage in exploring the option because of age or religious or cultural beliefs; (d) concern that aggressiveness of the disease requires immediate treatment; (e) belief that the type of disease is associated with risk of infertility at the time of diagnosis; (f) discomfort in discussing the topic; (g) lack of availability of preservation options in the community (Magnan & Reynolds, 2006); or (h) belief that the patient's prognosis is poor (Lindsey, 2005) (see Figure 21-8). One of the easiest methods of providing a male patient the option of fertility after treatment is the use of sperm banking, and yet 87% of physicians do not offer this option to their patients (Fertile Hope, n.d.-a).

The risk of infertility can be caused by reasons unrelated to cancer, such as age and environmental factors. Fifteen percent to 30% of healthy couples have difficulty conceiving a child. Many women focus on establishing their career and thus delay child-bearing (Knobf, 2006; Plante & Roy, 2006). Environmental factors of smoking, radiation, and chemotherapy decrease ovarian follicles (Davis, 2006). The decrease in number of follicles is called *atresia*. *Spermatogenesis* is the process by which male spermatogonia develop into mature spermatozoa; the entire process takes approximately 64 days. Similar to with infertility in women, environmental factors and age negatively affect sperm development in terms of quantity and/or quality of sperm. Spermatogenesis begins at puberty and usually continues uninterrupted until death.

The type of malignancy may affect male fertility. The three most common diagnoses that affect male fertility at the time of diagnosis are Hodgkin disease (HD), testicular cancer, and non-Hodgkin lymphoma (NHL). Of men diagnosed with HD, 70% have abnormal semen analyses (Lambert & Fisch, 2007) at the time of diagnosis. Sixty percent to 75% of patients with testicular cancer have low counts, poor motility, or low semen volume at diagnosis (Kaufman & Chang, 2007). Elevated follicle-stimulating hormone (FSH) level and/or advanced stage of disease increases the risk of infertility (Lambert & Fisch). However, the stage of testicular cancer does not affect sperm quality (Girasole et al., 2007).

Surgical interventions that can affect male fertility include bilateral orchiectomy and retroperitoneal lymph node dissection (RPLND), which can cause retrograde ejaculation (Lambert & Fisch, 2007). Surgeries that can affect female fertility include hysterectomy, bilateral salpingo-oophorectomy, and radical cystectomy.

The dose, treatment field, and schedule of radiation therapy affect male fertility in a dose-dependent manner; the greater the dose, the longer the time needed for spermatogenesis to return. If the man has a radiation

FIGURE 21-8	**Reasons Why Healthcare Staff May Not Offer Fertility Preservation Techniques**

- Lack of knowledge about fertility preservation techniques
- Concerns about affordability
- Concerns about availability
- Judgments based on age of patient and personal religious or cultural beliefs
- Fear of causing increased anxiety or invasion of privacy
- Belief that immediate treatment is required, precluding fertility options
- Belief that low sperm count at time of diagnosis precludes fertility preservation
- Discomfort in discussing the topic
- Work environment barriers (e.g., workload or lack of support)

Note. Based on information from King et al., 2008; Lindsey, 2005; Nieman et al., 2006.

dose less than 1 Gy, return to fertile levels will take 9–18 months (Girasole et al., 2007); with doses greater than 4 Gy, spermatogenesis can take five years or longer to return. Doses greater than 4 Gy and total body irradiation result in complete sterility (Bashore, 2007; Nieman et al., 2006).

For women older than age 40, doses of 4 Gy can result in infertility. Previously, it was reported that radiation would not be a great risk to prepubertal females. However, preliminary data indicate that the same number of oocytes are damaged, but the effect on the patient's fertility may be delayed because young females have a large number of oocytes (Leonard, 2006). Of all radiation treatments, total body irradiation carries the highest risk of infertility for both sexes (Davis, 2006). Even when the field of therapy is not near the genitals, such as with cranial radiation therapy, fertility can be affected (Thaler-DeMers, 2006).

If a woman is treated with radiation therapy and is able to conceive, she is at risk of not carrying the fetus to full term. Abdominal radiation of preadolescent and adolescent females can affect growth and development of the uterus, preventing full uterine growth and affecting blood flow to the uterus (Davis, 2006). Even if the woman is postpubertal, radiation to the pelvis will affect the uterus so that it may be unable to enlarge enough for the growing fetus, thus increasing the risk of miscarriage or premature birth (Breerendonk & Braat, 2005). Cranial-spinal radiation can increase the risk of miscarriage by 3.6 times (Alvarez et al., 2007).

Chemotherapy can be a significant threat to fertility depending on the age of the person being treated, type of chemotherapy given, dose of treatment, and length of treatment. For example, infertility occurs in 15%–55% of women ages 30–40 years old who receive alkylating chemotherapy for a diagnosis of breast cancer and in 90% of women who receive high-dose chemotherapy by chemically inducing menopause (Knobf, 2006). Androgen deprivation therapy, whether done medically or surgically, will affect fertility by preventing spermatogenesis (see Table 21-2).

Pathophysiology of Symptom

Why It Happens

The pathophysiology of infertility in patients diagnosed with cancer is not clearly understood. It may be caused by the tumor itself, the cytokine response, or disruption of the hypothalamic-pituitary axis (Lambert & Fisch, 2007).

What Causes It

Surgically induced infertility depends on the type of surgical procedure. Removal of reproductive organs in both men and women has an obvious impact on infertility, as well as consequences of surgery, such as retrograde ejaculation or failure of emission in men.

Cancer therapies have direct and indirect effects on fertility in men and women. The pathophysiology of chemotherapy-induced infertility for women is because of ovarian reserve reduction on the number and quality of oocytes in the ovaries (Schover, 2008). Chemotherapy-induced male infertility is caused by damage to the germinal epithelium (Girasole et al., 2007). Alkylating agents (busulfan, cyclophosphamide, chlorambucil, ifosfamide, melphalan), nitrosoureas (carmustine, lomustine), platinum agents, and others (procarbazine, nitrogen mustard, cytarabine, temozolomide, thiotepa, vinblastine) affect the gonads. Follicles are affected, and ovaries decrease in size and fibrose; somatic and germ cell function is disrupted, affecting spermatogenesis (Bashore, 2007; Knobf, 2006). Chemotherapy can affect both Sertoli cell and Leydig cell functions, which serve to nurture the cell through spermatogenesis and secrete androgens, respectively (Lambert & Fisch, 2007). The amount of DNA damage depends on the patient's age, amount of drug given, and length of treatment.

TABLE 21-2	Possible Threats to Fertility
Threats	**Threat Variables**
Non-cancer-related reasons	Age History of a sexually transmitted disease and/or pelvic inflammatory disease Extremes in body weight Environmental factors
Diagnosis of malignancy	Malignant diagnosis affects male fertility more. The three most common diagnoses to affect male fertility are Hodgkin disease, testicular cancer, and non-Hodgkin lymphoma.
Surgical interventions	Male fertility • Retroperitoneal lymph node dissection • Bilateral orchiectomy Female fertility • Hysterectomy • Bilateral salpingo-oophorectomy • Radical cystectomy
Radiation therapy	Dose given Treatment field Schedule of radiation therapy
Chemotherapy	Patient's age Type of chemotherapy given Dose of treatment Length of treatment
Androgen deprivation therapy	May reverse if chemically induced

Note. Based on information from Kelly-Weeder & O'Connor, 2006; Nieman et al., 2006; Paduch, 2006.

Men diagnosed with malignancies tend to have sperm with a higher rate of DNA damage, which is associated with lower fertility; however, this does not result in higher rates of birth defects in children born to these men following treatment (Schover, 2006). It is unknown if the newer treatments (i.e., monoclonal antibodies) will affect fertility.

Radiation therapy can affect fertility. Radiation to the pituitary gland affects production of FSH, LH, and testosterone. XRT to the brain impairs the hypothalamus and reduces the production of gonadotropin-releasing hormone. Radiation to the brain or spinal cord interferes with functioning of the hypothalamic-pituitary axis, which also affects the gonadotropin-releasing hormone (Davis, 2006). Patients who are at highest risk for infertility are young females within two years of menarche (before or after menarche) (Davis). Cranial-spinal irradiation infertility prior to the advancements in radiation equipment probably is caused by scattering of radiation to the ovaries (Davis). Total body irradiation creates the highest risk of infertility of all radiation treatments (Davis). Combination chemotherapy and XRT can cause spermatogonia destruction or spermatogenesis arrest (Thaler-DeMers, 2006).

Assessment

When cancer is first diagnosed, the pressing issue often is how quickly can treatment be started. Although fertility is not always the automatic first concern when a person is confronted with a new potentially life-threatening diagnosis, it must be considered when treatment decisions are being made.

A timely assessment of the meaning of fertility for the individual, couple, and/or family needs to occur, often before treatment options are chosen. Unfortunately, this is a time of great stress. However, responsible professionals will consider fertility for all patients, young and old, who are newly diagnosed with cancer. The assessment of fertility should query the values and belief systems of the patient and/or partner and include a discussion of prediagnosis expectations of parenting. Sensitivity to social, cultural, religious, financial, and legal considerations also should be included in the assessment.

Laboratory Tests

Multiple tests can be used to assess fertility (Lambert & Fisch, 2007). Nurses can help to explain the purpose of the tests and provide additional information when requested. For men, semen analysis examines the volume, sperm concentration, motility, and morphology. For women, decreased levels of inhibin B, a reproductive hormone, may be a marker for atresia, a decrease in ovarian follicles (Davis, 2006). Hormonal analysis of elevated serum FSH, estradiol level, low estrogen level, LH, anti-Müllerian hormone (AMH) concentration, testosterone, and prolactin can be performed (Davis). AMH concentration can be used as an early indicator of ovarian aging (Anderson, Themmen, Al-Qahtani, Groome, & Cameron, 2006).

Radiologic studies can include scrotal ultrasound and transrectal ultrasound. If scrotal varicoceles are present, color flow duplex ultrasonography can be performed. Pelvic ultrasounds of women may show decreased ovarian volume (Anderson et al., 2006) and a decreased number of antral follicles (Schover, 2008).

Physical Examination

For men, examination of the penis, scrotum, and testicular volume or examination for prostate abnormalities can be performed (Lambert & Fisch, 2007). The scrotal sac should be evaluated for varicoceles. These are found in about 40% of men without a history of cancer who are undergoing evaluation for infertility.

If a woman has had abdominal XRT as a child, an examination of uterine size can be performed. As with all fertility evaluations, a complete gynecologic examination, including size, shape, and position of the reproductive organs, should be done (see Table 21-3).

Evidence-Based Practice Recommendations for Infertility

The American Society of Clinical Oncology conducted a systematic review of the fertility preservation literature for patients with cancer, including literature from 1987 through 2005 (Lee et al., 2006). This sentinel reference will be used as the basis for the practice recommendations with the addition of recent supporting studies for each sex (see Figures 21-9 and 21-10).

The literature regarding preservation of male fertility is more robust than for other sexuality problems faced by patients with cancer. Currently, sperm cryopreservation after masturbation and prior to treatment and gonadal shielding during radiation therapy are supported in the literature and recommended for practice. Timely referral for sperm banking also is supported in the literature because no known relationship exists between a history of cancer and congenital abnormalities in offspring (Lee et al., 2006). Cryopreservation of sperm col-

TABLE 21-3	Laboratory, Radiologic, and Physical Examination Factors in Fertility Assessment		
Population	**Physical Examination**	**Radiologic Tests**	**Laboratory Tests**
Women (Davis, 2006)	Size, shape, and position of female reproductive organs	Pelvic ultrasound if female had abdominal external radiation therapy before puberty	Hormonal analysis: follicle-stimulating hormone, estradiol, luteinizing hormone, testosterone, and prolactin. Decreased levels of inhibin B may be a marker for atresia, a decrease in ovarian follicles.
Men (Quallich, 2006)	Examination of penis, scrotum, and testicular volume, or examination for prostate abnormalities. Varicoceles in the scrotal sac. Digital rectal examination	Ultrasound: Transrectal or scrotal. If there are scrotal varicoceles: Color flow duplex ultrasonography	Semen analysis × 2 examines the volume, sperm concentration, motility, and morphology. Follicle-stimulating hormone, luteinizing hormone, total and free testosterone, prolactin, and estradiol if high body mass index

FIGURE 21-9	Evidence-Based Practice Interventions for Male Fertility Preservation

Recommended for Practice
- Sperm cryopreservation after masturbation prior to treatment (Lee et al., 2006; van den Berg et al., 2007)
- Timely referrals for sperm banking (Chapple et al., 2006; Girasole et al., 2006; Lee et al., 2006)
- Gonadal shielding during radiation therapy (Dauer et al., 2007; Lee et al., 2006; Mazonakis et al., 2006)

Likely to Be Effective
- Sperm cryopreservation from alternative methods of sperm collection (masturbation, percutaneous or open sperm cell extraction methods, or postcoital urine extraction) (Keros et al., 2007; Lee et al., 2006; Paduch, 2006; van den Berg et al., 2006)

Benefits Balanced With Harms
- Intracytoplasmic sperm injection (Lee et al., 2006; Schover, 2006)

Effectiveness Not Established
- Testicular tissue cryopreservation and reimplantation (Lee et al., 2006)
- Grafting of human testicular tissue (Lee et al., 2006)

Effectiveness Unlikely
- No interventions at the time of publication

Not Recommended for Practice
- Hormonal gonadoprotection for highly sterilizing chemotherapy (Lee et al., 2006)
- Hypothalamic-pituitary-gonadal suppression plus testosterone (Lee et al., 2006)

lected from alternative methods is considered likely to be effective. Intracytoplasmic sperm injection is not considered standard treatment.

Female fertility preservation literature supports interventions of embryo cryopreservation, ovarian transposition, and trachelectomy. Oocyte cryopreservation is likely to be effective, and ovarian tissue cryopreservation may be beneficial.

FIGURE 21-10	Evidence-Based Practice Interventions for Female Fertility Preservation

Recommended for Practice
- Embryo cryopreservation (Lee et al., 2006)
- Ovarian transposition (Lee et al., 2006)
- Trachelectomy (Farthing, 2006; Lee et al., 2006; Matthews et al., 2007; Shepherd et al., 2006)

Likely to Be Effective
- Oocyte cryopreservation (Lee et al., 2006)

Benefits Balanced With Harms
- Ovarian tissue cryopreservation (Feigin et al., 2007; Lee et al., 2006)

Effectiveness Not Established
- Ovarian suppression (Davis, 2006; Lee et al., 2006)

Effectiveness Unlikely
- No interventions at the time of publication

Not Recommended for Practice
- No interventions at the time of publication

Other methods for fertility preservation are available to consider. Surrogate pregnancy, where another woman carries the patient's fertilized egg, requires discussion of the legal, ethical, and religious concerns. If embryo cryopreservation is selected, both members of the couple have equal rights to the embryo. Adoption also could be considered, but some adoption agencies will not select a family with a history of cancer or will require that the family wait for a period of time (e.g., five years) after completion of therapy (Fertile Hope, n.d.-b).

For young girls receiving abdominal radiation therapy, estrogen replacement therapy can help to prevent retardation of uterine growth (Davis, 2006). Even with replacement therapy, the uterus may grow to only 40% of the normal adult size (Davis).

Expected Outcomes Specific to Infertility

- Staff will feel comfortable discussing fertility issues with patients.
- Patients will feel comfortable discussing fertility concerns with staff.
- Fertility issues will be addressed in a culturally sensitive manner.
- Patients will be given options for fertility preservation if it is safe and can be done in a timely manner.
- When aggressiveness of tumor does not allow the initiation of treatment to be safely delayed, patients will be informed why fertility preservation cannot be done. When making this decision, keep in mind that it is no longer necessary to wait 36 hours between semen collections (Schover, 2006).
- Staff support is readily available for patients to ask questions about the cost of fertility preservation so that they can make informed decisions.
- Do not assume patients will not sperm bank because of poor finances. For sperm banking, only 7% of men gave cost as the reason for not choosing sperm banking (Schover, 2006).
- If patient is a minor, issues of fertility are addressed with guardians and the minor if he or she is mature enough to understand. Keep in mind that sexual maturation is an adolescent developmental task.
- Gonadal function is screened as a part of follow-up care (Huddart et al., 2005).
- Fertility will be discussed with the patient regardless of age, sex, ethnicity, sexual orientation, or marital status (Lee et al., 2006).

Patient Teaching Points Specific to Infertility

- A multidisciplinary and longitudinal approach, if possible, best serves the patient's fertility preservation decisions.

- Discussion about fertility preservation occurs at a time of great stress, which interferes with retention of information. Written handouts can help to reinforce complex information about options.
- Consider the patient's unique social, cultural, or religious characteristics.
- Female patients without partners have limited options, but available options are use of donor sperm, ovarian transposition, or cryopreservation of oocyte, embryo, or ovarian tissue.
- Two groups often overlooked when discussing fertility are older adults and adolescents. Older adults may be affected by the loss of fertility even when they are beyond their reproductive years. Adolescents are known to desire information about how their diagnosis and treatment might affect sexuality and fertility options (Bashore, 2007; Zebrack, Oeffinger, Hou, & Kaplan, 2006).
- Incorporate fertility preservation information into routine treatment checklists or protocols so that it is not overlooked.
- Discussion of fertility should include a section on the legal and cost implications of banking sperm, oocytes, or embryos. For example, if they should die, who "owns" the stored tissue, and if pregnancy occurs from use of the stored tissue after the death of the patient, what rights will the child have to insurance or other benefits (Davis, 2006).
- Resumption of regular menstruation is not an indicator of fertility (Sonmezer & Oktay, 2006).

Need for Future Research Specific to Infertility

Future studies regarding fertility should include physical issues of the possible effects of biologic agents such as interferons, interleukins, and monoclonal antibodies on fertility. Psychosocial and QOL issues also need to be investigated, such as how do fertility interventions affect fertility-related distress (Alfano & Rowland, 2006) and what are the QOL outcomes in patients who become infertile because of cancer treatments (Knobf, 2006).

Expected Outcomes for Altered Sexuality Patterns

Expected Outcomes for Providers

It is an expectation that providers will discuss sexual functioning, when possible, prior to treatment initiation. In the initial patient conversation, the nurse's focus is on reassuring the patients that even though their sexuality may change following diagnosis and treatment, sexuality can continue to be an enjoyable part of life (Junkin & Beitz, 2005). The nurse needs to be proactive and provide this information and not wait for patients to ask (Shell et al., 2008).

The expected outcome is that with experience, each staff member will feel more comfortable in discussing, in a culturally sensitive manner, topics of sexuality or fertility with patients regardless of age, sex, ethnicity, sexual orientation, partner status, or prognosis. It is important that providers not assume a heterosexual orientation, but rather ask patients about their sexual orientation (Boehmer et al., 2007).

For staff members who are not yet comfortable discussing sexuality, each staff member, at a minimum, must be able to raise the topic and then direct the patient to a team member who is more comfortable in discussing the topic and providing the patient with detailed information. This is not yet the standard practice, as evidenced in a 2006 study in which 87% of 126 women treated for cancer did not recall any of their healthcare providers talking with them about possible changes in sexual function caused by treatment (Huber et al., 2006).

FIGURE 21-11	Sexuality Assessment Models

PLISSIT Model
Permission
Limited **I**nformation
Specific **S**uggestions
Intensive **T**herapy

BETTER Model
Bring up the topic.
Explain that sex is part of quality of life.
Tell patients that resources are available to address their concerns.
Time the intervention for when patients are receptive.
Educate patients about treatment side effects.
Record the intervention.

ALARM Model
Activity
Libido/desire
Arousal/orgasm
Resolution
Medical history

Note. Based on information from Dixon & Dixon, 2006; Hordern, 2008; Katz, 2007.

When addressing altered sexual functioning issues, nursing care includes assessing the effectiveness of interventions. When the intervention is determined not to be helpful, the provider will consult with another professional for further options (Galbraith et al., 2005). It is expected that the provider will reinforce with patients that the discussion and assessment will continue through the cancer trajectory and even years after treatment (Pelusi, 2006), with tailored information provided as their experiences and circumstances change (Lauver, Connolly-Nelson, & Vang, 2007). Some of the more commonly used assessment tools include the PLISSIT, BETTER, and ALARM models (see Figure 21-11). These tools, although frequently used, have weaknesses. The ALARM model focuses on functional aspects of sexual activity; the PLISSIT model is viewed as paternalistic wherein the nurse/provider is the expert and imparts wisdom with little feedback from the client; and the BETTER model is viewed as the model with greater potential to communicate more openly with patients about intimacy and is not focused exclusively on function (Hordern, 2008). If nurses are aware of the potential limitations, they have the choice and ability to use any of the three models.

Expected Outcomes for Patients

Patients will develop a comfort level enabling them to ask nurses and physicians questions about sexuality and/or fertility. With knowledge, patients' awareness will increase and they will potentially avoid unsafe experimentation with folk remedies for sexual dysfunction because open discussion of the pros and cons of these strategies may limit their use. Patients will have access to and knowledge of resources to use at their discretion, such as books, journals, Web sites, and support groups. Patients and partners will be able to discuss changes in sexual functioning related to the disease and treatment, with the hope of resuming a more satisfying sex life (Stead, 2004).

Patient Teaching Points for Altered Sexuality Patterns

Patients can suffer from information overload during diagnosis and treatment. Therefore, written information with resources can be invaluable. An information-rich source of written information is available on the ACS Web site at www.cancer.org using a search for *sexuality*. This site also includes links to other helpful Web sites such as www.cancersymptoms.org/sexualdysfunction/index.shtml and http://cancercontrol.cancer.gov/ocs/index.html.

Following the crisis created by a diagnosis and treatment of cancer, a key role of the nurse is to reassure patients and their partners that counseling about marital/couple functioning during diagnosis and treatment has the potential to strengthen the patient and partner's relationship (Huber et al., 2006) rather than counseling being seen as a sign of weakness or marital discord (Kadmon et al., 2008). Patients should be informed that the oncology team is available to discuss sexual concerns throughout the cancer care trajectory because sexual functioning can change long after completion of therapy (Huber et al.). Because changes in sexuality affect both patient and partner, the patient should be encouraged to invite and include the partner in the conversations about possible side effects of diagnosis and treatments (McCorkle et al., 2007). Given that a partner may have different concerns than the patient, specific information may need to be provided to the partner (Sandham & Harcourt, 2007).

Need for Future Research for Altered Sexuality Patterns

Because patients are living longer, future research is needed in the form of longitudinal sexual effects of cancer treatment and diagnosis (Burwell et al., 2006; McCorkle et al., 2007). Most studies on sexual function focus on the first 24 months after treatment (Galbraith et al., 2005), notwithstanding evidence that sexual function tends to worsen in the second and third year after diagnosis (Pelusi, 2006). Present studies focus primarily on ED with little information about libido, body image, fertility, or everyday interactions with sexual partners (Galbraith et al.).

The focus of future research could be expanded beyond McCorkle et al.'s (2007) study on middle-class, educated, Caucasian men in heterosexual relationships. Studies are needed on other ethnicities, non-Caucasian men and women with grade school education, same-sex relationships, and men and women who have had more than one partner. Pelusi (2006) suggested including people who are single, widowed, or divorced to identify their possible unique concerns. In addition, studies that focus on partner issues would be helpful. Present studies seldom include the partners of patients (McCorkle et al.), even though sexual changes could be attributed to partner issues unrelated to the patient (Garos, Kluck, & Aronoff, 2007). Interventions are needed that improve partner understanding about the sexual impact of cancer diagnosis and treatment (Andersen, Carpenter, Yang, & Shapiro, 2007; Pelusi).

The design of future research may need to be reconsidered. More focused studies are needed and include (a) intervention studies that improve symptom management of sexual dysfunction (McCorkle et al., 2007), (b) randomized clinical trials on treatments (Alfano & Rowland, 2006), and (c) long-term outcomes of psychosocial interventions (Alfano & Rowland). The use of mixed research methods (Lauver et al., 2007) and multidisciplinary studies examining stressors and coping (Lauver et al.) would add to the richness of evidence.

Conclusion of Case Study

The oncology nurse recognizes that at the time she met with J.N. to talk about his chemotherapy, he was focused on his diagnosis and prognosis and how it would affect his life.

In the beginning, J.N. did not plan to marry or to have children. Given his life plans, when the nurse initially suggested consideration of sperm banking because of the possibility of infertility, J.N. was not interested. Looking beyond what J.N. thought he needed, the nurse took the time to have him discuss his beliefs and values. This led him to reflect and reconsider his initial decision to not do sperm banking.

Seven months after completion of his chemotherapy, J.N. moves to another state and the nurse loses contact with him. Eight years later, an envelope addressed to the nurse is delivered to the hospital. The nurse is surprised to find a letter from J.N. and two pictures. He asks the nurse if she remembers him, and then tells her how he has been doing. He still enjoys his career, but now the focus of his life is his wife and their twin daughters, who are a part of their lives because the nurse took the time to encourage him to participate in sperm banking.

Conclusion

The goal of this chapter was to stimulate nurses' awareness that changes in sexual functioning and perceived risks to fertility can have both an immediate and future impact on patients. Although some evidence-based interventions are known, much still needs to be investigated that can lead to improvements in patient care. Nevertheless, nurses are in a perfect position to complete a comprehensive and thorough assessment and to share knowledge of effective interventions to improve the sexual health of their patients.

References

Akin-Olugbade, O., Parker, M., Guhring, P., & Mulhall, J. (2006). Determinants of patient satisfaction following penile prosthesis surgery. *Journal of Sexual Medicine, 3*(4), 743–748.

Alfano, C.M., & Rowland, J.H. (2006). Recovery issues in cancer survivorship: A new challenge for supportive care. *Cancer Journal, 12*(5), 432–443.

Alvarez, J.A., Scully, R.E., Miller, T.L., Armstrong, F.D., Constine, L.S., Friedman, D.L., et al. (2007). Long-term effects of treatment for childhood cancers. *Current Opinion in Pediatrics, 19*(1), 23–31.

American Association of Clinical Endocrinologists. (2003). American Association of Clinical Endocrinologists medical guidelines for clinical practice for the evaluation and treatment of male sexual dysfunction: A couple's problem—2003 update. *Endocrine Practice, 9*(1), 77–95.

American Cancer Society. (2006). *Desire diary.* Retrieved February 2, 2008, from http://www.cancer.org/docroot/MIT/content/MIT_7_2X_Keeping_Your_Sex_Life_Going.asp

American Psychiatric Association. (2000). *Diagnostic and statistical manual of mental disorders* (4th ed., text revision). Washington, DC: Author.

American Urological Association. (2006). *Erectile dysfunction guidelines.* Retrieved September 29, 2007, from http://www.auanet.org/content/guidelines-and-quality-care/clinical-guidelines.cfm?sub=ed

Amsterdam, A., & Krychman, M.L. (2006). Sexual dysfunction in patients with gynecologic neoplasms: A retrospective pilot study. *Journal of Sexual Medicine, 3*(4), 646–649.

Andersen, B.L., Carpenter, K.M., Yang, H., & Shapiro, C.L. (2007). Sexual well-being among partnered women with breast cancer recurrence. *Journal of Clinical Oncology, 25*(21), 3151–3157.

Anderson, R.A., Themmen, A.P., Al-Qahtani, A., Groome, N.P., & Cameron, D.A. (2006). The effects of chemotherapy and long-term gonadotrophin suppression on the ovarian reserve in premenopausal women with breast cancer. *Human Reproduction, 21*(10), 2583–2592.

Baker, F., Denniston, M., Smith, T., & West, M.M. (2005). Adult cancer survivors: How are they faring? *Cancer, 104*(Suppl. 11), 2565–2576.

Barton, D.L., Wender, D.B., Sloan, J.A., Dalton, R.J., Balcueva, E.P., Atherton, P.J., et al. (2007). Randomized controlled trial to evaluate transdermal testosterone in female cancer survivors with decreased libido; North Central Cancer Treatment Group protocol N02C3. *Journal of the National Cancer Institute, 99*(9), 672–679.

Barclay, L., & Vega, C.P. (2007). *New guidelines issued for treatment of vaginal atrophy.* Retrieved April 24, 2009, from http://cme.medscape.com/viewarticle/556471

Bashore, L. (2007). Semen preservation in male adolescents and young adults with cancer: One institution's experience. *Clinical Journal of Oncology Nursing, 11*(3), 381–386.

Baum, A. (2006). Eating disorders in the male athlete. *Sports Medicine, 36*(1), 1–6.

Boehmer, U., Linde, R., & Freund, K.M. (2007). Breast reconstruction following mastectomy for breast cancer: The decisions of sexual minority women. *Plastic and Reconstructive Surgery, 119*(2), 464–472.

Braunstein, G.D., Sundwall, D.A., Katz, M., Shifren, J.L., Buster, J.E., Simon, J.A., et al. (2005). Safety and efficacy of a testosterone patch for the treatment of hypoactive sexual desire disorder in surgically menopausal women: A randomized, placebo-controlled trial. *Archives of Internal Medicine, 165*(14), 1582–1589.

Breerendonk, C.C., & Braat, D.D. (2005). Present and future options for the preservation of fertility in female adolescents with cancer. *Endocrine Development, 8,* 166–175.

Browall, M., Gaston-Johansson, F., & Danielson, E. (2006). Postmenopausal women with breast cancer: Their experiences of the chemotherapy treatment period. *Cancer Nursing, 29*(1), 34–42.

Bruce, S.D. (2007). Sperm and egg banking give patients hope for parenthood after cancer treatment. *ONS Connect, 22*(6), 17.

Burnett, A.L. (2005). Erectile dysfunction following radical prostatectomy. *JAMA, 293*(21), 2648–2653.

Burwell, S.R., Case, L.D., Kaelin, C., & Avis, N.E. (2006). Sexual problems in younger women after breast cancer surgery. *Journal of Clinical Oncology, 24*(18), 2815–2821.

Buster, J.E., Kingsberg, S.A., Aguirre, O., Brown, C., Breaux, J.G., Buch, A., et al. (2005). Testosterone patch for low sexual desire in surgically menopausal women: A randomized trial. *Obstetrics and Gynecology, 105*(5, Pt. 1), 944–952.

Cavallini, G., Modenini, F., Vitali, G., & Koverech, A. (2005). Acetyl-L-carnitine plus propionyl-L-carnitine improve efficacy of sildenafil in treatment of erectile dysfunction after bilateral nerve-sparing radical retropubic prostatectomy. *Urology, 66*(5), 1080–1085.

Champion, V., Williams, S.D., Miller, A., Reuille, K.M., Wagler-Ziner, K., Monahan, P.O., et al. (2007). Quality of life in long-term survivors of ovarian germ cell tumors: A Gynecologic Oncology Group study. *Gynecologic Oncology, 105*(3), 687–694.

Chapple, A., & McPherson, A. (2004). The decision to have a prosthesis: A qualitative study of men with testicular cancer. *Psycho-Oncology, 13*(9), 654–664.

Chapple, A., Salinas, M., Ziebland, S., McPherson, A., & Macfarlane, A. (2007). Fertility issues: The perceptions and experiences of young men recently diagnosed and treated for cancer. *Journal of Adolescent Health, 40*(1), 69–75.

Colella, J., & Scrofine, S. (2004). High-dose brachytherapy for treating prostate cancer: Nursing considerations. *Urologic Nursing, 24*(1), 39–44, 52.

Dauer, L.T., Casciotta, K.A., Erdi, Y.E., & Rothenberg, L.N. (2007). Radiation dose reduction at a price: The effectiveness of a male gonadal shield during helical CT scans. *BMC Medical Imaging, 7*(5). Retrieved August 7, 2007, from http://www.pubmedcentral.nih.gov/articlerender.fcgi?artid=1831769

Davis, M. (2006). Fertility considerations for female adolescent and young adult patients following cancer therapy: A guide for counseling patients and their families. *Clinical Journal of Oncology Nursing, 10*(2), 213–219.

DeFrank, J.T., Mehta, C.B., Stein, K.D., & Baker, F. (2007). Body image dissatisfaction in cancer survivors [Online exclusive]. *Oncology Nursing Forum, 34*(3), E36–E41. Retrieved October 7, 2007, from http://ons.metapress.com/content/9x80v31855269085/fulltext.pdf

Dixon, K.D., & Dixon, P.N. (2006). The PLISSIT model: Care and management of patients' psychosexual needs following radical surgery. *Lippincott's Case Management, 1*(2), 101–106.

Donatucci, C.F., & Greenfield, J.M. (2006). Recovery of sexual function after prostate cancer treatment. *Current Opinion in Urology, 16*(6), 444–448.

Dyer-Smith, R., Woodcock, N.P., & Hartley, J.E. (2006). Does neo-adjuvant radiotherapy increase the risk of male sexual dysfunction following surgery for rectal cancer [Abstract]? *British Journal of Surgery, 93*(Suppl. S1), 220.

Esco, M.R., Olson, M., & Williford, H. (2006). Body image perception among active college-aged men [Abstract]. *Medicine & Science in Sports & Exercise, 38*(Suppl. 5), S207.

European Association of Urology. (2006). *Guidelines on erectile dysfunction.* Retrieved June 6, 2008, from http://www.uroweb.org/fileadmin/user_upload/Guidelines/2005ErectileDysfunction.pdf

Fahmy, A.K., Mitra, S., Blacklock, A.R., & Desai, K.M. (1999). Is the measurement of serum testosterone routinely indicated in men with erectile dysfunction? *BJU International, 84*(4), 482–484.

Farthing, A. (2006). Conserving fertility in the management of gynaecological cancers. *British Journal of Obstetrics and Gynaecology, 113*(2), 129–134.

Feigin, E., Abir, R., Fisch, B., Kravarusic, D., Steinberg, R., Nitke, S., et al. (2007). Laparoscopic ovarian tissue preservation in young patients at risk for ovarian failure as a result of chemotherapy/irradiation for primary malignancy. *Journal of Pediatric Surgery, 42*(5), 862–864.

Fertile Hope. (n.d.-a). *Community statistics.* Retrieved February 14, 2009, from http://www.fertilehope.org/participate/community-stats.cfm

Fertile Hope. (n.d.-b). *Parenthood options: Women: Adoption.* Retrieved February 14, 2009, from http://www.fertilehope.org/learn-more/cancer-and-fertility-info/parenthood-options-women.cfm#TID18

Fertility and pregnancy after cancer treatment. (2006). *Journal of Supportive Oncology, 4*(2), 67–68.

Frid, M., Strang, P., Friedrichsen, M.J., & Johansson, K. (2006). Lower limb lymphedema: Experiences and perceptions of cancer patients in the late palliative stage. *Journal of Palliative Care, 22*(1), 5–11.

Galbraith, M.E., Arechiga, A., Ramirez, J., & Pedro, L.W. (2005). Prostate cancer survivors' and partners' self-reports of health-related quality of life, treatment symptoms, and marital satisfaction 2.5-5.5 years after treatment [Online exclusive]. *Oncology Nursing Forum, 32*(2), E30–E41. Retrieved April 24, 2009, from http://ons.metapress.com/content/t128147q6u1684t8/fulltext.pdf

Gallagher, P., Horgan, O., Franchignoni, F., Giordano, A., & MacLachlan, M. (2007). Body image in people with lower-limb amputation. *American Journal of Physical Medicine Rehabilitation, 86*(3), 205–215.

Garos, S., Kluck, A., & Aronoff, D. (2007). Prostate cancer patients and their partners: Differences in satisfaction indices and psychological variables. *Journal of Sexual Medicine, 4*(5), 1394–1403.

Geiger, A.M., West, C.N., Nekhlyudov, L., Herrinton, L.J., Liu, I.L., Altschuler, A., et al. (2006). Contentment with quality of life among breast cancer survivors with and without contralateral prophylactic mastectomy. *Journal of Clinical Oncology, 24*(9), 1350–1356.

Girasole, C.R., Cookson, M.S., Smith, J.A., Jr., Ivey, B.S., Roth, B.J., & Chang, S.S. (2007). Sperm banking: Use and outcomes in patients treated for testicular cancer. *BJU International, 99*(1), 33–36.

Gontero, P., Fontana, F., Zitella, A., Montorsi, F., & Frea, B. (2005). A prospective evaluation of efficacy and compliance with a multistep treatment approach for erectile dysfunction in patients after non-nerve sparing radical prostatectomy. *BJU International, 95*(3), 359–365.

Gonzalgo, M.L., & Eastham, J. (2007). Wide excision radical prostatectomy: Indications and surgical technique. *Contemporary Urology, 19*(1), 30–37.

Heiman, J.R., Talley, D.R., Bailen, J.L., Oskin, T.A., Rosenberg, S.J., Pace, C.R., et al. (2007). Sexual function and satisfaction in heterosexual couples when men are administered sildenafil citrate (Viagra) for erectile dysfunction: A multicentre, randomised, double-blind, placebo-controlled trail. *BJOG: An International Journal of Obstetrics and Gynaecology, 114*(4), 437–447.

Hendren, S.K., O'Connor, B.I., Liu, M., Asano, T., Cohen, Z., Swallow, C.J., et al. (2005). Prevalence of male and female sexual dysfunction is high following surgery for rectal cancer. *Annals of Surgery, 242*(2), 212–223.

Herbenick, D., Reece, M., Hollub, A., Satinsky, S., & Dodge, B. (2008). Young female breast cancer survivors: Their sexual function and interest in sexual enhancement products and services. *Cancer Nursing, 31*(6), 417–425.

Hewitt, M., Greenfield, S., & Stovall, E. (Eds.). (2006). *From cancer patient to cancer survivor: Lost in transition.* Washington, DC: National Academies Press.

Hickey, M., Saunders, C., Partridge, A., Santoro, N., Joffe, H., & Stearns, V. (2008). Practical clinical guidelines for assessing and managing menopausal symptoms after breast cancer. *Annals of Oncology, 19*(10), 1669–1680.

Hopwood, P., Fletcher, I., Lee, A., & Al Ghazal, S. (2001). A body image scale for use with cancer patients. *European Journal of Cancer, 37*(2), 189–197.

Hordern, A. (2008). Intimacy and sexuality after cancer: A critical review of the literature. *Cancer Nursing, 31*(2), E9–E17.

Huber, C., Ramnarace, T., & McCaffrey, R. (2006). Sexuality and intimacy issues facing women with breast cancer. *Oncology Nursing Forum, 33*(6), 1163–1167.

Huddart, R.A., Norman, A., Moynihan, C., Horwich, A., Parker, C., Nicholls, E., et al. (2005). Fertility, gonadal and sexual function in survivors of testicular cancer. *British Journal of Cancer, 93*(2), 200–207.

Iacono, F., Giannella, R., Somma, P., Manno, G., Fusco, F., & Mirone, V. (2005). Histological alterations in cavernous tissue after radical prostatectomy. *Journal of Urology, 173*(5), 1673–1676.

Junkin, J., & Beitz, J.M. (2005). Sexuality and the person with a stoma: Implications for comprehensive WOC nursing practice. *Journal of Wound, Ostomy, and Continence Nursing, 32*(2), 121–128.

Kadmon, I., Ganz, F.D., Rom, M., & Woloski-Wruble, A.C. (2008). Social, marital, and sexual adjustment of Israeli men whose wives were diagnosed with breast cancer. *Oncology Nursing Forum, 35*(1), 131–135.

Katz, A. (2007). When sex hurts: Menopause-related dyspareunia. *American Journal of Nursing, 107*(7), 34–39.

Kaufman, M.R., & Chang, S.S. (2007). Short- and long-term complications of therapy for testicular cancer. *Urologic Clinics of North America, 34*(2), 259–268.

Kelly-Weeder, S., & O'Connor, A. (2006). Modifiable risk factors for impaired fertility in women: What nurse practitioners need to know. *Journal of the American Academy of Nurse Practitioners, 18*(6), 268–276.

Kendirci, M., Bejma, J., & Hellstrom, W.J.G. (2006). Update on erectile dysfunction in prostate cancer patients. *Current Opinion in Urology, 16*(3), 186–195.

Keros, V., Hultenby, K., Borgstrom, B., Fridstrom, M., Jahnukainen, K., & Hovatta, O. (2007). Methods of cryopreservation of testicular tissue with viable spermatogonia in pre-pubertal boys undergoing gonadotoxic cancer treatment. *Human Reproduction, 22*(5), 1384–1395.

King, L., Quinn, G.P., Vadaparamil, S.T., Gwede, C.K., Miree, C.A., Wilson, C., et al. (2008). Oncology nurses' perceptions of barriers to discussion of fertility preservation with patients with cancer. *Clinical Journal of Oncology, 12*(3), 467–476.

Knobf, M.T. (2006). Reproductive and hormonal sequelae of chemotherapy in women: Premature menopause and impaired fertility can result, effects that are especially disturbing to young women. *Cancer Nursing, 29*(Suppl. 2), 60–65.

Kritcharoen, S., Suwan, K., & Jirojwong, S. (2005). Perceptions of gender roles, gender power relationships, and sexuality in Thai women following diagnosis and treatment for cervical cancer. *Oncology Nursing Forum, 32*(3), 682–688.

Lambert, S.M., & Fisch, H. (2007). Infertility and testis cancer. *Urologic Clinics of North America, 34*(2), 269–277.

Lancaster, L. (2004). Preventing vaginal stenosis after brachytherapy for gynaecological cancer: An overview of Australian practices. *European Journal of Oncology Nursing, 8*(1), 30–39.

Lauver, D.R., Connolly-Nelson, K., & Vang, P. (2007). Stressors and coping strategies among female cancer survivors after treatments. *Cancer Nursing, 30*(2), 101–111.

Lee, S.J., Schover, L.R., Partridge, A.H., Patrizio, P., Wallace, W.H., Hagerty, K., et al. (2006). American Society of Clinical Oncology recommendations on fertility preservation in cancer patients. *Journal of Clinical Oncology, 24*(18), 2917–2931.

Leonard, M. (2006). Fertility preservation options for women with cancer. *Current Topics in Cancer Fertility for Oncology Nurses, 1*(1), 1–2, 6.

Lindsey, H. (2005). Discussions about preserving fertility overlooked in young breast cancer patients. *Oncology Times, 27*(9), 18–20.

Madsen, L.T., & Ganey-Code, E. (2006). Assessing and addressing erectile function concerns in patients postprostatectomy. *Oncology Nursing Forum, 33*(2), 209–211.

Magnan, M.A., & Reynolds, K. (2006). Barriers to addressing patient sexuality concerns across five areas of specialization. *Clinical Nurse Specialist, 20*(6), 285–292.

Matsumoto, T., Ohue, M., Sekimoto, M., Yamamoto, H., Ikeda, M., & Monden, M. (2005). Feasibility of autonomic nerve-preserving surgery for advanced rectal cancer based on analysis of micrometastases. *British Journal of Surgery, 92*(11), 1444–1448.

Matthews, K.S., Numnum, T.M., Conner, M.G., & Barnes, M., III. (2007). Fertility-sparing radical abdominal trachelectomy for clear cell adenocarcinoma of the upper vagina: A case report. *Gynecologic Oncology, 105*(3), 820–822.

Mazonakis, M., Damilakis, J., Varveris, H., & Gourtsouiannis, N. (2006). Radiation dose to testes and risk of infertility from radiotherapy for rectal cancer. *Oncology Reports, 15*(3), 729–733.

McCaffrey, C.N. (2006). Major stressors and their effects on the well-being of children with cancer. *Journal of Pediatric Nursing, 21*(1), 59–66.

McClement, S. (2005). Cancer anorexia-cachexia syndrome: Psychological effect on the patient and family. *Journal of Wound, Ostomy, and Continence Nursing, 32*(4), 264–268.

McCorkle, R., Siefert, M.L., Dowd, M.F., Robinson, J.P., & Pickett, M. (2007). Effects of advanced practice nursing on patient and spouse depressive symptoms, sexual function, and marital interaction after radical prostatectomy. *Urologic Nursing, 27*(1), 65–77.

Mok, K., Juraskova, I., & Friedlander, M. (2008). The impact of aromatase inhibitors on sexual functioning: Current knowledge and future research directions. *Breast, 17*(5), 436–440.

Morales, L., Neven, P., Timmerman, D., Christiaens, M.R., Vergote, I., Van Limbergen, E., et al (2004). Acute effects of tamoxifen and third-generation aromatase inhibitors on menopausal symptoms of breast cancer patients. *Anti-Cancer Drugs, 15*(8), 753–760.

Mulhall, J., Land, S., Parker, M., Waters, W.B., & Flanigan, R.C. (2005). The use of an erectogenic pharmacotherapy regimen following radical prostatectomy improves recovery of spontaneous erectile function. *Journal of Sexual Medicine, 2*(4), 532–540.

Mydlo, J.H., Viterbo, R., & Crispen, P. (2005). Use of combined intracorporal injection and a phosphodiesterase-5 inhibitor therapy for men with a suboptimal response to sildenafil and/or vardenafil monotherapy after radical retropubic prostatectomy. *BJU International, 95*(6), 843–846.

Nandipati, K., Raina, R., Agarwal, A., & Zippe, C.D. (2006). Early combination therapy: Intracavernosal injections and sildenafil following radical prostatectomy increases sexual activity and the return of natural erections. *International Journal of Impotence Research, 18*(5), 446–451.

Ng, C., Kristjanson, L.J., & Medigovich, K. (2006). Hormone ablation for the treatment of prostate cancer: The lived experience. *Urologic Nursing, 26*(3), 204–212.

Nieman, C.L., Kazer, R., Brannigan, R.E., Zoloth, L.S., Chase-Lansdale, P.L., Kinahan, K., et al. (2006). Cancer survivors and infertility: A review of a new problem and novel answers. *Journal of Supportive Oncology, 4*(4), 171–178.

Nishimoto, P.W. (2008). Sexuality. In R.A. Gates & R.M. Fink (Eds.), *Oncology nursing secrets* (3rd ed., pp. 448–501). St. Louis, MO: Mosby.

Paduch, D.A. (2006). Testicular cancer and male infertility. *Current Opinion in Urology, 16*(6), 419–427.

Pelusi, J. (2006). Sexuality and body image: Research on breast cancer survivors documents altered body image and sexuality. *American Journal of Nursing, 106*(Suppl. 3), 32–38.

Plante, M., & Roy, M. (2006). Fertility-preserving options for cervical cancer. *Oncology, 20*(5), 479–488.

Ponholzer, A., Oismuller, R., Somay, C., Buchler, F., Maier, U., Hawliczek, R., et al. (2005). The effect on erectile function of 103palladium implantation for localized prostate cancer. *BJU International, 95*(6), 847–850.

Quallich, S. (2006). Examining male infertility. *Urologic Nursing, 26*(4), 277–288.

Raina, R., Agarwal, A., Allamaneni, S.S., Lakin, M.M., & Zippe, C.D. (2005). Sildenafil citrate and vacuum constriction device combination enhances sexual satisfaction in erectile dysfunction after radical prostatectomy. *Urology, 65*(2), 360–364.

Raina, R., Nandipati, K.C., Agarwal, A., Mansour, D., Kaelber, D.C., & Zippe, C.D. (2005). Combination therapy: Medicated urethral system for erection following nerve-sparing radical prostatectomy. *Journal of Andrology, 26*(6), 757–760.

Ralph, D., & McNicholas, T. (2000). UK management guidelines for erectile dysfunction. *BMJ, 321*(7259), 499–503.

Ralph, D.J., Garaffa, G., & Garcia, M.A. (2006). Reconstructive surgery of the penis. *Current Opinion in Urology, 16*(6), 396–400.

Ramsawh, H.J., Morgentaler, A., Covino, N., Barlow, D.H., & DeWolf, W.C. (2005). Quality of life following simultaneous placement of penile prosthesis with radical prostatectomy. *Journal of Urology, 174*(4, Pt. 1), 1395–1398.

Reed, S.D., Newton, K.M., LaCroix, A.Z., Grothaus, L.C., Grieco, V.S., & Ehrlich, K. (2008). Vaginal, endometrial, and reproductive hormone findings: Randomized, placebo-controlled trial of black cohosh, multibotanical herbs, and dietary soy for vasomotor symptoms: The Herbal Alternatives for Menopause (HALT) Study. *Menopause, 15*(1), 51–58.

Roberts, S., Livingston, P., White, V., & Gibbs, A. (2003). External breast prosthesis use: Experiences and views of women with breast cancer, breast care nurses, and prosthesis fitters. *Cancer Nursing, 26*(3), 179–186.

Rosen, R.C. (2007). Optimizing testosterone replacement therapy in hypogonadal men. *Contemporary Urology, 19*(5), 30–37.

Rosen, R.C., Fisher, W.A., Beneke, M., Homering, M., & Evers, T. (2007). The COUPLES-project: A pooled analysis of patient and partner treatment satisfaction scale (TSS) outcomes following vardenafil treatment. *BJU International, 99*(4), 849–859.

Rosen, R.C., Riley, A., Wagner, G., Osterloh, I.H., Kirkpatrick, J., & Mishra, A. (1997). The international index of erectile function (IIEF): A multidimensional scale for assessment of erectile dysfunction. *Urology, 49*(6), 822–830.

Rosen, R.C., Taylor, J.F., Leiblum, S.R., & Bachmann, G.A. (1993). Prevalence of sexual dysfunction in women: Results of a survey study of 329 women in an outpatient gynecological clinic. *Journal of Sex and Marital Therapy, 19*(3), 171–188.

Sandel, S.L., Judge, J.O., Landry, N., Faria, L., Ouellette, R., & Majczak, M. (2005). Dance and movement program improves quality-of-life measures in breast cancer survivors. *Cancer Nursing, 28*(4), 301–309.

Sandham, C., & Harcourt, D. (2007). Partner experiences of breast reconstruction post mastectomy. *European Journal of Oncology Nursing, 11*(1), 66–73.

Schover, L.R. (2006). The impact of cancer on men's fertility. *Current Topics in Cancer Fertility for Oncology Nurses, 1*(1), 3, 6–7.

Schover, L.R. (2008). Premature ovarian failure and its consequences: Vasomotor symptoms, sexuality, and fertility. *Journal of Clinical Oncology, 26*(5), 753–758.

Scott, J.L., Halford, W.K., & Ward, B.G. (2004). United we stand? The effects of a couple-coping intervention on adjustment to early stage breast or gynecological cancer. *Journal of Consulting and Clinical Psychology, 72*(6), 1122–1135.

Scott, J.L., & Kayser, K. (2009). A review of couple-based interventions for enhancing women's sexual adjustment and body image after cancer. *Cancer Journal, 15*(1), 48–56.

Segraves, R.T., Croft, H., Kavoussi, R., Ascher, J.A., Batey, S.R., Foster, V.J., et al. (2001). Bupropion sustained release (SR) for the treatment of hypoactive sexual desire disorder (HSDD) in nondepressed women. *Journal of Sex and Marital Therapy, 27*(3), 303–316.

Shah, K., & Montoya, C. (2007). Do testosterone injections increase libido for elderly hypogonadal patients? *Journal of Family Practice, 56*(4), 301–303.

Shell, J.A., Carolan, M., Zhang, Y., & Meneses, K.D. (2008). The longitudinal effects of cancer treatment on sexuality in individuals with lung cancer. *Oncology Nursing Forum, 35*(1), 73–79.

Shepherd, J.H., Spencer, C., Herod, J., & Ind, T.E. (2006). Radical vaginal trachelectomy as a fertility-sparing procedure in women with early-stage cervical cancer—Cumulative pregnancy rate in a series of 123 women. *BJOG: An International Journal of Obstetrics and Gynaecology, 113*(6), 719–724.

Sheppard, L.A., & Ely, S. (2008). Breast cancer and sexuality. *Breast Journal, 14*(2), 176–181.

Shifren, J.L., & Avis, N.E. (2007). Surgical menopause: Effects on psychological well-being and sexuality. *Menopause, 14*(3, Pt. 2), 586–591.

Sideris, L., Zenasni, F., Vernerey, D., Dauchy, S., Lasser, P., Pignon, J.P., et al. (2005). Quality of life of patients operated on for low rectal cancer: Impact of the type of surgery and patients' characteristics. *Diseases of the Colon and Rectum, 48*(12), 2180–2191.

Sonmezer, M., & Oktay, K. (2006). Fertility preservation in young women undergoing breast cancer therapy. *Oncologist, 11*(5), 422–434.

Spark, R.F. (2008). Evaluation of male sexual dysfunction [UpToDate]. Retrieved April 21, 2009, from http://www.utdol.com

Stead, M.L. (2004). Sexual function after treatment for gynecological malignancy. *Current Opinion in Oncology, 16*(5), 492–495.

Stephenson, R.A., Mori, M., Hsieh, Y.C., Beer, T.M., Stanford, J.L., Gilliland, F.D., et al. (2005). Treatment of erectile dysfunction following therapy for clinically localized prostate cancer: Patient reported outcomes from the Surveillance, Epidemiology and End Results Prostate Cancer Outcomes Study. *Journal of Urology, 174*(2), 646–650.

Styles, S.J., MacLean, A.B., Reid, W.M.N., & Sultana, S.R. (2006). Laser Doppler perfusion imaging: A method for measuring female sexual response. *BJOG: An International Journal of Obstetrics and Gynaecology, 113*(5), 599–601.

Sublett, C.M. (2007). Translating evidence into clinical practice: Critique of 'Effects of advanced practice nursing on patient and spouse depressive symptoms, sexual function, and marital interaction after radical prostatectomy'. *Urologic Nursing, 27*(1), 78–80.

Thaler-DeMers, D. (2006). Endocrine and fertility effects in male cancer survivors: Changes related to androgen-deprivation therapy and other treatments require timely intervention. *American Journal of Nursing, 106*(Suppl. 3), 66–71, 96–98.

Travison, T.G., Morley, J.E., Araujo, A.B., O'Donnell, A.M., & McKinlay, J.B. (2006). The relationship between libido and testosterone levels in aging men. *Journal of Clinical Endocrinology and Metabolism, 91*(7), 2509–2513.

van den Berg, H., Repping, S., & van der Veen, F. (2007). Parental desire and acceptability of spermatogonial stem cell cryopreservation in boys with cancer. *Human Reproduction, 22*(2), 594–597.

Wahlgren, T., Nilsson, S., Ryberg, M., Lennernas, B., & Brandberg, Y. (2005). Combined curative radiotherapy including HDR brachytherapy and androgen deprivation in localized prostate cancer: A prospective assessment of acute and late treatment toxicity. *Acta Oncologica, 44*(6), 633–643.

Windahl, T., Skeppner, E., Andersson, S.O., & Fugl-Meyer, K.S. (2004). Sexual function and satisfaction in men after laser treatment for penile carcinoma. *Journal of Urology, 172*(2), 648–651.

Witt, M.E., Haas, M., Marrinan, M.A., & Brown, C.N. (2003). Understanding stereotactic radiosurgery for intracranial tumors, seed implants for prostate cancer, and intravascular brachytherapy for cardiac restenosis. *Cancer Nursing, 26*(6), 494–502.

Zebrack, B.J., Oeffinger, K.C., Hou, P., & Kaplan, S. (2006). Advocacy skills training for young adult cancer survivors: The Young Adult Survivors Conference at Camp Māk-a-Dream. *Supportive Care in Cancer, 14*(7), 779–782.

CHAPTER 22

Skin and Nail Alterations

Megan Dunne, RN, MA, ANP-BC, AOCN®

Case Study

M.R. is a 70-year-old Caucasian man who recently was diagnosed with stage IV non-small cell lung cancer (NSCLC) with malignant pleural effusion (fluid in the pleural lining of the lung). The pathology revealed a bronchoalveolar carcinoma. The patient consented to a clinical trial of erlotinib 150 mg oral daily as first-line therapy and began the medication. Seven days after initiating therapy, M.R. presents to the clinic with grade 1 minimal rash over his face, chest, and back, and rare pustules are noted. The patient continued the erlotinib and returned for evaluation one week later, after 14 days of therapy. He continues to complain of pruritic, bothersome rash (grade 2 intolerable rash related to erlotinib). He comments, "I don't even want to see my friends."

Overview

Skin and nail bed changes related to treatment with chemotherapeutic agents have always existed. These alterations are now occurring with increasing frequency as novel agents that target specific pathways critical to tumor growth, such as erlotinib, sunitinib, and sorafenib, gain wider use (see Table 22-1). Over the past 10 years, the approach to cancer has changed because of an improved understanding of how tumors develop and grow. There are now anticancer strategies, such as epidermal growth factor receptor tyrosine kinase inhibitors (EGFR-TKIs), that inhibit growth and metastasis and yet do not affect the immune system. These drugs have gained notoriety because many toxicities (e.g., neutropenia and emesis) are avoided with these new agents; however, they encompass their own adverse side effects, including dermatologic toxicities. With proper management, patients often can manage to tolerate these agents quite well.

Dermatologic toxicities can range from localized non-bothersome changes to serious generalized alterations that are so severe that they lead to dose reductions or even abandonment of a therapy. Skin and nail alterations often are reversible within a few weeks to months of withdrawal of the causative agent (Dasanu, Vaillant, & Alexandrescu, 2007). Anticipation of and comprehensive symptom management for these changes may lead to prolonged therapy and improved tolerance of treatment regimens. This, in turn, may lead to a better chance for cure of patients' respective cancers.

Chemotherapy-induced dermatologic toxicity can significantly affect patients' quality of life (Hackbarth, Haas, Fotopoulou, Lichtenegger, & Sehouli, 2007). The cosmetic changes

TABLE 22-1	Dermatologic Adverse Events		
Adverse Event	**Causative Agents**	**Management**	**Comments**
Rash—Macular, papular, or erythemic rash may present on face, neck, scalp, torso, buttocks, or extremities.	Gefitinib, erlotinib, cetuximab, gemcitabine, dactinomycin, pemetrexed, high-dose methotrexate, long-term steroids (Perez-Soler et al., 2005)	Hypoallergenic cleanser twice daily, emollients to prevent dryness (leads to pruritus), sunscreen with sun protection factor ≥ 15 (Oishi, 2008; Perez-Soler et al., 2005)	Macular hyperpigmentation may persist long after papules have disappeared. Cosmetic cover-up may be used; over-the-counter (OTC) acne medications should be avoided (Perez-Soler et al., 2005).
Rash—follicular or pustular lesions present	Gefitinib, erlotinib, cetuximab, dactinomycin (usually the result of secondarily infected rash) (Perez-Soler et al., 2005; Robert et al., 2005)	Oral antibiotics (tetracyclines) for 1–2 weeks (Perez-Soler et al., 2005)	Dose interruption or reduction may be necessary to effectively control rash to a level that is tolerable for the patient (Perez-Soler et al., 2005; Robert et al., 2005).
Hyperpigmentation (asymptomatic)	Gefitinib, erlotinib, cetuximab, gemcitabine (Aapro et al., 1998; Robert et al., 2005)	Cosmetic cover-up (Robert et al., 2005)	This asymptomatic change in skin coloration can be bothersome in appearance. It can continue for months after discontinuation of the causative agent (Robert et al., 2005).
Dry skin/xerosis with accompanying pruritus	Gefitinib, erlotinib, cetuximab, pemetrexed, dactinomycin (Robert et al., 2005; Socinski, 2005)	Emollient OTC moisturizers or prescription Biafine® (OrthoNeutrogena) (TID or more frequently) (Robert et al., 2005)	Affected area may be local or generalized; moisturizing is key to management (Robert et al., 2005).
Acral erythema—may initially present with dysesthesia in hands and feet that can progress to pain. Characterized by areas of edematous erythema on palms, soles, or fingers.	High-dose cytarabine, sunitinib, sorafenib, cyclophosphamide, doxorubicin, methotrexate, mitoxantrone, taxanes, vinorelbine (Cetkovska et al., 2002; Rose et al., 2001; Wood, 2006)	Cold compresses, cushioning of soles, skin and wound care to prevent secondary infection (Wood, 2006)	Symptoms resolve within 7 days of discontinuation of causative agent (Wood, 2006).
Paronychia/periungual inflammation—inflammation of the nail fold with pyogenic painful lesions. Can affect any toenail or fingernail.	Gefitinib, erlotinib, cetuximab (Busam et al., 2001; Robert et al., 2005)	Often infection with *Staphylococcus aureus* is present, so antibiotics, silver nitrate, and antiseptic soaks may help (Robert et al., 2005).	Symptom can resolve spontaneously and always resolves with discontinuation of causative agent.

can interfere with body image and can be painful enough to limit one's ability to perform usual activities. A study of 91 patients receiving chemotherapeutic agents including taxanes, polyethylene glycol (PEG) doxorubicin, other anthracyclines (epirubicin and doxorubicin), topotecan, and other agents found that the overall incidence of dermatologic side effects (including skin, nail, and hair side effects) was 87% (Hackbarth et al.). This study utilized the Health-Related Quality of Life score, and skin changes were the most frequently reported bothersome side effect (34%). Yet, although hematologic toxicity of cancer agents is well documented, the incidence and severity of dermatologic morbidity are not well studied or reported.

Nail Bed Changes

A number of anticancer agents are known to produce pigmentary changes affecting the skin or nails. Nail changes are reported in up to 40% of patients receiving docetaxel therapy (Robert et al., 2005). Nail bed changes also commonly occur with the chemotherapeutic agents 5-fluorouracil (5-FU), doxorubicin, paclitaxel, docetaxel, and bleomycin. Nail and nail bed abnormalities usually are not serious. These changes in appearance range from cosmetic changes, such as Beau's lines (transverse white lines or grooves), which signal a cessation of nail growth (see Figure 22-1), to severe deformities in the appearance of fingers and toes. Nails can appear ridged, and cuticles and periungual areas (areas surrounding fingernails or toenails) can become dry enough to cause fissures or splitting. This can lead to paronychias characterized by inflammation of the tissues adjacent to the nail, usually accompanied by infection and pus formation (see Figure 22-2). Paronychias can cause patients significant pain and become dose-limiting. Dry skin or xerosis is very common in patients receiving EGFR inhibitors. For treatment, frequent application of emollients with 5%–10% urea can substantially improve skin dryness (Robert et al.). *Onycholysis* refers to a condition in which nails are separated partially or completely

FIGURE 22-1	Beau's Lines

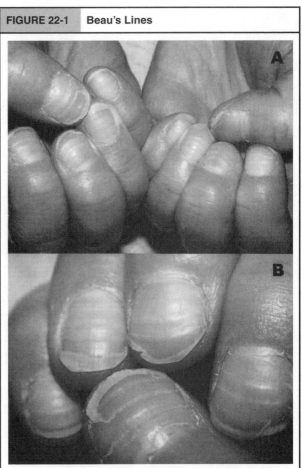

Beau's lines affecting all fingernails. The presence of multiple lines in each nail indicates repetitive exposure to the drug.

Note. From "Taxane-Induced Nail Changes: Incidence, Clinical Presentation and Outcome," by A.M. Minisini, A. Tosti, A.F. Sobrero, M. Mansutti, B.M. Piraccini, C. Sacco, et al., 2003, *Annals of Oncology, 14*(2), p. 335. Copyright 2003 by European Society for Medical Oncology. Reprinted with permission.

FIGURE 22-2   **Paronychial Inflammation**

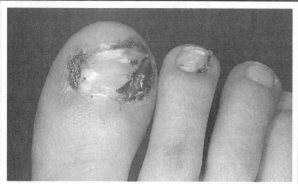

Paronychial inflammation with pyogenic granuloma-like lesions around the first two toenails in patient given gefitinib.

Note. From "Cutaneous Side-Effects of Kinase Inhibitors and Blocking Antibodies," by C. Robert, J.C. Soria, A. Spatz, A. Le Cesne, D. Malka, P. Pautier, et al., 2005, *Lancet Oncology, 6*(7), p. 495. Copyright 2005 by Elsevier. Reprinted with permission.

FIGURE 22-3   **Hemorrhagic Onycholysis**

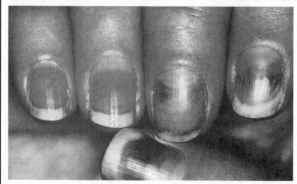

Development of the nail lesions was associated with intense pain.

Note. From "Taxane-Induced Nail Changes: Incidence, Clinical Presentation and Outcome," by A.M. Minisini, A. Tosti, A.F. Sobrero, M. Mansutti, B.M. Piraccini, C. Sacco, et al., 2003, *Annals of Oncology, 14*(2), p. 335. Copyright 2003 by European Society for Medical Oncology. Reprinted with permission.

from the nail bed (see Figure 22-3). A variety of antineoplastic agents, including the anthracyclines, bleomycin, dactinomycin, mitomycin, and mitoxantrone, have been reported to cause this alteration (Daniel & Scher, 1984; Flory et al., 1999).

Subungual splinter hemorrhage forms within the epidermis of the nail bed and consists of a mass of blood in a layer of squamous cells that adhere to the underlying surface of the nail (see Figure 22-4). This condition usually is not associated with pain or change in nail integrity (Robert et al., 2005). However, hemorrhagic onycholysis and subungual abscesses can lead to substantial discomfort with negative impact on patients' quality of life. Morbidity associated with these alterations can lead to dose reductions or even discontinuation of treatment with the causative agent because of patients' intolerance of these effects.

Pemetrexed is a multitargeted antifolate and is active as a single agent or in combination with cisplatin or carboplatin in both NSCLC and malignant pleural mesothelioma (Adjei, 2004). Current research also supports its usefulness in other solid tumors such as colorectal cancer (CRC) (Hochster, 2002), small cell lung cancer (Socinski, 2005), and breast cancer (Llombart-Cussac et al., 2007). Skin rash is one of the principal toxicities of pemetrexed. Routine use of prophylactic oral dexamethasone appears to lessen the frequency of severe rash (Socinski). A typical dose regimen of dexamethasone is 4 mg administered twice daily for three days beginning the day prior to pemetrexed administration.

Taxanes include paclitaxel and docetaxel, which were both introduced in the late 1980s. Both drugs have proven efficacy in solid tumors such as lung, breast, ovarian, and bladder cancers. Unfortunately, both drugs also cause nail abnormalities, including changes in nail pigmentation, splinter hemorrhage, subungual hematoma, Beau's lines, acute paronychia, and onycholysis. Paclitaxel has been documented to lead to toxicities of discoloration or ridging of nails in approximately 17% of patients treated (Minisini et al., 2003) (see Figure 22-5). Grade 2 of the National Cancer Institute Cancer Therapy Evaluation Program's Common Terminology Criteria for Adverse Events (CTCAE) toxicities of onycholysis (separation or loosening of a nail from its bed) or paronychia occurs in 3% of those treated with paclitaxel. The incidence of onycholysis and dyschromia related to docetaxel may be as high as 44%. Possible explanations for these occurrences include taxane-induced thrombocytopenia (low platelet level) and vascular abnormalities. However, more studies are necessary to understand the pathogenesis of taxane-induced nail changes (Minisini et al.).

Hyperpigmentation

Hyperpigmentation refers to asymptomatic darkening of the skin or nails that can occur within two weeks of treatment with a causative agent and last for several months after the agent has been discontinued. This can occur in nail beds or over the joints of fingers (interphalangeal) or hands (metacarpophalangeal) as a result of chemotherapeutic agents such as doxorubicin, capecitabine, and 5-FU. Hyperpigmentation occurs in less than 2% of patients treated with paclitaxel (Bristol-Myers Squibb Co., 2000). Hyperpigmentation also can occur with novel targeted therapies like EGFR-TKIs after a papulopustular eruption has resolved (Lacouture, Boerner, & LoRusso, 2006). The under-

| FIGURE 22-4 | Hemorrhagic Onycholysis and Subungual Hyperkeratosis in a Patient Treated With Docetaxel |

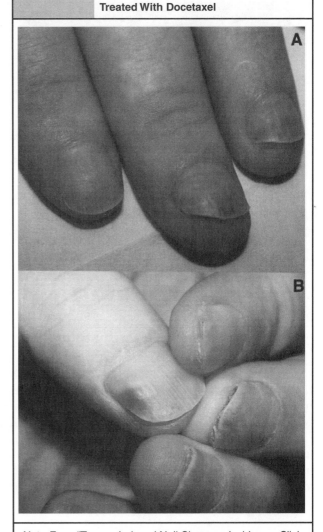

Note. From "Taxane-Induced Nail Changes: Incidence, Clinical Presentation and Outcome," by A.M. Minisini, A. Tosti, A.F. Sobrero, M. Mansutti, B.M. Piraccini, C. Sacco, et al., 2003, *Annals of Oncology, 14*(2), p. 334. Copyright 2003 by European Society for Medical Oncology. Reprinted with permission.

lying mechanism is not known, but inhibitor-induced functional alterations of melanocytes may increase pigment transfer to basal keratinocytes or dermal macrophages (Chang et al., 2004). No treatment is currently known, but sun exposure may worsen the condition; therefore, patients should use broad-spectrum sunscreen (Segaert & Van Cutsem, 2005).

Hyperpigmentation is strictly cosmetic, without discomfort, and often reversible once treatment is completed. It is more common in patients of Mediterranean descent and may be the result of melanocyte stimulation by chemotherapeutic agents.

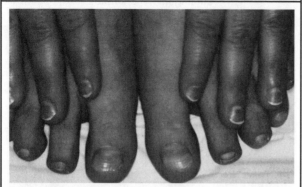

| FIGURE 22-5 | Paclitaxel-Induced Nail Toxicities |

Diffuse fingernail orange discoloration due to hemorrhagic suffusion of the nail bed and toenail onycholysis with subungual suppuration of the left great toenail in a patient treated with paclitaxel.

Note. From "Taxane-Induced Nail Changes: Incidence, Clinical Presentation and Outcome," by A.M. Minisini, A. Tosti, A.F. Sobrero, M. Mansutti, B.M. Piraccini, C. Sacco, et al., 2003, *Annals of Oncology, 14*(2), p. 335. Copyright 2003 by European Society for Medical Oncology. Reprinted with permission.

Paronychia and Onycholysis

Both paronychia (Robert et al., 2005) and onycholysis (Minisini et al., 2003) can occur with EGFR inhibitors like erlotinib and gefitinib. Associated periungual inflammation can cause pain and difficulty with usual activities of hands and feet. These changes occur four weeks to several months after initiation of EGFR inhibitor therapy. They can affect any finger or toe but most often are seen in the thumb or great toe (O'Keeffe, Parilli, & Lacouture, 2006). The reason why some nails are affected and others are not is not known. Paronychias can be painful and prevent patients from performing certain activities or wearing shoes other than sandals. Paronychias can resolve spontaneously and always disappear within a few days of discontinuation of the causative agent. The pathogenesis of paronychia is unknown. When the appearance suggests presence of infection with pus or erythema, a culture should be obtained. Paronychia does not seem to have an infectious origin, although superinfection with *Staphylococcus aureus* is common. For infectious cases, treatment with antibiotics may prove helpful. Infection with *Candida albicans* has not been reported (Lacouture et al., 2006). Patients should be advised to avoid paronychial trauma (e.g., nail or cuticle biting, restrictive shoes, use of nonsterile nail care equipment at nail salons during manicures or pedicures) (Robert et al., 2005). In the presence of infection, oral cephalexin can be helpful. Topical agents that may be of benefit include mupirocin ointment, ketoconazole, or silver nitrate. Minor surgical excisions of ingrown nails also can prevent recurrences of paronychia (Robert et al.).

Palms and Soles

Palmar-plantar erythrodysesthesia syndrome (PPES) refers to skin changes on the hands and feet (hand-foot syndrome). Incidence of PPES depends on the agent, dose, and route of drug delivery. Hand-foot syndrome was first reported in 1982 and occurred in 34% of patients receiving 5-FU continuous infusion therapy (Lokich & Moore, 1984). In patients receiving 5-FU as an IV bolus, incidence was 13%. In a study of patients with CRC receiving daily capecitabine oral chemotherapy (a prodrug of 5-FU that converts enzymatically to 5-FU in vivo), the incidence of hand-foot syndrome was 68%, and 11%–17% of patients experienced severe grade 3 toxicity with moist desquamation, ulceration, blistering, and severe pain interfering with activities of daily living (Abushullaih, Saad, Munsell, & Hoff, 2002). Fifty-six percent of patients with breast cancer experienced PPES associated with capecitabine in a study by Blum, Jones, Buzdar, and Fleishman (1999).

PPES incidence is highest in patients receiving PEG doxorubicin (doxorubicin encapsulated in PEG-coated liposomes), estimated at 37%, with highest grade 3 to 4 severity occurring in 16% of patients (Alza Pharmaceuticals, 1999). Liposomal daunorubicin has been cited to cause PPES when given in higher doses with infusion rates longer than commonly used (Hui & Cortes, 2000).

Acral erythema is characterized by cutaneous macules and patches that are painful, symmetrical, and erythematous, and edematous areas on palms and soles, commonly preceded or accompanied by paresthesias (tingling sensations). Painful sole involvement can produce functional disturbances with walking (Wood, 2006). Acral erythema (see Figure 22-6) also can affect the lateral fingers or periungual zones (surrounding area of nail beds). Hyperkeratosis (skin thickening) and desquamation often occur simultaneously. Patients who are at risk for plantar hyperkeratosis can benefit from a preventive pedicure prior to treatment to remove callous and dry skin (Rob-

FIGURE 22-6	Acral Erythema in a Patient Given Sorafenib

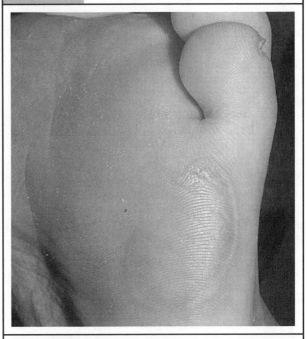

Note. From "Cutaneous Side-Effects of Kinase Inhibitors and Blocking Antibodies," by C. Robert, J.C. Soria, A. Spatz, A. Le Cesne, D. Malka, P. Pautier, et al., 2005, *Lancet Oncology, 6*(7), p. 496. Copyright 2005 by Elsevier. Reprinted with permission.

ert et al., 2005). Fingers can have symmetric areas of well-demarcated redness versus blanching, suggesting vascular involvement. In a study of patients with leukemia, incidence was noted to be about 20% in those who received cytosine arabinoside and anthracycline antibiotics. Acral erythema can be confused with PPES or even graft-versus-host disease in this population of patients who receive bone marrow transplantations (Demircay et al., 1997). Acral erythema also can arise after two to four weeks of treatment with sunitinib or sorafenib. Both agents are effective for treatment of renal cell carcinoma. Although the true incidence related to these agents is not yet known, sorafenib-related incidence of acral erythema may be as high as 30% (Wood). Although this syndrome can mimic PPES, when induced by kinase inhibitors, acral erythema is more localized with hyperkeratotic lesions that are distinct from classic hand-foot syndrome (Robert et al.). Areas of hyperkeratosis, especially on the soles, are more common with sorafenib. This may result in thick calluses, and treatment includes use of topical exfoliants, such as Kerasal® (Alterna) and Keralac® (Bradley Pharmaceuticals) (Wood).

Incidence of Rash: Epidermal Growth Factor Receptor Tyrosine Kinase Inhibitors

Next, this chapter will discuss oral agents that target members of the human epidermal growth factor receptor (HER) family. EGFR-TKIs, such as gefitinib and erlotinib, have demonstrated improved overall survival in patients with lung, colorectal, and pancreatic cancers. Generally, the rash appears one to two weeks after treatment with an EGFR inhibitor (Albanell et al., 2002; Hidalgo et al., 2001).

The incidence of rash with gefitinib is 43% with a dose of 250 mg daily and 54% with dose of 500 mg daily (Perez-Soler et al., 2005). EGFR-TKIs are associated with dermatologic toxicity of varying severity. The Br.21 trial of erlotinib (N = 731) revealed skin toxicity as the most common adverse event, with an incidence of any grade rash in 76% of patients treated. The most severe grade 3 or 4 rash occurred in 9% of patients. Twelve percent of patients had rash severe enough to warrant dose reduction, and erlotinib dosing was interrupted in 14% of patients because of intolerable rash (Shepherd et al., 2005).

Cetuximab is an EGFR antibody given by IV infusion. Rash with cetuximab is commonly called acneform rash and is defined as any event of acne, rash, maculopapular rash, pustular rash, dry skin, or exfoliative dermatitis (see Figure 22-7). Rash occurred in 88% of patients treated with cetuximab in combination with irinotecan and in 90% of patients treated with cetuximab monotherapy (ImClone Systems Inc., 2004).

Sorafenib and sunitinib are TKIs that target two different signaling pathways. The first pathway is vascular endothelial growth factor, which plays a critical role in the proliferation, migration, and survival of endothelial cells involved in angiogenesis. The second pathway is platelet-derived growth factor. By blocking this pathway, sorafenib and sunitinib disrupt the stability and maturation of existing blood vessels around tumors. Rash and desquamation related to sunitinib occurs in 40% of patients receiving this therapy. For those receiving sorafenib, hand-foot skin reaction occurs in 30% of patients (Wood, 2006).

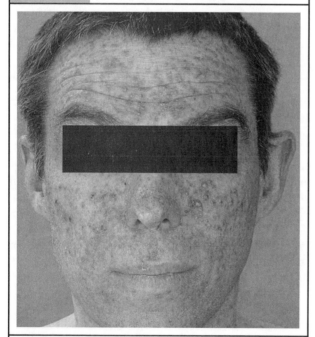

| FIGURE 22-7 | Facial Folliculitis in a Patient Given Cetuximab Over Two Weeks |

Note. From "Cutaneous Side-Effects of Kinase Inhibitors and Blocking Antibodies," by C. Robert, J.C. Soria, A. Spatz, A. Le Cesne, D. Malka, P. Pautier, et al., 2005, *Lancet Oncology, 6*(7), p. 491. Copyright 2005 by Elsevier. Reprinted with permission.

Pathophysiology

A study by Busam et al. (2001) presented data of rash with 10 patients treated with cetuximab. These patients were examined clinically, and immunohistochemical and in situ hybridization studies were performed on skin biopsies from these patients. The researchers concluded that rash was characterized by lymphocytic perifolliculitis or suppurative superficial folliculitis but had no infectious underlying etiology. Suppurative inflammation may occur in response to follicular rupture, but the inflammation in the surrounding areas of the follicles may be a response to change in cutaneous microflora attributable to altered follicular growth and differentiation (Busam et al.).

Several studies have reported cases of folliculitis with erlotinib, gefitinib, and cetuximab. Some studies stated that the rash was sterile, whereas others concluded that microorganisms were present, particularly when follicular plugs were present. Most studies have shown that unlike acne vulgaris, the sebaceous glands are not affected. The stratum corneum of the epidermis also has been noted to be thinner and without the characteristic basket-weave pattern in the skin of patients treated with cetuximab or gefitinib (Perez-Soler et al., 2005).

Assessment

Nurses must accurately describe skin and nail alterations. A familiarity with common dermatologic descriptive terms is imperative in order to accomplish this. Many terms will be defined further in this chapter, but the following are some commonly used descriptive terms for rash or skin changes.
- Skin lesion—localized, pathologic change in skin
- Macule—flat lesion
- Papule—raised, conical lesion
- Pustule—lesion with inflamed base, lesion that contains pus
- Discrete—refers to a single lesion with well-defined borders
- Confluent—refers to multiple lesions with ill-defined borders that are conjoined
- Erythema—redness, inflammation (often painful)
- Follicular—lesion of or surrounding a hair follicle in skin

Skin alterations should be described as either localized to one small area or generalized over a broader area of skin.

Although other grading systems for rash exist, nurses should be familiar with the CTCAE, a grading system used by clinicians to describe adverse effects of cancer therapies (see Table 22-2).

EGFR-TKIs are novel treatments for cancer, and, therefore, their associated dermatologic side effects have not yet been rigorously studied and evaluated. The current lack of evidence-based recommendations to manage this distressing and often chronic side effect makes rash management and etiology investigation high priorities for clinicians. Accurate clinical assessment is difficult at present because terminology and grading systems are not consistent among healthcare providers.

The pathology and etiology of rash associated with EGFR-TKIs are not yet clear, but this rash is certainly distinct from acne vulgaris, which has a unique pathology. Therefore, terms such as *acneform* or *acne* should be avoided when describing rash associated with EGFR-TKIs. Many EGFR-HER targeted agents are being developed, mainly TKIs or monoclonal antibodies. The current main indications for these agents are for NSCLC, pancreatic cancer, or CRC, but they are being tested in numerous other populations, including patients with glioblastoma and head and neck cancers. As routine use of these agents becomes more common, the etiology and management of rash will take precedence (Perez-Soler et al., 2005).

Rash generally is mild (grade 1) to moderate (grade 2), with severe rash (grade 3 or 4) occurring less commonly. Inconsistent use of various scales to grade rash and terms to describe rash makes it difficult to compare severity of rash among trials and agents.

Skin rash typically presents initially as dry skin within a week or two of beginning treatment (Shepherd et al., 2005; Soulieres et al., 2004). Grade 1 rash appears sooner with scattered maculopapular lesions that may have slight erythema occurring on the patient's face, neck, scalp, anterior chest, or back. Discomfort at this stage typically is minimal, with patients reporting mild, localized pruritus.

TABLE 22-2	National Cancer Institute Common Terminology Criteria for Adverse Events				

	Grade				
Adverse Event	**1**	**2**	**3**	**4**	**5**
Rash maculo-papular	Macules/papules covering < 10% BSA with or without symptoms (e.g., pruritus, burning, tightness)	Macules/papules covering 10%–30% BSA with or without symptoms (e.g., pruritus, burning, tightness); limiting instrumental ADL	Macules/papules covering > 30% BSA with or without associated symptoms; limiting self care ADL	–	–
Palmar-plantar erythrodys-esthesia syndrome	Minimal skin changes or dermatitis (e.g., erythema, edema, or hyperkeratosis) without pain	Skin changes (e.g., peeling, blisters, bleeding, edema, or hyperkeratosis) with pain; limiting instrumental ADL	Severe skin changes (e.g., peeling, blisters, bleeding, edema, or hyperkeratosis) with pain; limiting self care ADL	–	–
Dry skin	Covering < 10% BSA and no associated erythema or pruritus	Covering 10%–30% BSA and associated with erythema or pruritus; limiting instrumental ADL	Covering > 30% BSA and associated with pruritus; limiting self care ADL	–	–
Skin hyperpig-mentation	Hyperpigmentation covering < 10% BSA; no psychosocial impact	Hyperpigmentation covering > 10% BSA; associated psychosocial impact	–	–	–
Nail discoloration	Asymptomatic; clinical or diagnostic observations only; intervention not indicated	–	–	–	–
Nail loss	Asymptomatic separation of the nail bed from the nail plate or nail loss	Symptomatic separation of the nail bed from the nail plate or nail loss; limiting instrumental ADL	–	–	–
Nail ridging	Asymptomatic; clinical or diagnostic observations only; intervention not indicated	–	–	–	–

ADL—activities of daily living; BSA—body surface area

Note. From *Common Terminology Criteria for Adverse Events* (Version 4.0), by National Cancer Institute Cancer Therapy Evaluation Program, 2009. Retrieved July 24, 2009, from http://ctep.cancer.gov/protocolDevelopment/electronic_applications/docs/ctcaev4.pdf.

Interventions for Epidermal Growth Factor Receptor Tyrosine Kinase Inhibitor Rash

Over-the-Counter Emollients and Cleansers

Patients should be encouraged to cleanse skin with mild, hypoallergenic emollient soaps like Basis® (Beiersdorf, Inc.) or Cetaphil® (Galderma Laboratories) (Morse & Calarese, 2006).

Regular skin cleansing can diminish the potential for secondary infection of skin lesions. Products with perfumes, alcohol, benzoyl peroxide, or salicylic acid should be avoided because they can increase skin dryness or cause further irritation. To prevent rash-associated pruritus, dry skin generally is effectively managed with use of a gentle cleanser and frequent application of any emollient, a product that maintains skin moisture and does not irritate skin or nails. Lotions containing aloe vera or dimethicone may be of benefit. Recommended products include Curel® (Kao Brands Company), Aveeno® (Johnson & Johnson Consumer Companies, Inc.), Eucerin® (Beiersdorf, Inc.), and Aquaphor® (Beiersdorf, Inc.). Shower gel and liquid cleansers are recommended. Nail and nail bed moisture may be maintained with products such as tea tree oils and Bag Balm® (Dairy Association Co., Inc.) (Morse & Calarese; Perez-Soler et al., 2005; Wood, 2006).

If pruritus persists, systemic antihistamines may relieve symptoms (Halpern & Thomas, 2005). The rash can cause distress regarding body image and appearance. A dermatologist-approved cover-up like Dermablend™ (Dermablend) may be helpful cosmetically, although any type of foundation that does not cause irritation may be used to cover erythema or lesions. Rash may be aggravated by sunlight, so patients should be advised to use sunscreen like Anthelios® (La Roche-Posay) or a nonirritating sunscreen with a sun protection factor (SPF) of 15 or higher (Perez-Soler et al., 2005). Female patients should be encouraged that coverage make-up can be safely applied and improve appearance (Robert et al., 2005) (see Figure 22-8).

Topical Corticosteroids

Topical corticosteroids are largely ineffective in patients with severe grade 3 or 4 rash. They may have a role if utilized early in therapy for mild rash or after antibiotics to abate inflam-

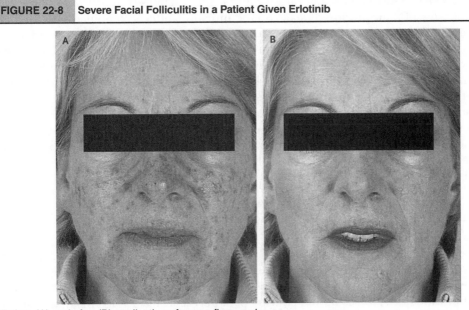

FIGURE 22-8   **Severe Facial Folliculitis in a Patient Given Erlotinib**

Before (A) and after (B) application of camouflage make-up.

Note. From "Cutaneous Side-Effects of Kinase Inhibitors and Blocking Antibodies," by C. Robert, J.C. Soria, A. Spatz, A. Le Cesne, D. Malka, P. Pautier, et al., 2005, *Lancet Oncology, 6*(7), p. 493. Copyright 2005 by Elsevier. Reprinted with permission.

mation and prevent infection. No clinical trials have been conducted thus far to prove this hypothesis. Current evidence does support the relative safety of using intermittent cortico-steroids on the face, as the risk of skin thinning or atrophy occurs only after prolonged use and reverses once treatment has stopped (Perez-Soler et al., 2005). Topical immunomodu-latory agents, such as pimecrolimus (Elidel®, Novartis Pharmaceuticals Corp.), warrant fur-ther investigation, considering the inflammatory nature of the rash. However, use of retin-oids such as Differin® gel (Galderma Laboratories) should be avoided because they may ex-acerbate skin dryness and pruritus (Perez-Soler et al.).

Antihistamines

Rash-associated pruritus is often bothersome to patients, and unfortunately no effective alleviating regimen is available. Antihistamines such as diphenhydramine or hydroxyzine hy-drochloride can be used, but their effectiveness is considered marginal (Perez-Soler et al., 2005). These drugs block histamine response and may relieve the itching associated with rash caused by EGFR-TKIs.

Antibiotics

Patients who develop a rash related to any agent may develop secondary infection with as-sociated pustules, inflammation, and worsening erythema. These can worsen the rash, partic-ularly in appearance. To reduce the likelihood of secondary infection of nasal mucosa, con-sider twice-daily application of intranasal mupirocin. Secondarily infected rash that is con-fined to a localized area (e.g., chin or paranasal area) may be effectively managed with topical agents such as clindamycin. Generalized infected rash over larger areas or follicular pustules may respond well to a short course of oral antibiotics. Tetracyclines (minocycline) have been suggested because of their proposed weak anti-inflammatory effects combined with their ac-tivity against *Staphylococcus aureus*. However, many different oral antibiotics may be effective. Because no clinical trials exist to support the use of one agent over another, effectiveness should be evaluated after one week of treatment and only continued for another week if the rash does not worsen. The agent should be continued for a total of two weeks, and if no im-provement occurs, it should be considered ineffective (Perez-Soler et al., 2005).

Skin rash can rapidly deteriorate to grade 2 or 3. Patients may report severe generalized pruri-tus or itching, with acute areas of painful breakout on their face, neck, or scalp. Patients may feel overwhelmed by the change in their appearance and require support to continue with their treat-ment. Patients with grade 3 toxicity may have generalized erythroderma with associated macular and vesicular eruptions that are accompanied by pain and/or fever (Busam et al., 2001).

Patient Teaching Points

Patient education prior to the initiation of a drug that causes dermatologic toxicity is im-perative. Nurses provide this education so that patients can recognize the early signs of skin rash and seek timely intervention with management to minimize the progression to a high-grade, bothersome rash. Nurses should educate patients receiving EGFR-TKIs that rash may be an indication of response to therapy. This reinforcement may encourage patients to re-main on a therapy despite experiencing low-grade, cosmetically challenging skin changes. It may help for patients to decide what degree of rash is tolerable in relation to a positive outcome in their response to treatment (Oishi, 2008). Nurses should teach patients the elements of skin care as discussed in this chapter, including regular use of mild cleansers and emollient moisturizers. Skin irritants, for example, alcohol-based cleansers, should be avoided. Nurses should educate patients regarding the increased risk of sun exposure associated with these agents and the necessity of using products with SPF 15 or greater.

Need for Future Research

Randomized clinical trials are needed to test these interventions and determine those that best manage EGFR-TKI rash. Oncology nurses are an important part of the treatment team and can lead the way to future research. The cosmetic challenges encountered by patients with facial and body rash can be daunting. Nurses use evidence-based techniques of active and empathetic listening to patients while they convey their psychological concerns (Oishi, 2008). No studies have examined the impact of nursing interventions or measured the effectiveness of the guidelines recommended by clinical experts in this chapter.

Conclusion of Case Study

M.R.'s case illustrates the importance of considering nursing interventions that can positively affect the patient's ability to tolerate cancer therapies despite adverse side effects. Nurses assess and grade rash and provide recommendations for management. Techniques that nurses should teach patients regarding skin care while they are receiving EGFR-TKIs are discussed earlier in this chapter. M.R. returns to the clinic after two weeks on erlotinib. The nurse assesses his rash and finds him to have a scattered papulopustular rash on his face, neck, scalp, chest, and back. Erythemic inflammation accompanies the rash, particularly on his face and chest. The nurse's treatment plan should include patient education regarding cleansing with mild, nonirritating products and frequent application of emollient moisturizer to the skin. The nurse also should encourage the patient to adhere to the treatment plan despite the presence of rash. The nurse should consult with a physician or nurse practitioner to prescribe a tetracycline antibiotic, such as oral minocycline 100 mg BID. The nurse is part of the treatment team that decides whether a dose reduction of erlotinib to 100 mg daily is warranted at this time. The nurse will be able to convey the patient's feelings to the team, and this may influence the decision. The team decides to dose-reduce the patient. His rash improves but remains present and more tolerable for him. He returns to the clinic for regular follow-up and has an excellent response to treatment. But after six months, persistent bothersome grade 2 rash is present. The decision is made to further dose-reduce M.R.'s erlotinib to 50 mg daily. His rash improves and was far more tolerable, and he continues on therapy for four years after an initial excellent response to erlotinib. His disease remains stable at this time.

Conclusion

These novel agents have unique dermatologic side effects. Only limited research has been conducted to help nurses in developing strategies for treating rash and changes associated with targeted agents. More randomized clinical trials are necessary to develop new strategies to discern the optimum treatment for skin effects of HER1/EGFR-TKIs. Until then, current interventions are based on prior clinical experience and patient response. As previously stated, maintaining skin moisture with alcohol-free, bland emollients may alleviate dryness and associated itching, but no evidence-based recommendations are available for effectively treating rash because of a lack of randomized controlled clinical trials to investigate efficacy of techniques. The recommendations contained here are based on knowledge of the rash's inflammatory nature and the experience of nurses and oncologists. As the use of these agents becomes more widespread, evidence-based guidelines for rash management will be imperative.

Nursing education for patients prior to initiation of treatments that may alter their skin or nails is imperative. This helps patients to recognize early onset of these changes and ensure prompt intervention to prevent worsening or intolerable skin changes. This, in turn, may enable patients to tolerate higher doses of cancer therapies for longer durations, thus leading to better control of their illness.

References

Aapro, M., Martin, C., & Hatty, S. (1998). Gemcitabine—a safety review. *Anti-Cancer Drugs, 9*(3), 191–201.

Abushullaih, S., Saad, E.D., Munsell, M., & Hoff, P.M. (2002). Incidence and severity of hand-foot syndrome in colorectal cancer patients treated with capecitabine: A single-institution experience. *Cancer Investigation, 20*(1), 3–10.

Adjei, A.A. (2004). Pemetrexed (Alimta): A novel multitargeted antineoplastic agent. *Clinical Cancer Research, 10*(12, Pt. 2), 4276s–4280s.

Albanell, J., Rojo, F., Averbuch, S., Feyereislova, A., Mascaro, J.M., Herbst, R., et al. (2002). Pharmacodynamic studies of the epidermal growth factor receptor inhibitor ZD1839 in skin from cancer patients: Histopathologic and molecular consequences of receptor inhibition. *Journal of Clinical Oncology, 20*(1), 110–124.

Alza Pharmaceuticals. (1999). Doxil [Package insert]. Palo Alto, CA: Author.

Blum, J.L., Jones, S.E., Buzdar, A.U., & Fleishman, S. (1999). Multicenter phase II study of capecitabine in paclitaxel-refractory metastatic breast cancer. *Journal of Clinical Oncology, 17*(2), 485–493.

Bristol-Myers Squibb Co. (2000). Taxol [Package insert]. Princeton, NJ: Author.

Busam, K.J., Capodieci, P., Motzer, R., Kiehn, T., Phelan, D., & Halpern, A.C. (2001). Cutaneous side-effects in cancer patients treated with the antiepidermal growth factor receptor antibody C225. *British Journal of Dermatology, 144*(6), 1169–1176.

Cetkovska, P., Pizinger, K., & Cetkovsky, P. (2002). High-dose cytosine arabinoside-induced cutaneous reactions. *European Academy of Dermatology and Venereology, 16*(5), 481–485.

Chang, G.C., Yang, T.Y., Chen, K.C., Yin, M.C., Wang, R.C., & Lin, Y.C. (2004). Complications of therapy in cancer patients: Case 1. Paronychia and skin hyperpigmentation induced by gefitinib in advanced non-small-cell lung cancer. *Journal of Clinical Oncology, 22*(22), 4646–4648.

Daniel, C.R., III, & Scher, R.K. (1984). Nail changes secondary to systemic drugs or ingestants. *Journal of the American Academy of Dermatology, 10*(2, Pt. 1), 250–258.

Dasanu, C.A., Vaillant, J.G., & Alexandrescu, D.T. (2007). Distinct patterns of chromonychia, Beau's lines, and melanoderma seen with vincristine, Adriamycin, dexamethasone therapy for multiple myeloma. *Dermatology Online Journal, 12*(6). Retrieved September 20, 2007, from http://dermatology.cdlib.org/126/case_reports/nail/dasanu.html

Demircay, Z., Gurbuz, O., Alpdogan, T.B., Yucelten, D., Alpdogan, O., Kurtkaya, O., et al. (1997). Chemotherapy-induced acral erythema in leukemic patients: A report of 15 cases. *International Journal of Dermatology, 36*(8), 593–598.

Flory, S.M., Solimando, D.A., Jr., Webster, G.F., Dunton, C.J., Neufeld, J.M., & Haffey, M.B. (1999). Onycholysis associated with weekly administration of paclitaxel. *Annals of Pharmacotherapy, 33*(5), 584–586.

Hackbarth, M., Haas, N., Fotopoulou, C., Lichtenegger, W., & Sehouli, J. (2007). Chemotherapy-induced dermatological toxicity: Frequencies and impact on quality of life in women's cancers. Results of a prospective study. *Supportive Care in Cancer, 16*(3), 267–273.

Halpern, A.C., & Thomas, M. (2005). *Anti EGFR therapy-related rash and other adverse events: Etiologies, prevention, and management* [Teleconference]. Available at http://www.academycme.org

Hidalgo, M., Siu, L.L., Nemunaitis, J., Rizzo, J., Hammond, L.A., Takimoto, C., et al. (2001). Phase I and pharmacologic study of OSI-774, an epidermal growth factor receptor tyrosine kinase inhibitor, in patients with advanced solid tumor malignancies. *Journal of Clinical Oncology, 19*(13), 3267–3279.

Hochster, H. (2002). The role of pemetrexed in the treatment of colorectal cancer. *Seminars in Oncology, 29*(6, Suppl. 18), 54–56.

Hui, Y.F., & Cortes, J.E. (2000). Palmar-plantar erythrodysesthesia syndrome associated with liposomal daunorubicin. *Pharmacotherapy, 20*(10), 1221–1223.

ImClone Systems Inc. (2004). Erbitux [Package insert]. New York: Author.

Lacouture, M.E., Boerner, S.A., & LoRusso, P.M. (2006). Non-rash skin toxicities associated with novel targeted therapies. *Clinical Lung Cancer, 8*(Suppl. 1), S36–S42.

Llombart-Cussac, A., Martin, M., Harbeck, N., Anghel, R.M., Eniu, A.E., Verrill, M.W., et al. (2007). A randomized, double-blind, phase II study of two doses of pemetrexed as first-line chemotherapy for advanced breast cancer. *Clinical Cancer Research, 13*(12), 3652–3659.

Lokich, J.J., & Moore, C. (1984). Chemotherapy-associated palmar-plantar erythrodysesthesia syndrome. *Annals of Internal Medicine, 101*(6), 798–799.

Minisini, A.M., Tosti, A., Sobrero, A.F., Mansutti, M., Piraccini, B.M., Sacco, C., et al. (2003). Taxane-induced nail changes: Incidence, clinical presentation and outcome. *Annals of Oncology, 14*(2), 333–337.

Morse, L., & Calarese, P. (2006). EGFR-targeted therapy and related skin toxicity. *Seminars in Oncology Nursing, 22*(3), 152–162.

Oishi, K. (2008). Clinical approaches to minimize rash associated with EGFR inhibitors. *Oncology Nursing Forum, 35*(1), 103–110.

O'Keeffe, P., Parrilli, M., & Lacouture, M. (2006). Toxicity of targeted therapy. *Cancer Network Oncology Supplement, 20*(13). Retrieved January 20, 2009, from http://www.cancernetwork.com/display/article/10 165/60568?pageNumber=2

Perez-Soler, P., Delord, J.P., Halpern, A., Kelly, K., Krueger, J., Sureda, B.M., et al. (2005). HER1/EGFR inhibitor-associated rash: Future directions for management and investigation outcomes from the HER1/EGFR inhibitor rash management forum. *Oncologist, 10*(5), 345–356.

Robert, C., Soria, J.-C., Spatz, A., Le Cesne, A., Malka, D., Pautier, P., et al. (2005). Cutaneous side-effects of kinase inhibitors and blocking antibodies. *Lancet Oncology, 6*(7), 491–500.

Rose, P.G., Maxson, J.H., Fusco, N., Mossbruger, K., & Rodriguez, M. (2001). Liposomal doxorubicin in ovarian, peritoneal, and tubal carcinoma: A retrospective comparative study of single-agent dosages. *Gynecologic Oncology, 82*(2), 323–328.

Segaert, S., & Van Cutsem, E. (2005). Clinical signs, pathophysiology, and management of skin toxicity during therapy with epidermal growth factor receptor inhibitors. *Annals of Oncology, 16*(9), 1425–1433.

Shepherd, F.A., Pereira, J.R., Ciuleanu, T., Tan, E.H., Hirsh, V., Thongprasert, S., et al. (2005). Erlotinib in previously treated non-small-cell lung cancer. *New England Journal of Medicine, 353*(2), 123–132.

Socinski, M.A. (2005). Pemetrexed (Alimta) in small cell lung cancer. *Seminars in Oncology, 32*(2, Suppl. 2), S1–S4.

Soulieres, D., Senzer, N.N., Vokes, E.E., Hidalgo, M., Agarwala, S.S., & Siu, L.L. (2004). Multicenter phase II study of erlotinib, an oral epidermal growth factor receptor tyrosine kinase inhibitor, in patients with recurrent or metastatic squamous cell cancer of the head and neck. *Journal of Clinical Oncology, 22*(1), 77–85.

Wood, L.S. (2006). Managing the side effects of sorafenib and sunitinib. *Community Oncology, 3*(9), 558–562.

CHAPTER 23

Sleep-Wake Disturbances

Jeanne Erickson, PhD, RN, AOCN®,
and Ann M. Berger, PhD, RN, AOCN®, FAAN

Case Studies

Adult Case Study

P.L. is a 50-year-old woman, married, and the mother of three children, ages 16, 14, and 11. She works as an accountant 20 hours per week and is very involved in her children's lives and activities. She was diagnosed with stage IIB breast cancer and has recovered from a mastectomy with reconstruction. Based on the pathology of the tumor, she has been prescribed four cycles of dose-dense chemotherapy (every 14 days) with doxorubicin and cyclophosphamide (AC), followed by four cycles of docetaxel. She is perimenopausal, having had irregular periods for the past six months, and has been experiencing frequent hot flashes.

P.L. comes to the clinic today for her second dose of AC. Using 0–10 visual analog scales, she reports her pain as a 2 and her fatigue as a 5. She has missed 4 days of work in the past 14 days related to problems of not getting enough sleep and feeling that she could not carry out her work because of daytime fatigue and sleepiness. She reports feeling distressed that she has "not been a very good wife or mother" since her first treatment. Her most frequent problem has been sleep maintenance. She reports waking up at least 8–10 times a night and having problems falling back to sleep almost every time. On the days she has called in sick and on weekends, she has stayed in bed until after 9 am, which is three hours later than her usual time. She also has started taking daytime naps when she feels sleepy and fatigued.

Factors contributing to P.L.'s sleep disturbances include
- Caucasian, perimenopausal, female
- Stimulating home environment with three adolescents
- Daytime naps
- Feelings of low self-worth and distress
- Recent mastectomy with reconstruction surgery; started chemotherapy three weeks later
- Highly emetogenic chemotherapy regimen associated with abrupt onset of menopause.

Adolescent Case Study

K.D. is an 18-year-old woman and a senior in high school who was diagnosed with chronic myeloid leukemia two and a half months ago. Her treatment is imatinib 300 mg PO daily, which she will continue until her bone marrow cytogenetics show remission. K.D. was hospitalized for several weeks at the time of diagnosis because of complications related to myelosuppression, but she is now at home with stable blood counts. She is trying to resume some schoolwork and hopes to be back in school soon so that she can graduate.

Currently, K.D.'s most troubling symptoms include fatigue and trouble sleeping, and she admits she had these problems before her diagnosis of leukemia. She is most bothered by difficulty falling asleep. She typically goes into her bedroom around 11 pm, turns on a movie, and lies in bed, hoping to feel sleepy. After the movie ends, however, she usually does not feel sleepy. She frequently sees the clock at 2 am before she eventually falls asleep. She sleeps through the night without many awakenings. Because she is not yet back in school, K.D. usually wakes up naturally around 11 am, but upon arising, she feels tired and not refreshed. During the day, she admits she is extremely bored and lonely. She feels too tired to concentrate much on school work, and she watches a lot of television because there is nothing else to do. She frequently falls asleep during the day, sometimes sleeping for more than an hour. She is "annoyed" at being idle and bored, and her mother describes her mood as irritable.

Factors contributing to K.D.'s sleep disturbances include
- Lack of daytime activity
- Long daytime naps
- Worry
- Use of the bed for activities other than sleep
- Watching late-night stimulating movies
- Lying in bed at night when she is not sleepy.

Overview

A sufficient amount of quality sleep is essential for the health and well-being of every person. Insufficient or disrupted sleep can lead to a number of negative health, safety, cognitive, and psychosocial outcomes. Unfortunately, sleep problems and their daytime consequences, especially those related to insufficient sleep, commonly affect many healthy adults and children in today's 24/7 culture (Berger, 2006). A diagnosis of cancer, its associated symptoms, various treatments, and side effects add further disruptions to a patient's quantity and quality of sleep. Troubling cancer-related symptoms and difficult and time-consuming therapies, as well as the emotional distress caused by cancer, frequently keep patients from getting a good night's sleep and feeling rested upon awakening. Sleep difficulties also add to the distress caused by other symptoms and compromise daily functioning and quality of life (Davidson, MacLean, Brundage, & Schulze, 2002). Although sleep problems are common in people with cancer, these symptoms have only recently become the focus for evidence-based prevention and management strategies by oncology caregivers (Roscoe et al., 2007).

Oncology care providers across all settings need adequate knowledge about sleep physiology and sleep-wake disturbances so that they can effectively assess their patients for these troubling symptoms. Primary sleep disorders are medical diagnoses defined by the American Academy of Sleep Medicine (AASM) in the *International Classification of Sleep Disorders*

(AASM, 2005), whereas sleep-wake disturbances are more general complaints that can be assessed and addressed by all providers. Oncology clinicians need to add emerging evidence from sleep research to practice so that they can prescribe interventions to promote sleep and enable patients to achieve optimal rest, energy levels, and function. Likewise, sleep researchers need to partner with oncology clinician colleagues when designing interventions to reduce sleep disturbances.

This chapter provides an overview of sleep physiology and the sleep-wake disturbances that are most prevalent in people with cancer. Chapter content includes strategies and instruments for clinical sleep screening and assessment, as well as diagnostic approaches when medical sleep disorders are suspected. Finally, evidence-based interventions for sleep-wake disturbances from the Oncology Nursing Society (ONS) Putting Evidence Into Practice (PEP) project are recommended to improve sleep-wake outcomes (Page, Berger, & Johnson, 2006). Although the focus of the chapter is on symptom management of patients with cancer, the authors recognize that family members, caregivers, and direct care providers also may experience sleep disturbances.

Sleep Physiology

Functions of Sleep

Sleep is an active, behavioral state of disengagement and unresponsiveness to the environment and is associated with physiologic processes vital to life (Carskadon & Dement, 2005). Although the exact purposes of sleep remain unknown, ongoing research finds that sleep plays a critical role in a variety of physiologic processes that include energy conservation, memory consolidation and learning, regulation of metabolism, hormone production, and immune function (Bonnet, 2005). Sleep is a basic drive to restore and rejuvenate the individual to achieve an optimal state of alertness, ability to function, and well-being during waking hours (Dement & Vaughn, 1999).

Sleep Architecture

The sleep-wake cycle in humans follows a diurnal circadian rhythm of approximately 24 hours (Turek, Dugovic, & Laposky, 2005). Sleep alternates with a state of wakefulness, characterized by readiness of the brain to respond to outside stimuli. Individual variances in circadian rhythms lead some individuals to possess a preference for early bedtimes and wake times (early birds or larks), whereas others prefer later bedtimes and wake times (night owls) (Lee, Cho, Miaskowski, & Dodd, 2004).

Sleep is divided into two general states: non–rapid eye movement (REM) sleep and REM sleep. During sleep, periods of non-REM sleep alternate with periods of REM sleep. Non-REM sleep is further divided into four stages, which vary from light sleep (stage I) to deep sleep (stage IV). The slower electroencephalogram (EEG) waves of deep sleep are most associated with the restorative function of sleep (Berger, 2006). Non-REM sleep is associated with minimal brain activity and a moderate amount of body activity. REM sleep includes bursts of rapid brain waves associated with dreaming and muscle atonia interrupted with episodes of muscle twitching. A typical night of sleep begins with the onset of sleep in stage I, followed by several alternating cycles of various stages of non-REM and REM sleep, which average 90–110 minutes in length (Carskadon & Dement, 2005). Early episodes of REM sleep are short but become longer as the night progresses. Figure 23-1 illustrates the alternating sleep stages

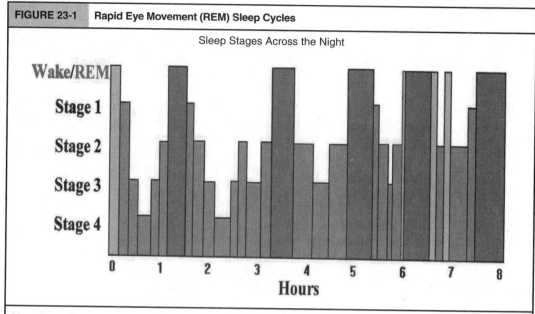

FIGURE 23-1   **Rapid Eye Movement (REM) Sleep Cycles**

Note. From "The Regulation of Sleep and Circadian Rhythms," by T.E. Scammell, 2004, *Sleep Medicine Alert,* 8(1), p. 2. Copyright 2004 by National Sleep Foundation. Reprinted with permission.

during an eight-hour period of sleep. Deep sleep (stages III and IV) occurs and cycles more frequently early in the sleep period. Lighter sleep (stages I and II) and more frequent periods of REM sleep occur later in the sleep period.

Model of Sleep Regulation

The two-process model of sleep regulation proposes that individual sleep and wake times are determined by the interaction of a circadian timing system (process C) and a sleep-wake homeostasis process (process S), each controlled by separate mechanisms (Borbely & Achermann, 2005). Process C is controlled by an internal "clock" located in the suprachiasmatic nucleus in the anterior hypothalamus, which synchronizes an elaborate feedback system of multiple oscillators located in tissues throughout the body. The process C system incorporates stimuli from the environment, especially related to lightness and darkness, and regulates the production of neuropeptides, which promote feelings of sleepiness in the evenings and wakefulness in the mornings. Process S is influenced by the individual's sleep-wake behaviors, including the duration and quality of prior episodes of wakefulness and sleep. Homeostatic sleep propensity, or the drive to sleep, rises during the waking hours and peaks just prior to bedtime, followed by a steady decline during sleep to its lowest level at wake time.

When the two regulatory processes of sleep-wake homeostasis and circadian timing are ideally coordinated, outcomes include robust rhythms of sleeping and waking associated with optimal wake-time performance and better-quality sleep and bodily functions (Berger, 2006; Dijk & Franken, 2005). Changes that affect processes C and S occur as a result of normal aging and as a result of lifestyle behaviors, such as rotating shift work and changing sleep and nap schedules. These changes influence the timing of sleep and wakefulness as well as the duration and structure of sleep and may result in problems such as difficulty falling asleep (sleep latency), difficulty staying asleep (sleep maintenance), and excessive daytime sleepiness.

The Conceptual Model of Impaired Sleep (Lee, 2003) emphasizes the effects of health-related issues as well as developmental and lifestyle factors that result in sleep deprivation and sleep disruption. This model, illustrated in Figure 23-2, identifies the adverse health outcomes associated with insufficient sleep, including impairments in immune function, metabolism,

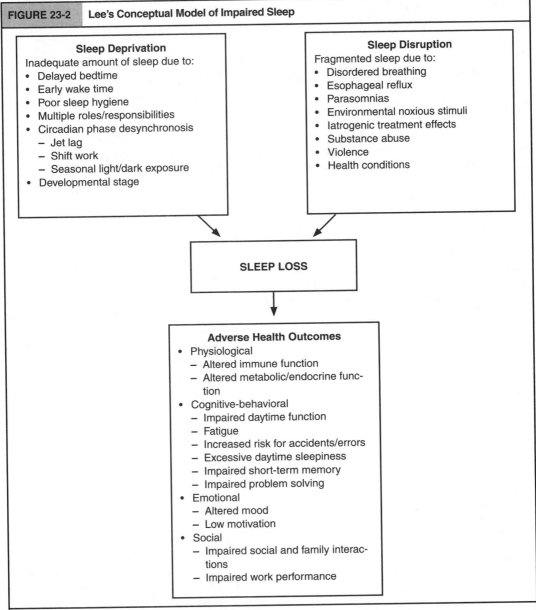

FIGURE 23-2   Lee's Conceptual Model of Impaired Sleep

Sleep Deprivation
Inadequate amount of sleep due to:
- Delayed bedtime
- Early wake time
- Poor sleep hygiene
- Multiple roles/responsibilities
- Circadian phase desynchronosis
  - Jet lag
  - Shift work
  - Seasonal light/dark exposure
- Developmental stage

Sleep Disruption
Fragmented sleep due to:
- Disordered breathing
- Esophageal reflux
- Parasomnias
- Environmental noxious stimuli
- Iatrogenic treatment effects
- Substance abuse
- Violence
- Health conditions

SLEEP LOSS

Adverse Health Outcomes
- Physiological
  - Altered immune function
  - Altered metabolic/endocrine function
- Cognitive-behavioral
  - Impaired daytime function
  - Fatigue
  - Increased risk for accidents/errors
  - Excessive daytime sleepiness
  - Impaired short-term memory
  - Impaired problem solving
- Emotional
  - Altered mood
  - Low motivation
- Social
  - Impaired social and family interactions
  - Impaired work performance

Note. From "Impaired Sleep," by K.A. Lee in V. Carrieri-Kohlman, A.M. Lindsey, and C.M. West (Eds.), *Pathophysiological Phenomena in Nursing: Human Response to Illness* (3rd ed., p. 364), 2003, St. Louis, MO: Saunders. Copyright 2003 by Elsevier. Reprinted with permission by Elsevier and Kathryn Lee.

daytime functioning, mood, and social interactions. Lee's model is especially useful for clinicians and researchers who are interested in patients with sleep problems. Nurses can use the model to conceptualize and organize the multiple factors that may contribute to a patient's sleep problems as well as to consider the multiple consequences of insufficient sleep on the patient's health and well-being. For example, the nurse may assess a 50-year-old woman with newly diagnosed colon cancer and find existing causes of insufficient sleep, such as family and work responsibilities and perimenopausal symptoms, which cause nighttime awakenings. The patient's recent diagnostic tests and anxiety about her health contribute further disruptions to her activity and sleep schedules. The nurse considers the effects of insufficient sleep on the patient's complaints of increased fatigue, depressed mood, and irritability.

Sleep-Wake Disturbances in Patients With Cancer

Pathogenesis of Sleep-Wake Disturbances

Potential etiologic factors for sleep-wake disturbances in patients with cancer are numerous because cancer is not a single disease, but rather many different disease processes that cause a variety of symptoms. Additionally, various cancer treatments, including surgery, chemotherapy, and radiation therapy, may increase a person's likelihood of having risk factors for sleeping problems. These factors have been organized by experts into demographic, lifestyle, psychological, disease-related, and treatment-related categories (Vena, Parker, Cunningham, Clark, & McMillan, 2004) (see Figure 23-3).

Demographic factors that increase the risk for problems sleeping include being older, female, and Caucasian (Savard & Morin, 2001). Lifestyle factors that increase risk include daytime napping patterns and excessive environmental stimulation. Sleep patterns are influenced by psychological health threatened by ongoing concerns and worries about the disease. Anxiety and depression are common and are believed to affect sleep in patients with cancer. Disease-related factors include the presence of other symptoms, such as pain and fatigue, changes in activity and rest patterns, and alterations in hormone and cytokine production. Treatments such as chemotherapy and hormonal therapy create estrogen deficiency and often result in premature menopause or aggravated menopausal symptoms, particularly hot flashes, that interfere with sleep (Carpenter, Johnson, Wagner, & Andrykowski, 2002; Savard et al., 2004). Cancer and cancer treatment also influence circadian

FIGURE 23-3	Factors That Increase the Risk of Sleeping Problems in People With Cancer

Demographic Factors
- Older age
- Female sex
- Caucasian

Lifestyle and Environmental Factors
- Poor sleeping habits
- Excessive stimulation
- Psychological responses
- Anxiety
- Depression

Disease-Related Factors
- Comorbidities
- Advanced stage of cancer
- Cancer-related symptoms, such as pain, cough, dyspnea, and fever

Treatment-Related Factors
- Postoperative symptoms, such as pain and nausea
- Chemotherapy side effects, such as nausea, fever, and hot flashes
- Radiation side effects, such as nausea

Note. Based on information from Berger et al., 2005.

rhythms (Mormont & Levi, 1997). Blunted or erratic production of cortisol, melatonin, and other substances has been identified in patients with cancer and affects sleep (Payne, Piper, Rabinowitz, & Zimmerman, 2006; Spiegel, Leproult, & Van Cauter, 2003). Cancer and medical, surgical, and radiation treatments are known to increase the production of inflammatory cytokines, including interleukin-1, that may be related to daytime sleepiness and longer sleep times (Dunlop & Campbell, 2000; Payne et al.). Increased knowledge about the relationships among sleep and neuroendocrine and metabolic patterns associated with various types of cancer and treatment is needed (Payne, 2004).

Common Sleep-Wake Disturbances

Common sleep disorders in adults include insomnia, sleep-related breathing disorders, sleep-related movement disorders, and parasomnias (AASM, 2005) (see Table 23-1). The term *insomnia* refers to complaints of difficulty initiating or maintaining sleep or nonrestorative sleep that lasts for at least one month and causes clinically significant distress or impairment in social, occupational, or other important areas of functioning (AASM). Primary insomnia, for which no other cause is known, has been termed *psychophysiologic* (heightened arousal and learned sleep-preventing associations), *physiologic* (subjective reports confirmed

TABLE 23-1	Common Sleep Disorders in Adults	
Sleep Disorder	**Definition**	**Presenting Symptom**
Insomnia	Difficulty initiating or maintaining sleep that causes significant impairment or distress for one month or more	Patient complains of difficulty falling asleep, staying asleep, or early morning awakening that impairs daytime function.
Obstructive sleep apnea-hypopnea syndrome	Recurrent episodes of partial or complete upper airway obstruction despite ongoing respiratory effort during sleep	Bed partner notices that patient stops breathing while asleep; often associated with snoring.
Narcolepsy	Uncontrollable sleepiness and intermittent signs of rapid eye movement sleep that interrupt normal wakefulness	Patient reports suddenly falling asleep during usual activities.
Restless legs syndrome	Unpleasant sensations in legs at night relieved by movement of limbs	Patient describes feelings of creeping, tingling, or cramping pain in legs that is worse when patient is lying down.
Periodic limb movement disorder	Periodic or random kicking or arm movements during sleep	Bed partner reports kicking or arm movements by patient during sleep.
Circadian rhythm disorder	Major sleep episode is advanced or delayed in relation to desired clock time and results in undesired insomnia or sleepiness	Patient reports inability to fall asleep or awaken relative to conventional sleep-wake times, but reports normal sleep.
Parasomnias	Undesirable physical events or behaviors that occur during sleep	Bed partner reports behaviors by patient such as sleepwalking, sleep talking, or sleep terrors.

Note. Based on information from National Sleep Foundation, 2006.

by objective sleep measures), or *idiopathic* (linked to childhood onset and a chronic inability to obtain adequate sleep). The prevalence of each type of primary insomnia has not been routinely assessed or reported in patients with newly diagnosed cancer, with recurrent disease, or at the end of life (Davidson et al., 2002).

Another group of insomnias, referred to as secondary or comorbid insomnias, are associated with other medical disorders, including cancer (National Institutes of Health, 2005). Because cancer is more prevalent in individuals older than 60 years of age, they are likely to have one or more medical or psychological conditions that increase their risk for insomnia (Extermann & Hurria, 2007). Depression is a frequent condition seen in the cancer population and is accompanied by complaints of changes in sleep patterns and fatigue (Alfano & Rowland, 2006; Bardwell et al., 2007). Insomnia can be transient (occasional nights), transient recurring (occasional nights whenever stress level is high), or chronic in nature (lasts six months or longer) (AASM, 2005). Problems with sleep latency and sleep maintenance are common complaints of people with cancer (Lee et al., 2004; Savard, Simard, Blanchet, Ivers, & Morin, 2001).

Daytime sleepiness has been described as the likelihood of a person falling asleep during eight phases of daily life (Johns, 1991). A healthy person is unlikely to fall asleep during usual daytime activities such as eating or reading, but illness can increase the likelihood of increased sleepiness while performing these activities. Patients with cancer frequently report daytime sleepiness to clinicians, but few studies have described the prevalence and consequences of daytime sleepiness in these patients (Berger et al., 2005).

Associated Symptoms and Clusters

Several symptoms have been reported to be associated with sleep-wake disturbances in people with cancer (Berger et al., 2005). Fatigue is the most commonly reported symptom, representing the daytime consequences of nonrestorative sleep (Ancoli-Israel, 2005; Ancoli-Israel, Moore, & Jones, 2001; Roscoe et al., 2007). Higher fatigue levels have been found to be associated with more disturbed sleep in people with cancer prior to (Ancoli-Israel et al., 2006; Berger, Farr, Kuhn, Fischer, & Agrawal, 2007), during (Berger & Farr, 1999; Hinds, Hockenberry, Rai, Zhang, Razzouk, McCarthy, et al., 2007; Kuo, Chiu, Liao, & Hwang, 2006), and after (Barton-Burke, 2006; Bower et al., 2000; Servaes, Verhagen, & Bleijenberg, 2002) the completion of chemotherapy. When sleep-wake disturbances are present, there is a high likelihood that they are part of symptom clusters (Dodd, Miaskowski, & Lee, 2004). Symptom clusters have been defined as "two or more symptoms that are related to each other and that occur together" (Kim, McGuire, Tulman, & Barsevick, 2005, p. 278). In addition to fatigue, the symptoms most frequently identified as clustering with sleep disturbances are depressed mood and pain. Recent articles have described the occurrence of symptom clusters that include pain, fatigue, and depression in addition to sleep disturbances in women with breast cancer at various times along the cancer trajectory (Beck, Dudley, & Barsevick, 2005; Donovan & Jacobsen, 2007).

Assessment of Sleep-Wake Disturbances

Because sleep-wake disturbances may bother up to half of all patients with cancer at some time in their disease trajectory (Davidson et al., 2002; Savard et al., 2001), oncology caregivers in all settings need to incorporate routine screening and assessment of sleep-wake disturbances into their practices. When patients complain of "difficulty sleeping," care providers need to conduct a comprehensive sleep assessment, with knowledge of which sleep variables to measure and how to access the information. To guide oncology clinicians and researchers in sleep assessment, a panel of oncology sleep experts proposed measurement of nine sleep parameters that provide a common language to use in symptom management discussions and comprehensive evaluations of sleep-wake disturbances (Berger et al., 2005). These sleep parameters and their definitions are listed in Table 23-2.

Self-Report Instruments for Clinical Use

Several helpful tools are available for nurses to use in assessing patients for sleep-wake disturbances. One tool recommended for use is the Clinical Sleep Assessment for Adults (Lee & Ward, 2005), which screens for sleep disturbances with seven questions that address the parameters of sleep quality, total sleep time, sleep latency, awakenings, daytime sleepiness, and use of sleep aids. The assessment can be shortened to four questions to use as a brief screening tool, and a children's version also is available. Results of the assessment indicate when referral to a sleep specialist should be considered, and the tool can be scored for research purposes.

The "BEARS" is another practical guide recommended for sleep screening and assessment that includes questions that assess five major sleep domains: **B** is for bedtime problems, **E** is for excessive daytime sleepiness, **A** is for awakenings, **R** is for regularity of sleep, and **S** is for sleep-disordered breathing (Owens & Dalzell, 2005). It also includes age-appropriate questions about sleep for children and parents.

Nurses can assess for specific sleep disturbances by using more focused assessment tools. For example, the Insomnia Severity Index (Savard, Savard, Simard, & Ivers, 2005) is a seven-item instrument that assesses for insomnia. The Epworth Sleepiness Scale (eight items) (Johns, 1991) can be used to identify patients who have excessive daytime sleepiness. For some patients, clinicians may need to obtain sleep information (e.g., snoring) from bed partners or parents, although these proxy reports will vary in reliability. Nurses also can obtain helpful sleep data from patients by suggesting that they keep a daily sleep diary in which they re-

TABLE 23-2	Nine Sleep Parameters Recommended for Evaluation of Sleep-Wake Disturbances
Sleep Parameter	**Definition**
Total sleep time	Number of minutes of sleep in bed
Sleep latency	Number of minutes between getting into bed and falling asleep
Awakenings	Number of awakenings during the sleep period
Wake after sleep onset	Number of minutes awake after initial sleep onset
Daytime napping	Number of minutes of sleep during daytime naps
Daytime sleepiness	Number of episodes of falling asleep without intention
Quality of perceived sleep	Subjective assessment of quality
Circadian rhythm	Biobehavioral phenomenon that repeats approximately every 24 hours
Sleep efficiency	Number of minutes of sleep divided by the number of minutes in bed

Note. Based on information from Berger et al., 2005.

cord selected sleep parameters, such as bedtime, wake time, number of nighttime awakenings, and number and length of daytime naps (Berger et al., 2005).

Objective Sleep Evaluation

Patients who complain of more severe sleep-wake disturbances may need a referral to a sleep disorders center, a medical facility staffed by trained sleep specialists that offers a multidisciplinary approach to the diagnosis and treatment of sleep disorders. The gold standard of objective sleep measurement is the comprehensive physiologic monitoring of polysomnography (Chervin, 2005). Polysomnography is an assessment usually performed in an overnight sleep laboratory and includes neurologic and neuromuscular measurements recorded by EEG, electrooculogram, and electromyelogram, as well as assessment of cardiac and respiratory parameters (see Figure 23-4). Polysomnography is necessary to diagnose sleep-related breathing disorders and unusual sleep-related behaviors or parasomnias and to examine stages of sleep (Kushida et al., 2005).

A second approach to objective sleep measurement is actigraphy, which uses a small portable device that can estimate sleep and activity parameters over extended periods of time outside of a laboratory setting. An actigraph is a wristwatch-like device that senses and records movements in short periods of time during sleep and/or wake periods (see Figure 23-5). Computer algorithms then translate the movement data into numeric and graphic values (Cole, Kripke, Gruen, Mullaney, & Gillin, 1992). Actigraphy does not analyze sleep stages, but it is helpful to evaluate patients with circadian rhythm disorders, to describe sleep patterns in healthy populations, and to document responses to sleep therapy (Morgenthaler et al., 2007). Actigraphy commonly is used for clinical and research purposes to objectively measure patients' responses to sleep interventions. For example, Hinds and colleagues used actigraphy to measure sleep outcomes in hospitalized children with cancer after an enhanced physical activity intervention (Hinds, Hockenberry, Rai, Zhang, Razzouk, Cremer, et al., 2007).

Self-report and objective measures of sleep may not always give the same results. For example, patients who report few nighttime awakenings may show evidence of multiple awakenings from a sleep-related breathing disorder when monitored with polysomnography. Because each subjective and objective measurement approach has a unique set of benefits and limitations and yields complementary information, a combination of sleep measures using subjective and objective approaches is recommended for a comprehensive sleep evaluation (Lashley, 2004; Vena et al., 2004). Some sleep measures can be particularly useful for clinical research or quality improvement projects, such as the Pittsburgh Sleep Quality Index (Buysse, Reynolds, Monk, Berman, & Kupfer, 1989). Additional information about measurement of sleep-wake disturbances can be found at www.ons.org/outcomes/measures/summaries.shtml.

Evidence-Based Interventions

Oncology nurses' scope of practice includes assessment and management of symptoms that are present with cancer and cancer treatment (Gobel, Beck, & O'Leary, 2006). ONS has identified patient outcomes that are sensitive to nursing intervention, known as nursing-sensitive patient outcomes (NSPOs) (Given & Sherwood, 2005). The ONS PEP process has rated the interventions that have been tested to reduce sleep-wake disturbances in people with cancer (Page et al., 2006; see www.ons.org/outcomes/volume1/sleep.shtml). Clinical nurses can use this information to determine the strength of the evidence for various interventions.

FIGURE 23-4	Polysomnography

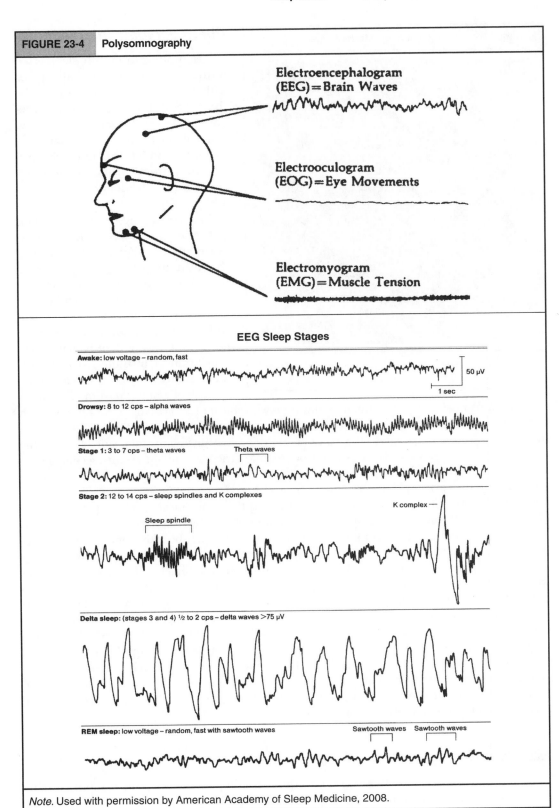

Electroencephalogram
(EEG)=Brain Waves

Electrooculogram
(EOG)=Eye Movements

Electromyogram
(EMG)=Muscle Tension

EEG Sleep Stages

Awake: low voltage – random, fast

50 µV

1 sec

Drowsy: 8 to 12 cps – alpha waves

Stage 1: 3 to 7 cps – theta waves   Theta waves

Stage 2: 12 to 14 cps – sleep spindles and K complexes

K complex

Sleep spindle

Delta sleep: (stages 3 and 4) ½ to 2 cps – delta waves >75 µV

REM sleep: low voltage – random, fast with sawtooth waves   Sawtooth waves   Sawtooth waves

Note. Used with permission by American Academy of Sleep Medicine, 2008.

FIGURE 23-5	Octagonal Basic Motionlogger

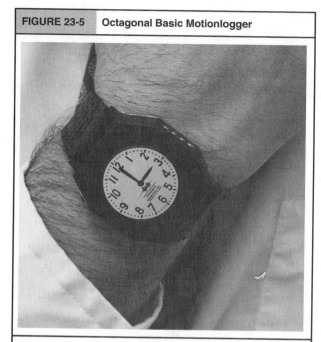

Note. Image courtesy of Ambulatory Monitoring, Inc., Ardsley, New York. Used with permission.

Pharmacologic Interventions

Attempting to modify sleep-wake disturbances in patients with cancer with medications has been rated by the ONS PEP resource in the category of *Benefits Balanced With Harms.* This category instructs clinicians and patients to weigh the beneficial and harmful effects of medications according to individual circumstances and priorities.

In spite of widespread prescribing of hypnotics to improve sleep, no experimental design study was found that examined the efficacy of using these drugs in patients with cancer. The drugs most commonly prescribed for short- and long-term use are in the benzodiazepine and nonbenzodiazepine groups and vary in their half-lives (National Cancer Institute [NCI], 2006). Medications with longer half-lives pose the risk of causing daytime sleepiness and may impair daytime functioning. Medications with shorter half-lives may wear off and result in problems with sleep maintenance during the second half of the night. The NCI Sleep Disorders (PDQ®) Web site lists agents that must be individually evaluated for their side effect profile (see Table 23-3). Benzodiazepines, nonbenzodiazepines, tricyclic antidepressants, second-generation antidepressants, and antihistamines may be considered when attempting to improve sleep. Newer agents such as eszopiclone (Lunesta®, Sepracor Inc.), ramelteon (Rozerem®, Takeda Pharmaceuticals North America), zaleplon (Sonata®, King Pharmaceuticals), and zolpidem (Ambien®/Ambien CR®, Sanofi-Aventis) are commonly prescribed. The risks for potential interactions between these medications and other medications the patient may be taking, including prescription, over-the-counter, and herbal agents, must be weighed with the potential benefits.

Herbal supplements, such as valerian, passionflower, kava, black cohosh, and St. John's wort, have also been assigned to the category *Benefits Balanced With Harms* based on the evidence. Studies have shown potential interactions between herbal agents and chemotherapy and other common drugs, making herbal agents potentially dangerous for use in patients with cancer (Berger et al., 2005). Unless they consult and receive approval from the oncology team, patients receiving chemotherapy should not use these herbal supplements for sleep problems (Block, Gyllenhaal, & Mead, 2004). Oncology nurses are advised to routinely review each patient's use of herbal agents. Assessing for use of prescription, over-the-counter, and herbal agents should be integrated into routine oncology clinical practice. For more information, refer to ONS PEP resources.

Nonpharmacologic Interventions

Growing evidence shows that several nonpharmacologic interventions promote quality sleep and daytime functioning in patients with cancer. These interventions have been or-

TABLE 23-3	Common Sleep Medications		
Drug	**Hypnotic Dose**	**Onset (Duration of Action)**	**Notes**
Benzodiazepines			
Diazepam (Valium®, Roche Pharmaceuticals)	5–10 mg (capsule, tablet)	30–60 minutes (6–8 hours)	May need to decrease opioid levels
Lorazepam (Ativan®, Wyeth Pharmaceuticals)	0.5–2 mg (tablets, liquid)	30–120 minutes (6–12 hours)	Dose-related effects: The larger the dose, the stronger and longer-lasting the effects.
Temazepam (Restoril®, Mallinckrodt Pharmaceuticals)	15–30 mg (capsule)	60 minutes minimum (6–8 hours)	Biphasic half-life can cause residual daytime sleepiness and dysfunction.
Triazolam (Halcion®, Pharmacia & Upjohn Co.)	0.125–0.5 mg (tablet)	30 minutes (peaks 1–1.5 hours)	Patients may have anterograde amnesia and rebound insomnia.
Clonazepam (Klonopin®, Roche Pharmaceuticals)	0.5–2 mg (tablet)	30–60 minutes (8–12 hours)	May be used during concomitant treatment of seizure disorder
Nonbenzodiazepine Hypnotics (Z Drugs)			
Zolpidem tartrate (Ambien®, Sanofi-Aventis)	5–20 mg (tablet)	30 minutes (4–6 hours)	Because of rapid onset, advise patient to go to bed immediately after taking zolpidem.
Zolpidem tartrate extended-release (Ambien CR®, Sanofi-Aventis)	6.25–12.5 mg (tablet)	15–30 minutes (6–8 hours)	Do not chew, crush, or divide tablets. Biphasic absorption, which results in rapid initial absorption then provides extended plasma concentrations.
Zaleplon (Sonata®, King Pharmaceuticals)	10–20 mg (capsule)	30 minutes (4–6 hours)	Do not give with or immediately after a meal.
Eszopiclone (Lunesta®, Sepracor Inc.)	1–3 mg (tablet)	30 minutes (5–7 hours)	Approved by the U.S. Food and Drug Administration for long-term use, unlike almost all other hypnotic sedatives
Tricyclic Antidepressants (TCAs)			
Doxepin (Sinequan®, Pfizer Inc.)	10–150 mg (capsule, liquid)	30 minutes	One of the most sedating TCAs
Amitriptyline (Elavil®, Merck Sharp & Dohme Ltd.)	10–15 mg (tablet, injectable)	30 minutes	Good for concomitant depression or neuropathic pain

(Continued on next page)

| TABLE 23-3 | Common Sleep Medications *(Continued)* | | |

Drug	Hypnotic Dose	Onset (Duration of Action)	Notes
Nortriptyline (Pamelor®, Mallinckrodt Pharmaceuticals)	10–50 mg (capsule)	30 minutes	Narrow therapeutic index (i.e., very small changes in dose can cause toxic results)
Antihistamines			
Diphenhydramine (Benadryl®, Pfizer Inc.)	25–100 mg (tablet, capsule, syrup)	10–30 minutes (4–6 hours)	Available over-the-counter and inexpensive; can increase digoxin and levodopa levels because of delayed gastric emptying
Hydroxyzine (Vistaril®, Atarax®, Pfizer Inc.)	10–100 mg (tablet, capsule, syrup)	15–30 minutes (4–6 hours)	Numerous other effects (antipruritic, muscle relaxant, bronchodilator, and antiemetic); can potentiate central nervous system depressants; may interact with other drugs, caution in hepatic impairment
Melatonin Receptor Agonist			
Ramelteon (Rozerem®, Takeda Pharmaceuticals)	8 mg (tablet)	30–90 minutes (2–5 hours)	Ramelteon is not addictive, is not a controlled substance, and does not cause withdrawal symptoms or rebound insomnia when it is stopped.

Note. Based on information from National Cancer Institute, 2006.

ganized into the categories of cognitive behavioral therapy (CBT), complementary therapies, psychoeducation/information, and exercise. These interventions have been classified as *Effectiveness Not Established* based on the evidence. This category indicates that insufficient supportive data currently exist to implement these interventions into practice (Page et al., 2006).

The most frequently tested interventions to improve patients' sleep have been CBTs and complementary therapies, but many of these studies have limitations. Study samples were small (N < 100), mostly Caucasian, and recruited from outpatient settings; interventions often were tested without using a comparison group; and outcomes may not have focused primarily on sleep. The knowledge base on sleep-wake disturbances will be advanced when results from several large (N > 100) randomized controlled trials (RCTs) are reported using sleep measurements with established reliability and validity and whose primary outcome variables are sleep-wake disturbances.

A variety of psychological and CBT interventions can be used alone or in combination to improve sleep. They are used to change negative thought processes—attitudes and behaviors related to one's ability to fall asleep, stay asleep, get enough sleep, and function during the day. CBT interventions that have been tested in patients with cancer include stimulus control, sleep restriction, relaxation therapy, sleep hygiene, profile-tailored cognitive-based therapy, and cognitive restructuring strategies (see Table 23-4). Overall results have shown several positive trends in sleep variables with CBTs, includ-

TABLE 23-4	Nonpharmacologic Interventions That Have Been Tested for Disturbed Sleep in Patients With Cancer

Cognitive Behavioral Therapy (CBT)—Effectiveness Not Established*	Outcomes on Sleep From CBT
Instruct patients in the following stimulus control techniques: • Go to bed only when sleepy and at approximately the same time each night • Get out of bed and go to another room whenever unable to fall asleep; return to bed only when sleepy again. • Use the bedroom for sleep and sex only. Instruct patients in the following sleep restriction techniques: • Maintain a regular bedtime and rising time each day. • Avoid daytime napping. If needed, limit to 30–45 minutes. Instruct patients in the following relaxation techniques: • Use preferred relaxation technique within two hours of going to bed, such as a warm bath or shower, reading, or listening to music. Instruct patients in the following sleep hygiene techniques: • Avoid caffeine and other stimulants after noon; complete dinner three hours before bedtime; do not go to bed hungry. • Replace mattress every 10–12 years and pillows more frequently; keep the bedroom cool and use light covers; do not watch television in the bedroom, etc.	• Improved sleep quality (Davidson et al., 2001; Epstein & Dirksen, 2007; Savard, Simard, et al., 2005) • Longer sleep duration (Allison, Edgar, et al., 2004; Allison, Nicolau, et al., 2004; Davidson et al., 2001; Epstein & Dirksen, 2007; Quesnel et al., 2003) • Higher sleep efficiency (Davidson et al., 2001; Epstein & Dirksen, 2007; Espie et al., 2008; Quesnel et al., 2003) • Maintenance of normal sleep patterns (Berger et al., 2002, 2003) • Improved insomnia (Arving et al., 2007; Davidson et al., 2001; Savard, Simard, et al., 2005) • Shorter sleep latency (Epstein & Dirksen, 2007; Espie et al., 2008) • Shorter waking after sleep onset (Davidson et al., 2001; Epstein & Dirksen, 2007; Espie et al., 2008) • Improved time in bed (Epstein & Dirksen, 2007) • Less sleep disturbances (Viela et al., 2006)
Complementary Therapies (CTs)—Effectiveness Not Established*	**Outcomes on Sleep From CTs**
• Encourage patients to decrease stress by selecting relaxation techniques that suit them, including massage, individual muscle relaxation, meditation, mindfulness-based stress reduction, yoga, and autogenic training. • Encourage patients to keep a journal in which they document their deepest thoughts and feelings about their illness and treatment. • Encourage patients to decrease stress by focusing on and isolating various muscle groups while moving progressively up and down the body. Encourage focused breathing, with all attention centered on the sensations of breathing, including the rhythm and rise and fall of the chest. • Provide referral to appropriate practitioners as needed.	• Improved sleep quality (Carlson et al., 2003, 2004, Carlson & Garland, 2005; Cohen et al., 2004; de Moor et al., 2002; Fobair et al., 2002; Shapiro et al., 2003; Soden et al., 2004) • Longer sleep duration (Cohen et al., 2004; de Moor et al., 2002; Simeit et al., 2004; Weze et al., 2004) • Higher sleep efficiency (Simeit et al., 2004) • Shorter sleep latency (Cannici et al., 1983; Cohen et al., 2004; Simeit et al., 2004; Wright et al., 2002) • Less need for sleeping medication (Cohen et al., 2004; Simeit et al., 2004) • Less daytime dysfunction (de Moor et al., 2002; Simeit et al., 2004) • Less sleep difficulties (Cohen & Fried, 2007) • Improved insomnia (Bozcuk et al., 2006; Carlson & Garland, 2005; Cohen et al., 2004; Weze et al., 2004) • Less sleep disturbance (Carlson et al., 2003, 2004)

(Continued on next page)

TABLE 23-4	Nonpharmacologic Interventions That Have Been Tested for Disturbed Sleep in Patients With Cancer *(Continued)*
Education/Information—Effectiveness Not Established*	**Outcomes on Sleep From Education**
• Provide patients with information regarding specifics of treatment and expected side effects, including sleep-wake disturbances. • Repeat this information throughout the treatment. • Teach patients basic information about sleep hygiene.	• Fewer problems sleeping (Kim et al., 2002)
Exercise—Effectiveness Not Established*	**Outcomes on Sleep From Exercise**
• Rule out bone metastasis or exercise contraindications. • Have patient complete moderate exercise (e.g., brisk walking 20–30 minutes four to five times per week) at least three hours before bedtime. • Encourage patients to perform strength and resistance training.	• Improved sleep quality (Mock et al., 1997; Young-McCaughan et al., 2003) • Longer sleep duration and improved sleep efficiency (Coleman et al., 2003)

* Level of evidence from Oncology Nursing Society Putting Evidence Into Practice. More information can be found at www.ons.org/outcomes.

ing higher sleep quality, longer sleep duration, and higher sleep efficiency. Berger and colleagues (Berger et al., 2002, 2003) demonstrated that intervention with the individual sleep promotion plan maintained normal ranges of sleep variables except for excessive nighttime awakenings.

Complementary therapies are a diverse group of medical and healthcare practices and products that are not generally considered to be part of conventional medicine. Several complementary therapy interventions have been tested in patients with cancer, including massage, individual muscle relaxation, meditation, mindfulness-based stress reduction, yoga, autogenic training, aromatherapy, music intervention, healing touch, expressive therapy, and expressive writing (see Table 23-4). Improvements in sleep disturbances that occurred when one or more of the previously mentioned complementary therapies strategies were employed include higher sleep quality, shorter sleep latency, longer sleep duration, higher sleep efficiency, less daytime dysfunction, and use of fewer sleep medications. Swedish techniques of therapeutic massage did not result in any improvements in sleep quality (Smith, Kemp, Hemphill, & Vojir, 2002). The strongest study thus far testing a complementary therapy intervention in an RCT was conducted by Shapiro, Bootzin, Figueredo, Lopez, and Schwartz (2003) using meditation and yoga to improve sleep quality in patients with breast cancer.

Psychoeducation/information interventions provide patients with structured education and information about treatment and side effects via the use of a variety of media. These interventions also may include strategies to decrease psychological mood, such as anxiety, in order to help the patient learn. An RCT using a single-item sleep measure reported increased sleep duration using an educational, informational tape in men receiving radiation for localized prostate cancer (Kim, Roscoe, & Morrow, 2002). Another RCT showed no change in sleep disturbances as measured by a daily sleep diary when using informational audiotapes in women with breast cancer undergoing chemotherapy (Williams & Schreier, 2005).

Exercise interventions include any planned, structured, and repetitive bodily movement that is performed to improve or maintain physical fitness, performance, or health. Three aerobic, strength, and resistance training interventions have been tested in people with cancer in an attempt to improve exercise tolerance and decrease fatigue; a secondary outcome was to improve sleep (Coleman et al., 2003; Mock et al., 1997; Young-McCaughan et al., 2003). Mock et al. used a one-group experimental study to test a self-paced progressive home-based exercise program in people with cancer that resulted in participants reporting less difficulty sleeping at the end of the study. Another one-group experimental study used exercise and education classes twice a week in people with cancer that resulted in improved self-reported sleep patterns (Young-McCaughan et al.). A third study (Coleman et al.) found a home-based aerobic and resistance training program intervention was feasible for patients who were receiving high-dose chemotherapy and peripheral blood stem cell transplant for multiple myeloma. Nurse clinicians are urged to work with other interdisciplinary members who have expertise regarding exercise in patients with cancer to tailor these interventions for patients. The ONS PEP resources are available to learn about how interventions were designed to improve sleep-wake disturbances in patients with cancer.

Expected Outcomes

When nurses intervene with evidence-based interventions to improve sleep in patients with cancer, positive outcomes are anticipated (Page et al., 2006). Positive sleep outcomes for patients include the ability to fall asleep easily, to stay asleep through the night, and to awaken feeling refreshed and rejuvenated with the use of fewer sleep aids. Other measurable outcomes during waking hours include less daytime sleepiness and napping, and fewer sick days from work. Because insufficient sleep can coexist with and exacerbate other symptoms, such as pain and mood disturbances, in patients with cancer, improving sleep may lead to improvement in these symptoms. Improved symptom management can then lead to increased physical, emotional, social, and mental functioning and overall quality of life. Nurses are in an excellent position to help patients to deal with their disturbed sleep.

Patient and Family Teaching Points

Many opportunities exist to teach patients and families about how to improve sleep. Teaching begins by influencing the values that adults have regarding the need to schedule seven to nine hours per night for sleep. For example, many parents do not value or know about the age-adjusted amount of sleep time suggested for their children or themselves (National Sleep Foundation, 2006). Chronic partial sleep loss in adolescents has been associated with dysregulation of neuroendocrine control of appetite and changes in glucose metabolism suggestive of an increased risk for diabetes (Van Cauter et al., 2007). Clinicians demonstrate the value of obtaining quality sleep for their patients by routinely screening them for sleep-wake disorders. Nurses are encouraged to use the ONS PEP resources to suggest evidence-based interventions that patients find acceptable and are willing to try to relieve insomnia. Nurses can then coach patients to increase adherence to the intervention and evaluate the outcomes of the intervention after six to eight weeks in that individual.

Need for Future Research

Although many recent studies have focused attention on sleep-wake disturbances in patients with cancer, more knowledge is needed to better understand the broad nature of sleep-wake disturbances related to cancer and their consequences (Berger et al., 2005). More research is needed into the pathophysiology of sleep difficulties related to specific types and stages of cancer, especially in high-risk groups such as older adults; in understudied populations such as adolescent and young adults; and at the end of life, where the evidence base is critically limited. More information also is needed about how sleep problems interact with other cancer-related symptoms, including fatigue, mood disturbances, and pain (Lee et al., 2004). Nurses are in an optimal position to explore other factors related to cancer treatment, such as schedules and settings, that contribute to sleep-wake disturbances and could be modified to promote improved sleep. Nurses can identify patients who are at high risk for sleep problems and intervene early in the treatment process to prevent and manage the distress attributed to these clusters of symptoms.

Additional work needs to be done to identify the most effective screening and assessment strategies for various oncology populations and in diverse clinical and research settings. Efficient screening techniques will enable nurses to identify common sleep problems that may go unrecognized or untreated in their patients. Although patients may volunteer reports of difficulty falling asleep, nurses may need to ask further questions to detect other common sleep-wake disturbances, such as excessive sleepiness or restless legs. Research is needed to test various sleep-promoting interventions for their effectiveness during the many phases of cancer treatment, including the early diagnosis and treatment phase and during the years of survivorship, as well as at the end of life. The research agenda is full of opportunities to advance knowledge about the importance of refreshing and restorative sleep in this population of patients. Because sleep is an excellent example of a clinical issue that crosses many disciplines and specialties, teams consisting of nurses, physicians, and other therapists are essential to maximize efforts in research and clinical care (Colten & Altevogt, 2006).

Conclusion of Case Studies

Adult Case Study

Recall that P.L. is a patient with stage IIB breast cancer who has been prescribed four cycles of dose-dense chemotherapy (every 14 days) with doxorubicin and cyclophosphamide, followed by four cycles of docetaxel, and is having difficulty sleeping. P.L.'s nurse in the clinic recommends a number of interventions from the ONS PEP resources on sleep-wake disturbances and fatigue to address P.L.'s complaints of difficulty maintaining sleep at night and daytime sleepiness, fatigue, and distress.

Recommendations to relieve P.L.'s sleep-wake disturbances include
- Use the bedroom for only sleep and sexual activity.
- If unable to fall back to sleep when awake during the night, go to a dark and quiet place to relax and return to bed only when sleepy; repeat if needed.
- Set 10 pm as bedtime and 6 am as wake time seven nights per week. Keep this schedule as much as possible. Ask husband to parent teenagers after 10 pm.
- Get up even if sleepy at 6 am, and take 20–30-minute power naps during the day.
- Maintain daytime activity at the same level it was prior to starting chemotherapy unless febrile, experiencing lower blood counts, or vomiting. Choose a pleasant place to walk.
- Take a warm bath or shower and enjoy a relaxing activity within two hours of bedtime.
- Discuss interventions for hot flashes with the oncology team. Avoid herbal remedies.
- Control other related symptoms (pain, fatigue, depression, nausea, and vomiting).

Adolescent Case Study

Recall that K.D. is a teenager with chronic myeloid leukemia diagnosed two and a half months ago. Her treatment is imatinib 300 mg PO daily, which she will continue until her bone marrow cytogenetics show remission. K.D. was hospitalized for several weeks at the time of diagnosis because of complications related to myelosuppression and is experiencing difficulty sleeping. K.D.'s nurse in the oncology clinic recommended a number of interventions from the ONS PEP resources on sleep-wake disturbances and fatigue to address K.D.'s complaints of difficulty falling asleep, daytime sleepiness, fatigue, and mood disturbances.

Recommendations to relieve K.D.'s fatigue and sleep-wake disturbances include
- Increase daytime activity to include two 15-minute walks each day with a family member, friend, or neighbor. Increase activity as tolerated.
- If sleepy during the day, go to bed for a 45-minute nap.
- Watch movies earlier in the evening with a friend or family member. Sit in a chair or on the bedroom floor.
- Set midnight as bedtime and 9 am as wake time until returning back to school. Keep this schedule as much as possible.
- For relaxation, take a bath, listen to music, and write in a journal before selected bedtime.
- If unable to fall asleep in 20 minutes, go into the living room and read English homework. Return to bed when feeling sleepy.

Conclusion

Sleep-wake disturbances are common and distressing symptoms for many patients throughout the cancer trajectory and can negatively affect their physical, social, and emotional health. With knowledge about sleep physiology, sleep assessment, and common sleep disorders, nurses can effectively intervene with patients with cancer who have problems with disrupted and insufficient sleep. Patients who are determined to be at increased risk for primary sleep disorders should be referred to a sleep disorders center for evaluation. For other patients with more general sleep-wake disturbances, nurses can implement a number of pharmacologic and nonpharmacologic interventions based on current evidence-based recommendations for practice. Nurses need to efficiently translate evidence from ongoing research to new clinical interventions for optimal sleep-wake outcomes.

References

Alfano, C.M., & Rowland, J.H. (2006). Recovery issues in cancer survivorship: A new challenge for supportive care. *Cancer Journal, 12*(5), 432–443.

Allison, P.J., Edgar, L., Nicolau, B., Archer, J., Black, M., & Hier, M. (2004). Results of a feasibility study for a psycho-educational intervention in head and neck cancer. *Psycho-Oncology, 13*(7), 482–485.

Allison, P.J., Nicolau, B., Edgar, L., Archer, J., Black, M., & Hier, M. (2004). Teaching head and neck cancer patients coping strategies: Results of a feasibility study. *Oral Oncology, 40*(5), 538–544.

American Academy of Sleep Medicine. (2005). *International classification of sleep disorders: Diagnostic and coding manual* (2nd ed.). Westchester, IL: Author.

Ancoli-Israel, S. (2005). Sleep and fatigue in cancer patients. In M.H. Kryger, T. Roth, & W.C. Dement (Eds.), *Principles and practice of sleep medicine* (pp. 1218–1224). Philadelphia: Elsevier Saunders.

Ancoli-Israel, S., Liu, L., Marler, M.R., Parker, B.A., Jones, V., Sadler, G.R., et al. (2006). Fatigue, sleep, and circadian rhythms prior to chemotherapy for breast cancer. *Supportive Care in Cancer, 14*(3), 201–209.

Ancoli-Israel, S., Moore, P.J., & Jones, V. (2001). The relationship between fatigue and sleep in cancer patients: A review. *European Journal of Cancer Care (English Language Edition), 10*(4), 245–255.

Arving, C., Sjoden, P.O., Bergh, J., Hellbom, M., Johansson, B., Glimelius, B., et al. (2007). Individual psychosocial support for breast cancer patients: A randomized study of nurse versus psychologist interventions and standard of care. *Cancer Nursing, 30*(3), E10–E19.

Bardwell, W.A., Profant, J., Casden, D.R., Dimsdale, J.E., Ancoli-Israel, S., Natarajan, L., et al. (2007). The relative importance of specific risk factors for insomnia in women treated for early-stage breast cancer. *Psycho-Oncology, 17*(1), 9–18.

Barton-Burke, M. (2006). Cancer-related fatigue and sleep disturbances. *Cancer Nursing, 29*(Suppl. 2), 72–77.

Beck, S.L., Dudley, W.N., & Barsevick, A. (2005). Pain, sleep disturbance, and fatigue in patients with cancer: Using a mediation model to test a symptom cluster. *Oncology Nursing Forum, 32*(3), 542.

Berger, A.M. (2006). Sleep and wakefulness. In K. Dow (Ed.), *Nursing care of women with cancer* (pp. 327–352). Philadelphia: Elsevier.

Berger, A.M., & Farr, L. (1999). The influence of daytime inactivity and nighttime restlessness on cancer-related fatigue. *Oncology Nursing Forum, 26*(10), 1663–1671.

Berger, A.M., Farr, L.A., Kuhn, B.R., Fischer, P., & Agrawal, S. (2007). Values of sleep/wake, activity/rest, circadian rhythms, and fatigue prior to adjuvant breast cancer chemotherapy. *Journal of Pain and Symptom Management, 33*(4), 398–409.

Berger, A.M., Parker, K.P., Young-McCaughan, S., Mallory, G.A., Barsevick, A.M., Beck, S.L., et al. (2005). Sleep/wake disturbances in people with cancer and their caregivers: state of the science. *Oncology Nursing Forum, 32*(6), E98–E126. Retrieved January 19, 2009, from http://ons.metapress.com/content/7244v4525u2j6408/fulltext.pdf

Berger, A.M., VonEssen, S., Kuhn, B.R., Piper, B.F., Agrawal, S., Lynch, J.C., et al. (2003). Adherence, sleep, and fatigue outcomes after adjuvant breast cancer chemotherapy: Results of a feasibility intervention study. *Oncology Nursing Forum, 30*(3), 513–522.

Berger, A.M., VonEssen, S., Khun, B.R., Piper, B.F., Farr, L., Agrawal, S., et al. (2002). Feasibility of a sleep intervention during adjuvant breast cancer chemotherapy. *Oncology Nursing Forum, 29*(10), 1431–1441.

Block, K.I., Gyllenhaal, C., & Mead, M.N. (2004). Safety and efficacy of herbal sedatives in cancer care. *Integrative Cancer Therapies, 3*(2), 128–148.

Bonnet, M.H. (2005). Acute sleep deprivation. In M.H. Kryger, T. Roth, & W.C. Dement (Eds.), *Principles and practice of sleep medicine* (4th ed., pp. 51–66). Philadelphia: Elsevier Saunders.

Borbely, A.A., & Achermann, P. (2005). Sleep homeostasis and models of sleep regulation. In M.H. Kryger, T. Roth, & W.C. Dement (Eds.), *Principles and practice of sleep medicine* (4th ed., pp. 405–417). Philadelphia: Elsevier Saunders.

Bower, J.E., Ganz, P.A., Desmond, K.A., Rowland, J.H., Meyerowitz, B.E., & Belin, T.R. (2000). Fatigue in breast cancer survivors: Occurrence, correlates, and impact on quality of life. *Journal of Clinical Oncology, 18*(4), 743–753.

Bozcuk, H., Artac, M., Kara, A., Ozdogan, M., Sualp, Y., Topcu, Z., et al. (2006). Does music exposure during chemotherapy improve quality of life in early breast cancer patients? A pilot study. *Medical Science Monitoring, 12*(5), CR200–CR205.

Buysse, D.J., Reynolds, C.F., III, Monk, T.H., Berman, S.R., & Kupfer, D.J. (1989). The Pittsburgh Sleep Quality Index: A new instrument for psychiatric practice and research. *Psychiatry Research, 28*(2), 193–213.

Cannici, J., Malcolm, R., & Peek, L.A. (1983). Treatment of insomnia in cancer patients using muscle relaxation training. *Journal of Behavior Therapy and Experimental Psychiatry, 14*(3), 251–256.

Carlson, L.E., & Garland, S.N. (2005). Impact of mindfulness-based stress reduction (MBSR) on sleep, mood, stress and fatigue symptoms in cancer outpatients. *International Journal of Behavioral Medicine, 12*(12), 278–285.

Carlson, L.E., Speca, M., Patel, K.D., & Godey, E. (2003). Mindfulness-based stress reduction in relation to quality of life, mood, symptoms of stress, and immune parameters in breast and prostate cancer outpatients. *Psychosomatic Medicine, 65*(4), 571–581.

Carlson, L.E., Speca, M., Patel, K.D., & Godey, E. (2004). Mindfulness-based stress reduction in relation to quality of life, mood, symptoms of stress and levels of cortical, dehydroepiandrosterone sulfate (DHEAS) and melatonin in breast and prostate cancer outpatients. *Psychoneuroendocrinology, 29*(4), 448–474.

Carpenter, J.S., Johnson, D., Wagner, L., & Andrykowski, M. (2002). Hot flashes and related outcomes in breast cancer survivors and matched comparison women. *Oncology Nursing Forum, 29*(3), E16–E25. Retrieved January 19, 2009, from http://ons.metapress.com/content/6616786818742847/fulltext.pdf

Carskadon, M.A., & Dement, W.C. (2005). Normal human sleep: An overview. In M.H. Kryger, T. Roth, & W.C. Dement (Eds.), *Principles and practice of sleep medicine* (4th ed., pp. 13–23). Philadelphia: Elsevier Saunders.

Chervin, R.D. (2005). Use of clinical tools and tests in sleep medicine. In M.H. Kryger, T. Roth, & W.C. Dement (Eds.), *Principles and practice of sleep medicine* (4th ed., pp. 602–614). Philadelphia: Elsevier Saunders.

Cohen, M., & Fried, G. (2007). Comparing relaxation training and cognitive-behavioral group therapy for women with breast cancer. *Research on Social Work Practice, 17*(3), 313–323.

Cohen, L., Warneke, C., Fouladi, R.T., Rodriguez, M.A., & Chaoul-Reich, A. (2004). Psychological adjustment and sleep quality in a randomized trial of the effects of a Tibetan yoga intervention in patients with lymphoma. *Cancer, 100*(10), 2253–2260.

Cole, R.J., Kripke, D.F., Gruen, W., Mullaney, D.J., & Gillin, J.C. (1992). Automatic sleep/wake identification from wrist activity. *Sleep, 15*(5), 461–469.

Coleman, E.A., Coon, S., Hall-Barrow, J., Richards, K., Gaylor, D., & Stewart, B. (2003). Feasibility of exercise during treatment for multiple myeloma. *Cancer Nursing, 26*(5), 410–419.

Colten, H.R., & Altevogt, B.M. (Eds.). (2006). *Sleep disorders and sleep deprivation: An unmet public health problem.* Washington, DC: National Academies Press. Retrieved August 28, 2007, from http://www.iom.edu/CMS/3740/23160/33668.aspx

Davidson, J.R., MacLean, A.W., Brundage, M.D., & Schulze, K. (2002). Sleep disturbance in cancer patients. *Social Science and Medicine, 54*(9), 1309–1321.

Davidson, J.R., Waisberg, J.L., Brundage, M.D., & MacLean, A.W. (2001). Nonpharmacologic group treatment of insomnia: A preliminary study with cancer survivors. *Psycho-Oncology, 10*(5), 389–397.

de Moor, C., Sterner, J., Hall, M., Warneke, C., Gilani, Z., Amato, R., et al. (2002). A pilot study of the effects of expressive writing on psychological and behavioral adjustment in patients enrolled in a Phase II trial of vaccine therapy for metastatic renal cell carcinoma. *Health Psychology, 21*(6), 615–619.

Dement, W.C., & Vaughn, C. (1999). *The promise of sleep.* New York: Random House.

Dijk, D.J., & Franken, P. (2005). Interaction of sleep homeostasis and circadian rhythmicity: Dependent or independent systems? In M.H. Kryger, T. Roth, & W.C. Dement (Eds.), *Principles and practice of sleep medicine* (4th ed., pp. 418–434). Philadelphia: Elsevier Saunders.

Dodd, M.J., Miaskowski, C., & Lee, K.A. (2004). Occurrence of symptom clusters. *Journal of the National Cancer Institute Monographs, 2004*(32), 76–78.

Donovan, K.A., & Jacobsen, P.B. (2007). Fatigue, depression, and insomnia: Evidence for a symptom cluster in cancer. *Seminars in Oncology Nursing, 23*(2), 127–135.

Dunlop, R.J., & Campbell, C.W. (2000). Cytokines and advanced cancer. *Journal of Pain and Symptom Management, 20*(3), 214–232.

Epstein, D.R., & Dirksen, S.R. (2007). Randomized trial of a cognitive-behavioral intervention for insomnia in breast cancer survivors [Online exclusive]. *Oncology Nursing Forum, 34*(5), E51–E59. Retrieved January 19, 2009, from http://ons.metapress.com/content/l13681kwjk712374/fulltext.pdf

Espie, C.A., Fleming, L., Cassidy, J., Samuel, L., Taylor, L.M., White, C.A., et al. (2008). Randomized controlled clinical effectiveness trial of cognitive behavioral therapy compared with treatment as usual for persistent insomnia in patients with cancer. *Journal of Clinical Oncology, 26*(15), 1–9.

Extermann, M., & Hurria, A. (2007). Comprehensive geriatric assessment for older patients with cancer. *Journal of Clinical Oncology, 25*(14), 1824–1831.

Fobair, P., Koopman, C., DiMiceli, S., O'Hanlan, K., Butler, L.D., Classen, C., et al. (2002). Psychosocial intervention for lesbians with primary breast cancer. *Psycho-Oncology, 11*(5), 427–438.

Given, B.A., & Sherwood, P.R. (2005). Nursing-sensitive patient outcomes—A white paper. *Oncology Nursing Forum, 32*(4), 773–784.

Gobel, B.H., Beck, S.L., & O'Leary, C. (2006). Nursing-sensitive patient outcomes: The development of the Putting Evidence Into Practice resources for nursing practice. *Clinical Journal of Oncology Nursing, 10*(5), 621–624.

Hinds, P.S., Hockenberry, M., Rai, S.N., Zhang, L., Razzouk, B.I., Cremer, L., et al. (2007). Clinical field testing of an enhanced-activity intervention in hospitalized children with cancer. *Journal of Pain and Symptom Management, 33*(6), 686–697.

Hinds, P.S., Hockenberry, M., Rai, S.N., Zhang, L., Razzouk, B.I., McCarthy, K., et al. (2007). Nocturnal awakenings, sleep environment, interruptions, and fatigue in hospitalized children with cancer. *Oncology Nursing Forum, 34*(2), 393–402.

Johns, M.W. (1991). A new method for measuring daytime sleepiness: The Epworth sleepiness scale. *Sleep, 14*(6), 540–545.

Kim, H.J., McGuire, D.B., Tulman, L., & Barsevick, A.M. (2005). Symptom clusters: Concept analysis and clinical implications for cancer nursing. *Cancer Nursing, 28*(4), 270–282.

Kim, Y., Roscoe, J.A., & Morrow, G.R. (2002). The effects of information and negative affect on severity of side effects from radiation therapy for prostate cancer. *Supportive Care in Cancer, 10*(5), 416–421.

Kuo, H.H., Chiu, M.J., Liao, W.C., & Hwang, S.L. (2006). Quality of sleep and related factors during chemotherapy in patients with stage I/II breast cancer. *Journal of the Formosan Medical Association, 105*(1), 64–69.

Kushida, C.A., Littner, M.R., Morgenthaler, T., Alessi, C.A., Bailey, D., Coleman, J., Jr., et al. (2005). Practice parameters for the indications for polysomnography and related procedures: An update for 2005. *Sleep, 28*(4), 499–521.

Lashley, F.R. (2004). Measuring sleep. In M. Frank-Stromborg & S.J. Olsen (Eds.), *Instruments for clinical health-care research* (3rd ed., pp. 293–314). Sudbury, MA: Jones and Bartlett.

Lee, K., Cho, M., Miaskowski, C., & Dodd, M. (2004). Impaired sleep and rhythms in persons with cancer. *Sleep Medicine Reviews, 8*(3), 199–212.

Lee, K.A. (2003). Impaired sleep. In V. Carrieri-Kohlman, A.M. Lindsey, & C.M. West (Eds.), *Pathophysiological phenomena in nursing* (3rd ed., pp. 363–385). St. Louis, MO: Saunders.

Lee, K.A., & Ward, T.M. (2005). Critical components of a sleep assessment for clinical practice settings. *Issues in Mental Health Nursing, 26*(7), 739–750.

Mock, V., Dow, K.H., Meares, C.J., Grimm, P.M., Dienemann, J.A., Haisfield-Wolfe, M.E., et al. (1997). Effects of exercise on fatigue, physical functioning, and emotional distress during radiation therapy for breast cancer. *Oncology Nursing Forum, 24*(6), 991–1000.

Morgenthaler, T., Alessi, C., Friedman, L., Owens, J., Kapur, V., Boehlecke, B., et al. (2007). Practice parameters for the use of actigraphy in the assessment of sleep and sleep disorders: An update for 2007. *Sleep, 30*(4), 519–529.

Mormont, M.C., & Levi, F. (1997). Circadian-system alterations during cancer processes: A review. *International Journal of Cancer, 70*(2), 241–247.

National Cancer Institute. (2006, February 16). *Sleep disorders (PDQ®).* Retrieved September 18, 2007, from http://www.nci.nih.gov/cancertopics/pdq/supportivecare/sleepdisorders/HealthProfessional

National Institutes of Health. (2005). National Institutes of Health State of the Science Conference statement on Manifestations and Management of Chronic Insomnia in Adults, June 13–15, 2005. *Sleep, 28*(9), 1049–1057.

National Sleep Foundation. (2006). *Sleep-wake cycle: Its physiology and impact on health.* Retrieved September 17, 2007, from http://www.sleepfoundation.org/atf/cf/%7BF6BF2668-A1B4-4FE8-8D1A-A5D39340D9CB%7D/Sleep-Wake_Cycle.pdf

Owens, J.A., & Dalzell, V. (2005). Use of the 'BEARS' sleep screening tool in a pediatric residents' continuity clinic: A pilot study. *Sleep Medicine, 6*(1), 63–69.

Page, M.S., Berger, A.M., & Johnson, L.B. (2006). Putting evidence into practice: Evidence-based interventions for sleep-wake disturbances. *Clinical Journal of Oncology Nursing, 10*(6), 753–767.

Payne, J., Piper, B., Rabinowitz, I., & Zimmerman, B. (2006). Biomarkers, fatigue, sleep, and depressive symptoms in women with breast cancer: A pilot study. *Oncology Nursing Forum, 33*(4), 775–783.

Payne, J.K. (2004). A neuroendocrine-based regulatory fatigue model. *Biological Research for Nursing, 6*(2), 141–150.

Quesnel, C., Savard, J., Simard, S., Ivers, H., & Morin, C.M. (2003). Efficacy of cognitive-behavioral therapy for insomnia in women treated for nonmetastatic breast cancer. *Journal of Consulting and Clinical Psychology, 71*(1), 189–200.

Roscoe, J.A., Kaufman, M.E., Matteson-Rusby, S.E., Palesh, O.G., Ryan, J.L., Kohli, S., et al. (2007). Cancer-related fatigue and sleep disorders. *Oncologist, 12*(Suppl. 1), 35–42.

Savard, J., Davidson, J.R., Ivers, H., Quesnel, C., Rioux, D., Dupere, V., et al. (2004). The association between nocturnal hot flashes and sleep in breast cancer survivors. *Journal of Pain and Symptom Management, 27*(6), 513–522.

Savard, J., & Morin, C.M. (2001). Insomnia in the context of cancer: A review of a neglected problem. *Journal of Clinical Oncology, 19*(3), 895–908.

Savard, J., Simard, S., Blanchet, J., Ivers, H., & Morin, C.M. (2001). Prevalence, clinical characteristics, and risk factors for insomnia in the context of breast cancer. *Sleep, 24*(5), 583–590.

Savard, J., Simard, S., Ivers, H., & Morin, C.M. (2005). Randomized study on the efficacy of cognitive-behavioral therapy for insomnia secondary to breast cancer, part II: Immunologic effects. *Journal of Clinical Oncology, 23*(25), 6097–6106.

Savard, M.H., Savard, J., Simard, S., & Ivers, H. (2005). Empirical validation of the Insomnia Severity Index in cancer patients. *Psycho-Oncology, 14*(6), 429–441.

Servaes, P., Verhagen, C., & Bleijenberg, G. (2002). Fatigue in cancer patients during and after treatment: Prevalence, correlates and interventions. *European Journal of Cancer, 38*(1), 27–43.

Shapiro, S.L., Bootzin, R.R., Figueredo, A.J., Lopez, A.M., & Schwartz, G.E. (2003). The efficacy of mindfulness-based stress reduction in the treatment of sleep disturbance in women with breast cancer: An exploratory study. *Journal of Psychosomatic Research, 54*(1), 85–91.

Simeit, R., Deck, R., & Conta-Marx, B. (2004). Sleep management training for cancer patients with insomnia. *Supportive Care in Cancer, 12*(3), 176–183.

Smith, M.C., Kemp, J., Hemphill, L., & Vojir, C.P. (2002). Outcomes of therapeutic massage for hospitalized cancer patients. *Journal of Nursing Scholarship, 34*(3), 257–262.

Soden, K., Vincent, K., Craske, S., Lucas, C., & Ashley, S. (2004). A randomized controlled trial of aromatherapy massage in a hospice setting. *Palliative Medicine, 18*(2), 87–92.

Spiegel, K., Leproult, R., & Van Cauter, E. (2003). [Impact of sleep debt on physiological rhythms]. *Revue Neurologique, 159*(Suppl. 11), 6S11–6S20.

Turek, F.W., Dugovic, C., & Laposky, A.D. (2005). Master circadian clock, master circadian rhythm. In M.H. Kryger, T. Roth, & W.C. Dement (Eds.), *Principles and practice of sleep medicine* (4th ed., pp. 318–320). Philadelphia: Elsevier Saunders.

Van Cauter, E., Holmback, U., Knutson, K., Leproult, R., Miller, A., Nedeltcheva, A., et al. (2007). Impact of sleep and sleep loss on neuroendocrine and metabolic function. *Hormone Research, 67*(Suppl. 1), 2–9.

Vena, C., Parker, K., Cunningham, M., Clark, J., & McMillan, S. (2004). Sleep-wake disturbances in people with cancer part I: An overview of sleep, sleep regulation, and effects of disease and treatment. *Oncology Nursing Forum, 31*(4), 735–746.

Viela, L.D., Nicolau, B., Mahmud, S., Edgar, L., Hier, M., Black, M., et al. (2006). Comparison of psychosocial outcomes in head and neck cancer patients receiving a coping strategies intervention and control subjects receiving no intervention. *Journal of Otolaryngology, 35*(2), 88–96.

Weze, C., Leathard, H.L., Grange, J., Tiplady, P., & Stevens, G. (2004). Evaluation of healing by gentle touch in 35 clients with cancer. *European Journal of Oncology Nursing, 8*(1), 40–49.

Williams, S.A., & Schreier, A.M. (2005). The role of education in managing fatigue, anxiety, and sleep disorders in women undergoing chemotherapy for breast cancer. *Applied Nursing Research, 18*(3), 138–147.

Wright, S., Courtney, U., & Crowther, D. (2002). A quantitative and qualitative pilot study of the perceived benefits of autogenic training for a group of people with cancer. *European Journal of Cancer Care (English Language Edition), 11*(2), 122–130.

Young-McCaughan, S., Mays, M.Z., Arzola, S.M., Yoder, L.H., Dramiga, S.A., Leclerc, K.M., et al. (2003). Research and commentary: Change in exercise tolerance, activity and sleep patterns, and quality of life in patients with cancer participating in a structured exercise program. *Oncology Nursing Forum, 30*(3), 441–454.

CHAPTER 24

Spiritual Care From the Oncology Nurse

Susan Tinley, PhD, RN

Case Study

M.L. comes to the cancer genetics clinic for an evaluation and possible genetic testing. The nurse obtains a fairly extensive family history of cancer, inclusive of M.L.'s history of breast cancer seven years previously and her youngest sister's recent diagnosis of stage IV ovarian cancer. As she is providing the information about her sister's diagnosis, M.L. talks about how unfair it is that her sister will not survive the ovarian cancer, when M.L. is doing so well after her own treatment. Her sister still has children in the primary and middle grades, but M.L.'s children are raised and independent.

Overview

"What do we live for, if not to make the world less difficult for each other?"
—Mary Ann Evans (George Eliot), *Middlemarch: A Study of Provincial Life*

Spiritual care by the oncology nurse involves the process of making the world of cancer (physical, social, psychological, spiritual) less difficult for patients. Yet, spiritual care often is not experienced or at least recognized by patients, nor even by the nurses themselves. The reasons for this lack of recognition or experience are many, but one of the major ones is definitional.

Meaning of Spirituality

In our diverse society, the human spirit is defined quite differently by Christians, Jews, Muslims, agnostics, new age followers, Native Americans, and so on. Therefore, what is meaningful to a new age follower may not be meaningful to a Christian unless there is a willingness to look for the common ground while respecting the differences. This is what makes spiritual care challenging and also rewarding. The oncology nurse may reap the rewards if willing and able to meet the challenge.

A definition of *spirit* that would probably be acceptable for most is the essence of a human being, the source of life, what makes an individual uniquely human. It is all that a human person is except for the physical body and yet is inextricably united with the body. It is what connects one human with all others. For those who believe in God or a higher power, the spirit is defined first as what connects with God or that higher power. Opposed to popular portrayal of the heart as the seat of love, it is the spirit that connects one with another and with God in love. The differing beliefs about a connection with a higher power mandate that nursing care for the human spirit be based on a respect for both the patient's and the nurse's beliefs.

Because of the inextricable union of spirit and body, the pain of the body can be the source of pain of the soul and vice versa. Therefore, care for the body and care for the spirit are not separable in spiritual care. Within the realm of nursing, the activities of this care renew, uplift, comfort, heal, and inspire patients, their families, and the nurses themselves. Among others, these activities include a focus on the individuality of the patient, supportive activities, advocacy, and referral. All nurses should be competent to assess the need for and provide these interventions.

What Patients Have to Say About the Spirit

A brief review of what patients with cancer, survivors, and high-risk individuals have said about their experience is an essential starting point for a consideration of spirituality. At the time of diagnosis, women with breast cancer experienced shock, fear of dying, and a frightening sense of vulnerability and aloneness while trying to maintain self-identity (Coward & Kahn, 2004). The women turned inward to mobilize their inner resources. Reliance on God and their own internal resources increased their hope for survival. They reached outward to connect with family, friends, caregivers, and faith communities for support to relieve the fear and isolation. Helping others and meeting their commitments at home and work helped to maintain their sense of identity. As the women passed through the cancer trajectory toward survivorship, they regained a sense of normalcy, but it was different than before diagnosis; their bodies were different and their life values had changed (Coward & Kahn).

Isolation has been identified in the experience of women newly diagnosed with breast cancer, but it was a self-imposed isolation in which the women focused their attention on what was happening and mustering up their inner strength (Logan, Pinto, & De Grasse, 2006). They sought comfort selectively from those who could provide it. For many, this search for comfort included prayer and their relation with God and the prayers of others. For others, nature was a source of comfort. Some wanted the offer of a referral to a chaplain in the outpatient setting and others did not, but as one participant said, "Someone needs to ask the questions" (Logan et al., p. 124).

Families have described the support from church communities in many forms, including assistance in meeting the daily needs for meals, transportation, and child care, as well as prayer chains and healing services. One woman with breast cancer described her experience of physical and spiritual support from her church community that continued after moving to another part of the country.

> "We had more food than we could eat. Some women came and packed my entire kitchen and did a lot of other packing because I couldn't lift any weight. They were supportive in every sense of the word: prayer, person, visiting, bringing food. After I moved, it was a very lonely time, but I could feel the wave up from Texas. I was still in their thoughts and prayers there and I was very aware of that. I could feel it." (Tinley, 2006, pp. 89–90)

In contrast with the experience of women, Kronenwetter et al. (2005) found that men with early-stage prostate cancer rarely discussed spirituality in relation to their cancer diagnosis. When they did, they were equally likely to view the diagnosis as having no change or as having a positive relationship with their spirituality. However, others have found that prayer was highly valued by African American prostate cancer survivors (Jones et al., 2007). This may reflect a difference in the cancer trajectory or a difference in ethnicity. Krupski et al. (2005) found that among low-income men with prostate cancer, African American and Hispanic men scored significantly higher than Caucasian men did on the Functional Assessment of Chronic Illness Therapy–Spiritual Well-Being. The implication from these studies is that nurses should be aware of variances among ethnicities and between the sexes, and generalities cannot be assumed with any one patient.

Among parents of children with cancer, the support of their ministers was an important source of support. These parents found that the act of having faith in God and prayer were essential sources of support and comfort throughout their child's illness, despite occasional periods of doubt. They described their confidence in God's presence and how that bolstered their ability to keep going. Those who were part of a church appreciated and found the prayers of their faith communities to be a source of comfort and hope. Parents with theistic beliefs and those without them also found spiritual comfort and a source of strength in the beauty of nature (Schneider & Mannell, 2006).

A Gallup poll indicated that 78%–86% of Americans expressed a firm belief in God (Newport, 2007). A belief in God is not universal among patients or providers. An awareness and appreciation of how alternative beliefs affect coping with potential, existing, and past cancer experiences is essential to providing spiritual care. A young woman with a *BRCA1* mutation identified her spirituality as a belief in a balance in life with a purpose for everything that happens, but not belief in a god. In describing how that belief has helped her to cope with her family history, she said the following.

> "I think it helps to know that maybe there is a reason for this. This might open another door and I am one of those annoying people that always say there has got to be a silver lining. I believe that out of the bad things, something good could happen, so you just have to deal with it and hope that something good comes along. So I think that helps me cope with it." (Tinley, 2006, p. 91)

Prerequisites and Self-Care for Engagement in Spiritual Care

"Be at peace with yourself first and then you will be able to bring peace to others."
—Thomas à Kempis

Many nurses have a desire to be active, to make a difference, and to apply the skills they possess to make a difference for their patients. When a patient needs undivided attention and time, nurses must be able to quiet the need for activity and the chatter in their mind (Miller & Cutshall, 2001). To provide this kind of caring presence, nurses have identified the need to develop and care for their own internal space: a space where the nurse can examine beliefs, resolve personal issues, cultivate a desire to connect with others, and develop a comfort with the spiritual (Kirkham, Pesut, Meyerhoff, & Sawatzky, 2004).

The nurse's tools for spiritual care are personal. They include sensitivity, intuition, presence, altruism, openness, genuineness, and vulnerability. These tools require a depth of personal knowledge and comfort with one's past journey and with the uncertainty of the future. In a study with nurses who provide spiritual care, additional requisites to providing spiritual care that were identified included a willingness to connect, comfort with spiritual matter, a conviction that spiritual care is part of nursing care, integration of spiritual care with all aspects of patient care, and a sincere desire to understand another's spiritual beliefs (Kirkham et al., 2004). Although some knowledge of different religious practices and beliefs, especially as they relate to health, illness, and treatment, can be beneficial, mostly there is a need for respect for others' beliefs and an openness to being taught by patients while being true to the nurse's own beliefs. It is not a kind of expert care in which the nurse teaches or advises; most of the time, there will be as much, if not more, for the nurse to learn from the patient.

For nurses to develop competency in spiritual care, they must also be aware of potential barriers to this care. External barriers can include the emphasis on cure even when beyond the possible, the secularism of our society, an institutional focus on financial matters, and the dilution of specific religious beliefs by trying to accommodate everyone in the same way, thus meeting no one person's needs. Depending on the setting, these barriers can be more or less of a problem. When problematic, they require nurses to be an advocate for the care that the patient deserves and to be creative in care delivery.

The nurse's internal barriers include the chatter of one's mind and burnout. The Oncology Nursing Society's (ONS's) Spiritual Care Special Interest Group (SIG) Toolkit (ONS, 2005b) has identified a need for oncology nurses to intervene on behalf of themselves to prevent compassion fatigue and replenish their resources. This self-care needs to be provided within the work environment and on the individual level of the nurse. It should include meditation and prayer. Although not mentioned in the toolkit, nurses may additionally benefit from a relationship with a certified spiritual director. The development of an internal space and the ability to quiet the mental chatter also can be enhanced by a spiritual retreat. The retreat may or may not be religious in nature, can be somewhere else or in one's own backyard, may be conducted by another or alone, and can occur over a weekend or during whatever time the participant or participants can afford. The retreat allows for nurses to reexamine what is happening internally and replenish resources. Innumerable sites on the Web are available to assist in the process just by searching for *spiritual retreat* or *online spiritual retreat.*

General consensus in the nursing literature recognizes that spiritual care is an essential part of the nurse's role (Cavendish et al., 2004; Pesut, 2003; Taylor, 2002). However, the opinion of the patient in this matter always takes precedence, especially when considering the theistic aspects of spiritual care. In the words of one group of patients, spiritual care requires that the nurse have an established relationship with the patient and have some training in spiritual care. It was less important to these patients that they and the nurse share similar spiritual or religious beliefs or similar life experiences (Taylor, 2007). Patients in other studies have clearly indicated that they do not perceive nurses as having any role in their spiritual care. In a survey about what patients with cancer and family caregivers want from nurses, the desires varied widely. The greatest agreement among patients and families was for interventions that allowed personal spiritual development in independent ways and not wanting overtly religious interventions or those that involved a very personal approach by the nurse (Taylor & Mamier, 2005). Clearly, one of the prerequisites to providing spiritual care is that the nurse be open to and honor the wishes of the individual patient.

Assessment of Spiritual Needs

Religion is a widely understood term among patients, but *spirituality* is not. For many, the distinction between religion and spirituality will be not only artificial but perhaps offensive.

When nurses are attempting to assess patients' needs and desires especially related to the theistic aspect of spirituality, the nurse and the patient must ensure they are talking about the same concepts.

Who can define another's spiritual needs related to that individual's connection with God? Is a Jewish nurse competent to assess the spiritual needs of a Lutheran or Catholic, Muslim, or agnostic patient? For that matter, are most nurses competent to assess the spiritual needs of a patient, especially those that relate to another's connection with a higher being? If this is so, then spiritual assessment has to be open-ended, allowing the patient to tell the nurse what he or she needs. Does this mean that nurses have no role in spiritual care beyond being open to what patients choose to share and making referrals to the appropriate minister, rabbi, shaman, new age therapist, etc.? No, there is a role in nursing care for supporting the spirit of all patients, no matter what their religious views.

For the sake of clarity, an artificial line can be drawn between spiritual care for the "human" and the "theistic" needs of the patient. The *human needs* refer to those that can be met through human connections, one spirit to another, and the connections made through nature and the environment. These needs generally are less sensitive, and nurses feel more competent in assessing them. Human needs are not always seen by nurses or patients as being spiritual. They include the fears, anxieties, pain, and discomforts that are associated with cancer and its treatment. Although these needs are almost universally recognized as part of the cancer experience, they often are overlooked in the busyness of an oncology unit or are treated with the latest and greatest drugs.

The *theistic needs* refer to those needs related to the patient's connection with God or a higher power. In addition to being uniquely couched in the patient's beliefs, theistic needs are personal and private. Because of the patient's vulnerability, spiritual care designed to meet these needs has the potential to be harmful, ranging from being intrusive to being destructive to the patient's belief system (Pesut, 2006; Pesut & Sawatzky, 2006; Winslow & Winslow, 2003).

The nurse utilizes the self more than any other kind of assessment tool when assessing the patient's spiritual needs. This use of self includes intuition, active listening, and an ability to communicate empathy, trustworthiness, and acceptance that allows the patient to feel safe and free to share.

Without ever overtly discussing a patient's theistic needs, a nurse often can gather information from the admission page about religious affiliation and visual cues in the patient's room, such as the presence of a Bible, prayer book, icons, prayer shawl, or other items. The level of rapport established with the patient and the nurse's intuition also should be components in the nurse's decision about how direct to be in assessing the patient's needs that might be met by theistic spiritual care.

Competency in assessing and meeting the theistic needs will be variable among nurses and the degree to which they and their patients are open to each other because the nurse relies primarily on the subjective perspective of the patient. Pesut and Sawatzky (2006) advocated for the use of an open-ended assessment tool that allows the patients to decide what to reveal. Another important element of the assessment is an inquiry about how patients want the nurse to support their beliefs and practices (Taylor & Mamier, 2005).

Pulchaski (2006) has defined a mnemonic, FICA, to assist healthcare providers in conducting an open-ended spirituality assessment that will help to identify religious preferences in a nonthreatening manner. *Faith* signifies whether patients have religious or spiritual beliefs that help with coping and, if not, what does help them with coping. *Important* refers to how important their belief system is and how they see it relating to their health and decisions for treatment. *Community* relates to a church or spiritual community or group of individuals that are important in patients' lives and provide support for them. *Address* represents a discussion of how patients want healthcare providers to address these issues while caring for them.

Application of FICA to Case Study

A return to the case study presented at the beginning of this chapter can demonstrate the application of FICA. As the nurse completes the family history, she asks M.L. how she has coped with all of the cancers, her own and her sister's. M.L. explains that after years of being away, she had resumed regular church attendance when she was diagnosed with breast cancer. She says that she thought her religion had been an important support for her at that time. However, she describes herself as a "CEO"—Christmas and Easter only—Christian for the past few years. She expresses feelings of anger at God for allowing her sister to suffer. The nurse asks if M.L. thinks it is OK for her to be angry with God, and M.L. laughs and says yes, she thinks he is big enough to bear her anger without retribution. As M.L. discusses her sorrow over her sister's diagnosis, she also expresses a desire to have half the faith that her sister has. She talks of her sister's faith and participation in a church community as a source of a calm and trusting acceptance of her future.

The nurse is constantly aware of M.L.'s responses and is cautious to never push, but to allow M.L. to reveal what she wants to discuss. With just a couple of open-ended questions following M.L.'s lead, the nurse learns that her belief system includes a <u>faith</u> in God that had been a source of support in the past. Her faith has not been so <u>important</u> in recent years, but she expresses a desire to possess a faith and trust in God similar to her sister's. She also had derived support from participation in a church <u>community</u> in the past but not recently. Yet, she expresses an admiration for her sister's consistent participation in her church community. Because of M.L.'s potential ambivalence about her faith in God and church attendance, the nurse assesses how M.L. wants her to <u>address</u> her spiritual care by allowing M.L. to take the lead in their discussion and by asking if she wanted a referral to a minister.

Interventions

"We can make our minds so like still water that beings gather about us that they may see, it may be, their own images, and so live for a moment with a clearer, perhaps even with a fiercer life, because of our quiet."
—William Butler Yeats, *The Celtic Twilight: Faerie and Folklore*

Interventions in spiritual care in nursing often are supportive in nature. It can be ethically problematic for nurses to go beyond that role to one of actively intervening in the theistic aspect of a patient's spirituality (Pesut & Sawatzky, 2006). The exception would be those few nurses who have the additional education that allows them to be spiritual directors, and even with that educational preparation, the nurse/spiritual director needs to be totally transparent as to which role is being offered to a patient.

Spiritual care has been described as having four attributes: intuitive, interpersonal, altruistic, and integrative (Sawatzky & Pesut, 2005). The *intuitive* attribute requires a way of knowing beyond rational thought and a connection between the patient and nurse that allows the nurse to intuitively discern when the patient provides the opportunity for discussion. The nurse's intuition always requires validation by the patient. The *interpersonal* attribute refers to the nurse's therapeutic use of self. It means that the nurse needs to accept a degree of personal vulnerability in engaging with the patient. The characteristics for this attribute include warmth, nonjudgmental acceptance, compassion, and the ability to communicate those qualities. *Altruism* implies a willingness to place the patient first. Altruism in spiritual care is necessary to avoid even an inadvertent taking advantage of the patient's vulnerability to meet the nurse's agenda. Lastly, spiritual care is *integrative* in that physical, social, psychological, and spiritual realms are integrated.

In an ethnographic study of spiritual care, nurses described the need to keep spiritual care in the forefront while interacting with the patient in order to be open to the patient's cues (Kirkham et al., 2004). Without such a conscious effort, it was too easy for the nurses to get caught up with everything else and lose sight of the patient as a whole. The nurses also described a purposeful avoidance of imposing one's own beliefs and maintenance of awareness of the potential for harm.

Presence

> *"The only gift is a portion of thyself."*
>
> —Ralph Waldo Emerson

Presence has been identified as the bedrock of spiritual care in the ONS Spiritual Care SIG Toolkit (ONS, 2005a). It is an intervention in and of itself, but it also is an essential component of every other spiritual intervention. One nurse described her intentional and purposeful presence:

> "The challenge and the discipline of that was to go in and leave my own self outside the door, just walk in, available . . . it's discipline and hard work to really be in tune. You leave the room realizing if you believed your traditional things, I didn't provide spiritual care because we didn't talk about God, read any Bible verses, and I didn't even pray with him. So how did I provide spiritual care? Well, I was aware of his spirituality. I was present for him." (Kirkham et al., 2004, p. 158)

Miller and Cutshall (2001) have identified the following seven steps in the art of being present.

- Preparation of self as provider by being open to yourself, being honest and accepting of your history
- Intentional aspiration to be present with the patient
- Preparation of a physical space if possible and a mental space within yourself, clearing out your own needs, expectations, and the chatter in your mind
- Honor and respect for the one to whom your presence is being offered
- The gift of what you have to offer, with no strings attached and a sincere realization that it is the patient's choice whether to accept it
- Gratitude and acceptance of any gifts that flow from being present to your patient such as a new relationship, lessons learned from their stories, joy, and laughter
- Replenishment of your spirit, especially when there is grief, disappointment, failure, or an inability to connect. The last step requires acknowledgment of your own needs and allowing others to be a healing presence to you.

Sometimes there is only a moment for presence, and other times, there may be an opportunity to be truly present for longer periods of time. The nurse's full and undivided attention is focused on the patient, and yet the nurse also may be performing routine cares at the same time. Listening and really focusing on what the patient has to say, not on how to respond and not jumping ahead or making assumptions, is part of being present. Sometimes it is not easy to be truly present, and nurses need to be able to acknowledge when it is not possible and never try to fake it.

Human Connections

Oncology nurses can foster human connections directly with the patient or indirectly through family members and friends. As noted previously, in some of the research, there may be times when patients need to focus on their own inner resources (Coward & Kahn, 2004; Logan et al., 2006). However, at many other times, the connections with friends and family are essential. Nurses can play an important role in coaching and encouraging family members to provide those connections. Among other interventions, nurses caring for older adult patients have identified the intervention of assisting patients to connect with family or significant others by encouraging these individuals to visit frequently and helping the patient to complete unfinished business (Narayanasamy et al., 2004). Often, older adult patients are eager to share the story of their life. Asking about photos, cards, or memorabilia in the room can serve as an encouragement. A written or recorded history can provide an important legacy for the family while also providing the impetus for the patient to recollect his or her life's history.

Humor

Humor produces physiologic, psychological, social, and spiritual effects (James, 1995). Most people can identify with the positive effects that laughter can have by relieving tension and providing or deepening a connection between people. In describing how spirituality affected her adjustment to breast cancer, one woman described how she and her two sisters, also affected with breast cancer, laughed at and with each other as they experimented with various prosthesis. She questioned if this was spiritual and then answered her own question affirmatively because it strengthened the bond between the sisters and aided in their acceptance of a drastically altered body image (Tinley, 2006). The daughter of another patient with breast cancer described how her mother incorporated humor as part of her spirituality when she uplifted herself, her family, and the staff at the cancer center with the clown wigs and silly hats she would wear while going through chemotherapy (Tinley). Sometimes, the nurse's humor intervention may be merely connecting with the patient as they share in laughter about something one has said or done. Nurses can intervene more actively by sharing jokes, cartoons, and amusing tales with their patients. Oncology units or clinics can make available humorous tapes, DVDs, and reading materials. Carefully encouraging patients to find humor in some of the disruptions in their lives can facilitate their ability to cope. For some patients with a theistic view, the connection between spirituality and humor may not be as apparent, but for others, attribution of humor to their god can demystify and encourage a more intimate relationship. As with other forms of spiritual care, the nurse needs to assess the patient's receptivity, the timing, and the content prior to using humor as an intervention.

Hope

The ability to look with confidence to the future is a sign of spiritual well-being. Hope can be elusive but is vital to coping for patients with cancer. Times when it may be especially difficult for the patient to maintain hope include the time of diagnosis, when the side effects of treatment cannot be adequately managed, when metastasis or other signs of disease progression are present, and when the patient is dying. Oncology nurses can help their patients to cultivate a realistic sense of hope during any of these times with presence, humor, listening, helping them to establish and use support systems, affirming personal worth, recalling positive memories, or providing information in an honest, respectful, and compassionate manner. There should always be a sense of hope. Even when cure is no longer realistic, patients can have hope for time to do those things they always wanted to do, to make peace with loved ones, or to have a peaceful death (Pulchaski, 2006). Hope can be supported and enhanced through religious ritual and prayer when appropriate to the patient.

Prayer and Ritual

For many individuals, prayer and ritual are important aids to coping with health issues. In a national poll conducted by Columbia Broadcasting System/New York Times, 60% of Americans reported they pray at least once a day (Tu, 2004). However, the treatment of cancer, including hospitalizations, surgeries, and medications, can present challenges in the patient's ability to focus attention on prayer. There may be times when patients would welcome the assistance of their nurses in praying. If, in the process of caring for a patient, the nurse assesses a commonality in religious beliefs through the presence of a religious symbol or based on something said by the patient, it is appropriate for the nurse to offer, with no hint of persuasion, to share in a religious practice. Nurses must always take care when intervening with a religious practice or discussion. First of all, evangelization of a patient by a nurse is unethical because of the imbalance of power in their relationship and the potentially offensive nature of this type of approach. The ethical considerations of praying with a patient can be subsumed under two broad categories, respectful care of the patient and the integrity of the nurse (Winslow & Winslow, 2003). Respect for the patient includes a constant awareness that the patient is a unique individual with his or her own values. A nurse always asks for permission before introducing prayer and never urges or pressures the patient in any way. If the patient requests the nurse's assistance or company in a religious practice, the nurse can accommodate the patient as long as the action is acceptable within the nurse's belief system. Spiritual care also requires the integrity of the nurse. If participation in prayer that is meaningful to the patient is not meaningful to the nurse, the nurse should refer to a chaplain or offer to contact the appropriate clergy, rabbi, shaman, or another individual.

A nursing student wrote about the following experience in her clinical journal. She was caring for an older adult female patient who was becoming increasingly anxious the morning she was to go to surgery. The student assessed her patient's increasing anxiety as having a potentially negative impact on her physical state going into surgery. The student noticed that the patient had a rosary laid out on her bedside stand. Being a Catholic herself, the student offered to pray with the patient. The patient indicated that praying a portion of the rosary would be nice if the student knew how. The student then led the patient through the prayers of the rosary. The patient became visibly more relaxed as they prayed. When they had completed the prayers, the patient thanked the student and expressed a readiness to go to surgery.

Chaplains

Professional healthcare chaplains are individuals who have graduate education in theology or divinity, have postgraduate training in clinical pastoral education, and have demonstrated competency in chaplaincy. Their role includes providing supportive spiritual care that crosses religious boundaries. They lead nondenominational ceremonies of worship and ritual and participate on healthcare teams and ethics committees. They are an excellent resource for nurses, especially when the patient's spiritual needs exceed the competency of the nurse. Chaplains also can cross disciplinary lines to provide care for staff members experiencing the stress of patient care (VandeCreek & Burton, 2001).

Community-Based Spiritual Care

A community-based intervention was organized and conducted by oncology providers from a secular healthcare system and interdenominational community clergy (Dann, Higby, & Mertens, 2005). Physicians, nurses, patients, survivors, and caregivers participated; the services were structured around the themes of fear, hope, peace, feeling God's love, and importance of community. The authors identified the benefit of the collaborative effort in the message to patients that "the religious community supports their pursuit of physical well-being and the medical community supports their effort to bring spirituality into the healing process" (p. 140). The Web site indicates that materials for the service can be downloaded from www.baystatehealth.com/forms/pastoral_pdf/sacred_gathering.pdf and adapted as appropriate for a given community.

Spirituality/religion may be an essential resource for families just as it is for individuals. Sometimes it can be the vehicle for resolving rifts within a family and leading to cohesion, but there is also the possibility that individual members may have differing views of spirituality that result in disagreements or isolation. Nurses need to carefully assess whether conflicts exist among members of a family because of differing views of religion or spirituality (Tanyi, 2006). It also can be helpful to patients if the nurses provide opportunities for spouses and family members to meet their needs so that they, in turn, are in a better position to meet the needs of the patients. Nurses may need to offer family members reassurance or encouragement to leave so that they can get the rest and nourishment they need.

Interventions in the Case Study

The nurse's assessment and interventions on M.L.'s behalf require the nurse's openness and respect for M.L.'s vulnerability. The nurse is able to assess M.L.'s needs and at the same time provide the intervention of presence, by attending solely to what M.L. had to say and conveying a sense of acceptance and understanding. This provides an opportunity for M.L. to express her response to her sister's diagnosis in a way that helped her to sort out some of her spiritual ambivalence. Although the nurse does not introduce humor as an intervention, she shares in M.L.'s laughter as well as her distress. Because M.L. has expressed a desire to have a faith like her sister's, the nurse offers a referral to a chaplain or minister. M.L. decides to go back to the minister who had helped her in the past. At the end of her time with the nurse, M.L. says it was not something she would choose, but she thought it would be a privilege to accompany her sister in the journey ahead.

Conclusion

Spiritual care can enable coping, diminish negative feelings, provide connection between nurses and patients, reduce suffering, and promote growth and greater self-understanding. "Spirituality, then, must be acknowledged, appreciated, and included. It may not be the law, but it is the ethically appropriate course of action" (Pulchaski, 2006, p. 38). However, not all patients want a theistic type of spiritual care from nurses, nor are all nurses comfortable or competent in providing it. The nurse who is to provide spiritual care needs to tread lightly, always keeping the patient's needs and values in the forefront. Nurses may not be able to provide spiritual care within a religious framework, but they can always be open to connecting with their patients on the plane of one human spirit to another. It is imperative that oncology nurses provide this latter type of care to their patients regardless of the patient's spiritual outlook, age, language, or culture. Without the spiritual connection, patients will be deprived of the best that nurses have to offer—themselves.

References

Cavendish, R., Luise, B.K., Russo, D., Mitzeliotis, C., Bauer, M., Bajo, M.A.M., et al. (2004). Spiritual perspectives of nurses in the United States relevant for education and practice. *Western Journal of Nursing Research, 26*(2), 196–221.

Coward, D.D., & Kahn, D.L. (2004). Resolution of spiritual disequilibrium by women newly diagnosed with breast cancer [Online exclusive]. *Oncology Nursing Forum, 31*(2), E24–E31. Retrieved June 25, 2005, from http://ons.metapress.com/content/e80687q677404626/fulltext.pdf

Dann, N.J., Higby, D.J., & Mertens, W.C. (2005). Can a cancer program-sponsored spiritual event meet with acceptance from patients and other attendees? *Integrative Cancer Therapies, 4*(3), 230–235.

James, D.H. (1995). Humor: A holistic nursing intervention. *Journal of Holistic Nursing, 13*(3), 239–247.

Jones, R.A., Taylor, E.J., Bourguignon, C., Steeves, R., Fraser, G., Theodorescu, D., et al. (2007). Complementary and alternative medicine modality use and beliefs among African American prostate cancer survivors. *Oncology Nursing Forum, 34*(2), 359–364.

Kirkham, S.R., Pesut, B., Meyerhoff, H., & Sawatzky, R. (2004). Spiritual caregiving at the juncture of religion, culture and state. *Canadian Journal of Nursing Research, 36*(4), 148–169.

Kronenwetter, C., Weidner, G., Pettengill, E., Marlin, R., Crutchfield, L., McCormac, P., et al. (2005). A qualitative analysis of interviews of men with early stage prostate cancer. *Cancer Nursing, 28*(2), 99–107.

Krupski, T.L., Sonn, G., Kwan, L., Maliski, S., Fink, A., & Litwin, M.S. (2005). Ethnic variation in health-related quality of life among low-income men with prostate cancer. *Ethnicity and Disease, 15*(3), 461–468.

Logan, J., Pinto, R.H., & De Grasse, C.E. (2006). Women undergoing breast diagnostics: The lived experience of spirituality. *Oncology Nursing Forum, 33*(1), 121–126.

Miller, J., & Cutshall, S.C. (2001). *The art of healing presence: A guide for those in caring relationships.* Fort Wayne, IN: Willowgreen Publishing.

Narayanasamy, A., Clissett, P., Parumal, L., Thompson, D., Annasamy, S., & Edge, R. (2004). Responses to the spiritual needs of older people. *Journal of Advanced Nursing, 48*(1), 6–16.

Newport, F. (2007). *Americans more likely to believe in God than the devil, heaven more than hell.* Gallup News Service. Retrieved January 2, 2008, from http://www.gallup.com/poll/27877/Americans-More-Likely-Believe-God -Than-Devil-Heaven-More-Than-Hell.aspx

Oncology Nursing Society. (2005a). Presence. In *Spiritual Care SIG toolkit.* Retrieved August 15, 2007, from http://www.new.towson.edu/sct/presence.htm

Oncology Nursing Society. (2005b). Spiritual self-care for oncology nurses. In *Spiritual Care SIG toolkit.* Retrieved August 15, 2007, from http://www.new.towson.edu/sct/selfcare.htm

Pesut, B. (2003). Developing spirituality in the curriculum: Worldviews, intrapersonal connectedness, interpersonal connectedness. *Nursing Education Perspectives, 24*(6), 290–294.

Pesut, B. (2006). Fundamental or foundational obligation? Problematizing the ethical call to spiritual care in nursing. *Advances in Nursing Science, 29*(2), 125–133.

Pesut, B., & Sawatzky, R. (2006). To describe or prescribe: Assumptions underlying a prescriptive nursing process approach to spiritual care. *Nursing Inquiry, 13*(2), 127–134.

Pulchaski, C.M. (2006). *A time for listening and caring.* New York: Oxford University Press.

Sawatzky, R., & Pesut, B. (2005). Attributes of spiritual care in nursing practice. *Journal of Holistic Nursing, 23*(1), 19–33.

Schneider, M.A., & Mannell, R.C. (2006). Beacon in the storm: An exploration of the spirituality and faith of parents whose children have cancer. *Issues in Comprehensive Pediatric Nursing, 29*(1), 3–24.

Tanyi, R.A. (2006). Spirituality and family nursing: Spiritual assessment and interventions for families. *Journal of Advanced Nursing, 53*(3), 287–294.

Taylor, E.J. (2002). *Spiritual care: Nursing theory, research and practice.* Upper Saddle River, NJ: Pearson Education, Inc.

Taylor, E.J. (2007). Client perspectives about nurse requisites for spiritual caregiving. *Applied Nursing Research, 20*(1), 44–46.

Taylor, E.J., & Mamier, I. (2005). Spiritual care nursing: What cancer patients and family caregivers want. *Journal of Advanced Nursing, 49*(3), 260–267.

Tinley, S.T. (2006). Spirituality and the experience of being a member of a family with hereditary breast and ovarian cancer (Doctoral dissertation, University of Utah, 2006). *Dissertation Abstracts International, 67,* 3710.

Tu, J.I. (2004). *Times poll: More than half of us pray daily.* Retrieved January 9, 2008, from http://community.seattletimes.nwsource.com/archive/?date=20040411&slug=pollprayer11m

VandeCreek, L., & Burton, L. (Eds.). (2001). *Professional chaplaincy: Its role and importance in healthcare.* Retrieved January 9, 2008, from http://www.healthcarechaplaincy.org/publications/publications/white_paper_05.22.01/index.html

Winslow, G.R., & Winslow, B.W. (2003). Examining the ethics of praying with patients. *Holistic Nursing Practice, 17*(4), 170–177.

Index

The letter f *after a page number indicates that relevant content appears in a figure; the letter* t, *in a table.*